Good Design Practices for GMP Pharmaceutical Facilities

Second Edition

DRUGS AND THE PHARMACEUTICAL SCIENCES
A Series of Textbooks and Monographs

Series Executive Editor
James Swarbrick
PharmaceuTech, Inc.
Pinehurst, North Carolina

Recent Titles in Series

Good Design Practices for GMP Pharmaceutical Facilities, Second Edition,
Terry Jacobs and Andrew A. Signore

Handbook of Bioequivalence Testing, Second Edition, *Sarfaraz K. Niazi*

Generic Drug Product Development: Solid Oral Dosage Forms, Second Edition,
edited by Leon Shargel and Isadore Kanfer

Drug Stereochemistry: Analytical Methods and Pharmacology, Third Edition,
edited by Krzysztof Jozwiak, W. J. Lough, and Irving W. Wainer

Pharmaceutical Powder Compaction Technology, Second Edition,
edited by Metin Çelik

Pharmaceutical Stress Testing: Predicting Drug Degradation, Second Edition,
edited by Steven W. Baertschi, Karen M. Alsante, and Robert A. Reed

Pharmaceutical Process Scale-Up, Third Edition, *edited by Michael Levin*

Sterile Drug Products: Formulation, Packaging, Manufacturing and Quality,
Michael J. Akers

Freeze-Drying/Lyophilization of Pharmaceutical and Biological Products,
Third Edition, *edited by Louis Rey and Joan C. May*

Oral Drug Absorption: Prediction and Assessment, *edited by Jennifer B. Dressman
and Christos Reppas*

Generic Drug Product Development: Specialty Dosage Forms, *edited by
Leon Shargel and Isadore Kanfer*

Generic Drug Product Development: International Regulatory Requirements
for Bioequivalence, *edited by Isadore Kanfer and Leon Shargel*

Active Pharmaceutical Ingredients: Development, Manufacturing, and
Regulation, Second Edition, *edited by Stanley Nusim*

Pharmaceutical Statistics: Practical and Clinical Applications, Fifth Edition,
edited by Sanford Bolton and Charles Bon

Biodrug Delivery Systems: Fundamentals, Applications and Clinical
Development, *edited by Mariko Morishita and Kinam Park*

Biodrug Delivery Systems: Fundamentals, Applications and Clinical
Development, *edited by Mariko Morishita and Kinam Park*

Handbook of Pharmaceutical Granulation Technology, Third Edition,
edited Dilip M. Parikh

*A complete listing of all volumes in this series
can be found at **www.crcpress.com***

Good Design Practices for GMP Pharmaceutical Facilities

Second Edition

Edited by

Terry Jacobs, AIA
JacobsWyper Architects
Philadelphia, PA, USA

Andrew A. Signore, PE
ISG-Institute for Strategic Growth
Wayne, PA, USA

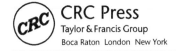
CRC Press
Taylor & Francis Group
Boca Raton London New York

CRC Press is an imprint of the
Taylor & Francis Group, an **informa** business

CRC Press
Taylor & Francis Group
6000 Broken Sound Parkway NW, Suite 300
Boca Raton, FL 33487-2742

First issued in paperback 2022

© 2017 by Taylor & Francis Group, LLC
CRC Press is an imprint of Taylor & Francis Group, an Informa business

No claim to original U.S. Government works

ISBN-13: 978-1-482-25890-5 (hbk)
ISBN-13: 978-1-03-233996-2 (pbk)
DOI: 10.1201/9781315372242

Library of Congress Cataloging-in-Publication Data

Names: Signore, Andrew A., author. | Jacobs, Terry (Architect), author.
Title: Good design practices for GMP pharmaceutical facilities / Terry Jacobs and Andrew A. Signore.
Other titles: Drugs and the pharmaceutical sciences.
Description: Second edition. | Boca Raton : Taylor & Francis, 2017. | Series: Drugs and the pharmaceutical sciences | Author's names reversed on the first edition. | Includes bibliographical references and index.
Identifiers: LCCN 2016007232 | ISBN 9781482258905 (alk. paper)
Subjects: | MESH: Technology, Pharmaceutical | Facility Design and Construction | Quality Control
Classification: LCC RS192 | NLM QV 778 | DDC 615.1/9--dc23
LC record available at http://lccn.loc.gov/2016007232

Visit the Taylor & Francis Web site at
http://www.taylorandfrancis.com

and the CRC Press Web site at
http://www.crcpress.com

Dedication

This publication is dedicated to all professionals who help bring life-altering medical solutions to the world, including but not limited to industry innovators, supporters, suppliers, educators, and regulators.

Contents

Preface

Good design yields better-functioning facilities and better performance for pharmaceutical manufacturers. In particular, good design leads to shorter delivery cycles; lower costs to build and operate; better facility performance, resulting in lower costs of goods; and fewer compliance infractions. The effective application of good design practices (GDPs) offers an advantage to operators and is an essential skill for professionals. GDPs are a set of sound design approaches that offer powerful tools to help professionals develop and build facilities that efficiently and safely meet the commercial and regulatory challenges of current Good Manufacturing Practices (cGMPs). The GDPs are not to be confused with cGMPs. The application of GDPs also encourages the effective accommodation of evolving technologies, which offer novel processes and the means of producing high-quality products for a global marketplace.

Design may be defined, for our purposes, as the process of developing "intentional functionality" for a challenging set of operational requirements. Design for the pharmaceutical industry incorporates planning and delivering special purpose facilities, using cGMPs, and involves architectural, engineering, and other compliance activities to conceive and document the physical solutions to specific functional requirements. Design drawings and specifications are used to direct vendors, suppliers, equipment fabricators, and construction firms. Design documents also address operational, maintenance, and compliance requirements for commissioning and validation. Notable observations on design include the following:

- "Design is a funny word. Some people think design means how it looks [and feels]. But, of course, if you dig deeper, it is really how it works" (Steve Jobs, founder of Apple).
- "Good design is good business" (Thomas J. Watson, former CEO of IBM).
- "Simple is good" (Jim Henson, originator of the Muppets).
- "A designer knows he has achieved perfection, not when there is nothing left to add but when there is nothing left to take away" (Antoine de Saint Exubery).
- "Almost all quality improvement comes via simplification of design manufacturing layout processes and procedures" (Tom Peters, coauthor of *In Search of Excellence*).
- "We shape our buildings; thereafter they shape us" (Winston Churchill).
- "I don't build in order to have clients. I have clients in order to build" (Ayn Rand, from *The Fountainhead*).
- "Form follows function" (Lewis Sullivan, architect).
- "A doctor can bury his mistakes, but an architect can only advise clients to plant vines" (Frank Lloyd Wright).
- "Simplicity is the ultimate sophistication.... I have been impressed with the urgency of doing. Knowing is not enough; we must apply. Being willing is not enough. We must do" (Leonardo da Vinci).
- "The greater danger for most of us lies not in setting our aim too high and falling short but in setting our aim too low in achieving a mark" (Michelangelo).

The cGMPs are a series of widely recognized, legally binding rules, regulations, and guidelines promulgated by local drug regulatory agencies. They are typically defined by authorized governmental bodies and are diligently followed by professional practitioners. The cGMPs have the force of law. The objectives of all cGMPs, as well as GDPs, are the delivery and operation of facilities used to manufacture regulated drug substances and products that meet specified requirements for fitness for their intended use. They provide for systems that ensure proper design, monitoring, and control of manufacturing processes and facilities.

The cGMPs require that processes, procedures, and methods be written down through the creation of standard operating procedures. Regulatory authorities view the most critical areas of compliance as validation, record keeping, environmental monitoring, notation of equipment failures, and failure to investigate adequately "out-of-specification" results and deviations. All manufacturing and testing facilities of pharmaceutical products, biologics, diagnostics, and devices are controlled by the U.S. Food and Drug Administration and by respective authorities overseas. These facilities are subject to inspections before approval of new products and routinely thereafter. In addition, the manufacturer is required to perform regular self-inspections to ensure that compliance with cGMPs is current throughout the facility.

The buildings, and the equipment and systems within, are designed and operated in compliance with applicable statutes, codes, and regulatory requirements. These facilities process, pack, store, and distribute regulated substances and products intended for sale. These substances may be characterized as active pharmaceutical ingredients, drugs, biologics, and medical devices. The cGMPs apply to clinical development operations supplying materials for phase 1, 2, or 3 trials, as well as full-scale production operations and commercial testing laboratories.

GDPs, on the other hand, are planning and design approaches that encourage the achievement of complex manufacturing challenges. There is no official, legally recognized definition of GDPs. Application of GDPs involves a design process that is robust, repeatable, and approved by stakeholders and interested parties. The implications of formality and clarity of the GDPs can be defended and taught to practitioners.

Harnessing GDPs will help the professional to address the many challenges arising with modern cGMP facilities and to deliver high-quality products safely, in an effective, sustainable manner. In other words, GDPs help us to respond to cGMPs, encourage risk-based solutions by promoting the application of recognized solutions, and address prudent design and engineering concepts; they observe standards of care statutes as they apply to professional conduct and the generally accepted level of competence expected from designers and builders. In addition, GDPs embrace value engineering practices and offer acceptable ways to conceive and appraise project scope.

GDPs comprise practical approaches employed to address a set of challenges. GDPs address such considerations as

- Risk management: Sustainable production methods
- Quality: Consistent product output, design reviews, and peer assessments
- Performance: Capacity and flexibility of output
- Technology: Processes and control
- Scope: Vision, objectives, and boundaries
- Cost: First cost of the facility, operating costs, and costs of goods
- Time: Cycle time to deliver the facility
- Drug regulatory compliance: Global perspective
- Safety, health, and environment
- Team: Project execution roles, responsibilities, and protocols

GDPs include formal processes for quality management to verify completeness and appropriateness of solutions against stated goals. Similar review techniques are used by architects for formal building code reviews to ensure a design will comply with applicable local building code requirements.

Acknowledgments

We are exceptionally fortunate to have a wonderful team of chapter authors who have given their time, expertise, and insights for this book and to this profession, while maintaining their full-time endeavors. They truly represent the best of this industry and their profession. We are sure the readers will appreciate their contributions and insights in their chapters. In this edition, we have included more graphics and diagrams and hope they will help illustrate and simplify the concepts discussed.

On the production side, we owe a deep debt and gratitude to a few dedicated individuals who helped produce the work. Our sincerest thanks are due to Cassidy Hobbs, the book's project editor and chapter author, who brought her exceptional organizational abilities to the whole team, as well as her writing, editing, and graphic skills. This book would not have been possible without her effort, which included many hours outside of the normal workday. We also want to acknowledge Julia Ewing, Aubrey Kessler, and Tori Williams, who have greatly improved our diagrams and illustrations, and Jennifer Bielecki, Melanie Mauer, and Kimberly Goodman, who provided administrative support in compiling the text. We owe a great debt to our friend Jane, who brought our writing and editing to a new level. And of course, we would be remiss without thanking our dear wives and life sponsors, Annemarie and Sally, for their understanding and loving support.

Editors

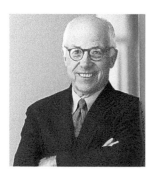

Terry Jacobs is a principal with JacobsWyper Architects, an architectural, planning, and interior design firm founded in 1981 in Philadelphia, Pennsylvania. The firm's practice focuses in part on large, complex projects for corporate and educational clients, including research laboratories and manufacturing facilities for the biotech, pharmaceutical, and research universities. Jacobs's extensive experience with pharmaceutical projects led him to coedit the first edition of *Good Design Practices for GMP Pharmaceutical Facilities* in 2005, and the second edition in 2015. Jacobs was an adjunct professor at both Temple University and Drexel University and a visiting critic at the University of Pennsylvania, all in Philadelphia. He has won design awards from the American Institute of Architects and the Pennsylvania Society of Architects. Jacobs earned his BA from Dartmouth College and his master's in architecture from the University of Pennsylvania. He was chairman of ISPE's Continuous Advancement Subcommittee and was president of the Delaware Valley Chapter of ISPE. He has been a course leader and speaker at numerous IPSE courses, and a member of the ISPE since 1981.

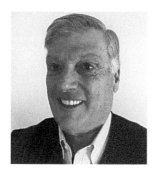

Andrew A. Signore is president of the Institute for Strategic Growth (ISG), Wayne, Pennsylvania, where he provides advisement and consulting to professional service firms. He is also cofounder of Integrated Project Services (IPS), Blue Bell, Pennsylvania, a project delivery firm focused on health care and pharmaceutical facilities. Andy has held engineering management positions at SmithKline Beckman (now Glaxo), Pfizer, and Merck. He earned his BSChemEng from Manhattan College and an MBA from Pace University, both of New York. He is a registered professional engineer in Pennsylvania, New York, and New Jersey. He is currently an adjunct professor in the School of Engineering in the Construction Management Division at Drexel University, Philadelphia. Andy was founding president of Design Build Institute of America's (DBIA) Delaware Valley Chapter and is a charter holder of a DBIA designation. He is past president of the New Jersey Chapter of the Project Management Institute (PMI). In addition, he has earned the CPIP designation, is a past president of the International Society for Pharmaceutical Engineering (ISPE) and of ISPE Delaware Valley Chapter, and is a frequent course leader. He has received ISPE's Distinguished Achievement Award in recognition for his many professional contributions to the industry. Andy remains a student of the pharmaceutical industry, has had more than a dozen articles published, and lectures on pharmaceutical industry technology and management topics.

Contributors

Eric Bohn
JacobsWyper Architects
Philadelphia, PA

Mark A. Butler
Seniro Vice President, IPS
Blue Bell, PA

Jack C. Chu, PE/MBA
Vice President of Life Science Engineering,
    RPA Associates
Wyomissing, PA

Christina Meyer Dell Cioppia
Senior Vice President
Validation Amec Foster Wheeler
Power and Process Americas Division
Philadelphia, PA

Rose Mary Dollard
Senior Director of Regulatory Compliance
Johnson & Johnson
New Brunswick, NJ

Samuel Halaby
Senior Director of Global Strategy and
    Technology
IPS-Integrated Project Services, LLC
Blue Bell, PA

Cassidy Hobbs
JacobsWyper Architects
Philadelphia, PA

John S. Holton, PE
Teva Pharmaceuticals/Director
Americas Engineering
Mohnton, PA

Terry Jacobs
JacobsWyper Architects
Philadelphia, PA

Joe Maida, PE
President of Maida Engineering
Philadelphia, PA

David M. Marks, PE
Principal, DME
Allentown, PA

Art Meisch
Senior Project Director (Retd.), CE&IC, Inc.
Burlington, NJ

George Petroka
Director, IES
Blue Bell, PA

Hank Rahe, MSE
Director of Technology
Containment Technologies Group, Inc.
Indianapolis, IN

Michael Rooney
Senior Technology Manager – OSD
Jacobs Engineering
Conshohocken, PA

Leonid Shnayder, PhD/PE
Industry Professor, Stevens Institute of
    Technology
Hoboken, NJ

Andrew A. Signore, PE
Institute for Strategic Growth
Wayne, PA

Asif Syed
Partner, STE Engineers
New York, NY-Princeton, NJ

Edward J. Tannebaum
AIA President
Strategic Planning Initiatives, LLC
Huntingdon Valley, PA

Brian G. Ward, PhD, CChem, FRSC
Containment Engineering Technology Center
    of Eli Lilly (Retd.)
Indianapolis, IN

George Wiker
Executive Director
AES Clean Technology, Inc.
Montgomeryville, PA

Gary V. Zoccolante
Pharmaceutical Technical Director
Evoqua Water Technologies LCC,
Lowell, MA

Introduction

This publication is an expansion and revision of the original edition released in 2005. This edition has been completely revised to include updated information and new graphics. The dynamic pharmaceutical industry continues to evolve and respond to global market forces. Exciting technologies and research productivity are ushering in a potential new golden age of life-altering medicines for the world. The safe and effective production of these products occupies a significant seat at the table of global quality of life considerations. The enlightened professional engaged in the manufacture of pharmaceutical products must maintain constant vigilance for the application of new techniques, which offer effective ways to bring new products to market quickly and cost-effectively. The first chapter of this book paints a vivid picture of the industry, including the strategic drivers that comprise the business landscape. Additional chapters are devoted to specific areas of focus to the manufacturer and those who support production with technical services, equipment, and system solutions and supplies.

Industry technical professionals are deeply aware of the challenges to deliver products to market where conformance and performance are essential imperatives. Those engaged in bringing new products to market are consistently struggling to navigate these turbulent times for the pharmaceutical industry. Balancing the age-old business challenges of cost and value continues to drive the pharmaceutical industry to innovate and deliver affordable medicines to an ever-increasing population.

Factories of the future will no doubt be remarkably efficient and incorporate stunning new technologies to enable production of high-quality, technically complex products, while conforming to world-class safety and quality standards. Future plants will incorporate green chemistry developments, sustainable processing techniques, energy-conserving systems, smart computer–assisted integrated control systems, online diagnostic and real-time inspection systems, enhanced security and safety, final dosage serialization approaches, and a host of other evolving technologies. The professional of the future will be expected to master the arts and sciences involved in delivering new facilities. This publication is offered as a convenient and effective tool for interested parties to investigate the modern challenges and approaches in delivering facilities that must *perform* to ever-demanding new market requirements and *conform* to evolving, harmonized regulatory demands.This publication is intended to serve as a helpful tool for professionals (both expert and evolving) engaged in planning, designing, constructing, validating, and operating modern current Good Manufacturing Practice (cGMP) pharmaceutical facilities. In the academic setting, this text is intended to serve as an introduction to the pharmaceutical industry for students who are majoring in related fields of engineering and science. Business development professionals may find this publication of interest, as it provides much insight into industry dynamics and likely avenues for future opportunity identification. This book may also serve as support material for active training and development programs delivered to industry through corporate in-house programs or by outside consulting training providers. Essential background information is presented, as well as suggested approaches to common issues met in the practice of conceiving and delivering facilities.

Every chapter of this publication has been prepared by accepted subject matter experts recognized in their respective fields. Special attention has been given to defining the challenges of a successful facility, as well as noting state-of-the-art approaches. This publication is not intended to substitute for detailed texts where professionals will find more comprehensive, handbook-style data and information.

This subject material was first addressed in a publication of the same title in 2005 and is now offered in a second edition. Over the past decade, the industry environment and responses to evolving challenges have made it appropriate to take a fresh look and review the dynamic changes, and herein offer refreshed insights for the coming decade.

We recommend that this book serves as an introduction or a confirmation source for the reader. Each author has presented his or her chapter's content with the intent to provide a solid overview of the subject matter. Each chapter is designed to stand alone. The publication includes virtually all significant content necessary to gain a good appreciation and insight into current challenges and approaches to delivering modern compliant pharmaceutical manufacturing facilities.

The reader is urged to address this material with an open mind. References are given for extended investigation. Extensive reference citations are generally not provided. The reader is encouraged to inquire directly with the many organizations listed, as they are regularly issuing updates and new editions of their standards and guidance materials. We recommend the external sources be searched as interest exists for deeper understanding and additional information. The information provided in this publication is limited to generally available published data and the opinions and experiences of each contributor. All compliant facilities must follow published legal guidelines applicable to the facility, and nothing presented herein is intended to override or compete with applicable laws, statutes, or generally recognized practices. Following any guidance and recommendations provided within this publication should be done so with keen consideration and recognition that these materials are offered as information and are for the benefit of the readers' appreciation and awareness, and not to be followed strictly, and possibly in conflict with local prevailing practices.

The publication does not present original research or extensive technical backup. Rather, it offers a collection of approaches in practice today as offered by veteran professionals. The collection is intended to serve as a general introduction or reminder of key concepts and approaches, and does not present a set of detailed instructions and procedures.

The reader is urged to consider additional technical sources, which will extend and supplement the materials provided in this publication. All chapter contributors are available for direct contact. Their contact information is provided in the Contributors section.

Depending on your professional pursuits, you will find this publication addresses some of your information needs.

1. The practicing pharmaceutical professional will find this material of interest when seeking to refresh or update one's understanding of current issues being confronted in the planning, design, and construction or commissioning of regulated new and renovated facilities.
2. The student will find this information to be excellent background data for gaining awareness and understanding of key issues confronting the delivery of modern pharmaceutical facilities.
3. The instructor will find this material to be easily assigned for reading and as a source of awareness and stimulation for the aspiring student, whether in a matriculated program of science and engineering or in an industrial training and orientation program.
4. The technical professional seeking deeper understanding of an allied profession will find this material valuable as part of his or her research and discovery process.
5. The pharmacist seeking advanced knowledge of industrial approaches will find this material to be helpful in his or her study of commercial approaches to modern manufacturing.
6. The marketing professional will see this publication as a handy source of insights into conditions and dynamics confronting his or her potential prospects and sales targets.

The editors believe this collection of manufacturing-related insights is valuable. We trust the readers will benefit from an expanded awareness and appreciation of the many dynamics and evolving technologies being applied to cGMP-compliant manufacturing facilities as they are planned, designed, constructed, and commissioned around the world for contributions of significant social value to the global market.

1 Pharmaceutical Industry Profile

Andrew A. Signore

CONTENTS

INDUSTRY OVERVIEW: INTRODUCTION

The pharmaceutical industry of today is experiencing unprecedented challenges and rapid transformation. For the purposes of this text, the pharmaceutical industry includes the producers of pharmaceutical products and their chain of service providers, including professional consultants, material and equipment suppliers, contract manufacturers, and any other entities that are involved in delivering regulated medicines (e.g., drug substance and products, whether chemically or biologically based, supplied as tablets, liquids, or injectables, or delivered by a medical device as defined by the U.S. Food and Drug Administration [FDA]).

The pharmaceutical industry is facing disruptive changes as headwinds continue from many sources, such as cost containment and accessibility initiatives by payers, governments, and health care insurance organizations. These forces are creating a challenging business environment by controlling pricing and promoting generic alternatives, as well as presenting obstacles to bringing innovative drugs to market. Cost pressures are mounting at the same time as remarkable scientific innovation and technology applications are offering significant opportunities to develop new therapies.

Change has been constant for the pharmaceutical industry, which has steadily evolved from a multinational base (1950s and 1960s) through global (1970 to 1990s) to international (2000 to present). The pharmaceutical industry has transformed from a strong product-based, local presence

1

to an increasingly international presence, seeking cost advantages by leveraging parent company capabilities through worldwide adoption and a partner-friendly "health solution" focus. Rapidly evolving science and engineering innovations have also provided steady opportunities to modernize and transform manufacturing platforms to gain economic advantages and deliver greater levels of product differentiation and quality.

A new business model is emerging for the pharmaceutical industry, which includes growth opportunities gained through partnering in novel ways. Companies seeking competitive advantages are increasingly collaborating with other players, such as information technology companies, medical technology companies, food companies, and retailers, to deliver "patient-centric" products and services. Future collaborations and partnerships will be aimed at helping patients manage their health and expand their access to products and services that address yet unmet medical challenges. The pharmaceutical industry, however, faces many challenges, including (1) setting and enforcing globally accepted manufacturing standards; (2) rapid patent expiration of widely used brand drugs; (3) unregulated parallel trades, including reimportation; (4) intellectual property rights protection; (5) highly fluid and unregulated Internet sales; (6) shortage of pharmaceutical scientists; (7) biotechnology drugs and genetically engineered products; (8) ineffective postmarketing surveillance; (9) foreign manufacturing, regulatory, and pricing challenges; and (10) counterfeit products.

Research and development expenditures for new drugs often do not yield an acceptable return on investment. Over the last decade, the costs to develop novel compounds rose, while the useful market life shrunk as a result of innovative competitors. The number of future blockbuster drugs may be unable to support the industry as they have done in the past. Blockbuster drugs (i.e., primary care drugs that bring in more than $1 billion in revenue) have been the centerpiece of industry success. Compounding these challenges are regulatory requirements to ensure drug safety that have grown more stringent, bringing increased scrutiny and greater hurdles for reaching the market.

During the past decade, the industry has countered by diversifying around product lines. Some companies have elected to spend less on research and development (R&D), while seeking research partnerships and pursuing product acquisitions to fill the pipeline. Such strategic behaviors are changing the landscape for in-house R&D manufacturing capabilities and shifting these functions increasingly to outsourced contractors, known as contract development and manufacturing organizations (CDMOs).

The strategic implications for timely and cost-effective delivery of new facilities are growing. As margins continue to be squeezed, an organization's capital deployment capacity becomes more prominent. In addition, these strategic implications put pressure on the manufacturing organization to anticipate and implement quality and capacity improvements to support business objectives. New facilities, whether owned by innovator companies or operated through contractors, are being forced to be highly efficient while balancing the need to meet quality requirements and the ability to deliver product sustainably.

The current Good Manufacturing Practice (cGMP) manufacturing operations typically follow a hierarchical structure where corporate strategy drives business strategy, which, in turn, drives manufacturing strategy and therefore cGMP facilities' expectations. Supply chain and plant networking strategies have grown more important in recent years in response to globalization and customer expectations for speed and access. While designing and delivering cGMP pharmaceutical facilities have always been a challenge, the challenges are growing. Dynamic global developments are raising the bar of strategic implications for manufacturers as they consider appropriate responses, which affect the mission, size, configuration, cost, and location of new cGMP production facilities.

The productive life expectancy of cGMP facilities is decreasing as a result of advancements in technology and market conditions, which include increasing use of CDMOs and rationalization of facilities due to mergers and acquisitions. Contract manufacturers face similar challenges as they

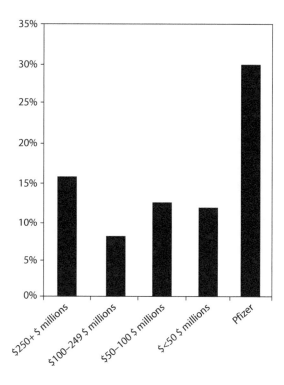

FIGURE 1.1 Average profitability profile: contract manufacturers by enterprise size. (From Contract Pharma, "Pharma Source Research". www.contractpharma.com)

seek to maintain a competitive advantage for their services, which may include adoption of the latest processes, equipment, and approaches that ensure high-quality production levels, while maintaining a reasonable cost structure and worker safety (Figure 1.1).

Outsourcing Contract Development and Manufacturing

The pharmaceutical industry is increasingly turning to outside, third-party organizations, or CDMOs, to help develop and manufacture their products. By some estimates, 25%–30% of current pharmaceutical development and production is now through CDMOs. These contractors specialize as developers and producers for small-molecule active pharmaceutical ingredients (APIs), oral dosages, and emerging biologic products. Many industries use this approach, including aerospace, defense, computer, semiconductor, food, and others. The strategic objectives for producer organizations, regardless of the industry, are to speed up development time, lower costs, and enhance quality. Drugs developed and made by CDMOs must meet all of the quality expectations, including compliance with all applicable cGMP guidelines.

The trend toward outsourcing development and production has accelerated over the last 10 years, largely in response to market pressures on innovator firms to manage costs and gain access to new technologies. Benefits to innovator firms for using CDMOs include reduction in capital costs for equipment and facilities, speed to market, and access to advanced skills. Outsourcing high-volume, low-margin drugs and older drugs also allows innovator companies to focus on core competencies in development and production and newer, complex processes kept in-house. Potential risks inherent in contracting include reduced control and responsiveness, quality management complexity, and loss of intellectual capital.

Partnering with CDMOs is now a well-established strategic approach for the pharmaceutical industry. Establishing and managing relationships with CDMOs will continue to be a critical organizational imperative. Technical innovations in packaging, filling, and high-volume production will increasingly originate from CDMOs. Current challenges for CDMOs include adding value through process optimization; expanding use of green, sustainable chemistry to reduce the use of solvents; and decreasing the number of processing steps. High-volume, oral dose production has moved steadily toward and will likely expand further with CDMOs. Costly capital investment and expensive production, such as sterile filling, will likely move to CDMOs, especially for biosimilars (generic products), which are expected to gain more approvals as patents expire. Cost efficiency will likely drive many innovators toward outsourcing decisions and more partnering with CDMOs.

The CDMO industry is experiencing consolidation as pressure rises due to pricing competition, lower profit margins, and the lack of organic growth potential. Typical profit margins for CDMOs are lower (about half) than those for the pharmaceutical industry. Mergers and acquisition activity are up, and consolidation is occurring. There are many hundreds of globally based CDMOs, but it has been estimated that 70% of world CDMO production is handled by 30 companies [1]. Outsourcing of API processing and drug product development and manufacturing is a significant economic driver. In 2014, the pharmaceutical industry spent approximately $140 billion on formulation, development, and manufacturing, with $40 billion outsourced to CDMOs [2].

Biotech innovators are increasingly turning to CDMOs since bioderived products are particularly challenging and costly to formulate and produce in commercial quantities. Biotech products typically comprise large molecules, including proteins, which need protection as stable products. Large molecules are more difficult to make, ship, store, and deliver to patients. The CDMOs are increasingly partnering with innovators for new drug applications (NDAs). Formulation programs include challenging work with physiochemical characteristics of the biologics of interest. Most biological products are delivered as parenteral drugs, and many of these are lyophilized, reconstituted, and shipped as liquids. They are filled under aseptic conditions, which is challenging and expensive. Advances in barrier isolation approaches to aseptic processing have been embraced by CDMOs.

SUPPLY CHAIN LOGISTICS AND SECURITY

The pharmaceutical industry relies heavily on a complex system of suppliers and distributors. Security and brand integrity are primary operating concerns. The Drug Supply Chain Security Act (initiated in January 2015) has set requirements for serialization and traceability to be implemented in three phases over a 10-year period. Traceability techniques are aimed at improving product integrity and reducing the counterfeiting through brand security measures, including microprinting, holograms, invisible inks, and other printing and mechanical methods. To implement these techniques, additional capital investments, up to $250,000–$500,000 per packaging line, additional floor space, and line efficiencies are necessary. Computer-assisted processing will proliferate with these new systems and may be implemented through cloud-based platforms. Below is a list of interesting statistics that concern the projected direction of the pharmaceutical industry:

- The National Association of Boards of Pharmacy reported that "the growth of global counterfeit piracy activities is estimated to range up to 10% of the global drug supply and could seriously threaten the economic well-being of international pharmaceutical companies" [3].
- Pharmaceutical industry employment in the United States includes 810,000 direct employees and more than 3.4 million indirect employees.
- From 2004 to 2013, more than 400 medicines were approved.
- There are currently 900 biological medicines in development.
- The generic market share (prescription volume) increased from 49% in 2000 to 86% in 2013.
- The growth rate for R&D spending declined from 10% from 1985 to 2003 to 4.2% from 2004 to 2013.
- The annual sales growth of pharmaceutical companies declined from 10.8% from 1985 to 2003 to 3.3% from 2004 to 2013.

- The approval rate for research candidate drugs entering phase 3 is 16%.
- Only 2 of 10 approved drugs recover their R&D costs [4].
- Worldwide prescription drug sales in 2013 were flat as industry patents tapered off.
- Oncology drugs are set to record the highest worldwide sales growth of all major therapy categories, with projections for an 11.2% compounded annual growth rate from 2013 to 2020.
- Within the top 100 prescription products in 2020, biological products are expected to account for 50% of sales [5].
- Generics were 84% of all prescriptions filled in 2012, up from 63% in 2007, and are projected to grow to 87% in 2017.
- More than 7,000 rare diseases have been identified, affecting an estimated 25 to 30 million people. To date, only 470 therapies have been approved for these rare diseases [6].

RISK MANAGEMENT

The cost of cGMP failures to society and to the responsible producing enterprise is significant and increasing. Some organizations have reported remediation costs totaling $500 million or more. Managing the risks presented by the manufacture of globally sourced products is a major business activity and presents significant responsibilities to technical professionals charged with the sustainable production of compliant products. Patient injuries; shortages of key medicines, resulting from production restrictions; and economic losses to producers barred from the marketplace are clearly undesirable situations demanding attention and oversight. Manufacturing professionals are confronted daily with such challenges and play a vital role in offering solutions.

Risk-based approaches are being employed wherein production quality methods incorporate up-to-date science and encourage new scientific advancements. Quality by design (QbD) initiatives have emerged on product development programs and provide some useful structured approaches for the facility designer. QbD is described in International Conference of Harmonisation (ICH) guidelines Q8, Q9, Q10, and Q11, and is defined as a science-based approach to pharmaceutical development and manufacturing, intending to ensure product quality. The approach includes defining target performance metrics and control strategies. The FDA and the European Medicines Agency (EMA) jointly launched a pilot program in 2012 to allow joint evaluation of QbD elements. Applying this approach to facility and process support systems offers a solid foundation for facility design. Conducting risk assessments is also encouraged by QbD approaches.

Harmonization of global production regulations has increased over the last decade to include quality risk management (QRM) and other approaches promulgated by the ICH organization. The development of the regulatory initiative led by the FDA, design space verification, is another design-focused approach that seeks to demonstrate that a combination of input process parameters and material attributes ensures the manufacturing of a quality product on a commercial scale.

High-risk manufacturing challenges are being raised by recent product developments, including customized controlled release, dividable tablets, advanced soft gels, nanodose formulations, self-administered delivery forms, combination therapies, and uniform ratios for antibody drug conjugates (ADCs). Also known as immunotherapies, ADCs are a new class of therapeutic agent that is gaining worldwide attention. The marriage of an antibody with a cytotoxic drug is known as a conjugate. ADCs are thought to be more efficient and effective in the treatment of disease. Safe processing of cytotoxic materials presents considerable challenges to the manufacturer to ensure reliable protection for workers and the community.

Delivering facilities that serve the global marketplace presents many risks and challenges to technical professionals. Diverse consumer preferences and regional business practices complicate the objectives to plan, design, construct, and operate cGMP facilities successfully. These plants must deliver a globalized product subject to evolving technologies and compliance requirements, emanating from several influential regulatory authorities, such as the U.S. FDA, Medicine and Healthcare Products Regulatory (United Kingdom), Ministry of Health, Labor, and Welfare (Japan), China Food and Drug Administration, Central Drugs Standard Control Organization (India), and World Health Organization (United Nations), among others around the globe. Despite recent progress with regulatory harmonization, global regulatory requirements remain discontinuous, especially in remote locations where there are questionable capabilities of local suppliers and support industries.

Pharmaceutical innovator companies (those who invest extensively in R&D programs) typically devote 5%–10% of their annual sales each year toward capital spending for plant and equipment. This is a relatively low rate of capital investment when compared to other industries that typically commit 15%–40% of annual revenues to capital investment in such groups as infotech, semiconductors, chemicals, and mining. Innovator companies do invest heavily in R&D where typically up to 20% or more of annual sales is spent toward innovation.

Operating costs are increasing as a result of rising energy costs, environmental management, and demands to minimize waste. Technical professionals are deeply involved in the project management and delivery of facilities that must adhere to dynamic business requirements and conform to evolving regulatory demands. The application of good design practices offers assistance for an organization to achieve needed efficiencies and strong performance.

STRATEGIC ENVIRONMENTAL FORCES

The pharmaceutical manufacturing landscape comprises a wide range of entities, including global innovators, generics, CDMOs, providers of professional services and equipment and system solutions, and suppliers of specialty materials. Pharmaceutical manufacturing includes the production of small-molecule (traditional chemical processes) and large-molecule (newer biological processes) drugs. For manufacturing and related cGMP facilities, the industries' production lies largely with global innovator companies; however, over the last decade, a growing level of production, approximately 10%–15%, is outsourced to CDMOs.

Pharmaceutical manufacturers are typically large, complex enterprises. There are more than 700 companies operating in the pharmaceutical industry in the United States. The leading 10 firms account for more than 40% of industry sales. Interestingly, pharmaceutical industries remain quite decentralized. Many large industries consolidate over time, so that the top three or four firms own 60%–75% of the respective markets. While some highly public pharmaceutical industry consolidations are occurring, the market share of the top 10 enterprises has remained steady at less than 50% of the total market for the last 20 years. There appears to be much more room for consolidation in the future.

The implications of profound and accelerating market changes offer many future manufacturing challenges for all players, including operating companies, service, and solution providers. Technical professionals engaged in the planning, designing, constructing, commissioning, validating, and operating of pharmaceutical cGMP facilities occupy an increasingly strategic role within their organizations. Engineers, architects, scientists, and management professionals are assuming pivotal roles in supporting the successful implementation of manufacturing and supply chain strategies. Whether employed by an innovator company's in-house staff, a professional design and construction firm, a CDMO, or a specialty vendor or supplier, the built-environment professional, is deeply engaged in developing and delivering complex facilities. Being fully skilled in the application of good design practices is a vital capability for technical professionals who contribute daily to their organization's success.

Industry manufacturing costs are increasing as solutions are becoming more complex in response to increasing demands for quality and sustainable practices, including imperatives to address global standards for responsible energy and environmental management. Technical professionals are deeply involved in the project management and delivery of facilities, which are required to "perform" in response to dynamic business requirements, while also expected to "conform" to evolving regulatory demands (Figure 1.2 and Tables 1.1 through 1.3).

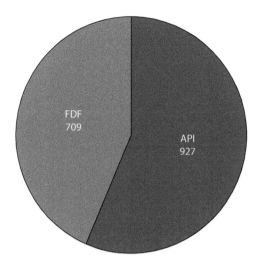

FIGURE 1.2 Global pharma manufacturing facilities. FDF, finished drug facilities; API, active pharma ingredients facilities.

TABLE 1.1
Global Pharmaceutical Market: 2013

	Total Global Sales		U.S. Sales Only	
Orals	55%	$542 bn	52%	
Parenterals	30%	$260 bn[a]	29%	
Topicals	5%	$45 bn		
Other	9%	$80 bn	19%	
Totals	100%	$972 bn	100%	$329 bn

Source: Kunst M, et al., A New Pharma Launch Paradigm, Bain & Co., www.bain.com/publications/articles/a-new-pharma-launch-paradigm.aspx.
Note: bn, billion.
[a] Biologics, $124 bn; small-molecule injectables, $100 bn; vaccines, $13 bn; and others, $33 bn [7].

TABLE 1.2
Total Global Manufacturing cGMP Facilities

	2015	2014
APIs	927	942
FDFs	709	685
API/FDF testing only	1,027	975

Source: Kunst M, et al., A New Pharma Launch Paradigm, Bain & Co., www.bain.com/publications/articles/a-new-pharma-launch-paradigm.aspx.
Note: APIs, active pharmaceutical ingredients; cGMP, current good manufacturing practice; FDF, finished dosage form [8].

TABLE 1.3

Manufacturing Countries: Number of Approved Facilities

	API 2015/2014	API/PDF Testing 2015/2014	FDF 2015/2014
Canada	16/16	45/43	30/30
China	170/168	71/63	43/43
Germany	38/40	62/53	31/28
India	235/238	11/206	154/142
Italy	68/69	34/32	22/23
Japan	29/23	7/5	5/3
Mexico	10/13	8/10	3/3
Spain	30/29	24/18	15/13
Switzerland	21/24	14/15	10/11
United States	123/136	350/353	283/281

Source: Kunst M, et al., A New Pharma Launch Paradigm, Bain & Co., www. bain.com/publications/articles/a-new-pharma-launch-paradigm.aspx.

Note: Of the 709 total registered global finished drug facilities, there were 370 (55%) solid dosage form production facilities and 339 (45%) injectable production facilities, of which 130 are in the United States [9]. PDF, pharmaceutical development facility; FDF, finished dosage form.

The pharmaceutical industry is a global business and subject to a complex landscape. The following discussions offer a summary of the major strategic forces at play that demand strong enterprise responses to navigate change successfully and deliver highly regulated products effectively to an increasingly diverse and expanding global market (Figure 1.3).

POLITICAL FORCES

Due to the rising costs of health care and especially the high prices of many new medications, governments are focusing on the pharmaceutical industry for solutions. Senior citizens consume considerably more medications than any other age group and have a progressively more powerful voice. As the population ages worldwide, so too does the influence of this demographic. The "gray vote" is driving discussions on the high cost of medications and the desired advocacy role of government in reimbursement, as well as control of the health care insurance industry.

The Affordable Care Act (ACA) of 2013 promises to have a prodigious effect on the pharmaceutical industry. With such critical issues as consumers' pay share of medical insurance, universal coverage, and promised cost reductions for health care coverage achieved through competition and efficiency, the ACA will likely affect the ability of companies to recover innovation investments and sustain profit margins.

Emerging and highly visible concerns for global climate change will also affect the industry through pressure to produce drugs, using environmentally sustainable processes. Government regulations will likely demand that future manufacturing activities incorporate state-of-the-art energy conservation and waste and emission reduction methods. Investors and local communities will also be watching as all manufacturers, not only in the pharmaceutical sector, respond with strategies that include greener, more sustainable approaches to their net impact on the environment. In the short run, these additional environmentally friendly processes will likely raise the cost of manufacturing. There are promises of net efficiencies and new technologies that

Pharmaceuticals industry: strategic environmental factors			
External factors	Macro trends	Industry impact	Manufacturing facility response
Social	Aging population ↑ Greening ↑ Awareness ↑ Pharma public trust ↓ Supply shortages ↑ Pandemics ↑	Higher unit volume ↑ Focus on sustainability ↑ Home care ↑	Faster turnovers/high speed/more output ↑ Safety stock ↑ Redundancy ↑
Political	Gray vote ↑ ACA ↑ Climate change ↑	Publicity sensitive ↑ $ Cost of failure ↑	
Technology	Biotech ↑ Genome ↑ e-Based solutions ↑ Cloud ↑	Obsolescence ↑ New processes/tech transfer ↑ New dosage deliveries ↑ Complex manufacturing cold chain ↑ Management ↑	Flexible plant designs ↑ Modular unit ops EQ ↑ Single use systems ↑ Cloud based I/O ↑
Finance	Tax strategies ↑ Stock market/investors ↑ M&A ↑	Global site selection ↑ Country of operations ↑ Excess facilities ↑	Plant closure/ remodeling ↑ Off balance street deals ↑ Leasing ↑
Economics	Global ↑ Mid-classs ↑ Insurers role ↑	Higher unit volumes ↑ Prive sensitivity ↑ Lower margins ↑	COGS sensitivity ↑
Legal/ regulatory	Counterfeiting ↑ Regulatory aggression ↑ Whistle-blower class actions ↑ Patent expirations ↑	$ Cost of failures ↑ Shorter life cycles ↑ R&D spending ↑ Compliance costs ↑	$ Cost of quality management ↑ Commissioning ↑ Standardization ↑
Market	Generics ↑ Blockbusters ↓ Specialty small market drugs ↑ Global brands/ products ↑	Fewer customers/large volume buyers Reduced sales #'s ↑ Focus on health outcome vs. product only ↑ Speed to market ↑	Outsourcing CMO/CRO ↑ Partnering vendors ↑ Fasttrack CM ↑

Note: ↑ indicates trend

FIGURE 1.3 Pharmaceuticals industry: strategic environmental factors.

would reduce the negative impacts on the cost of goods. Below is a summary of some business activities within the pharmaceutical industry.

• The prices of drugs are increasing faster than any other patient expense.
• Pharmaceutical companies spend almost twice as much on marketing and administration than on research.
• Americans pay more for prescription medications than anyone else in the world.
• The average per capita number of prescriptions written in the United States is 12.2 per year, which is an annual increase of 1.7% in 2013. The average number of prescriptions for patients over 65 years old is 28 per year.
• Two-thirds of all new prescription drugs are identical to existing drugs and essentially are modified versions.

- Over the last few years, the FDA has sent warning letters about manufacturing and packaging violations to companies operating in Australia, Austria, Canada, Germany, Ireland, Japan, Spain, India, China, and others. Commonly cited problems are contamination and inadequate testing of medications.
- The FDA has pledged to increase foreign facility inspections and to do so as frequently as it does domestic plants, which is every 2 years, according to the FDA Safety and Innovation Act of 2012. The agency also announced beefing up the number of inspectors it has in India from 12 to 19 and in China from 8 to 27.
- According to the FDA, approximately 40% of finished drugs come from abroad, and 80% of APIs are also manufactured outside the United States.
- Spending on branded (patent-protected) drugs accounts for 71% of total consumer drug spending in the United States. Generic drugs account for 29% of domestic spending.
- Branded prescription drugs account for 14%.

Social Forces

Pharmaceutical manufacturing strategies are increasingly challenged to respond to evolving social forces that affect the scale of production and the nature of the products consumed by a growing, aging, and diverse global population. The industry also must respond effectively to actual and potential supply interruptions of critical medications, which threaten to harm dependent patients, as well as raise a public outcry for additional government intervention (Figure 1.4).

People are living longer and are seeking healthier outcomes for better lifestyles. The average life expectancy in the United States in 1900 was 47 years; in 2000, it was 80 years. Global literacy in 1970 was 47%, and today it is 84%. Global infant mortality in 1990 was 61 per 1,000; today it is 40 per 1,000. The global population is increasing, which raises the consumption of medical products, as well as the total cost of providing these products. The world population was 2.5 billion in 1950, 3.5 billion in 1970, and today it is more than 7 billion.

Consumption of medicine increases dramatically with age. Consumers over 65 years of age buy more than twice the number of prescriptions as the general population average and more than five times the number of prescriptions as those under 25 years of age. The impact on manufacturers is an increased demand from the marketplace and governments for greater access to cost-effective drugs. Providing specialty products for home care is a growing opportunity driven by an aging population. Pharmaceutical manufacturers see this trend as an opportunity to expand distribution channels with an accompanying drive to reduce the cost of goods. Custom medications, offered in safer and more stable ways, such as single-dose packaging, are clearly on the rise.

The once highly regarded pharmaceutical industry has recently suffered a reduction in public trust. Claims of price gouging, fraudulent research activities, and high-profile product failures are increasingly common headlines and provide significant challenges for industry leaders. The media label of "big pharma," similar to "big oil" and "big tobacco," is a popular pejorative reference to "big" industries that are increasingly characterized as powerful and greedy.

The continuing threat of a global disease pandemic also affects industry policy and practice. The potential spread of life-threatening disease across the world is in the headlines. Government leaders look to the health care system for solutions, including medications that can reduce or eliminate the spread of infectious diseases. The high level of public awareness drives government officials toward high-profile remedies, which will likely include the accelerated introduction of medications offering potential solutions. The pharmaceutical industry's role in this arena is prominent and offers significant potential for bolstering goodwill and driving manufacturing processes to deliver an adequate supply of medications in a timely manner.

Some industry observers claim that the high cost of health care is, in part, due to the lack of progress and low efficiencies in health care delivery. "Productivity improvements in health

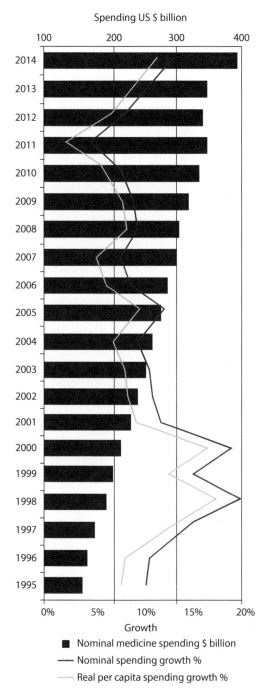

Spending US $ billion

FIGURE 1.4 Medicine Spending and Growth. (From IMS Health, National Sales Perspectives, December 2014; U.S. Census Bureau; U.S. Bureau of Economic Analysis. www.imshealth.com)

care industries have generally underperformed most other sectors. Incorporation of new process technologies has lagged other industries. Statistics from the Bureau of Economic Analysis and Centers for Medicine and Medicaid Services indicate that productivity improvements for health care have actually declined slightly over the last 20 years when compared to significant increases in sectors such as computers, Internet, telecom, retail trade, and wholesale trade" [10].

FINANCIAL FORCES

As one of the largest global industries, the pharmaceutical industry is a major economic force. Several hundred companies discover, develop, manufacture, and distribute thousands of unique pharmaceutical products globally. Over the last 50 years, investors have been choosing the pharmaceutical sector as a source of above-average growth potential. The pharmaceutical industry has earned the reputation as a well-managed group of companies that consistently offer favorable returns. In the last several years, however, there has been a mixed performance for many companies, resulting from competition from generic drugs and a loss of patent protection on blockbuster products. The ACA promises to accelerate the level of uncertainty and the rate of change confronting the industry, a rate that will require strategic responses; these responses, in turn, will affect manufacturing operations and the future mission of cGMP facilities.

The pharmaceutical industry has lost some of its shine from a once golden image for investors over the last decade. A review of the current top 500 corporations, as listed by *Fortune Magazine* in June 2015, notes that only one pharmaceutical company, Allergan, made the list of the top 20 leaders in returns to shareholders over the last year, and only one company, Biogen, made the list for the last 5 years. Two companies, Celgene and Gilead Sciences, are listed for a 10-year horizon. A ranking by market value yields two pharmaceutical companies on the list of the top 20 corporations: Pfizer and Johnson & Johnson. There are no pharmaceutical companies on the list of the top 20 corporations as measured by employees or equity. There are no pharmaceutical companies on the top 20 list as measured by return on shareholders' equity (Tables 1.4 and 1.5).

Increased drug approvals by the FDA in 2014 and the somewhat lessened effect of patent expirations are positively affecting pharmaceutical stock valuations, which are up approximately 50% in 2015 compared to 2014. Pharmaceutical stock values have doubled in the last 3 years, rebounding from a downturn starting in 2006, when values took a long slow slide to reach lows of 50% of the previous value.

The financial performance of pharmaceutical companies has also been challenged in the last decade by the number of layoffs due to mergers and acquisitions. In 2009 and 2010, for example, Pfizer merged with Wyeth, and Merck merged with Schering-Plough, which resulted in approximately 40,000 layoffs.

TABLE 1.4
Industry Comparisons: 2014

Industry Sectors	Number of Firms[a]	Revenue ($ bn)	Profits ($ bn)	Profit (% Revenue)
Pharma	11	284	65	22
Banks	18	630	103	21
Railroads	3	48	9	18
Semiconductors	9	137	20	12
Utilities	24	312	27	9
Chemicals	14	225	20	9
Mining	13	235	10	8
Airlines	6	151	7	6
General merchandizing	10	700	17	4
Petroleum	13	1107	66	3
Engineering/construction	6	67	2	3
Food/drug stores	8	450	11	2

Source: Selected Industries, 500 Largest US Firms, *Fortune Magazine*, May 2015.

[a] Biggest firms in sector.

TABLE 1.5

Pharma Industry Large Mergers and Acquisitions[a]: Highest Premium Price Paid

Acquirer	Acquired	Date	Deal Value ($ bn)	Premium[b]%
Gilead Sciences	Pharmasset	2011	11.0	89
Cardinal Health	Allegiance Corp.	1998	6.4	67
Takeda Pharma	Millennium	2008	8.4	53
Pfizer	Hospira	2015	17.0	39
Amgen	Onyx	2013	10.2	38
Roche	InterMune	2014	8.4	38
Merck	Cubist	2014	9.5	37
Merck	Schering-Plough	2009	53.9	34
Hologic	Cytyc Corp.	2007	6.0	33

Source: As reported in Dealogic, Fattest Deals in USA, *Fortune Magazine*, February 6, 2015.

Note: Acquisition price share value over stock price at announcement.

[a] U.S. pharma merger activity compared to other industries ("other" average multiple 34%).

[b] In 2014, 938 deals valued at $310 bn, up 57% over 2013.

Compared with other industries, health care has demonstrated poor productivity improvements. The Bureau of Economic Analysis's Center for Medicare and Medicaid Services estimates that during the period 1990–2007, the health care industry has actually registered a reduced annual productivity rate of 0.8%, while the average employment growth rate was 3%. This is the poorest productivity improvement rate and the highest average growth rate in employment among 15 major industry sectors [10] (Table 1.6).

Better manufacturing operations have increasingly been the industry's response to reduce the cost of goods in the current low-profit landscape. Sales volumes have been adversely affected in several ways in the last decade. An expanding consumer marketplace is demanding better access to low-cost medicine. Government and insurance actions have reduced prices for many popular brands that have lost patent protection. Manufacturers are seeking efficiencies, where possible, to protect profit margins. Strategies have included consolidation of manufacturing facilities; abandonment of small-volume, low-profit products; and mergers and acquisitions to improve scale and distribution potential. The CDMOs have grown considerably in the past 10 years and offer options to innovator companies that seek to rationalize their global production capacity.

The intensity of mergers and acquisitions, including consolidation of innovator companies, has continued over the last decade and promises to remain a potent strategy going forward. In 2013, there were 615 announced and closed transactions, involving targets in the pharmaceutical sector, compared to 456 in 2012 [11]. These activities continue to generate many plant closures, consolidations, renovations, and relocations of productive capacity for the posttransaction entity.

Globalization has also resulted in companies increasing the effectiveness of their investments in R&D, leveraging the productive life cycle of their medicines, and producing product with acceptable financial returns. Strategic tax management goals are also driving the deals, including so-called inversions where the newly merged entities enjoy lower business taxes by being headquartered outside the United States.

According to PricewaterhouseCoopers in their publication "Pharma 2020: The Vision," "the current pharmaceutical industry business model is both economically unsustainable and operationally incapable of acting quickly enough to produce the types of innovative treatments demanded by

TABLE 1.6

Top Merger and Acquisition Deals in 2014: Ranked on Deal Value

Rank	Target	Target Location	Target Focus	Acquirer	Completion Date	Deal Value ($ bn)
1	Forest Laboratories	United States	Specialty	Actavis	July 1, 2014	28
2	InterMune	United States	Biotechnology	Roche	September 29, 2014	8.3
3	Questcor Pharmaceuticals	United States	Specialty	Mallinckrodt Pharmaceuticals	August 14, 2014	5.6
4	BMS Diabetes Business[a]	United States	Specialty	AstraZeneca	February 1, 2014	4.3
5	ViroPharma	United States	Biotechnology	Shire	January 14, 2014	4.2
6	Idenix Pharmaceuticals	United States	Biotechnology	Merck & Co.	August 5, 2014	3.9
7	Galderma	Switzerland	Specialty	Nestle	July 8, 2014	3.6
8	Rottapharm	Italy	Specialty	Meda	October 10, 2014	3.1
9	Algeta	Norway	Biotechnology	Bayer	March 6, 2014	2.9
10	Aptalis Holdings	United States	Specialty	Forest Laboratories	February 3, 2014	2.9
11	CFR Pharmaceuticals	Chile	Specialty	Abbott Laboratories	September 26, 2014	2.9
	Other					49
	Total					115.8

[a] Bristol.

global markets. In order to make the most of future growth opportunities Pharma must fundamentally change the way it operates" [12]. Global pharmaceutical companies are known to strategically position their operations to maximize the positive effect on taxation rates. The global nature of the business offers significant potential to realize lower tax rates by incorporating and operating where local governments offer incentives for their presence. These practices have been observed for the last 40 years and will likely continue to be an option for companies to maximize their profit margins and their attractiveness to investors.

Plant location strategies affect manufacturing activities by decentralizing operations and requiring support for multiple facilities. Significant manufacturing densities can be observed in tax-haven locales, such as Puerto Rico, Singapore, and Ireland, where local governments entice jobs through tax reductions. Inversions, the controversial tactic of relocating corporate headquarters in the United States to a sovereign state with lower taxes, are popular strategies.

TECHNOLOGY AND MANUFACTURING

Pharmaceutical manufacturing operations are becoming more complex in response to rapidly changing markets. Growing global populations and increased standards of living have created a demand for affordable, effective pharmaceutical products, especially for millions of new customers in emerging markets, such as China, India, Indonesia, and Brazil. The demand for producing greater volumes of high-quality, high-cost compliant products is on the rise and is creating additional risks for the pharmaceutical manufacturer and the supply chain. In addition, the pharmaceutical industry is rapidly "offshoring" by establishing manufacturing, research, and clinical trials in India, China, Singapore, and elsewhere to lower costs and remain competitive. According to Elaine Pratt at Stevens Institute of Technology, "pharmaceutical operations are becoming more global than ever requiring a new mix of skills. Engineers, managers, and technicians in the field must be prepared to deal with cultural differences, management of manufacturing environments, and local methods" [13].

Manufacturing processes are advancing to meet the challenges to deliver high-precision formulations, including long-acting, time-released coatings, nanogranulations, and anticounterfeiting techniques. Evolving biochemical process technology is adding to the scope of pharmaceutical production, including the need for high-containment facilities for toxic component handling and sterile production facilities necessary for the many new, biologic, injectable, large-molecule, dosage forms, arising from new biotechnological developments.

Significant strategic business benefits can be secured through improved manufacturing and supply chain performance. Advantages may include reduction of cost, shortened manufacturing lead times, reduced inventory levels, and minimized product obsolescence. Drug shortages may also be reduced, thus increasing access for millions of patients in the emerging markets. Reduction in counterfeiting activity may also be achieved. By some estimates, the health care sector can improve margins by tens of billions of dollars and improve safety by improving its supply chain.

Advances in science and engineering have played a significant role in the development and delivery of modern medicine. The industry continues to be a major investor in R&D, using advanced science applied to innovation and product delivery to a growing world market. Advances in the application of biotechnology over the last several decades have significantly altered the industry's approach to new product development and the resulting effectiveness of disease management regimes.

Some observers note that pharmaceutical manufacturing practices are relatively low tech and have not developed as fast or as well as other technology-based industries. According to McKinsey & Company, "many other industries have adapted much more quickly. If engineers who had worked on a manufacturing system for an automotive company in the 1950s were to visit a state-of-the-art automotive plant today, the many changes would astonish them as they observe robots tirelessly spot welding car bodies where men once stood wearing welding masks. Their counterparts in the steel industry would observe a similar experience as highly automated, integrated mills turnout competitively priced products" [14].

Emerging sophisticated process techniques, including those for strict containment, sterile filling, and high-speed packaging, are increasingly being developed by third-party solution providers who have made the investments to advance the effectiveness and productivity of their offerings. The pharmaceutical shop floor now sees increased use of modular, prefabricated process unit operations, which support high-quality output, including effective measures to maintain controlled environments for sterility, product containment, and a safer workplace. Advances in plastics are now seen in the workplace through deployment of flexible single-use or disposable (SUD) systems, which promise to reduce capital investment and increase the use of existing plant space, while avoiding cleaning and maintenance expenses.

Advances in manufacturing technology offer opportunities to reenergize pharmaceutical production. The shape and scope of the manufacturing plant of the future is emerging with advancements in computing power, sensors, and connectivity. Future facilities will likely include larger numbers of embedded sensors, connected via cloud-based networks, enabling address through mobile devices. The so-called Internet of Things concept will support improvements in manufacturing efficiency and flexibility and greater autonomy of operations on the shop floor. As the marketplace demands more custom, personalized, and complicated medicines, evolving technology will enable elegant solutions, especially for biologically derived products, where manufacturing advances will reshape operations to include smaller campaign sizes, higher-value components, and demanding containment requirements. See Appendix II for Special Article 2, "Biopharmaceutical Factories of the Future," by Mark A. Butler.

As a consequence of accelerated technology advancement, the effective productive life of manufacturing facilities is shrinking, and obsolescence is a growing challenge to capital investment in plants and equipment. The industry has significant overcapacity in some geographic areas. Also, certain processes have a marginal ability to contribute to the organization's strategic program. Consequently, a significant number of plants are closing, consolidating, or renovating to realign the industry's productive capacity to meet new challenges. These activities have resulted in reduced employment and disfavor in the local community as the plants are closed or downsized.

The adoption of new innovative technologies within the pharmaceutical industry has been slowed to some extent by new regulatory requirements, which often demand voluminous documented evidence of sustainable practice. The time and cost of compliance activities required to validate new manufacturing processes tend to be an obstacle to change. It can take many months to demonstrate the organization's control of new processes. The documentation embedded in the standard operating procedures (SOPs) and in the qualification documents of new equipment and systems is considerable, often totaling thousands of pages.

Amending validation documents to accommodate process changes becomes a significant organizational challenge when innovative opportunities arise. Seasoned veterans admit that changing validated processes is difficult and often delayed in consideration of investment and risk management. Regulators are aware of the potential obstacles to modernization and collaborate with industry professionals in organizations such as the International Society for Pharmaceutical Engineering (ISPE), Parenteral Drug Association, American Association of Pharmaceutical Scientists, and Regulatory Affairs Professional Society.

Advances in novel dosage form delivery systems are also affecting the industry's production profile. Strategic partnering arrangements are also evolving to accommodate the blend of new combination products and medical device influences, arising from single-dose, convenient patient-centric delivery forms. The possibilities of using three-dimensional printing techniques for future nanoparticle dosage forms are accelerating to offer intriguing new opportunities in manufacturing and distribution. The industry is being driven by marketplace challenges to participate in holistic, disease prevention, and management solutions. Simply producing high-quality medicines is fading as an effective marketplace strategy. Rather, pharmaceutical companies of the future must partner in unique ways with health care providers and allied industries to produce cost-effective, highly accessible pharmaceutical products on a global scale.

New biotechnology-derived products and novel delivery schemes are adding diversity and new challenges to the manufacturing scene. Many new specialty products offer significant safety and production challenges. High-value, low-volume products also present risk management considerations for product quality, storage, and delivery. Value-based pricing for certain chronic and life-threatening disease management regimes is now emerging wherein the cost of these medicines is running in the hundreds of thousands of dollars a year. Life cycle, value-based pricing has produced oral dosage forms that cost $1,000 per dose, such as Sovaldi produced by Gilead Sciences [4]. Aside from the reimbursement implications of such pricing strategies, the manufacturing challenge to sustainably deliver these high-value products will drive future production strategies.

In the future, governments are likely to demand additional sustainability and low-energy consumption for all manufacturing facilities. This greening of new buildings will include increases in thermal insulation, window glazing and shading, rainwater collection, higher-efficiency equipment, and sophisticated building management systems to help provide detailed operating energy consumption data. State-of-the-art facilities for R&D, which often include cGMP production of early-stage materials, will incorporate "social" buildings that encourage team-based collaboration. Features may include both open and closed laboratory designs and flexibility to accommodate change through deployment of stand-alone equipment and electronic communication, as well as locations in science parks to facilitate partnerships between government and the private sector.

Research and Development

A widely recognized strategic success factor for the pharmaceutical industry is R&D productivity. A fiercely competitive marketplace mandates a robust pipeline of new innovative products. Recent merger activity and heightened rates of partnering programs attest to the need for consistent revenue generated from new products, as patent protection is lost and competition depletes sales. The cost to innovate in the pharmaceutical industry has risen dramatically in the past decade. Some estimates claim the cost to bring a new product to market can approach $2 billion [4]. Innovator companies are typically devoting 15% or more of their sales revenues to research programs. This spending rate is among the highest of any industry and well above typical industry averages of 3%–5%. The pharmaceutical industry devotes an average of 10–15 years of R&D to a new drug before it is approved for sale. For every 5,000–10,000 compounds tested, only one receives FDA approval. Patents provide protection for a total of 20 years. However, the average effective patent life of a prescription medicine is about 11 years due to the time lost during the R&D of the new medicine (Figure 1.5).

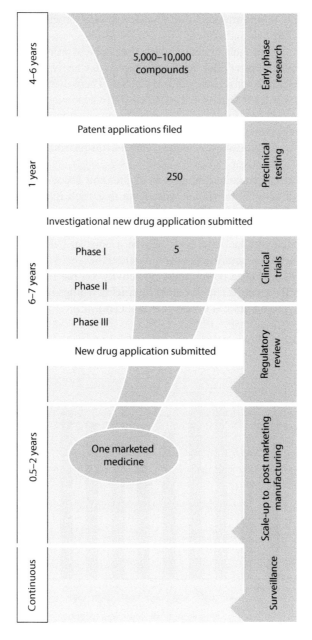

FIGURE 1.5 Drug research and regulatory approval process. (Adapted from 2011 PhRMa Industry Profile. www.phrma.org)

The Treaty of Marrakesh (2004) approved international trade in full patent protection for pharmaceutical products across industrial nations, as well as in the less developed nations. The industry boasts an investment rate of return that is four times the magnitude of that of a typical Fortune 500 company. The contract research organizations (CROs) are examples of outsourcing by innovator companies that enter into a contract for some or all aspects of development with a third party. Approximately 15%–20% of all research spending by innovator companies is now being executed through CROs. This trend has had a major impact in innovator company culture as historic R&D facilities have been sold or shuttered around the world. Innovator companies have reduced the scope of their research efforts as they focus on commercially attractive disease areas. Over the past decade, biotech, large-molecule research occupied a growing portion of new development programs. The cGMP regulations apply to research facilities that develop compounds for use in clinical phase 1 investigations (Figure 1.6).

Patent protection is often sought very early in the development process, making the length of patent protection for a product shorter after approval is received. Clearly, the economic stakes are high as costs rise and time shortens for recovery of investments. These dynamics are likely to continue to drive the industry to seek cost efficiencies, enhanced productivity measures gained through partnering, and new techniques, as well as a focus on commercially attractive products that address either large portions of global populations or specialty diseases where performance-based pricing is achievable. Below is a compilation of some business activities related to the pharmaceutical industry marketplace.

- International piracy and counterfeiting of medicines now account for an estimated 2%–7% of world trade, or about $500 billion, according to Zurich Insurance Group. Some estimates have higher rates (20%–40%) in the pharmaceutical business, especially in some developing countries.
- Emerging biosimilar product approvals will be a boon to CDMOs that are expected to handle 40% of the manufacturing of new biologics [15].
- The evolution of computing power and connectivity via the Internet is providing strong business support for growth. The so-called Internet of Things is anticipated to support the connection of 50 billion devices by the year 2025 [16].

Figures 1.7 through 1.10 show statistics on R&D spending in the United States and globally.

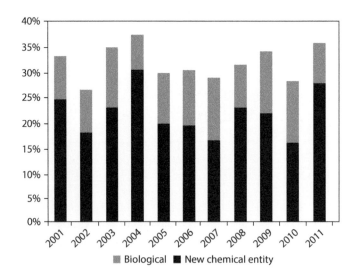

FIGURE 1.6 New chemical and biological entities approved by the U.S. FDA: 2001–2011. (From EvaluatePharma, World Preview 2012: Embracing the Patent Cliff. www.evaluategroup.com)

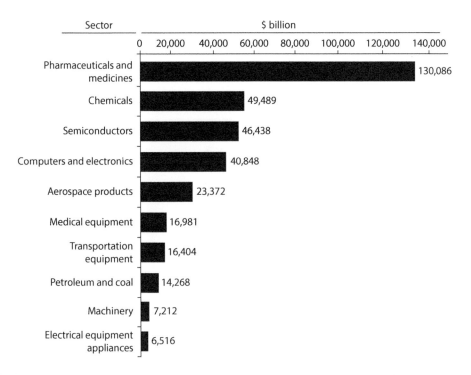

FIGURE 1.7 R&D expenditures per employee: U.S. manufacturing sectors 2000–2010. (From PhRMA, Biopharmaceutical Research Industry, 2015 Profile, PhRMA, April 2015. www.phrma.org/sites/default/files/pdf/2015_phrma_profile.pdf)

ECONOMICS

Pharmaceutical products are increasingly in demand around the world as global populations become more prosperous, especially in Asia, which produces a significantly larger consumer base. The emerging middle-class group presently number in the hundreds of millions. Among the growing expectations of this increasingly wealthy base of consumers is a higher standard of living, which includes improved access to affordable health care, which, in turn, becomes a main objective for governments as well as patients for greater access to pharmaceutical products. Thus, growing populations translate into potential growth in the pharmaceutical industry worldwide.

The rising cost of health care is a significant agenda item for the government. Today pharmaceutical products are reported to be 10%–15% of total health care costs. These costs are clearly a target for efficiencies and regulation as governments and consumers voice their concerns over affordability. Currently, more than 80% of all prescriptions filled around the world are generic products. The generic pharmaceutical industry has expanded significantly over the last decade and has benefited from patent losses of blockbuster drugs and a growing consumption trend.

The regulated pharmaceutical industry encompasses production of medicines originating from manufacturing facilities owned and operated by innovator companies, generic manufacturers, and CDMOs. The economic incentives of each of these producers vary considerably as their scale, scope, and incentive markets reflect the diverse global marketplace. Regardless of origin, all pharmaceutical production requires compliance with the cGMPs. While the rules are the same regardless of manufacturer, the risk management approach taken by each manufacturer varies, depending on cultural and geographical considerations. Conformance with cGMP quality standards also varies with the enforcement profile of the regulatory authorities who govern production within their boundaries. Risk-managed pharmaceutical operations can raise the cost of goods. Investments in redundant utility systems, flexible scale, local quality control units,

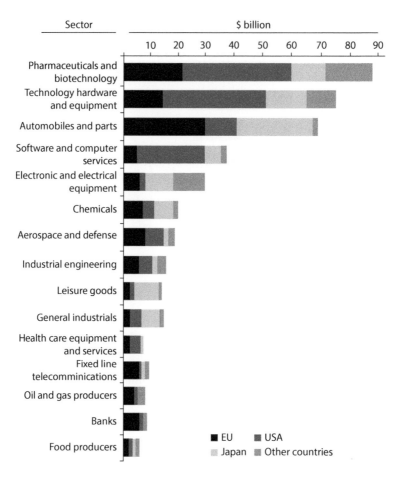

FIGURE 1.8 R&D investment: global industries: 2010. (From EvaluatePharma, World Preview 2012, Embracing the Patent Cliff. www.evaluategroup.com)

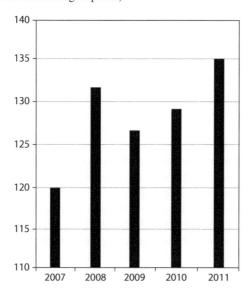

FIGURE 1.9 Global pharmaceutical R&D spending (in US$ billion). (From EvaluatePharma, World Preview 2012, Embracing the Patent Cliff. www.evaluategroup.com)

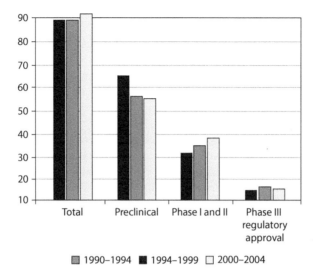

FIGURE 1.10 Pharmaceutical R&D failure rates.

	Proof of concept				Validation			Commercial
	Preclinical	P1	P2 A		P2 B	P3		
API	Process development, CTM			Go/no go/license	Tech transfer, scale-up, CTM		Regulatory approval	Market supply process improvement
Drug product		Powder in bottle/capsule			Preformation, commercial formulation, CTM, tech transfer			Market supply New formulations
Analytical	Characterization, API methods, CTM release and stability, raw materials				DP methods, CTM release and stability, reg. stability, validation, raw materials			Release, raw materials, new form. methods

FIGURE 1.11 Drug approval process.

size, configuration, maintenance of physical plant facilities, and other operational considerations contribute to the cost of goods (Figure 1.11).

Manufacturing strategies also vary in response to the forecasted sales and customer base for each product. Large-volume blockbuster innovator products can benefit from economies of scale achievable through high-volume approaches. High-volume generic products enjoy lower profit margins and also can be produced efficiently by large-scale, highly automated production techniques. Low-volume, high-priced specialty pharmaceutical markets can produce high rewards for innovator companies. Manufacturing considerations for these products include additional risk management investments to ensure stability of supply and high-quality output.

Competitive pressure for low-cost, highly accessible pharmaceutical products is likely to be a strong economic factor for the foreseeable future. Manufacturers are driven to balance the demands for high-quality, sustainable production facilities with total life cycle costs to operate modern facilities that meet strategic objectives and conform to challenging quality requirements embodied in cGMPs. According to industry experts, supply chain expenses now represent nearly 25% of pharmaceutical costs and 40% of medical device costs, which represent an annual spending of approximately $230 billion [14]. Up to $50 billion in inefficiencies exist in the pharmaceutical business [17].

LEGAL AND REGULATORY ISSUES

Pharmaceutical companies conduct their operations in a demanding legal environment. Successful operation includes high-priority responses to legal challenges. Originators of new drugs that seek regulatory permission through the NDA of the FDA are responsible for the entire production process until the drug reaches the consumer. The originator of the drug product holds ultimate market accountability. These responsibilities make it imperative that producers remain compliant throughout the market life of the product.

The health and safety of consumers are paramount. "Too costly to fail" is the strategic driving force behind the pharmaceutical industry's emphasis on quality and risk management. Regulatory authorities exercise their power to make certain cGMP violators cease production or submit to increased regulatory oversight as a result of quality failures. These legal actions are well-known and clearly understood risks to the business. Quality failures can end up as tragedies to consumers and as difficult business situations for the producers that face costly remedies and diminished public trust. The costs of production failures are rising and affecting risk management practices for manufacturing investments and operation.

Drug shortages are increasing and by some estimates have tripled since 2005. Typical annual drug shortages occur between 100 and 300 times as a result of production delays or stoppages due to quality problems and regulatory issues. The FDA reported 267 shortages in 2011, 204 shortages in 2012, and 140 shortages in 2013. According to the FDA, the United States had 5 drug recalls a week in 2005, but 19 recalls a week in 2011. Medication errors are on the rise, and it is thought that counterfeiting may account for some of this increase. Errors have been reported to affect 10%–20% of all inpatient hospital admissions, of which a third lead to adverse effects. One in 10,000 admissions dies from an adverse drug event [18].

Maintaining patent protection for the valuable intellectual property represented by innovative product developments has been a major business dynamic for research-based organizations for decades. The effective product market life span has been shrinking over the last decade as a result of several factors, which results in shorter time to recover development and market launch expenses. One factor is the trend to register for patent protection earlier in the R&D cycle to seek protection of the promising molecule, but in effect shortening the market life protection for the remaining life of the patent.

Patents for pharmaceutical products are generally granted for an exclusive market presence of 20 years. If, for example, an innovator company seeks and is granted a patent for a promising molecule that will require 4 or 5 more years of development and regulatory approval, the remaining market protection time after launch is 15 or so years. To make matters more pressing, accelerated innovation of competitive molecules is resulting in newer, often more effective therapies appearing more often and in shorter times, also having the effect of shortening the commercial life of the innovative product. These dynamics add to the challenges of sustainable innovation, investment recovery, and enhanced legal activities to protect new intellectual property. The effects of shortening product life cycles on manufacturing decisions, capacity investments, and outsourcing contracts are deepening and clearly are major challenges for long-term planning and manufacturing managers who are charged with anticipating and supplying the products of the future. Figures 1.12 through 1.14 show statistics relating to patents.

High-profile fines, fraudulent research data, whistle-blower cases, and class action suits because of product failure have broken down the high regard and goodwill with which the public has historically regarded the pharmaceutical industry. Shortages of certain medicines have also contributed to public concerns and increased the calls for government intervention. The cost of legal defense and the loss of market share are mounting at a time when profit margins have diminished and the cost of innovation has increased. Manufacturing operations are increasingly regarded as a strategic activity in their abilities to minimize quality failures and drug shortages.

Pharmaceutical companies have been experiencing rising costs of litigation. According to KPMG International, "over the past decade, pharmaceutical companies have paid billions of dollars

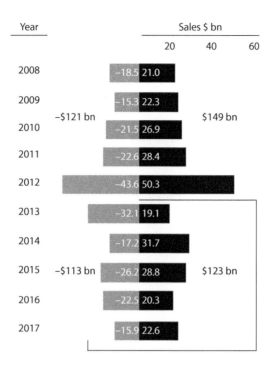

FIGURE 1.12 Developed markets' patent exposure and impact. (From EvaluatePharma, World Preview 2015, Outlook to 2020, 8th ed., EvaluatePharma, June 2015. www.evaluategroup.com)

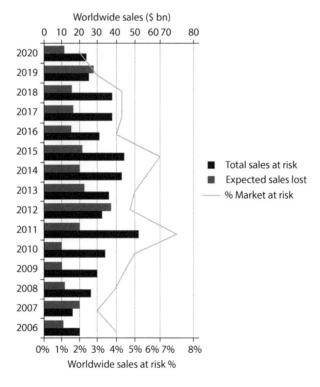

FIGURE 1.13 Worldwide sales at risk from patent expiration: 2006–2020. (From EvaluatePharma, World Preview 2012, Embracing the Patent Cliff. www.evaluategroup.com [May 22, 2015].)

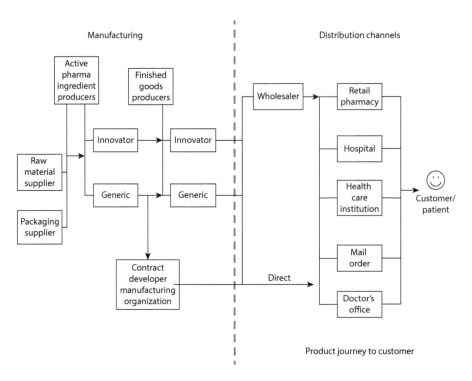

FIGURE 1.14   Pharmaceutical supply landscape.

to settle U.S. federal lawsuits. In fact, the global pharmaceutical industry surpassed the defense industry in the number of violations of the False Claims Act. From 2001 to 2010 pharmaceutical companies have accounted for about 25% of all False Claim Act settlements compared to 11% for the defense industry. From 1991 to 2010, the number of settlements and financial penalties attributed to the pharmaceutical industry has risen from an average of 15 a year during the 1990s to 200 a year on average during the first decade of the 21st century" [19].

The issues that most often drive legal settlements are drug safety, off-label promotion, and inflated prices. Over the last 20 years, more than 165 cases of civil and criminal actions have been settled in the United States by pharmaceutical companies with a total penalty of nearly $20 billion (e.g., Merck, $4.8 billion for Vioxx; Pfizer, $2.3 billion for Bextra; Eli Lilly, $1.4 billion for Zyprexa; and GlaxoSmithKline, $1 billion for Paxil). In addition to fines, the cost of litigation can be significant. AstraZeneca announced in 2010 that it had spent $656 million to defend itself in numerous cases, involving Seroquel, which was in addition to the company's $520 million agreement to settle a U.S. investigation.

Worldwide regulatory harmonization of cGMP guidelines is helping to address the need for standard approaches to manufacturing, quality control, and operations management. The costs of compliance with multiple governing organizations can be mitigated through approaches to shared risk oversight. According to the FDA leadership, they recognize the need to streamline and modernize their processes and work with industry and patients to identify appropriate goals. The FDA has been criticized for being a barrier to progress.

The uniform application of cGMPs across the globe is a challenge for regulators; it also provides risks for consumers and significant costs for global manufacturers for compliance. Understanding the requirements imposed by local regulatory authorities requires a strong organizational commitment and a powerful quality organization to interpret, apply, and execute designs and operational processes that meet or exceed local inspectors' challenges.

The emergence of global generic manufacturers and CDMOs has placed significant burdens on regulatory authorities to monitor and inspect regularly the several hundred facilities in the United States alone. Currently, there are several thousand cGMP manufacturing facilities spread throughout the world requiring regular inspection. In the United States, the FDA has been addressing this challenge with increased inspections of foreign manufacturing facilities, especially in China and India, that import to the United States and are therefore subject to FDA oversight.

FOOD AND DRUG ADMINISTRATION

Gaining timely and frequent approval for market drug products is a major business dynamic in the pharmaceutical industry. The FDA is charged with securing scientific confidence that new proposed products meet reasonable standards for safety and efficacy. Recently, the economic advantages of new medicines have played a role in the approval process, whereby the FDA has shown sensitivity to the cost of certain new medicines as it considers the advantages of market approval. The annual level of approvals for new molecular entities (NMEs) by the FDA has been generally accepted as too few to support the historic growth of the industry. The R&D productivity was a hot-button issue in the last decade and promises to be a top concern for the industry in the years ahead. Innovator companies have begun to use CROs for enhancing the efficiency of R&D programs.

The FDA was formed in 1902 and charged with protecting the safety of pharmaceutical consumers. The control of this agency, which now includes far-reaching controls, makes pharmaceuticals the most regulated products in the United States. These regulations have been instituted in response to highly publicized tragedies among consumers. For example, in 1937 the solvent diethylene glycol, which is used in antifreeze, was mistakenly mixed in an antibiotic drug liquid elixir, sulfanilamide, which resulted in the death of 107 people, mostly children. This tragedy led to the Food, Drug, and Cosmetic Act of 1938 that requires drugs to be proven safe before marketing. In another infamous tragedy, more than 10,000 European babies were born deformed when mothers took thalidomide to treat morning sickness. This led to the Kefauver Harris Amendments of 1962, which required that the efficacy of new drugs be proven before marketing. The list that follows presents statistics concerning new drug approvals and pricing:

- New drug and biologic approvals totaled 41 in 2014, which is the most since 1996. This rate of approvals compares with 39 approvals received in 2012 and 27 in 2013. In the period of 2012–2014, 44% of new drug approvals were totally new classes of medicines, compared to 27% for the period 1987–2001.
- Predictions are for 30–35 new drug approvals in the next 3 years. The average drug approval rate was 25 for the period 2000–2013. By some estimates, the number of new drug approvals for NMEs may not be enough to carry the 12 large global drug companies forward; thus, further consolidation and shrinkage in the number of independent large pharmaceutical companies (and the number of small pharmaceutical manufacturing facilities) should be expected.
- Inflation for drug products outpaces consumer inflation. The price of 5,000 popular drugs increased 11% in the United States, which was 14 times more than consumer inflation in the United States.

"From a scientific standpoint, it has never been a more exciting time. But how are we going to pay for it?" [20].

MARKETS

The global marketplace for pharmaceutical products continues to expand. The pharmaceutical industry is a global powerhouse producing more than $300 billion in revenue annually in the United States alone and nearly $1 trillion in revenue worldwide. The pharmaceutical market in the United States and Europe is stable and has been growing modestly over the last decade.

Expanding economies within China, Brazil, Indonesia, and other developing areas have increased their demands for low-cost accessible therapies. Volumes of drug production have increased accordingly, not only as a result of population demand but also in response to government reimbursement practices, which favor generic therapies that are cost-effective and tend to reduce national health care expenditures. Over the last decade, supply chain purchasing groups have emerged in the United States and Europe. These organizations, such as Walgreens, McKesson, and Cardinal Health, are leveraging their buying power, especially with generic producers, as they are buying billions of dollars of drugs and driving down prices (Figure 1.14).

The market share of generics has increased from 40% only 10 years ago to more than 85% of all global medicine prescriptions written today. Generic products are typically less than half the price to consumers of the previously patent-protected medicine. Generic manufacturers typically do not invest heavily in innovation for NMEs, thus raising the issue of from where new innovation will come and be supported through economic return. Generic biotech-derived products promise to grab sizable market share at lower prices. Expanded CDMOs in the biotech industry are anticipated (Tables 1.7 through 1.9).

TABLE 1.7
Top 20 Global Corporation Sales: 2013

	2013 Rank	2013 Sales (US$ mn)	2013 Growth (LC$ %)	2012 Sales (US$ mn)
Global market		874,611	4.5	857,710
Novartis	1	50,576	1.9	50,521
Pfizer	2	44,330	–2.6	46,707
Sanofi	3	38,181	1.4	38,531
Merck & Co., Inc.	4	36,350	–7.0	39,891
Roche	5	36,146	5.3	34,958
GlaxoSmithKline	6	32,544	1.5	32,736
Johnson & Johnson	7	30,784	12.2	27,717
AstraZeneca Pharmaceuticals LP	8	30,257	–2.9	31,704
Teva	9	24,258	–1.8	24,762
Lilly	10	23,045	8.4	21,583
Amgen	11	18,621	8.7	17,103
AbbVie	12	18,150	2.0	17,881
Boehringer Ingelheim	13	17,375	5.7	16,889
Bayer	14	17,276	8.3	16,431
Novo Nordisk	15	14,300	15.0	12,576
Takeda	16	13,399	–9.5	15,909
Actavis	17	12,742	2.9	12,375
Mylan	18	11,087	7.4	10,325
Bristol-Myers Squibb	19	11,023	–12.9	12,756
Gilead Sciences	20	11,011	14.8	9,540

Source: IMS Health MIDAS, December 2013.

Note: mn, million; US$, sales and rank in U.S. dollars with quarterly exchange rates; LC$, growth in constant dollars to normalize for exchange rate fluctuations. Growth rates in U.S. dollars are not recommended due to fluctuations in the value of the dollar. Sales cover direct and indirect pharmaceutical channel wholesalers and manufacturers. The figures above include prescription and certain over-the-counter data and represent manufacturer prices.

TABLE 1.8
Top 20 Global Products: 2013

Product	2013 Rank	2013 Sales (US$ mn)	2013 Growth (LC$ %)	2012 Sales (US$ mn)
Global market		874,611	4.5	857,710
Humira	1	9,851	18.5	8,318
Seretide	2	9,213	4.5	8,907
Crestor	3	8,149	1.5	8,215
Enbrel	4	7,949	8.7	7,370
Lantus	5	7,935	23.3	6,472
Nexium	6	7,863	7.0	7,407
Abilify	7	7,832	14.6	6,879
Remicade	8	7,678	7.8	7,259
Cymbalta	9	6,464	13.6	5,734
Mabthera	10	6,263	5.7	5,950
Avastin	11	5,719	8.9	5,364
Spiriva	12	5,318	7.0	4,998
Herceptin	13	5,170	3.4	5,024
Lyrica	14	5,123	14.9	4,531
Copaxone	15	4,698	5.6	4,432
Januvia	16	4,462	10.5	4,181
Lucentis	17	4,415	8.1	4,135
Neulasta	18	4,409	3.3	4,253
Glivec	19	4,136	0.9	4,149
Atripla	20	4,017	2.0	3,924

Source: IMS Health MIDAS, December 2013.

Note: mn, million; US$, sales and rank in U.S. dollars with quarterly exchange rates; LC$, growth in constant dollars to normalize for exchange rate fluctuations. Growth rates in U.S. dollars are not recommended due to fluctuations in the value of the dollar. Sales cover direct and indirect pharmaceutical channel wholesalers and manufacturers. The figures above include prescription and certain over-the-counter data and represent manufacturer prices. Product names shown are IMS International Product names. Products marketed around the world with different names or marketing companies are grouped together. The names generally reflect the name in the country where the product was first launched. A match on two of three criteria (local brand name, marketing corporation, and active ingredient) were grouped together.

Innovator companies are responding to market challenges with several strategies. Some are producing generic versions of their previously branded medicines. Others are contracting for production of their branded medicines as they near the end of patent protection with high-volume contract producers. Recently, there has been an increase in research and product licensing directed toward specialty disease categories where there are relatively low numbers of patients with high-cost treatments required for disease management and life extension. These are referred to as orphan drugs. Pricing for these new products has been set by pharmaceutical companies to highlight the value of the therapy compared to the health care costs for that disease. In some cases, new therapies will cost patients more than $100,000 a year and more than $1,000 a dose. The government and the public are beginning to pay attention to these pricing strategies (Figure 1.15).

TABLE 1.9
Top 20 Global Therapy Areas: 2013

	2013 Rank	2013 Sales (US$ mn)	2013 Growth (LC$ %)	2012 Sales (US$ mn)
Global market		874,611	4.5	857,710
Oncologics	1	67,132	8.5	63,082
Pain	2	57,293	4.7	56,230
Antidiabetics	3	54,369	10.2	50,352
Antihypertensives, plain and combined	4	49,609	−1.7	52,664
Antibacterials	5	40,248	2.6	40,244
Mental health	6	39,495	−2.6	41,214
Respiratory	7	38,115	−1.8	39,357
Autoimmune diseases	8	31,080	14.4	27,473
Lipid regulators	9	28,938	−10.8	33,301
Dermatologics	10	26,778	11.3	24,815
Antiulcerants	11	25,583	1.7	26,022
Anticoagulants	12	24,076	−2.5	25,420
GI products	13	23,530	7.4	22,650
Other cardiovasculars	14	21,943	6.2	21,279
HIV antivirals	15	20,609	8.7	18,936
Nervous system disorders	16	20,170	9.7	18,758
Other central nervous system	17	18,584	6.4	17,952
Cough and cold, including flu antiviral	18	14,500	10.1	13,697
Vaccines (pure, combined, other)	19	14,076	4.5	13,851
Hematopoietic growth factors	20	13,475	5.0	12,833

Source: IMS Health MIDAS, December 2013.

Note: mn, million; US$, sales and rank in U.S. dollars with quarterly exchange rates; LC$, growth
in constant dollars to normalize for exchange rate fluctuations. Growth rates in U.S. dollars
are not recommended due to fluctuations in the value of the dollar. Sales cover direct and
indirect pharmaceutical channel wholesalers and manufacturers. The figures above include
prescription and certain over-the-counter data and represent manufacturer prices.

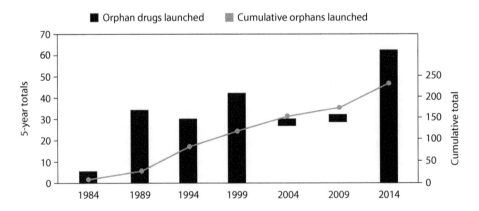

FIGURE 1.15   Number of orphan drugs launched in the United States: 1983–2014.

Large-volume purchasing through health care organizations and governments has transformed sales strategies over the last decade. In response to pressures to lower the cost of health care, insurers and government agencies have been following several strategies, including limiting the number of approved drugs on their formularies, thereby reducing the choices physicians have when they prescribe; this increases the purchasing leverage of the buying organization. During the past decade, the number of physicians employed by health care organizations has grown dramatically. By some estimates, more than 40% of physicians are now employed by health care organizations that direct the prescription habits of their patients and further concentrate purchasing decisions among fewer buyers. The pharmaceutical industry has responded by focusing on sales to these larger accounts and reducing the number of sales representatives. The number of pharmaceutical sales representatives has been reduced from 100,000 ten years ago to 65,000 today. Companies are now pursuing large-volume marketing and sales strategies to the highly focused buying community and increasingly do not deploy representatives to call on independent physicians and low-volume purchasers.

In the coming years, experts expect the focus of the pharmaceutical industry will be to achieve more healthy outcomes for patients who will be increasingly under the care of large health care provider organizations. Energies will be increasingly directed to data management and quality of life outcomes where treatments will also include lifestyle management and combination therapies that promise to reduce health care costs to governments and patients. Below is a summary of some market activities in the United States (Figures 1.16 and 1.17).

- The FDA estimates that roughly 80% of APIs and 40% of finished drugs sold in the United States are now made from foreign sources.
- The FDA estimates that since 2009, there have been approximately 300 warning letters issued globally; for example, India received 75 such warning letters and China 84.
- The India Chamber of Commerce estimates that there were 120 Indian FDA-approved API drug manufacturing plants in 2011. Italy has 55, China has 27, and Spain has 10 such plants.
- Consumers in the United States seldom know who has made their drugs or where they were made. The package very seldom provides the identity of the actual manufacturer. Even physicians and pharmacists do not know where the drugs are made, facts that are disclosed only to the FDA or other regulatory authorities (Figure 1.18).

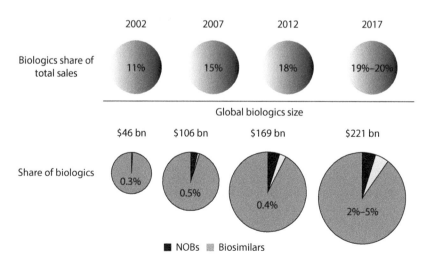

FIGURE 1.16 The biologics market. (From IMS Health, Thought Leadership, September 2013. www.imshealth.com)

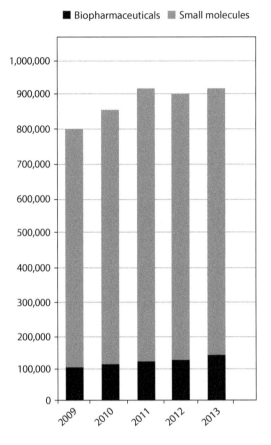

FIGURE 1.17   Traditional (small molecules) vs. biopharma product sales profile. (From Moorcroft M [Presenter], The Resurgence of the Small-Molecule API Market, an Industry Primer, March 5, 2015, Cambrex Corp.)

- A common myth is that generic drugs are cheaper to make. Generics are only equal to branded drugs if they are made and tested properly, using high-quality standards. This requires similar facilities and equipment and similar active ingredients and packaging.
- Compounding laboratories are challenged to make generic drugs safely and at low cost. The FDA reported in 2009 that there are high rates of contamination from drugs sourced from these labs. Many foreign labs, including Indian and Chinese suppliers that currently export to the United States and Europe, have never been inspected, making the probability of detecting a problem very low. For the fiscal year ending 2013, the FDA inspected 23% of domestic drug and device facilities, but only 9% of registered foreign drug and device facilities [21].
- According to the India Brand Equity Foundation (March 2013), India now accounts for more than 10% of the world's pharmaceutical production, where more than 60,000 generic brands are produced spanning 60 therapeutic categories and manufactured in more than 400 API plants. The current market for pharmaceuticals consumed in India was estimated to be $15.6 billion in 2011 and is expected to grow to $35.9 billion in 2016.
- Consumers may be under the impression that the vitamins and supplements industry is regulated like drugs. Under the Dietary Supplement Health and Education Act of 1994, all

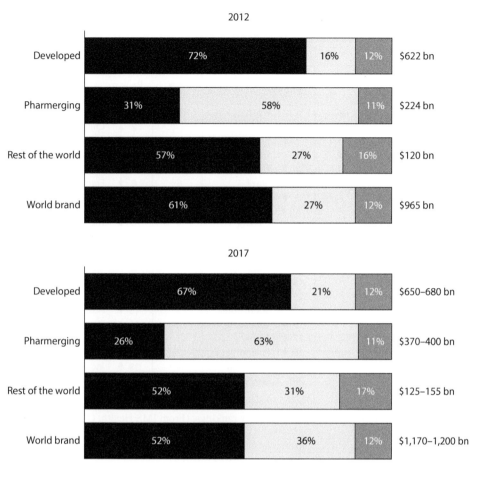

2012

Developed	72%	16%	12%	$622 bn
Pharmerging	31%	58%	11%	$224 bn
Rest of the world	57%	27%	16%	$120 bn
World brand	61%	27%	12%	$965 bn

2017

Developed	67%	21%	12%	$650–680 bn
Pharmerging	26%	63%	11%	$370–400 bn
Rest of the world	52%	31%	17%	$125–155 bn
World brand	52%	36%	12%	$1,170–1,200 bn

FIGURE 1.18 Pharmaceuticals: global spending 2012. (From IMS Health, Global Use of Medicines Outlook, 2013. www.imshealth.com)

supplements, including minerals, medicinal herbs, and protein powders, were categorized as food rather than drugs; thus, supplement manufacturers can sell their products without proving their safety or efficacy so long as the labels do not claim to prevent or treat any specific disease. "If vitamins were a regulated industry, megavitamins would have a black box warning on them," said public health specialist Dr. Paul Offit [22].

- Patients covered more than 90% of their medicine costs out of pocket in 1965. As recently as 1991, Americans still bore more than 50% of their drug costs directly. By 2012, consumers were paying just 18%, with private insurers and Medicare picking up the difference. U.S. taxpayers have a lot at stake since the government pays 37% of America's $300 billion prescription drug bill, which is expected to rise to $450 billion by 2018.
- Contract sales organizations sold 11% of U.S. pharmaceutical markets in 2014, which is up from 8% in 2011.
- "No-see" sales representative policies are now reported at 53% of U.S. physician offices, up from 28% in 2008.
- Advertising directly to the consumer is allowed in the United States and only one other country in the world.

Figures 1.19 through 1.22 show data on pharmaceutical spending worldwide.

| Pharmaceutical sales: global country rankings | | | | | | | | |
| 2007 | | | 2012 | | | 2017 | | |
Rank	Country	Index	Rank	Country	Index	Rank	Country	Index
1	U.S.	100	1	U.S.	100	1	U.S.	100
2	Japan	27	2	Japan	27	2 ▲	China	45
3 ▲	France	13	3 ▲	China	25	3 ▼	Japan	29
4 ▼	Germany	13	4	Germany	13	4 ▲	Brazil	13
5 ▲	China	11	5 ▼	France	11	5 ▼	Germany	13
6 ▼	Italy	8	6 ▲	Brazil	8	6 ▼	France	10
7	U.K.	7	7 ▼	Italy	8	7	Italy	8
8 ▲	Spain	7	8 ▼	U.K.	7	8 ▲	Russia	7
9 ▼	Canada	7	9 ▼	Canada	7	9 ▼	U.K.	7
10	Brazil	5	10	Spain	6	10 ▼	Canada	7
11	Mexico	4	11	Russia	5	11 ▲	India	6
12	Australia	4	12	Australia	4	12 ▼	Spain	5
13	South Korea	3	13	India	4	13 ▲	Mexico	4
14 ▲	Russia	3	14 ▼	Mexico	4	14 ▲	South Korea	4
15 ▲	Turkey	2	15	South Korea	3	15 ▼	Australia	4
16 ▼	India	2	16 ▲	Venezuela	3	16 ▲	Turkey	3
17 ▼	Netherlands	2	17 ▼	Turkey	3	17 ▼	Venezuela	2
18 ▲	Greece	2	18 ▲	Poland	2	18 ▲	Argentina	2
19 ▼	Poland	2	19	Argentina	2	19 ▲	Indonesia	2
20 ▼	Belgium	2	20	Belgium	2	20 ▼	Poland	2

FIGURE 1.19 Pharmaceutical sales: global country rankings. (From IMS Health, Global Use of Medicines Outlook, 2013.)

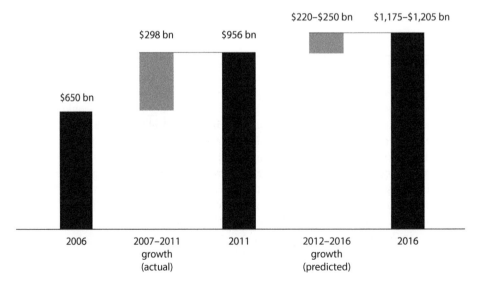

FIGURE 1.20 Global spending on medicines. (From IMS Institute for Healthcare Informatics, 2012.)

Rank	Company	Worldwide generic sales ($ bn)		% Growth	Worldwide market share (%)		Change (+/−)	Rank change (+/−)
		2013	2014		2013	2014		
1	Teva Pharmaceutical Industries	9.2	9.1	−1	13.3	12.2	−1.0 pp	−
2	Novartis	8.2	8.5	+4	11.8	11.5	−0.3 pp	−
3	Activis	6.3	6.6	+6	9.0	8.9	−0.1 pp	−
4	Mylan	5.9	6.5	+10	8.5	8.8	+0.3 pp	−
5	Sun Pharmaceutical Industries	2.7	4.5	+68	3.8	6.0	+2.2 pp	+1
6	Aspen Pharmacare	2.7	3.0	+13	3.9	4.1	+0.2 pp	−1
7	Hospira	2.4	2.6	+12	3.4	3.6	+0.2 pp	−
8	Sanofi	2.2	2.4	+11	3.1	3.2	+0.1 pp	+1
9	Fresenius	2.3	2.3	+0	3.3	3.1	−0.2 pp	−1
10	Lupin	1.7	2.0	+19	2.4	2.7	+0.3 pp	+1

Worldwide unbranded generic drug sales in 2014: Top 10 companies

FIGURE 1.21 Worldwide unbranded generic drug sales in 2014: top 10 companies. (From EvaluatePharma, May 22, 2015.)

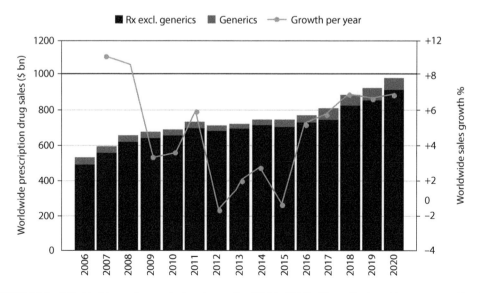

FIGURE 1.22 Worldwide total prescription drug sales (2006–2020). (From EvaluatePharma, May 22, 2015. www.evaluategroup.com)

THE LOOK AHEAD

Predicting the future of the pharmaceutical industry has always been a challenge, especially when considering its turbulent past and a likely politically charged future. As the built-environment professional strives to make sense of the swirling changes, it is recommended that professions make persistent examination a foundational approach. Pharmaceutical facilities and operations will continue to respond to the powerful driving forces of innovation and safety and react swiftly to calamities, failures, and the political responses that typically follow.

A recent survey of pharmaceutical manufacturing professionals offers some insights into what senior industry practitioners see as priorities ahead. A mail survey was taken of senior industry manufacturing executives in the fall of 2013. Out of a total of 75 survey requests, 23 were returned; the results are summarized below. The developments described below may affect how future facilities are planned and delivered. Items noted have been taken from recent news and current professional press, a recent survey of manufacturing executives, and discussions with industry professionals. The complete survey is included as Appendix 1.B at the end of this chapter.

- Larger payers of medical expenses are seeking leverage from bulk purchasing. Governments are not the only big purchasers. Most pharmaceuticals sold in the United States are purchased by managed care organizations (MCOs), hospitals, and governments. The large organizational buyers use their market power to negotiate better prices. The MCOs typically do not take physical possession, as most medicines are passed to the market through wholesalers to pharmacies and then to patients.
- More mergers and acquisitions are likely with resulting plant closures, job displacement, and asset rationalization.
- Cost pressures for manufacturers will continue, requiring organizations to stay lean.
- Marketing challenges will demand better product development and manufacturing speed to design compliant facilities, as well as capacity flexibility to adapt to dosage and presentation evolution.
- Risk management strategies will grow in response to rising costs of failure. Adding redundancy to processes and utility systems is a likely response to the rising challenges of risk management.
- Supply chain consistency will grow in strategic importance, and partner stability will remain a strong risk management initiative.
- The market will demand more specialties in pharmaceutical products, which have relatively high costs with more high-value and smaller-volume product runs.
- Increased approvals of biosimilar products are expected. The Biologics Price Competition and Innovation Act of 2009, enacted as part of the Patient Protection and ACA in March 2010, amended the Public Health Services Act to include an abbreviated pathway for approval of biosimilar products. Increased manufacturing volumes will demand new and advanced production facilities, including additional sterile-filling capacity.
- One potential solution to future production demands may include large, multiproduct centers of manufacturing excellence, which promise greater economies of scale and more uniform meeting of worldwide minimum quality standards.
- Professionals will conduct more benchmarking to learn about and adopt successful process techniques from other high-tech industries.
- Contracting for design and construction services will include more risk-sharing partnerships with project team members (designers and builders) to encourage better performance. Wide adoption of standardized contracts for design and construction services will be seen.

- Small, highly classified production spaces will be built to increase environmental control and reduce operating costs.
- A greater adoption of innovative manufacturing solutions can be expected, including the use of more closed systems, SUD plastic systems for piping and components, modular buildings, and proprietary skid-mounted equipment systems.
- Single-use systems offer advantages, such as reduction of cleaning costs and smaller footprints, because of smaller equipment size and ease of movement; smaller amounts of classified space may also result. Flexibility might be the single biggest advantage, including accommodation of process changes. Speed and flexibility, along with adaptability and mobility, are becoming more important. A higher degree of use for SUD technologies, including those for bioreactors, centrifuges, filtration chromatography, and transfer systems, will be seen.
- Modularization, the use of standardized components and systems, has been used by other industries for decades and is fast becoming an essential component of the pharmaceutical facility design. Modularization offers the industry reduced cost, accelerated construction schedules, and high-quality construction. Local or regional issues, such as labor availability, labor rates, and logistics, could be favorably addressed by modularization.
- A continued drive to minimize human presence in critical operating areas to allow lower costs of operation and greater control of the environment can be expected.
- The lyophilization process is likely to remain, especially for extended shelf life applications.
- The wider use of commercial leveraging techniques by major buyers may be expected to include volume buying of project building components, such as utility systems (e.g., boilers, HVAC equipment, and related system components).
- A greater role will be played by system solution providers, including proprietary providers of innovative product development and specialized process solutions provided by high-tech manufacturing equipment.
- Use of prefabrication of mechanical and electrical components, skid-mounted processes, and utility systems can be expected. Driving forces include future construction labor skill shortages, pressures to compress schedules, increased demand for field productivity, requirements for applying lean construction techniques, improved quality, reduction of field and operating costs, field simplification, uniformity, and greater ease of maintenance and future replacement.
- The market will drive the quest to realize continued productivity gains in process yields for bioderived bulk materials, as well as greater efficiencies and capacities for downstream processing systems.
- Future manufacturing spaces for evolving bioprocessing schemes will include greater use of large, undeveloped, nonspecified floor spaces and building shells, accommodating flexible fit-outs and innovative process solutions.
- Continued progress toward harmonization of worldwide regulatory policies, including cGMP and sustainability compliance, can be expected.
- Expanded use of emerging e-based techniques is expected, including cloud-based process control, visualization, data storage, and retrieval.
- Greater use of smart project management tools, including mobile technologies for live status reporting and monitoring of field activities, can be expected.
- Recent activity has seen some manufacturing being sourced back to the United States. This onshoring for new or renovated plants may be countering a trend in offshoring over the last decade. Healthy labor costs and productivities, as well as political stability and security of supply chain risks in the United States, may be contributing to this trend.

- Emerging pharmaceutical manufacturing technologies promise to benefit U.S. competitiveness and society as a whole through use of less energy and raw materials, creating less waste, potentially decreasing effects on the environment, and reducing manufacturers' footprint [23].
- The capacity for sterile injectable manufacturing may not be adequate to accommodate the growing volume of biological pharmaceutical product introductions. Key players and contract manufacturers have had troubles over the last 5 years with plant shutdowns and resulting shortages of critical drugs and cancer therapies. Mistakes and compliance slips are bringing attention to the industry [24].

PROJECT DELIVERY ISSUES

Most cGMP production facilities are complicated and expensive and present challenging capital projects to execute. Technical professionals are challenged to support their organizations with the delivery of facilities that meet current business expectations and standards, as well as accommodating the dynamic changes likely to be experienced. How is a built-environment professional to maximize impact for his or her organization? What is the best way to approach the challenges to deliver professional services for the design, construction, commissioning, and validation services needed to achieve project goals and deliver well-functioning, compliant (performing and conforming) facilities? The project manager of the future will truly be a master integrator, able to merge a complex series of equipment and solution providers, as well as designers, builders, and validators.

Project management challenges of restricted budgets, tight schedules, and project team dynamics can stifle innovation and reduce project success. Evolving regulatory and marketing realities can impose a changing scope and expectations for facilities, either in design or, worse, in construction. Scope changes and redirections are inevitable and often essential to be certain that the facility will meet strategic business objectives. Given a choice, it is more preferable that a facility meets strategic success than simply offers a technical achievement that misses the mark by providing limited production skills and capacity.

Incorporating innovative project delivery schemes, including use of risk-sharing contracts and cloud-based support, can offer advantages in delivering new facilities quicker and with good response to cost and quality demands. Modern cGMP facilities typically take between 2 and 3 years to design and deliver and can cost several hundred millions of dollars. Virtually all design and construction services are now delivered by outside technical consulting and contracting organizations.

Project management expertise is highly valued by sponsoring organizations as demands for integration and effective teamwork rise to meet challenging schedule and delivery imperatives for new cGMP facilities. The modern technical professional engaged in planning and delivering the "factory of the future" can now rely on solid support from evolving design and project management tools, as well as an increasingly sophisticated equipment and systems supply network. Integration of these many complex and interactive project pieces is essential and a highly valuable sought-after capability and differentiator when organizations consider their professional partners for capital project delivery.

APPENDIX 1.A: cGMP DESIGN AND CONSTRUCTION FACILITY FEATURES

The objective of cGMPs is to ensure the quality of the product for the safety, well-being, and protection of the patient; it is impossible to overemphasize the importance of the quality of medicinal products. Most defective medicinal products have resulted from human error or carelessness, not from technology failures, according to the Medicines Control Agency. Rules and guidance for pharmaceutical manufacturers and distributors define cGMPs and quality assurance to ensure that products are consistently produced under quality standards and the principles that are specified in the European Economic Community (EEC) Directive 91/356.

The following cGMP facility requirements are generally recognized as minimum responsibilities among both U.S. and global regulatory authorities [25]. Some authorities have added additional requirements, which are generally understood. This is not a comprehensive set of requirements but is offered here to make the reader aware of the types of requirements found in cGMP design and construction.

- Facilities should be of a suitable size, construction, and location to facilitate cleaning, maintenance, and proper operations.
- Emphasis is placed on providing adequate space for the storage of components and providing the means for moving all components through the plant with minimum risk of contamination and cross-contamination. Separate areas must be designated for quarantine and release materials and for in-process materials of the quarantined and released final product. A product that offers exceptional risk of cross-contamination is to be handled in a separate facility or unit provided with a separate air supply.
- Areas designated for aseptic operations must have walls, floors, and ceilings with smooth hard surfaces for easy cleaning and temperature and humidity control; a high-efficiency particulate air-filtered air supply; and positive pressure. These areas must be adequately monitored. This is where inspectors are commonly drawn, and citations are very frequent.
- There are commonly use designations for the air quality in specially purposed pharmaceutical facilities based on accepted FDA standards, which are, in turn, based on the standards of the International Organization for Standardization.
- The cGMP facilities also require adequate lighting in all areas, adequate ventilation, and provision of equipment for appropriate control of air pressure, microorganisms, dust, humidity, and temperature.
- All cGMP facilities require that the water supply to the facility be potable. These standards are in the U.S. Environmental Protection Agency's primary drinking water regulations. Some manufacturing requirements call for the installation of United States Pharmacopoeia (USP) purified water or water for injection. These systems require special scrutiny, especially for microbial organisms.
- Floor drains must be of adequate size and must be fitted with an air break to prevent back siphoning.
- All cGMP facilities must provide for the removal of sewage and refuse in a safe and sanitary manner. They must also provide washing and toilet facilities that are easily accessible.
- Written procedures must be in place for the maintenance of the entire facility in a clean and sanitary state. All buildings and facilities must be maintained in a good state of repair.
- Production and process controls are strongly regulated and monitored, as they cover the most critical areas of cGMP and deal with actual manufacturing packaging distribution and quality control processes. The manufacturer is expected to perform and monitor operations efficiently and effectively to demonstrate that a facility continuously meets its design and product performance objectives. Deviations cannot be allowed from validated processes as described in approved SOPs.
- It is mandated that SOPs shall be followed in the execution of production and process control functions and that procedures shall be documented with a time of performance.

APPENDIX 1.B: THE FUTURE OF PHARMA MANUFACTURING FACILITIES SURVEY SUMMARY

1. More use of new processing and novel delivery systems to accommodate new therapies that present challenges of high insolubility and potent/toxic processing exposure potential. Such evolving processing examples may include nanotechnology, combination dosages, hot melt extrusion, and spray drying, among others.

Answer Options	No Change in Likelihood	Less Likely	Strongly Less Likely	More Likely	Strongly More Likely	Rating Average
	0	2	0	16	5	4.04

1A. Same question, but considering its relevancy to manufacturers.

Answer Options	No Change for Manufacturers	Somewhat Important to Manufacturers	Very Important to Manufacturers	Rating Average
	0	10	13	2.57

2. Expand use of serialization approaches to assist in supply management and anticounterfeiting measures.

Answer Options	No Change in Likelihood	Less Likely	Strongly Less Likely	More Likely	Strongly More Likely	Rating Average
	3	0	0	9	11	4.09

2A. Same question, but considering its relevancy to manufacturers.

Answer Options	No Change for Manufacturers	Somewhat Important to Manufacturers	Very Important to Manufacturers	Rating Average
	1	8	14	2.57

3. Greater use of new/innovative processing to deliver large-molecule (biotech-based) products as modified presentations, such as oral solid doses, transdermals, and inhalants, to improve accessibility, including lower costs of goods, less complicated storage, and transportation factors.

Answer Options	No Change in Likelihood	Less Likely	Strongly Less Likely	More Likely	Strongly More Likely	Rating Average
	1	1	0	16	5	4.00

3A. Same question, but considering its relevancy to manufacturers.

Answer Options	No Change for Manufacturers	Somewhat Important to Manufacturers	Very Important to Manufacturers	Rating Average
	1	10	12	2.48

4. Greater adoption of standardized, risk-adjusted approaches to GMP excellence/compliance in plant design and equipment/systems deployed by innovator, generics, and contract manufacturers so as to blur/eliminate any production philosophy and operating differences.

Answer Options	No Change in Likelihood	Less Likely	Strongly Less Likely	More Likely	Strongly More Likely	Rating Average
	4	3	2	7	6	3.36

4A. Same question, but considering its relevancy to manufacturers.

Answer Options	No Change for Manufacturers	Somewhat Important to Manufacturers	Very Important to Manufacturers	Rating Average
	5	10	6	2.05

5. Increased value recognition of project leadership (management and technology) skills for pharmaceutical facility professionals as they design, build, and validate new and renovated facilities, since requirements of system integration and coordination of the many contributors (vendors, suppliers, contractors) to each project place higher demands on the project staffer.

Answer Options	No Change in Likelihood	Strongly Less Likely	Less Likely	Likely	More Likely	Strongly More Likely	Rating Average
↑	5	4	4	4	4	5	3.00

5A. Same question, but considering its relevancy to manufacturers.

Answer Options	No Change for Manufacturers	Somewhat Important to Manufacturers	Very Important to Manufacturers	Rating Average
↑	8	6	7	1.95

6. Wider deployment of single-use (plastic) processing systems for biopharma manufacturing.

Answer Options	No Change in Likelihood	Strongly Less Likely	Less Likely	Likely	More Likely	Strongly More Likely	Rating Average
↑	2	0	2	9	9	9	4.05

6A. Same question, but considering its relevancy to manufacturers.

Answer Options	No Change for Manufacturers	Somewhat Important to Manufacturers	Very Important to Manufacturers	Rating Average
↑	0	11	11	2.50

7. More pressures on manufacturers to meet the challenges of lower margin opportunities, therefore requiring constant attention to cost of goods through efficient deployment of capital, effective spending, capital spending, and lean efficient operations.

Answer Options	No Change in Likelihood	Strongly Less Likely	Less Likely	Likely	More Likely	Strongly More Likely	Rating Average
↑	0	0	1	11	9	9	4.38

7A. Same question, but considering its relevancy to manufacturers.

Answer Options	No Change for Manufacturers	Somewhat Important to Manufacturers	Very Important to Manufacturers	Rating Average
↑	2	3	17	2.68

8. Wider incorporation of sustainable design aimed to reduce to building's energy consumption, production wastes, and water consumption.

Answer Options	No Change in Likelihood	Strongly Less Likely	Less Likely	Likely	More Likely	Strongly More Likely	Rating Average
↑	3	2	2	11	5	5	3.59

8A. Same question, but considering its relevancy to manufacturers.

Answer Options	No Change for Manufacturers	Somewhat Important to Manufacturers	Very Important to Manufacturers	Rating Average
↑	2	14	6	2.18

9. More use of continuous processes for API and OSD (eventually BIO) manufacturing and online, real-time (PAT) process control.

Answer Options	No Change in Likelihood	Strongly Less Likely	Less Likely	Likely	More Likely	Strongly More Likely	Rating Average
↑	3	2	2	12	2	2	3.38

9A. Same question, but considering its relevancy to manufacturers.

Answer Options	No Change for Manufacturers	Somewhat Important to Manufacturers	Very Important to Manufacturers	Rating Average
↑	2	14	4	2.10

10. Wider use of "factory of the future" integrated active (smart) control (wireless?) systems that provide robust data flow and responsive control of building systems and processes.

Answer Options	No Change in Likelihood	Strongly Less Likely	Less Likely	More Likely	Strongly More Likely	Rating Average
↑	4	2	1	9	5	3.43

10A. Same question, but considering its relevancy to manufacturers.

Answer Options	No Change for Manufacturers	Somewhat Important to Manufacturers	Very Important to Manufacturers	Rating Average
↑	4	12	5	2.05

11. More risk-adjusted deployment of robots and other nonhuman operating support systems.

Answer Options	No Change in Likelihood	Strongly Less Likely	Less Likely	More Likely	Strongly More Likely	Rating Average
↑	7	4	2	6	2	2.62

11A. Same question, but considering its relevancy to manufacturers.

Answer Options	No Change for Manufacturers	Somewhat Important to Manufacturers	Very Important to Manufacturers	Rating Average
↑	7	9	4	1.90

12. Wider use of prefabricated/modular building and utility systems, such as skids for utility generation, water purification, processing unit operations such as bioreactors, chromatography, and filtration.

Answer Options	No Change in Likelihood	Strongly Less Likely	Less Likely	More Likely	Strongly More Likely	Rating Average
↑	3	0	2	14	2	3.57

12A. Same question, but considering its relevancy to manufacturers.

Answer Options	No Change for Manufacturers	Somewhat Important to Manufacturers	Very Important to Manufacturers	Rating Average
↑	4	14	3	1.95

13. Wider use of outsourced, full-service contractors who assume total responsibility for custom design, supply, and installation of unit operations, and also design, build, and commission/validation of future facilities to include the building and site.

Answer Options	No Change in Likelihood	Strongly Less Likely	Less Likely	More Likely	Strongly More Likely	Rating Average
↑	4	1	2	12	1	3.25

13A. Same question, but considering its relevancy to manufacturers.

Answer Options	No Change for Manufacturers	Somewhat Important to Manufacturers	Very Important to Manufacturers	Rating Average
↑	6	10	4	1.90

14. More value attributed to speed-to-market techniques that reduce the total cycle time to build and bring new facilities online, thus also supporting commitment decision delays in capital projects to reduce risk of premature funding.

Answer Options	No Change in Likelihood	Less Likely	Strongly Less Likely	More Likely	Strongly More Likely	Rating Average
	3	0	0	11	7	3.90

14A. Same question, but considering its relevancy to manufacturers.

Answer Options	No Change for Manufacturers	Somewhat Important to Manufacturers	Very Important to Manufacturers	Rating Average
	2	7	12	2.48

15. Greater use of automated design and data management tools for construction and operation, including BIM (building information management systems).

Answer Options	No Change in Likelihood	Less Likely	Strongly Less Likely	More Likely	Strongly More Likely	Rating Average
	5	1	2	8	5	3.33

15A. Same question, but considering its relevancy to manufacturers.

Answer Options	No Change for Manufacturers	Somewhat Important to Manufacturers	Very Important to Manufacturers	Rating Average
	7	11	3	1.81

16. Greater demand for high-volume, multiproduct (mega) facilities by innovators and contract manufacturers seeking economies of scale and more uniform methods, taking into consideration quality control/risk management issues arising for cross-contamination, mix-ups, and risks of supply disruptions.

Answer Options	No Change in Likelihood	Less Likely	Strongly Less Likely	More Likely	Strongly More Likely	Rating Average
	5	6	1	7	2	2.76

16A. Same question, but considering its relevancy to manufacturers.

Answer Options	No Change for Manufacturers	Somewhat Important to Manufacturers	Very Important to Manufacturers	Rating Average
	6	11	4	1.90

17. More strategic placement of future manufacturing facilities with high regard for securing benefits of presence in each local marketplace.

Answer Options	No Change in Likelihood	Less Likely	Strongly Less Likely	More Likely	Strongly More Likely	Rating Average
	4	3	1	11	2	3.19

17A. Same question, but considering its relevancy to manufacturers.

Answer Options	No Change for Manufacturers	Somewhat Important to Manufacturers	Very Important to Manufacturers	Rating Average
	4	12	5	2.05

FURTHER DISCUSSION

1. Considering the dynamic history of the pharmaceutical industry, what likely changes do you see happening in the next 5–10 years that will be driven by consumers and governments, which will have a significant effect on how drugs are manufactured, regulated, and distributed to the world markets.
2. What do you see as the future role and significance of CDMOs on the pharmaceutical industry over the next 5–10 years?
3. How do you see evolving biotechnology innovations, knowledge, and process advances driving future design and construction of manufacturing facilities?
4. What advice would you offer to future engineering students who are interested in working in the pharmaceutical industry on where to focus their education, in light of known and likely imminent advances in technology? What skills and experiences would prove to be the most valuable for career advancement with future employers?
5. How do you see the future of government regulation as it will likely affect the development and enforcement of future standards for pharmaceutical manufacturing operations, with special emphasis on global markets and intended safety and cost efficiency?

ABOUT THE AUTHOR

Andrew A. Signore is president of the Institute for Strategic Growth (ISG), Wayne, Pennsylvania, where he provides advisement and consulting to professional service firms. He is also cofounder of Integrated Project Services (IPS), Blue Bell, Pennsylvania, a project delivery firm focused on health care and pharmaceutical facilities. Andy has held engineering management positions at SmithKline Beckman (now Glaxo), Pfizer, and Merck. He earned his BSChemEng from Manhattan College and an MBA from Pace University, both of New York. He is a registered professional engineer in Pennsylvania, New York, and New Jersey. He is currently an adjunct professor in the School of Engineering in the Construction Management Division at Drexel University, Philadelphia and industry professor in the pharmaceutical manufacturing engineering, masters program at Stevens Institute of Technology, Newark New Jersey. Andy was founding president of Design Build Institute of America's (DBIA) Delaware Valley Chapter and is a charter holder of a DBIA designation. He is past president of the New Jersey Chapter of the Project Management Institute (PMI). In addition, he has earned the CPIP designation, is a past president of the International Society for Pharmaceutical Engineering (ISPE) and of ISPE Delaware Valley Chapter, and is a frequent course leader. He has received ISPE's Distinguished Achievement Award in recognition for his many professional contributions to the industry. Andy remains a student of the pharmaceutical industry, has had more than a dozen articles published, and lectures on pharmaceutical industry technology and management topics.

SOURCES OF ADDITIONAL INSIGHT

The pharmaceutical industry is widely covered by a number of reputable sources of information, both public and private. All information presented in this chapter was obtained from publicly available sources. The reader is encouraged to keep up with the dynamic industry by accessing the following sources, as well as other news sites and sources of industry events. The following list presents organizations that regularly prepare and publish information on the pharmaceutical industry business activity; these are recommended for students and industry observers.

International Society for Pharmaceutical Engineering*
Ernst & Young
IMS Health
EvaluatePharma
PricewaterhouseCoopers
Pharmaceutical Research and Manufacturers of America
Contract Pharma Magazine
BioPharm International
Fortune Magazine
Parenteral Drug Association
Stevens Institute of Technology
Bain and Company
KPMG
McKinsey & Company
FiercePharma Manufacturing
Wall Street Journal
New York Times
India Brand Equity Foundation
European Economic Community
World Health Organization
United Kingdom Ministry of Medicine

REFERENCES

1. Miller J, Changing Contract Services Landscape, PharmSource, March 19, 2014, www.pharmsource.com.
2. EvaluatePharma, World Preview 2014, Outlook to 2020, 7th ed., EvaluatePharma, April 2014, www.evaluategroup.com.
3. National Association of Boards of Pharmacy, Counterfeiting and Piracy in Pharma, National Association of Boards of Pharmacy, October 2008, www.nabp.net/publications/assets/Oct08NABP.pdf.
4. PhRMA, Biopharmaceutical Research Industry, 2015 Profile, PhRMA, April 2015, www.phrma.org/sites/default/files/pdf/2015_phrma_profile.pdf.
5. EvaluatePharma, World Preview 2015, Outlook to 2020, 8th ed., EvaluatePharma, June 2015, www.evaluategroup.com.
6. IMS Institute, Medicines Use and Spending Shifts: A Review of the Use of Medicines in the US in 2014, IMS Institute, April 2015, www.imshealth.com/en/thought-leadership/ims-institute/reports/medicines-use-in-the-us-2014.
7. IMS Institute, Global Outlook for Medicines through 2018, IMS Institute, November 2014, www.imshealth.com/en/thought-leadership/ims-institute/reports/global-outlook-for-medicines-through-2018.
8. U.S. Food and Drug Administration, www.fda.gov.
9. Kunst M, Natanek R, Plantevin L, Eliades G, A New Pharma Launch Paradigm, Bain & Co., www.bain.com/publications/articles/a-new-pharma-launch-paradigm.aspx.
10. Buscher B, Viquene P, How U.S. Healthcare Companies Can Thrive Amid Disruption, McKinsey & Company, June 2014, www.mckinsey.com/insights/health_systems_and_services/how_us_healthcare_companies_can_thrive_amid_disruption.
11. IMAP, Global Pharma and Biotech M and A Report 2014, IMAP, April 2015, www.IMAP.com.
12. PricewaterhouseCoopers, Pharma 2020: The Vision, PricewaterhouseCoopers, October 2014, www.pwc.com/gx/en/industries/pharmaceuticals-life-sciences/pharma-2020/pharma-2020-vision-path.html.

---

* There are various classification systems designed to identify the various types of process and utility equipment in a manufacturing facility and categorize them as to their criticality and effect on product quality. The ISPE has developed a series of pharmaceutical engineering guides, known as Baseline Guides, which present generally accepted approaches to designing and constructing modern pharmaceutical facilities. This group of professional guidance publications have generally been accepted and contributed to by the FDA and are in wide use among industry professionals.

13. Pratt E, Five Trends That Will Shape the Future of Pharmaceutical Manufacturing, Stevens Institute of Technology, June 2015, www.Stevens.edu/ses.

14. Ebel T, George K, Larsen E, Shah K, Ungerman D, Building New Strengths in the Healthcare Supply Chain, McKinsey & Company, January 2013, www.mckinsey.com/~/media/mckinsey/dotcom/client_service/Pharma%20and%20Medical%20Products/PMP%20NEW/PDFs/McKinsey%20white%20paper%20-%20building%20new%20strenghts%20in%20healthcare%20supply%20chain%20VF.ashx.

15. Pharmaceutical Industry 10th Annual Survey, *Contract Pharma Magazine*, February 2015.

16. PricewaterhouseCoopers, Convergence toward a Healthier Future, PricewaterhouseCoopers, www.pwc.com/us/en/health-industries/our-perspective/convergence.html.

17. Cremer P, Losch M, Schrader U, Driving a Transformation in Efficiency, McKinsey & Company, 2010, www.McKinsey.com

18. Poon EG, Keohane CA, Yoon CS, Ditmore M, Bane A, Levtzion-Korach O, Moniz T, et al., Effect of Bar-Code Technology on the Safety of Medication Administration, *New England Journal of Medicine*, 362, 1698–1707, 2010.

19. KPMG International, Issues Monitor, KPMG International, June 2011, www.kpmg.com/Global/en/IssuesAndInsights/ArticlesPublications/Issues-monitor-pharmaceuticals/Documents/issues-monitor-pharmaceuticals-june-2011.pdf.

20. Miller S, Pharmaceutical Manufacturing, Express Scripts, April 2015, www.pharmanufacturing.com.

21. Champion H, Ensuring Drug Quality on a Global Economy, *Contract Pharma Magazine*, May 2014.

22. Offit P, The Children's Hospital of Philadelphia, *Consumers Health Digest*, April 2015.

23. Jacoby R, Pernenkil L, Sabad A, Heim M, Advanced Biopharmaceutical Manufacturing: An Evolution Underway, Deloitte Life Sciences, April 2015, www2.deloitte.com/us/en/pages/life-sciences-and-health-care/articles/advanced-biopharmaceutical-manufacturing-paper.html.

24. Shanley A, Can Sterile Manufacturing Turn the Ship Around? *Pharmaceutical Technology*, 39(17), 2015.

25. U.S. Food and Drug Administration, Current Good Manufacturing Practices, U.S. Food and Drug Administration, Silver Spring, MD, www.fda.gov.

2 Current Good Manufacturing Practices

Rose Mary Dollard

CONTENTS

INTRODUCTION

This chapter provides an overview of the regulatory requirements of current Good Manufacturing Practices (cGMPs) and describes the importance of cGMPs when designing engineering processes within a pharmaceutical facility. All pharmaceutical manufacturing companies have similar objectives related to the planning, designing, building, validating, and maintenance of their facilities, including the following: (1) design, delivery, and maintenance of manufacturing support facilities, utilities, process equipment, and automation controls so that they perform as intended to meet business objectives, such as capacity, yield, operational efficiency, and reliability; (2) development of a production process that can repeatedly produce a quality product; (3) creation of a quality system necessary to meet regulatory as well as business requirements; and (4) project and process deliveries that are within budgets and schedules. These objectives need to comply with regulations while retaining a highly competitive position.

MANAGED AND INTEGRATED APPROACHES TO PROJECT DELIVERY

Achieving the objectives listed above requires both a managed and an integrated approach to project delivery. A managed approach uses written plans, schedules, budgets, definitions of responsibilities, and well-understood document structures to run a project successfully, while meeting objectives and regulatory expectations. An integrated approach considers regulatory, safety, environmental, operational, and project controls. Significant benefits of an integrated approach are realized when project teams apply this approach to all dimensions of a project. These benefits include (1) an increased focus on product and process knowledge, (2) the delivery of high-quality equipment, (3) an increase in project efficiency as risks are prioritized, (4) improvement in the equipment and system start-up, and (5) the results associated with the creation of regulatory compliance documentation.

RISK MANAGEMENT

A good understanding of the risks that equipment and systems present to product and process helps to ensure the development of adequate design, mitigation, and control plans that ultimately increase product quality. Product development, process development, and technology focus the information needed by the engineering design team. Understanding the relationship between equipment and system design facilitates conclusive troubleshooting if product quality defects occur (Figure 2.1).

All project risks need to be continuously assessed and controlled, including business risk, contractor performance risk, safety risk, environmental risk, and risk to the patient. Design and manufacturing practice regulations are the basis for controlling these risks. A pharmaceutical engineer focuses on analyzing, controlling, and managing the risks to the patient that may be present in the design of the manufacturing process, equipment, utilities, facilities, and automation.

GLOBAL REGULATORY ENVIRONMENT

The intention of global regulations is a harmonized approach, which has resulted in a better understanding of the expectations of various national authorities. Efforts by the International Conference on Harmonisation (ICH), the American Society for Testing and Materials (ASTM) International, and regional regulatory authorities, such as the Food and Drug Administration (FDA) and the European Medicines Agency (EMA), to align approaches toward regulatory compliance have been highly successful. The expectations of regulators are as follows: (1) Design, operating, and quality decisions are based on scientific knowledge of the product and process; that is, the attributes of the product necessary to deliver the desired effect to the patient are known. Scientific knowledge of the process means that the manufacturing process parameters necessary to achieve those product

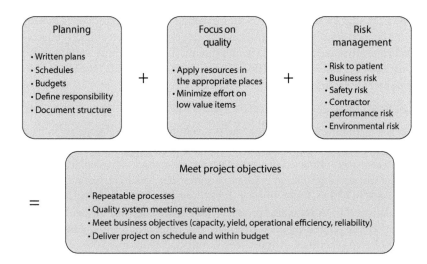

FIGURE 2.1   Integration of risk management principles.

attributes are also known. (2) Risks to the patient should be understood and managed, and this understanding should be used to drive the design, the operation, and the quality system of the manufacturing operation. (3) A comprehensive quality system should be implemented. For purposes of designing, verifying, and maintaining process, equipment, and systems, the processes defined by this chapter meet the expectations of a modern quality system.

For a project to meet regulatory deliverables, the following three aspects related to the impact on the patient need to be considered: (1) defining and verifying that critical quality attributes and critical process parameters can be met; (2) analyzing risks to the patient and verifying that they have been adequately controlled; and (3) planning, managing, and documenting qualification and validation efforts, with independent oversight by the quality unit at key points in the process. These three aspects should be the basis for how the specification, design, and validation life cycle process is to be implemented on different projects. A brief overview of several regulatory bodies and industry organizations that shape the requirements related to good pharmaceutical manufacturing design, build, and validation practices is provided below.

FOOD AND DRUG ADMINISTRATION

The FDA is an agency within the U.S. Department of Health and Human Services. It consists of the Office of the Commissioner and four directorates overseeing the core functions of the agency: medical products and tobacco, foods and veterinary medicine, global regulatory operations and policy, and operations.

The FDA is responsible for protecting public health by ensuring that foods (except for meat from livestock, poultry, and some egg products, which are regulated by the U.S. Department of Agriculture) are safe and properly labeled and by ensuring that human and veterinary drugs, vaccines, and other biological products and medical devices intended for human use are safe and effective. In addition, the FDA protects the public from electronic product radiation and ensures that cosmetics and dietary supplements are safe and properly labeled. The FDA is also responsible for advancing public health by helping to speed up innovations that make medicines effective, safe, and affordable and by helping the public get accurate, science-based information on medicines and foods to maintain and improve their health. Additionally, the FDA has the responsibility for regulating the manufacturing, marketing, and distribution of tobacco products to protect the public health and to reduce tobacco use by minors.

Finally, the FDA plays a significant role in the nation's counterterrorism capability by ensuring the security of the food supply and by fostering the development of medical products to respond to deliberate and naturally emerging public health threats. The FDA's responsibilities extend to all 50 states, the District of Columbia, Puerto Rico, Guam, the Virgin Islands, American Samoa, and other U.S. territories and possessions [1].

The FDA's Globalization Effort

Globalization is a fact of the economic life of the twenty-first century. Markets in the United States are now composed of myriad imported goods that consumers demand. In response to problems that have been associated with imported products over the years and the value derived from leveraging the activities and resources of foreign regulatory authorities, the FDA has established a permanent in-country presence in China, India, Europe, Latin America, and sub-Saharan Africa (Figure 2.2).

Global production of FDA-regulated products has quadrupled over the last decade and continues to grow. Today, FDA-regulated products originate from more than 150 countries, 130,000 importers, and 300,000 foreign facilities. Almost 40% of finished drugs and 80% of the manufacturing of active pharmaceutical ingredients (APIs) are located outside the United States. In addition, half of all medical devices are imported. The growth in imports has been rapid and promises to accelerate.

Globalization has fundamentally altered the economic and security landscape and demands a major change in the way the FDA fulfills its mission. The FDA has transformed from a domestically focused agency to a modern public health regulatory agency fully prepared for a complex globalized regulatory environment. The agency is already increasing transparency and accountability in the supply chain, developing better enforcement and regulatory tools, encouraging greater responsibility by industry, and enhancing collaboration with international regulatory counterparts [2].

The FDA and Pharmaceutical Manufacturing

Due to globalization, the pharmaceutical engineering professional needs to consider the countries where manufacturing occurs, where product is distributed, and the product labeling requirements

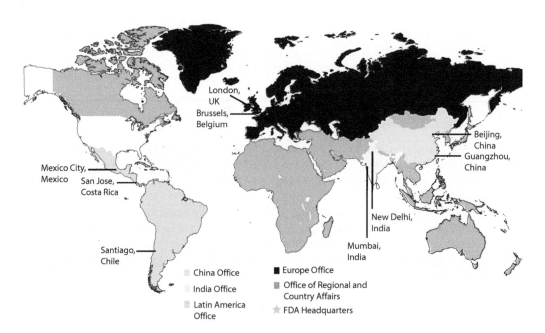

FIGURE 2.2 In-country presence of the Food and Drug Administration. (From U.S. Food and Drug Administration, FDA Globalization, U.S. Food and Drug Administration, Silver Spring, MD, May 1, 2015. http://www.fda.gov/InternationalPrograms/FDABeyondOurBordersForeignOffices/)

when designing facilities for pharmaceutical manufacturing. Various global requirements have a direct impact on project complexity, schedules, and costs. It is important for the pharmaceutical engineer to work with the regulatory and quality partners to define regulations that apply to projects, ensuring that the appropriate elements are built into the project definition and design phases. Additional information about the FDA can be found at http://www.fda.gov/.

European Medicines Agency

The main responsibility of the EMA is the protection and promotion of public and animal health, through the evaluation and supervision of medicines for human and veterinary use. The EMA works with a network of more than 4500 European experts and is the hub of a European medicine network comprising more than 40 national regulatory authorities. The EMA works closely with its European partners to build the best possible regulatory system for medicine in Europe and to protect the health of its citizens.

The EMA forges close ties with partner organizations around the world, including the regulatory authorities of non-European nations. These activities foster the timely exchange of regulatory and scientific expertise and the development of best practices in the regulatory field across the world [1]. Additional information about the EMA can be found at http://www.ema.europa.eu/ema/.

International Conference on Harmonisation

The mission of the ICH is to make recommendations toward achieving greater conformity in the interpretation and application of technical guidelines and requirements for pharmaceutical product registration, thereby minimizing the use of animal testing without compromising safety and effectiveness, streamlining the regulatory assessment process for new drug applications (NDAs), and reducing the development times and resources for drug development.

Launched in 1990, the ICH is a unique undertaking that brings together the drug regulatory authorities and the pharmaceutical industry of Europe, Japan, and the United States. Key to the success of ICH was the development and implementation of ICH Tripartite Guidelines, which were developed through scientific consensus with regulatory and industry experts. The current ICH Terms of Reference (2000) as they appear on the ICH website are listed below. Additional information about ICH can be found at http://www.ich.org/ [3].

- To maintain a forum for a constructive dialogue between regulatory authorities and the pharmaceutical industry on the real and perceived differences in the technical requirements for product registration in the EU, USA, and Japan to ensure a more timely introduction of new medicinal products, and their availability to patients;
- To contribute to the protection of public health from an international perspective;
- To monitor and update harmonized technical requirements, leading to a mutual acceptance of research and development data;
- To avoid divergent future requirements through harmonization of selected topics needed as a result of therapeutic advances and the development of new technologies for the production of medicinal products;
- To facilitate the adoption of new or improved technical research and development approaches which update or replace current practices, where these permit a more economical use of human, animal and material resources, without compromising safety;
- To facilitate the dissemination and communication of information on harmonized guidelines and their use to encourage the implementation and integration of common standards.

World Health Organization

The World Health Organization (WHO) is the directing and coordinating authority for health within the United Nations system. It is responsible for providing leadership on global health matters, shaping the health research agenda, setting norms and standards, articulating evidence-based policy options, providing technical support to countries, and monitoring and assessing health trends. Additional information about WHO can be found at http://www.who.int/en/ [4].

AMERICAN SOCIETY FOR TESTING AND MATERIALS INTERNATIONAL

ASTM International is a globally recognized leader in the development and delivery of international voluntary consensus standards. This organization has developed more than 12,000 ASTM standards, which are used around the world to improve product quality, enhance safety, facilitate market access and trade, and build consumer confidence. Additional information about ASTM International can be found at http://www.astm.org/ [5].

KEY PHARMACEUTICAL REGULATIONS RELATED TO DESIGN AND ENGINEERING

Different nations and different economic blocks follow regulations and guidance documents that can vary greatly in terms of specificity and detail regarding design, build, and validation expectations for pharmaceutical facilities. This section contains excerpts from the FDA, EU, ASTM International, and WHO regulations and guidance documents that relate to pharmaceutical design life cycle processes. This is not an all-inclusive list of global regulations, but it highlights the regulations that represent major global market segments. Pharmaceutical engineering professionals, with quality and regulatory personnel, should develop an understanding of the intent of the regulations and apply that to specific projects.

FOOD AND DRUG ADMINISTRATION

The FDA issues regulations in the Code of Federal Regulations (CFR) 21. The applicable regulations that include facility and equipment design requirements can be found in the following:

21 CFR 210, Subpart C: "Buildings and Facilities": cGMP regulations in manufacturing, processing, packaging, or holding of drugs

21 CFR 211, Subpart D: "Equipment": the cGMPs for finished pharmaceuticals [6]

DESIGN AND CONSTRUCTION FEATURES (§211.42)

(a) Any building or buildings used in the manufacture, processing, packing, or holding of a drug product shall be of suitable size, construction, and location to facilitate cleaning, maintenance, and proper operations.

(b) Any such building shall have adequate space for the orderly placement of equipment and materials to prevent mix-ups between different components, drug product containers, closures, labeling, in-process materials, or drug products, and to prevent contamination. The flow of components, drug product containers, closures, labeling, in-process materials, and drug products through the building or buildings shall be designed to prevent contamination.

(c) Operations shall be performed within specifically defined areas of adequate size. There shall be separate or defined areas for the firm's operations as are necessary to prevent contamination or mix-ups during the course of the following procedures:

   (1) Receipt, identification, storage, and withholding from use of components, drug product containers, closures, and labeling, pending the appropriate sampling, testing, or examination by the quality control unit before release for manufacturing or packaging;

   (2) Holding rejected components, drug product containers, closures, and labeling before disposition;

   (3) Storage of released components, drug product containers, closures, and labeling;

   (4) Storage of in-process materials;

   (5) Manufacturing and processing operations;

(6) Packaging and labeling operations;
(7) Quarantine storage before release of drug products;
(8) Storage of drug products after release;
(9) Control and laboratory operations;
(10) Aseptic processing, which includes as appropriate:
(i) Floors, walls, and ceilings of smooth, hard surfaces that are easily cleanable;
(ii) Temperature and humidity controls;
(iii) An air supply filtered through high-efficiency particulate air filters under positive pressure, regardless of whether flow is laminar or nonlaminar;
(iv) A system for monitoring environmental conditions;
(v) A system for cleaning and disinfecting the room and equipment to produce aseptic conditions;
(vi) A system for maintaining any equipment used to control the aseptic conditions.
(d) Operations relating to the manufacture, processing, and packing of penicillin shall be performed in facilities separate from those used for other drug products for human use.

LIGHTING (§211.44)

The paragraph on lighting states that adequate lighting shall be provided in all areas.

VENTILATION, AIR FILTRATION, AND AIR HEATING AND COOLING (§211.46)

- Adequate ventilation shall be provided.
- Equipment for adequate control over air pressure, microorganisms, dust, humidity, and temperature shall be provided when appropriate for the manufacture, processing, packing, or holding of a drug product.
- Air filtration systems, including prefilters and particulate matter air filters, shall be used when appropriate on air supplies to production areas. If air is recirculated to production areas, measures shall be taken to control recirculation of dust from production. In areas where air contamination occurs during production, there shall be adequate exhaust systems or other systems to control contaminants.
- Air-handling systems for the manufacture, processing, and packing of penicillin shall be completely separate from those for other drug products for human use.

EQUIPMENT DESIGN, SIZE, AND LOCATION (§211.63)

The regulations dealing with equipment requirements are written in a similar fashion.

Equipment used in the manufacture, processing, packing, or holding of a drug product shall be of appropriate design, adequate size, and suitably located to facilitate operations for its intended use and for its cleaning and maintenance.

EQUIPMENT CONSTRUCTION (§211.65)

- Equipment shall be constructed so that surfaces that contact components, in-process materials, or drug products shall not be reactive, additive, or absorptive so as to alter the safety, identity, strength, quality, or purity of the drug product beyond the official or other established requirements.

Any substances required for operation, such as lubricants or coolants, shall not come into contact with components, drug product containers, closures, in-process materials, or drug products so as to alter the safety, identity, strength, quality, or purity of the drug product beyond the official or other established requirements.

Summary

Since the above requirements can be satisfied using various methods, designers must be thoroughly knowledgeable of industry practices and systems related to pharmaceutical design. There are numerous courses sponsored by universities and professional and educational associations that introduce an individual to the requirements of facility design.

To complement the regulations, the FDA has drafted several guidance documents for industry. These guidance documents represent the FDA's current thinking on a topic. Guidance documents do not create or confer any rights for or on any person and do not operate to bind the FDA or the public. Alternative approaches from those described in the guidance can be applied if the approach satisfies the requirements of the applicable statutes and regulations. Two guidance documents related to good design practice are "Process Validation: General Principles and Practices" issued in January 2011 and "Quality Systems Approach to Pharmaceutical cGMP Regulations" issued in September 2006. The "Process Validation" document provides guidance for good design practices relating to pharmaceutical facilities and equipment, including recommendations on the team approach for process design and validation of utilities and equipment. It reinforces the expectation that project teams of subject matter experts (SMEs) from various disciplines define the project requirements and expectations throughout the project life cycle. The FDA also stresses the importance of having senior management sponsorship. Management awareness and accountability are critical for efficient decision making, removal of roadblocks, and escalation of key issues or risks. Several relevant topics within these guidance documents are outlined below.

Process Qualification

During the process qualification stage of process validation, the process design is evaluated to determine if it is capable of reproducible commercial manufacture. This stage has two elements: (1) design of the facility and qualification of the equipment and utilities and (2) process performance qualification. During process qualification, cGMP-compliant procedures must be followed. Successful completion of process qualification is necessary before commercial distribution. Products manufactured during this stage, if acceptable, can be released for distribution.

Design of a Facility and Qualification of Utilities and Equipment

Proper design of a manufacturing facility is required under part 211, Subpart C, of the cGMP regulations on buildings and facilities. It is essential that activities performed to ensure proper facility design and commissioning precede process performance qualification. Here, the term *qualification* refers to activities undertaken to demonstrate that utilities and equipment are suitable for their intended use and perform properly.

Qualification of utilities and equipment generally includes the following activities:

- Selecting utilities and equipment construction materials, operating principles, and performance characteristics based on whether they are appropriate for their specific uses.
- Verifying that utility systems and equipment are built and installed in compliance with the design specifications.
- Verifying that utility systems and equipment operate in accordance with the process requirements in all anticipated operating ranges. This should include challenging the equipment or system functions while under loads comparable to those expected during routine production. It should also include the performance of interventions, stoppage, and start-up as expected during routine production. Operating ranges should be capable of being held as long as would be necessary during routine production.

Qualification of utilities and equipment can be covered under individual plans or as part of an overall project plan. The plan should consider the requirements of use and can incorporate risk management to prioritize certain activities and identify a level of effort in both the performance and documentation of qualification activities. The plan should identify the following items: (1) the studies or tests to use, (2) the criteria appropriate to assess outcomes, (3) the timing of qualification activities, (4) the responsibilities of relevant departments and the quality unit, and (5) the procedures for documenting and approving the qualification.

The project plan should also include the firm's requirements for the evaluation of changes. Qualification activities should be documented and summarized in a report with conclusions that address criteria in the plan. The quality control unit must review and approve the qualification plan and report (§211.22).

The "Quality Systems Approach to Pharmaceutical cGMP Regulations" guidance provides a link to the regulations related to the design of facilities and equipment under Section IV: "The Quality Systems Model." The quality systems model is described according to four major factors: (1) management responsibilities, (2) resources, (3) manufacturing operations, and (4) evaluation activities. Appropriate allocation of resources is key to creating a robust quality system and complying with the cGMP regulations.

Facilities and Equipment

Under a quality system, the technical experts (e.g., engineers and development scientists), who have an understanding of pharmaceutical science, risk factors, and manufacturing processes related to the product, are responsible for defining specific facility and equipment requirements. Under the cGMP regulations, the quality unit must review and approve all initial design criteria and procedures that pertain to facilities and equipment and any subsequent changes (§211.22[c]). Under the cGMP regulations, equipment must be qualified, calibrated, cleaned, and maintained to prevent contamination and mix-ups (§211.63, 211.67, 211.68). The cGMP regulations require a higher standard for calibration and maintenance than most nonpharmaceutical quality system models. The cGMP regulations place as much emphasis on process equipment as on testing equipment (§211.160, 211.63, 211.67, and 211.68), while most quality systems focus only on testing equipment. The full text of 21 CFR 210 and 211, as well as the preamble, "Process Validation" guidance and "Quality Systems Approach to Pharmaceutical cGMP Regulations" guidance can be obtained from http://www.FDA.gov [7, 8].

AMERICAN SOCIETY OF TESTING AND MATERIALS INTERNATIONAL

The ASTM International has issued the "Standard Guide for Specification, Design, and Verification of Pharmaceutical and Biopharmaceutical Manufacturing Systems and Equipment" (ASTM E2500-13), which governs the specification, design, and verification process. This standard is based on understanding and managing risks to the patient that may be present in the manufacturing process equipment and facilities and also ensuring that process requirements are met. It also provides guidance on how to conduct verification activities. Figure 2.3 is an introductory overview of the process. The process has four major phases and is supported by four control programs applied throughout the project.

The process is to (1) identify, collect, and manage the product, process, and other quality requirements that form the basis of the design; (2) develop the design, and assess patient risk based on scientific knowledge; (3) establish risk mitigation controls and critical aspects; (4) verify that the critical aspects are in place and acceptance criteria are met as defined in the risk assessment and final design review; and (5) review the results and accept the systems and process equipment, formally releasing them for use in manufacturing operations.

The process is performed, using good design and engineering practices and risk management and change management principles. Additional traditional project controls, such as scheduling and purchasing, should also be considered and are addressed in subsequent chapters.

This risk-based approach to specification, design, and verification provides a number of opportunities to save time and money, while improving the overall quality of the delivered process equipment and systems. This approach can meet both the letter and the intent of various international cGMP regulations, regarding equipment suitability and formal qualification when applied appropriately. When using this approach, project teams should adapt it to their particular situations, using the ASTM E2500-13 2013 standard as a guide [9].

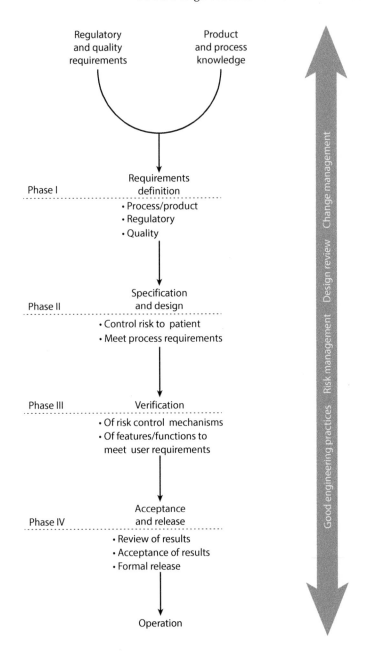

FIGURE 2.3 Risk-based specification, design, and verification process. (From ASTM International, ASTM Standard E2500-13, Standard Guide for Specification, Design, and Verification of Pharmaceutical and Biopharmaceutical Manufacturing Systems and Equipment, ASTM International, West Conshohocken, PA, 2013.)

EUROPEAN GOOD MANUFACTURING PRACTICE

The body of EU legislation for the pharmaceutical sector is compiled in *EU Pharmaceutical Legislation for Medicinal Products for Human Use*, Vol. 1, and *EU Pharmaceutical Legislation for Medicinal Products for Veterinary Use*, Vol. 5.

These rules govern medicinal products in the EU. The EU is an economic and political union of 28 countries. It operates a single market, which allows free movement of goods, capital, services, and people between member states. The EU countries are shown in Figure 2.4.

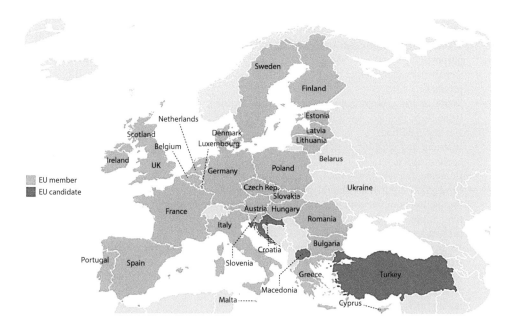

FIGURE 2.4 European Union countries: Austria, Belgium, Bulgaria, Croatia, Republic of Cyprus, Czech Republic, Denmark, Estonia, Finland, France, Germany, Greece, Hungary, Ireland, Italy, Latvia, Lithuania, Luxembourg, Malta, Netherlands, Poland, Portugal, Romania, Slovakia, Slovenia, Spain, Sweden, and United Kingdom. (From European Commission, Public Health, EU Pharmaceutical Information, European Commission, Brussels, July 26, 2015. http://ec.europa.eu/health/documents/eudralex/index_en.htm)

This basic legislation is supported by a series of guideline documents. *Good Manufacturing Practice (GMP) Guideline*, Vol. 4, contains guidance for the interpretation of the principles of GMPs for medicinal products for human and veterinary use. Chapter 3 is dedicated to premises and equipment. Several excerpts are included below.

PRINCIPLE

Premises and equipment must be located, designed, constructed, adapted, and maintained to suit the operations to be carried out. Their layout and design must aim to minimize the risk of errors and permit effective cleaning and maintenance to avoid cross-contamination, buildup of dust or dirt, and, in general, any adverse effect on the quality of products.

PREMISES

- Premises should be situated in an environment, which, when considered together with measures to protect the manufacture, presents minimal risk of causing contamination of materials or products.
- Premises should be carefully maintained, ensuring that repair and maintenance operations do not present any hazard to the quality of products. They should be cleaned and, where applicable, disinfected, according to detailed written procedures.
- Lighting, temperature, humidity, and ventilation should be appropriate so that they do not adversely affect, directly or indirectly, either the medicinal products during their manufacture and storage or the accurate functioning of equipment.
- Premises should be designed and equipped so as to afford maximum protection against the entry of insects or other animals.
- Steps should be taken to prevent the entry of unauthorized people. Production, storage, and quality control areas should not be used as a right of way by personnel who do not work in them.

EQUIPMENT

- Manufacturing equipment should be designed, located, and maintained to suit its intended purpose.
- Repair and maintenance operations should not present any hazard to the quality of the products.
- Manufacturing equipment should be designed so that it can be easily and thoroughly cleaned. It should be cleaned, according to detailed and written procedures, and stored only in a clean and dry condition.
- Washing and cleaning equipment should be chosen and used so as not to be a source of contamination.
- Equipment should be installed in such a way as to prevent any risk of error or of contamination.
- Production equipment should not present any hazard to the products. The parts of the production equipment that come into contact with the product must not be reactive, additive, or absorptive to such an extent that it will affect the quality of the product and, thus, present any hazard.
- Balances and measuring equipment of an appropriate range and precision should be available for production and control operations.
- Measuring, weighing, recording, and control equipment should be calibrated and checked at defined intervals by appropriate methods. Adequate records of such tests should be maintained.
- Fixed pipework should be clearly labeled to indicate the contents and, where applicable, the direction of flow.
- Distilled, deionized and, where appropriate, other water pipes should be sanitized, according to written procedures that detail the action limits for microbiological contamination and the measures to be taken.
- Defective equipment should, if possible, be removed from production and quality control areas or, at least, be clearly labeled as defective.

A complete copy of the EU legislation *Eudralex*, Vols. 1 and 4, can be found at http://ec.europa.eu/health/documents/eudralex/index_en.htm [10].

INTERNATIONAL CONFERENCE ON HARMONISATION

ICH Harmonised Tripartite Guideline Q10, "Pharmaceutical Quality System" (June 4, 2008), establishes a new guideline describing a model for an effective quality system for the pharmaceutical industry, referred to as the pharmaceutical quality system. This pharmaceutical quality system is based on International Organization for Standardization (ISO) quality concepts and includes applicable cGMPs. This quality system can be implemented throughout the different stages of a product life cycle. Much of the content of the ICH Q10 that is applicable to manufacturing sites is currently specified by regional cGMP requirements. The ICH Q10 is not intended to create any new expectations beyond current regulatory requirements. Consequently, the content of the ICH Q10 that is additional to current regional cGMP requirements is optional.

Within this guidance document, the "provision of facilities, utilities, and equipment" for commercial manufacturing is considered to be a technical activity for new and existing products in the product life cycle. Specific requirements include resource management and a process performance and product quality monitoring system.

Resource Management

Management should determine and provide adequate and appropriate resources (i.e., humans, finances, materials, facilities, and equipment) to implement and maintain the pharmaceutical quality system and continually improve its effectiveness.

Process Performance and Product Quality Monitoring System

Pharmaceutical companies should plan and execute a system for the monitoring of process performance and product quality to ensure a state of control is maintained. An effective monitoring system provides assurance of the continued capability of processes and controls to produce a product of desired quality and identify areas for continual improvement. The process performance and product quality monitoring system should

- Use quality risk management to establish the control strategy. This can include parameters and attributes related to drug substance and drug product materials and components, facility and equipment operating conditions, in-process controls, finished product specifications, and the associated methods and frequency of monitoring and control. The control strategy should facilitate timely feedback and feed-forward, appropriate corrective action, and preventive action.
- Provide the tools for measurement and analysis of parameters and attributes identified in the control strategy (e.g., data management and statistical tools) [11].

WHO VALIDATION GUIDELINE

The WHO Technical Report Series No. 937, 2006, Annex 4, "Supplementary Guidelines on Good Manufacturing Practices: Validation" provides guidance that may be helpful in defining validation and qualification for projects related to new or renovated facilities, equipment, utilities, and systems; specific principles of qualification and validation for various equipment and systems are addressed in the appendices.

IMPLICATIONS FOR PERFORMANCE AND COMPLIANCE

The scope and overall approach for the development of the regulatory and quality strategy throughout the project life cycle is dictated by the project scope and objectives. Integrating this strategy into the project management effort provides key input for the design approach and for overall project success.

The requirements delineated in the regulations require a disciplined approach to the design of pharmaceutical manufacturing facilities. The foundation of this approach is the manufacturing processes and the products that will be produced, tested, or held in the facility and the equipment or system being designed. The focus of design decisions and design criteria should be based on the critical quality attributes and critical process parameters of the product; environmental, health, and safety requirements; and operational requirements.

A designer must have knowledge of how the facility is to be validated, operated, and maintained. To integrate the design effort into the project, the project team needs to develop a structured approach to project management. The general project flow should include the following phases: requirements and design, build and test, and turnover.

REQUIREMENTS AND DESIGN

During the requirements and design phase, the engineering team develops the design from concept through "issued for construction/fabrication." The project team begins to define the approach to the cGMP aspects of the project life cycle and documents these in a project-specific validation plan, which is developed using current company processes and procedures. The validation plan is the document that details the validation life cycle approach; it will be used for the project and is developed in conjunction with the basis of design for the facility.

The basis of design is also developed and the manufacturing equipment, system, and facility requirements are defined during the requirements and design phase. These are developed through review of product development or validation reports and discussions with the end users, manufacturing, quality, research and development (R&D), engineering, and the validation groups.

Goals and objectives of the manufacturing unit also influence the project and depend on corporate philosophies, operating principles, and regulatory requirements.

Corporate philosophy on operational and financial management must be considered when defining the project approach. Operational requirements, such as the minimum level of finished goods inventory, directly affect the size of the warehouse, production equipment output rates, and associated design and project costs. Capital investments must meet certain criteria for return on investment (ROI) before a commitment of funds by the corporation can be made. The design of the facility, equipment, and systems (e.g., energy management and level of automation) may be dependent on the ROI.

The general company operating philosophy is an input into the design. The presence or absence of in-process material quarantine areas during the manufacturing operation, for example, will affect the physical size and layout of the new facility.

The cGMP regulations provide requirements for the design of the facility as noted above. These are considered part of an integrated design effort. Examples include the need for entry and exit gowning areas, material control during a batching operation, and easy equipment access for cleaning and maintenance operations. An understanding of these factors is essential in designing a compliant manufacturing facility.

User Requirements

To understand fully the expectations of the user of the manufacturing facility, it is necessary to develop user requirement specifications (URSs). These documents delineate the requirements and expectations of the end user of the facility, equipment, and system. The manner in which the facility, equipment, and systems are used forms the foundation for the manufacturing operation. These documents also are used as the starting point in the validation effort.

A constructive technique to assist in the understanding of all aspects of the manufacturing process is the preparation of process flow and operational flow diagrams. Process flow diagrams depict each unit operational step of the manufacturing process. In analyzing the overall production scheme, the operation can be broken down into its basic elements.

These elements are arranged in a facility operational flow diagram that depicts the relationships between the manufacturing process steps and other operating departments. The designer thus incorporates the entire operation into the layout of the facility.

Engineering Design Process

System design criteria need to be established for each production and support system required by the manufacturing process. The products being manufactured are the focus for establishing design criteria. An analysis of the manufacturing process conducted in each room or area must be completed to identify all systems that impact the quality of the product or the efficiency of operations. The process flow and operational flow diagrams, along with URS documents, are the basis for this analysis.

The activities leading to this point have resulted in the development of a design basis for the facility. Alternative concepts need to be explored and decisions made as to which are to be used. The conceptual designs of the manufacturing process are developed during the creation of the process flow diagrams. The concepts for the support utilities are derived when the quantity of the utility is known and a decision concerning the segregation of process and building utilities has been reached. Once the manufacturing process and support utility conceptual designs are completed, the facility layout is developed. The designs, drawings, schematics, and layouts are reviewed and approved as part of a formal design review process. This process should be followed throughout the full project life cycle.

The engineering and validation disciplines should also have an approved validation master plan at the end of the requirements and design phase of the project. Once the initial design reviews are complete and a validation plan is approved, a preoperational review with the FDA may be requested. Refer to the "Special Discussion" section for additional details.

Build and Test

During the build and test phase, a series of assessments are performed to confirm, using direct evidence, that a particular physical or functional specification has been met. These tests also highlight the maintenance procedures, which need to be implemented or modified early in the project life cycle. Testing activities must include verification of critical cGMP regulations, but also must examine other general requirements and specifications, such as safety and ergonomic, environmental, and general conformance to specifications. A key principle is that the scope, extent, level of effort, formality, and documentation of the verification process are commensurate with the level of patient risk. As a result, all verification work does not need to be treated with the same degree of control or documentation rigor. Those items that affect product quality and patient safety should receive the most attention. Testing can consist of different steps, such as (1) factory acceptance testing (FAT), (2) testing during construction that proves that construction is being satisfactorily executed, (3) prefunctional inspections used to confirm that the installation is ready for functional testing, (4) functional or operational testing that proves that functional or operational requirements are met, and (5) integrated system performance testing that confirms process user requirements have been met.

During the testing phase, project change management is an important supporting process to detect, describe, resolve, and track changes coming from design changes, field installation, and physical and functional changes during testing. Milestones should be defined during the testing activities to track and control progress.

To ensure proper control of the testing activities, they must be documented. SMEs should develop the particular inspections and test forms, scripts, procedures, or protocols. The approval authority may vary, but in all cases, it should be done by an appropriate SME. The SME may be part of a vendor organization, a third-party service provider, or an in-house technical expert. In most cases, an in-house technical expert should approve the testing documentation before its execution.

Persons with appropriate education, experience, and training should be used to execute the field tests, that is, fabrication, installation, operation, and performance. A separate SME should review the results of each inspection or test item and ensure that all tests were completed and appropriately documented. There may be different situations where the field result does not match the specifications from which the verification documentation was developed. The validation plan should specify the process by which departures from specification are satisfactorily addressed.

Turnover

The turnover phase is the point at which a formal review of all the testing work takes place, the systems and process equipment are deemed suitable for the intended use, and the systems and process equipment are approved for release to begin manufacturing operations. This review includes an appropriate SME and a representative from the department that will accept care, custody, and control of the item. If a system or piece of equipment includes critical aspects, then the quality unit must be part of the turnover formal review, focusing on those critical aspects. Turnover can take place system by system, on an "area" basis (e.g., all items within the component prep area), or for the entire facility or project. This depends on the turnover requirements defined by manufacturing.

The above provides a framework to the design of a cGMP facility. Input is provided by a multidisciplinary team, consisting of facilities professionals with backgrounds in manufacturing, quality, engineering, and validation. The approach includes a formal design review process at the appropriate time in the design cycle, as well as the inclusion of the testing requirements. A well-designed facility is by definition one that meets regulatory requirements and expectations. The key point is to create a fully integrated project approach with full understanding of the product, regulatory manufacturing process, and validation requirements. With this basis, an experienced designer can use his or her knowledge and experience to develop a cGMP-compliant and sustainable design.

Project Size Considerations

All other things being equal (i.e., nature of technology and purpose of facility), the larger the project, the more planning and coordination that will be necessary; for example, the validation plan may need to be developed as several plans (i.e., a high-level validation plan followed by a more detailed validation execution plan). The converse is also true: with small projects, the amount of effort needed to plan and coordinate the execution is less; for example, the validation plan could be combined into an overall project quality plan, which for very small projects could be combined with the project execution plan. Creation of such an integrated plan requires additional input from a broad set of participant groups.

Another impact of project size is the number of design reviews, who does them, and how they are scheduled. For a very small project with a straightforward use of known technology, there could be a single design review. For a very large project or one using complex, novel technology, simply scheduling and managing the design review effort could be significant.

The approach to qualification or validation is also typically a function of project size. For example, on a very large project, it may be advantageous to have a dedicated effort to inspect each item upon receipt at the job site and to initiate material tracking procedures. This helps identify nonconformance to requirements early. This is especially true if the material will not be installed immediately after receipt. For a very small project, the equipment may be received and installed immediately, and a single receipt and installation inspection may be most expedient. Large projects may use factory inspections and acceptance testing. The number of factory visits associated with a large project may require a dedicated coordination of effort.

Project Complexity Considerations

Project complexity occurs at many levels. A project could involve a complex process or a particularly complex piece of equipment or control system. The project itself could be complex in how it must be executed, perhaps shutting down an existing operation in stages or restarting in stages, for example. Complexity may affect planning, execution coordination, and management; how risks are assessed; attention to design; and the approach to qualification and validation.

A complex process requires additional effort to understand the process and capture all the product and process user requirements. The process control scheme may require additional engineering design to meet the challenges of a complex process. It may be more difficult to assess all of the risks to the patient that may be found in a complex process. Additional time may be required during start-up for full-scale process development or engineering studies.

A complex piece of equipment or control system may warrant additional dimensions of risk assessment. While the effort to analyze risks to the patient may not be more difficult, it may be desirable to use additional risk analysis methods to determine component or function failure modes from an operational perspective. The design and design review efforts for complex equipment or control systems require greater attention. There may be special expertise required to complete the design and review it properly. The approach and effort required for testing a complex piece of equipment or control system are also greater. There may be additional steps in the testing process, such as vendor fabrication, hold-point inspections, automation design reviews, and code walk-through exercises. There may be additional inspection steps during start-up and additional effort for operational or cleaning cycle development.

Existing Facility Upgrades, Retrofit Projects, and Expansion Projects

The objective for facility upgrades, retrofit, or expansion projects is to define a set of activities that challenge the new aspects of the facility and confirm that existing aspects have not changed within the project timeline and cost. Detailed planning is needed to achieve this objective. Plans need to consider the impact on existing equipment due to temporary storage, disconnection, movement, reconnection, and interface with new equipment or controls. The reinstallation and restart must be managed to reduce the possibility that equipment operation is affected. Any potential change as to how the equipment is configured, operates, or performs must be assessed, and appropriate inspections and tests must be performed to confirm fitness for purpose. The operations department should be consulted in developing the project execution and validation plans.

The project team should ensure that life cycle documentation (drawings, equipment manuals, calibration, and preventive maintenance programs) has been updated to reflect the new or modified process equipment and systems affected by the upgrade or retrofit project. This, along with the inspection and testing work for new or modified process equipment and systems, is the most important aspect of the project from a regulatory compliance perspective.

Unknown Product and Process Requirements

For some types of projects, the product or process user requirements may not be known; for example, projects where product or process development work is ongoing; in multiproduct facilities, contract manufacturing facilities, or other situations where the product to be manufactured has not yet been determined; in R&D facilities; and in clinical manufacturing facilities. There still needs, however, to be some basis for the design. For most projects, the user will be able to define a generic set of process requirements or performance capabilities that the equipment or systems should meet. These requirements become the basis for design and can serve as the process requirements. For some facilities, there may also be some general requirements that are derived from regulatory expectations; for example, aseptic filling will occur under ISO 14644-1 Class 5 conditions with unidirectional airflow.

Inspection and testing are based on engineering specifications and are carried out by SMEs. The verification work should include performance tests and determination of equipment operating capabilities so that future product and process requirements can be readily evaluated against the capabilities of the process equipment and systems. In many cases, it will be appropriate to evaluate the equipment suitability in the following terms: (1) confirm that the assessed risks to the patient are adequately controlled and (2) define equipment performance capabilities that are acceptable to the user. Since there are no defined product or process user requirements other than general requirements used as the basis for design, the acceptance criteria become what are acceptable and agreed on by the user and process SME. Once development work is complete and product or process user requirements are finalized, it is imperative that the project team confirms and documents that the general product or process user requirements defined are aligned with the final product or process requirements. Additional details for the application to oral solid dosages, APIs, biotechnology, sterile manufacturing facilities, and design practices in the validation life cycle can be found in subsequent chapters.

CROSS-FUNCTIONAL PROJECT TEAMS FOR INTEGRATION OF REGULATORY AND QUALITY STRATEGIES

The overall regulatory strategy addresses a wide array of requirements related to FDA, EU, local, and other worldwide regulatory requirements. These requirements and corresponding controls should be integrated into the overall project planning process for deliverables, schedules, costs, and defining roles and responsibilities, as well as design and engineering approaches.

The project team should perform assessments of regulatory filing requirements and their impact on the project schedule from the outset of the project and determine how to integrate the engineering deliverables and scheduling constraints into the earliest project plans. Once this scope is defined, the project team should plan for sufficient manpower, planning, preparation, expertise, and lead time focused on all regulatory and project requirements.

Key players on the regulatory strategy development team include the project lead, technical resources group, research and development, safety and industrial hygiene, quality lead, regulatory lead, process engineer, and manufacturing lead. During the project "kickoff" meeting, the overall regulatory strategy is defined. Key areas of focus include (1) defining the project's regulatory and compliance objectives and approach; (2) assigning project regulatory leadership responsibility; (3) identifying expected FDA, EU, or other regulatory agency filing milestones, constraints, and possible inspections, as required, within the overall project schedule; and (4) developing initial regulatory and compliance strategies based on available information. This information should be documented, including key assumptions and alternative strategies, and approved by the appropriate parties to ensure there is alignment and understanding across functions. Figure 2.5 represents one approach for the collection of regulatory information.

It is a cGMP requirement that individuals have appropriate education, training, and experience to perform the assigned functions. This holds true for each phase of the project. As stated above, it is critical to the success of the project to have the cross-functional team define a project's regulatory and quality strategy. However, an SME is required throughout the project life cycle for the team to function efficiently and effectively. For example, quality assurance professionals are SMEs with respect to formulation of a quality system, auditing, and oversight over the implementation of quality policies and plans. Engineers are SMEs with respect to the details of process equipment, systems, and automation installation, operation, and performance, and the inspection and testing thereof. Engineers are also SMEs with respect to evaluating different design alternatives and resolving departures from technical specifications. Process development scientists are SMEs with respect to the manufacturing process, in particular the critical process parameters and other key aspects of the process necessary to manufacture a quality product and control risks to the patient.

Product	Region or country	Governing regulatory agency	Expected submission date	Target submission date	Anticipated approval cycle	Anticipated approval date	Responsibility

FIGURE 2.5 Project regulatory strategy.

Engineers are primarily responsible for quality control. This includes defining system and equipment designs, determining inspections and tests necessary to verify conformance to specifications, conducting a given inspection or test, and determining when in the project delivery process it is most appropriate to perform each inspection or test, and whether the results are acceptable.

In addition, the cGMPs place special requirements on quality professionals. In the United States, an independent quality unit is responsible for approving the release of each lot or batch. In the EU, a qualified person who has undergone special training and certification performs this release. The cGMPs require that an independent quality unit "approve specifications and procedures impacting on the safety, quality, purity, identity, and strength of the drug product" [12]. The EU GMPs require a qualified person to verity processes to manufacture product are validated.

Integrated engineering and quality systems are designed to meet both the specific requirements for involvement of an independent quality unit or qualified person and the intent of the cGMPs regarding use of SMEs. Select key aspects and associated roles and responsibilities include the following:

- Obtaining product and process requirements from process development SMEs or appropriate product technology transfer reports or development reports
- Quality unit approval of the product and process requirements
- Quality unit approval of the overall project validation plan
- Using a multidisciplinary team to perform risk assessments
- Engineering review of design documents
- Quality unit approval of the risk assessments that document how each patient safety-related risk is being controlled, including the critical specifications (i.e., installation and operation) that serve to control those risks
- Quality unit approval of those functions that meet process requirements
- Engineering approval of appropriate inspection and test items, procedures, and acceptance criteria
- Engineering approval (independent of the person performing the commissioning or qualification work) of the results of testing and correction of departures from engineering specifications
- Quality unit involvement in any departure from specifications involving a critical aspect
- Quality unit approval of the suitability or fitness for use of each process equipment, system, or automation control, and release of that item for manufacturing purposes

It is not necessary to create new systems for determining who is qualified to be a particular SME, over and above that required by regulations. Project plans should list responsibilities for various groups on a given project; those responsibilities should be based on the project scope and SME required to meet project deliverables. Sample roles and a responsibility matrix are illustrated in Figure 2.6.

There are a variety of contractors, consultants, and other service providers used during the life cycle of a project that are integrated into project teams in key roles. These include, but are not limited to, functions such as engineering design, construction, testing, and validation. These firms can provide meaningful reviews, bring broader experience to a project or site, and provide objective evaluations. However, it is critical to evaluate the output from the contractors, consultants, and service providers to ensure that decisions are reviewed and approved by the quality unit, if cGMP relevant; that their qualifications are thought adequate before hiring; and that project needs are continuously met.

R = Responsible A = Approver C = Contribute I = Inform	Quality unit	User SME	Project manager	Engineering SME	Validation SME	Process science	Constructing/ engineering firm
Process/product requirements	A	A	A	C	C	A	I
General user requirments	I	A	A	C	C	I	I
Project change management	A	A	A	R	C	I	I
Project validation plan	A	A	A	A	R	I	I
Construction/vendor quality plan				A	A		R
Develop design		C		R	C	C	R
Vendor assessment	A	I	I	R	A		
Product risk assessment	A	A	I	A	A	R	I
Design review	A	A	I	A	R	C	I
Factory acceptance testing			I	A			I
Construction/vendor testing			I	A	A		R
Installation qualification			I	A	C	I	C
Operational qualification		C	I	A	R	I	C
Performance qualification	A	A	I		R	C	
Acceptance and release	A	A	I	R	C	I	I
Design review	A	A	I	A	R	C	I
Factory acceptance testing			I	A			I
Construction/vendor testing			I	A	A		R
Installation qualification			I	A	C	I	C
Operational qualification		C	I	A	R	I	C
Performance qualification	A	A	I		R	C	
Acceptance and release	A	A	I	R	C	I	I

FIGURE 2.6 Sample project roles and responsibility matrix.

PREOPERATIONAL REVIEW BY THE FDA AND IMPACT OF NONCOMPLIANCE

PREOPERATIONAL REVIEW

One important option to consider when designing, building, or renovating a pharmaceutical manufacturing technology, process, or facility is a preoperational review of the manufacturing facilities by the FDA. Field Management Directive (FMD) 135 provides guidance for conducting these reviews. Based on the process or technology, various reviews may be necessary. These include (1) design review, (2) preconstruction review, (3) construction or equipment installation and qualification review, and (4) preproduction review.

Providing the FDA with an opportunity for early review and comment on the design, construction, and validation may reveal issues or risks that can be addressed early in the process, thereby preventing costly design and construction errors. By addressing the agency's concerns early in the design process, corrective actions after construction can be eliminated. This review can expedite the certification of a facility and increase efficiency and timely processing of required FDA filings and applications.

It is important to note that the purpose of FDA reviews is to offer the best opinion as to whether the new or modified facilities and processing procedures would comply with cGMP regulations.

However, it is the manufacturer's responsibility to design, construct, qualify, validate, and operate a plant in a compliant manner.

The meeting with the FDA can include a review of the conceptual design of the facility and the validation master plan. While the FDA will not approve the design, the agency can indicate areas of concern. The project team should conduct an internal cGMP audit before the meeting with the FDA, the purpose of which is to determine whether the design of the facility meets cGMP requirements and accepted industry practices. The audit should be conducted by personnel who are familiar with cGMP design practices and who are not directly involved in the project.

IMPACT OF NONCOMPLIANCE

This section summarizes the implications of not complying with FDA regulations, including issuance of 483 citations, warning letters, seizures, and injunctions. Recent examples of FDA 483 citations related to the design of pharmaceutical equipment, systems, and facilities are provided. The objective of FDA regulatory programs is to ensure compliance with the Federal Food, Drug, and Cosmetic Act. For pharmaceutical companies who violate the law and regulations, specific enforcement activities are taken to correct and prevent violations, remove noncompliant products or goods from the market, and punish offenders. The enforcement activity used by the FDA depends on the degree and severity of the violation. The range of enforcement activities include issuing a letter notifying the individual or firm of a violation, and requesting correction, to criminal prosecution of the individual or firm. Several types of enforcement actions are noted below:

- At the conclusion of an inspection, if objectionable conditions are found, FDA Form 483 is presented and discussed with the company's senior management. Companies must respond to FDA Form 483 in writing with their corrective action plan and then implement that corrective action plan expeditiously.
- A warning letter is sent to the individuals or firms, advising them of specific violations. These letters request a written response as to the steps that will be taken to correct the violations.
- A seizure is an action brought against an FDA-regulated product because it is adulterated or misbranded within the meaning of the act. The purpose of such an action is to remove these goods from commerce.
- An order by a court (injunction) requires that an individual or corporation do or refrain from doing a specific act. The FDA may seek an injunction against individuals or corporations to prevent them from violating or causing violations of the act.
- Criminal prosecution may be recommended in appropriate cases for violation of Section 301 of the act. Misdemeanor convictions, which do not require proof of intent to violate the act, can result in fines or imprisonment up to 1 year. Felony convictions, which apply in the case of a second violation or intent to defraud or mislead, can result in fines or imprisonment for up to 3 years.

Any one of these enforcement actions can adversely impact the ability of a pharmaceutical company to manufacture or distribute product. Therefore, it is critical that everyone understands the impact of their actions as part of their role in quality within the organization.

Figure 2.7 represents the breakdown of the top 20 FDA 483 observations against 21 CFR 211: "Current Good Manufacturing Practices for Finished Pharmaceuticals" identified by the Center for Drug Evaluation and Research for fiscal year 2014. Of the top 20 observations, 4 are related to the design of pharmaceutical facilities. These include (1) 21 CFR §211.67(a) related to equipment cleaning and maintenance; (2) 21 CFR §211.68(a) related to automatic, mechanical, and electronic equipment calibration and maintenance; (3) 21 CFR §211.42(c)(10)(iv) related to design and construction features; and (4) 21 CFR §211.63 related to equipment design, size, and location.

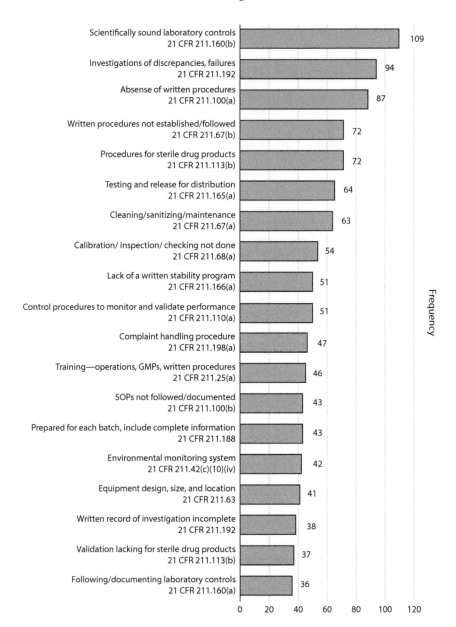

FIGURE 2.7 Top 20 FDA 483 observations for fiscal year 2014. (From U.S. Food and Drug Administration, Inspections, Compliance, Enforcement, and Criminal Investigations, Fiscal Year 2014 Inspectional Observation Summaries, U.S. Food and Drug Administration, Silver Spring, MD, November 28, 2014. http://www.fda.gov/ICECI/Inspections/ucm424098.htm#Drugs)

Many times the design of a process, equipment, or system can lead to deviations in cleaning, maintenance, or calibration processes or impact the ability of an operator to perform his or her job effectively. This can lead to regulatory observations well after the turnover of a project. Clearly defined, well-understood user requirements, a comprehensive inspection and testing process, and a robust maintenance program are critical to ensure processes, equipment, and systems maintain compliance with all applicable regulations for their lifetime.

The focus on the design, build, and maintenance of pharmaceutical facilities, equipment, and systems remains one of the highest areas of interest for regulators. Therefore, the need for pharmaceutical engineering professionals to maintain a working understanding of the new and changing regulatory requirements and a healthy partnership with quality control personnel is critical for the ongoing success of the pharmaceutical industry [13].

SPECIAL DISCUSSION

In July 2013, the FDA regulation for cGMP requirements for combination products (21 CFR 4) went into effect. As with all regulations, it is expected that pharmaceutical manufacturers are compliant with the stated requirements based on their product portfolio and the combination products' definition.

As defined in 21 CFR 3, a combination product is a product composed of any combination of drugs, devices, or biological products. The drugs, devices, and biological products included in combination products are referred to as constituent parts of the combination product. Under 21 CFR 3.2(e), a combination product includes

- A product comprised of two or more regulated components ... that are physically, chemically, or otherwise combined and produced as a single entity[, such as a prefilled syringe or drug-eluting stent];
- Two or more separate products packaged together in a single package or as a unit and comprised of drug and device products, device and biological products, or biological and drug products[, such as a surgical or first aid kit];
- A drug, device, or biological product packaged separately that according to its investigational plan or proposed labeling is intended for use only with an approved, individually specified drug, device, or biological product where both are required to achieve the intended use, indication, or effect and whereupon approval of the proposed product, the labeling of the approved product would need to be changed. e.g., to reflect a change in intended use, dosage form, strength, route of administration, or significant change in dose[, such as a light-emitting device and a light-activated drug]; or
- Any investigational drug, device, or biological product packaged separately that according to its proposed labeling is for use only with another individually specified investigational drug, device, or biological product where both are required to achieve the intended use, indication, or effect.

Manufacturers of combination products are required to understand the implications of the requirements of 21 CFR 4 and meet the applicable requirements of the drug cGMPs (21 CFR 211) and device quality system (21 CFR 820) regulations by designing and implementing a cGMP operating system that demonstrates compliance to the applicable regulations. The FDA recognizes that combination products may be complex but requires that each manufacturing site is responsible for compliance to the applicable cGMP [14]. For pharmaceutical projects that include combination products, the project team should include a combination product SME and a medical device quality system SME throughout the project life cycle to ensure accurate definition of user requirements, appropriateness of design reviews, and adequacy of validation plans.

In conclusion, the regulatory environment is ever changing and has a global reach. It is important for pharmaceutical engineering professionals to stay current with these changes by influencing regulations, getting involved with industry forums and associations, and engaging their regulatory and quality partners. The key benefit of these efforts is a continuous supply of high-quality pharmaceutical products for patients all over the world.

KEY WORDS

- **Quality system:** Formalized business practices that define management responsibilities for organizational structure, processes, procedures, and resources needed to fulfill product or service requirements, customer satisfaction, and continual improvement [15].

- **Current good manufacturing practices:** The cGMPs refer to the current Good Manufacturing Practice regulations enforced by the U.S. Food and Drug Administration (FDA). The cGMPs provide for systems that ensure proper design, monitoring, and control of manufacturing processes and facilities [16].
- **Quality risk management:** A systematic process for the assessment, control, communication, and review of risks to the quality of the drug (medicinal) product across the product life cycle [17].

FURTHER DISCUSSION

The following questions can be initiated during the scoping phase of the project and updated throughout the project life cycle. They incorporate aspects of the regulatory and quality strategy that should be included as part of the overall project management effort.

1. Have the products been identified, including forms, strengths, packaging configurations, and distribution? Is this product a combination product?
2. Are the manufacturing method, analytical method, raw materials, support systems, packaging method, and regulatory acceptance criteria understood?
3. What are the global regulatory requirements that must be met?
4. What changes to regulatory requirements are anticipated during the project? What effect might these changes have on the project's scope, design, costs, or schedule? How will the project be managed to mitigate their impact?
5. What quality assurance problems may impact the project? How will the project be managed to mitigate their impact?
6. What qualification or validation strategy will be employed?
7. Describe the parties responsible for addressing each of the questions above. How does the size and complexity of the project impact the process of addressing these questions?
8. Who are the various regulatory agencies with responsibility for establishing pharmaceutical regulations and requirements in the United States? How do they relate to each other and to their international equivalents?
9. What are the advantages of a preoperational review with the FDA?

ABOUT THE AUTHOR

Rose Mary Dollard is currently a senior director of regulatory compliance in Johnson & Johnson's enterprise compliance organization. She has more than 25 years of quality, compliance, and manufacturing experience in the pharmaceutical and medical device industries. Her broad range of experience includes various quality and compliance functions that support fast-paced manufacturing environments, with strengths in commissioning and qualification program development, as well as solid oral dose, solution, suspension, and packaging manufacturing technologies. She has been responsible for the design and deployment of several novel compliance solutions across global Johnson & Johnson businesses, including establishing robust compliance assessment and remediation programs and a progressive science and risk commissioning and qualification methodology. Rose Mary is involved with several industry organizations, including a chapter author of the International Society for Pharmaceutical Engineering (ISPE) Good Practice Guide *Applied Risk Management for Commissioning and Qualification* and past chair of the ISPE Commissioning and Qualification Community of Practice Steering Committee.

REFERENCES

1. U.S. Food and Drug Administration, What We Do, U.S. Food and Drug Administration, Silver Spring, MD, August 14, 2014, at http://www.fda.gov/AboutFDA/WhatWeDo/, accessed September 8, 2015.

2. U.S. Food and Drug Administration, FDA Globalization, U.S. Food and Drug Administration, Silver Spring, MD, May 1, 2015, http://www.fda.gov/InternationalPrograms/FDABeyondOurBordersForeign Offices/ (accessed September 1, 2015).

3. International Conference of Harmonisation, Welcome to the ICH Official Website, International Conference of Harmonisation, Geneva, n.d., http://www.ich.org/home.html (accessed September 8, 2015).

4. World Health Organization, About WHO, World Health Organization, Geneva, 2015, http://www.who.int/about/en/ (accessed September 8, 2015).

5. ASTM International, Detailed Overview, ASTM International, West Conshohocken, PA, 2015, http://www.astm.org/ABOUT/full_overview.html (accessed September 8, 2015).

6. U.S. Food and Drug Administration, CFR Title 21, U.S. Food and Drug Administration, Silver Spring, MD, April 1, 2015, https://www.accessdata.fda.gov/scripts/cdrh/cfdocs/cfCFR/CFRSearch.cfm?CFRPart=211 (accessed September 8, 2015).

7. U.S. Food and Drug Administration, Guidance for Industry Process Validation: General Principles and Practices, U.S. Food and Drug Administration, Silver Spring, MD, 2011, http://www.fda.gov/downloads/Drugs/Guidances/UCM070336.pdf (accessed September 8, 2015).

8. U.S. Food and Drug Administration, Guidance for Industry Quality Systems Approach to Pharmaceutical cGMP Regulations, U.S. Food and Drug Administration, Silver Spring, MD, September 1, 2006, http://www.fda.gov/downloads/Drugs/.../Guidances/UCM070337.pdf (accessed September 8, 2015).

9. ASTM International, ASTM E2500-13: Standard Guide for Specification, Design, and Verification of Pharmaceutical and Biopharmaceutical Manufacturing Systems and Equipment, ASTM International, West Conshohocken, PA, 2013.

10. European Commission, European Union Legislation: Eudralex, European Commission, Brussels, n.d., http://ec.europa.eu/health/documents/eudralex/index_en.htm (accessed September 1, 2015).

11. International Conference of Harmonisation, ICH Harmonised Tripartite Guideline Q10, Pharmaceutical Quality System, International Conference of Harmonisation, Geneva, June 4, 2008, http://www.ich.org/fileadmin/Public_Web_Site/ICH_Products/Guidelines/Quality/Q10/Step4/Q10_Guideline.pdf (accessed September 1, 2015).

12. Code of Federal Regulations, Title 21, vol. 4, 21 CFR 211.22, revised as of April 1, 2015.

13. U.S. Food and Drug Administration, Guidance, Compliance, and Regulatory Information, U.S. Food and Drug Administration, Silver Spring, MD, March 1, 2015, http://www.fda.gov/Drugs/GuidanceComplianceRegulatoryInformation/ (accessed September 1, 2015).

14. U.S. Food and Drug Administration, Combination Products, U.S. Food and Drug Administration, Silver Spring, MD, March 31, 2015, http://www.fda.gov/CombinationProducts/ (accessed September 1, 2015).

15. U.S. Food and Drug Administration, FDA Staff Manual Guides, Vol. III: General Administration, FDA Official Councils and Committees, FDA Quality System Framework for Internal Activities, SMG 2020, U.S. Food and Drug Administration, Silver Spring, MD, April 22, 2014.

16. U.S. Food and Drug Administration, Facts about the Current Good Manufacturing Practices (cGMPs), U.S. Food and Drug Administration, Silver Spring, MD, January 6, 2015, http://www.fda.gov/Drugs/DevelopmentApprovalProcess/Manufacturing/ucm169105.htm (accessed September 1, 2015).

17. International Conference of Harmonisation, ICH Harmonised Tripartite Guideline Q9: Quality Risk Management, International Conference of Harmonisation, Geneva, November 2005.

3 Legacy Facility Master Planning

Eric Bohn

CONTENTS

INTRODUCTION

The development of the modern pharmaceutical manufacturing facility is deeply entwined with the history of the twentieth century. After the Second World War, there was an explosion in drug development. In order to make these innovative lifesaving products available to patients, a corresponding eruption occurred in the construction of manufacturing plants. With each new drug, and new class of drug, additional manufacturing capacity was required and then built. As a consequence, today there are many of these older facilities still in use.

Due to their longevity and the need to continue to support the needs of patients, such established plants often have undergone numerous additions and renovations. Given their age, coming to terms with these existing legacy facilities is a challenge. A steel-framed structure can last upwards of 100 years. To avoid waste and the loss of capital that has been invested, in both building and human infrastructure, it is necessary to learn to revitalize these important assets.

Legacy facilities were built for Good Manufacturing Practices (GMPs) that existed at the time of their construction. Over time, these standards have evolved and changed. In the other chapters of this book, GMP issues are individually explored in depth. This chapter does not study the individual issues, but instead explores the legacy pharmaceutical facility as a complete entity. As such, this chapter touches on all aspects of facility design and all aspects of facility GMPs. To successfully design a new manufacturing facility, it is necessary to understand GMPs. The special conditions of a legacy facility also require knowledge of GMPs. However, in this chapter, we focus on describing a process that leads to making established, older facilities a sustainable link within the larger framework of the corporate supply chain.

This chapter's objective is to develop an understanding of the unique character of existing legacy facilities, their limitations, and the need to actively work to stay ahead of the curve in terms of industry changes in technology, quality assurance, and GMPs. In this chapter, we define legacy facilities, identify common issues and problems found in these facilities, and identify methodologies that can help manage legacy facilities for the long term. The intent is to enable management teams to maintain their facility as vital and sustainable now and into the future.

EXECUTIVE SUMMARY

Key Concepts

The following are key concepts that will be discussed in this chapter:

1. Legacy facility: An existing, older facility that has been successfully repurposed many times, over many years. Due to incremental changes and the pressures to act expeditiously, these facilities often face challenges staying current and sustainable.
2. Master plan: A comprehensive plan of action focused on a facility's process capability and physical plant. A master plan is a long-term planning document that establishes a framework for future changes that brings together a site's goals and aspirations and gives form and organization to define a realistic plan for action.

Definition of a Legacy Facility

Merriam-Webster defines legacy as "something transmitted by or received from an ancestor or predecessor or from the past." Legacy facilities are manufacturing plants that have been in use long enough that they have lived through several cycles of change. They develop over a period of time and, in the process, accrue incremental alterations that impact the integrity of the facility's original configuration and operational strategies. When new products, equipment, and processes are introduced, necessary steps must be taken to accommodate them.

Because of their success, profitability, and investment in infrastructure, the expansion of such facilities will logically follow. To provide for more capacity and new product lines, new processes and spaces are added and old spaces reconfigured. These modifications to the original plant arrangement create correspondingly new patterns of material and personnel movement. When such changes happen, they are often relatively small in scale and accommodated through solutions that emphasize cost-effectiveness. Over time, these individual changes accumulate, and eventually the original building configuration and operational strategies can be impacted.

Beyond the immediate boundaries of these facilities, there are additional pressures that mount. Unlike the physical structure of an existing facility, regulatory and business environments are not frozen in time. For instance, advances in technology cannot be stopped. Neither are Good Manufacturing Practices static. Over time, they evolve, which is why GMPs have acquired the moniker of "current" Good Manufacturing Practices (cGMPs). These differences develop gradually, and over many years they become significant. Contrasting the understanding of GMPs from 20 or 30 years ago to the science and risk-based approach of the present reveals how divergent they can become.

In terms of business trends, the environment in which the pharmaceutical industry operates is also continually under change. Generics, outsourcing, and new therapies, such as gene and protein therapies, have all exerted their influence. In the end, as a facility ages, its ability to reflect the most up-to-date and best industry practices degrades. As these changes accrue, such facilities become characterized by compromises. Eventually, legacy facilities become burdened with outmoded infrastructure, equipment, and production facilities due to their inability to keep pace with the current standards.

The pharmaceutical industry developed quickly at the beginning of the twentieth century. Initially, drugs were predominantly produced by small manufacturers with little control over their claims or the reality of efficacy and safety. Our modern, large-scale pharmaceutical industry emerged as part of the war effort to develop and commercialize penicillin during the Second World War. Throughout the 1950s, an explosion in the discovery of new classes of antibiotics and vaccines occurred. At this time, funding for medical and scientific research expanded from $161 million in 1950 to more than $2.5 billion in 1968 [1]. In 1962, drug development was modernized by the Kefauver–Harris Amendments, which for the first time required that drug manufacturers scientifically prove that a medication was both safe and effective. This act also provided that the U.S. Food and Drug Administration (FDA) set GMPs for industry and further mandated regular inspections of production facilities. Since then, drug discovery and development have continued unabated, with new drugs being developed every year.

The large-scale production of pharmaceuticals requires large buildings to support this activity. With the success of new drugs comes the need for additional capacity, and in turn, existing facilities are typically expanded to meet that demand. Historically, these buildings have followed a common pattern of successive cycles of expansion and retrofit as new products and technologies are incorporated. Today, such legacy facilities are found throughout the industry. After many decades of pharmaceutical development, it is not hard to find facilities that were first constructed 30–40 years ago, and in some cases, even longer.

Over this same period of time, changes in technology and regulations have been monumental. At the beginning of the twentieth century, Bayer AG's worldwide sales of aspirin attested to the industry's long-standing international character. However, this was the exception. Today globalization is a fundamental condition of the pharmaceutical industry, and a global supply chain is the norm.

GMPs have evolved and are instituted worldwide by numerous regional agencies. So too equipment and process advances have been enormous, and aided by the computer revolution of the same era, highly sophisticated controls have contributed to higher product quality and cost-effectiveness. As these and other forces of change continue, making sure that legacy facilities are up to current industry standards is a continual challenge.

LEGACY FACILITY ISSUES

As legacy facilities grow older, the development of certain traits is predictable. These identifiable characteristics are a hallmark of such facilities. Examples include

- Circuitous circulation
- Crossing of material, equipment, and personnel flows
- Excessive handling of materials
- Inconsistent gowning practices
- Inadequate segregation of unit operations, products, and batches
- Inefficient organization of environmental or hygienic zones

Incremental change in an existing facility is usually accompanied by the need to disturb as little of the current operations as possible. Building within the limits of a legacy structure restricts the options available and, if not carefully planned, will eventually end up with inappropriate placement of activities. If a holistic approach that considers the entire facility is not undertaken, the only way to resolve odd placements of function is with the introduction of circuitous and inefficient circulation patterns. Circuitous circulation, as the name implies, leads to flows that are not directionally linear and frequently places unit operations out of sequence.

Crossing and backtracking of in-process materials, along with equipment increases the risk of both product mix-ups and cross-contamination. Also, the lack of integration within the existing flows inevitably increases the handling and staging of material.

Excessive handling of material is counter to the fundamentals of lean manufacturing and erodes operational efficiency and escalates handling time, as well as staffing requirements and ultimately operational costs.

Gowning needs to be appropriate for the processes being accessed. Because the greatest source of contamination in a GMP environment is typically the operators, gowning is a critical strategy for protecting drug products from contamination. While gowning also serves to protect the operator, this aspect is generally considered to be secondary unless a potent compound is involved. Properly locating de-gowning operations is important to avoid transporting product residue to adjacent areas, which, of course, increases the risk of product cross-contamination. In older facilities, confused or muddled placement of process operations can result in inadequate gowning and de-gowning locations and protocols. Or, alternately, the older gowning strategies that the facility was previously designed for may simply not be appropriate any longer.

Another concern with gowning is operational effectiveness. Gowning and de-gowning are time-consuming and require an abundance of gowning supplies (gowns, hair nets, booties, etc.). If not strategically located, gowning can occur too frequently. Multiple gowning operations just to gain access to a single manufacturing task slows the operation, which leads to excessive operating costs due to the inefficient consumption of time and materials. For this reason, when possible, gowning should be centralized, located to provide access to aggregated areas of the same level of gowning. Such a configuration will result in maximizing the operators' time for actual production.

Segregation is another important GMP concept. Physical separation that creates autonomous spatial environments maintains isolation of different unit operations, raw materials, batches, and products. Keeping these materials from being exposed to each other prevents cross-contamination. In legacy facilities, after years of modifications, segregation can be poorly organized, inefficient, or ineffective. As a result, the risk of cross-contamination is increased. An alternative approach is to choose chronological segregation, which is to say careful timing and sequencing of the use of spaces and equipment, including cleaning. This approach is labor-intensive and not an efficient use of the building and its infrastructure, which is expensive to own and operate. A clear and simple physical segregation strategy is always the best approach and eliminates the human error that is possible when relying exclusively on procedures.

Related to segregation is the idea of hygiene zoning. This is a concept that goes by several different titles. Some organizations refer to it as cleanliness levels and some hygiene zones, while the International Society for Pharmaceutical Engineering (ISPE) refers to levels of protection. Regardless of the name, the idea revolves around the integration of several of the previous concepts. Working together, product quality is protected by the combined action of environmental control, segregation of product, segregation of unit operations, and appropriate gowning. These varying levels of operational zoning also require the design of clean room air systems, which minimize the risk of contamination through pressurization, air change rates, and air filtration. Like segregation, ill-defined and poorly organized hygiene zones that create isolated pockets of the same type of space almost always lead to increased staging and material handling, again leading to excessive operational costs. Grouping similar levels of protection together maintains the least amount of work from gowning and wiping down of materials that enter the area. In addition, air systems can realize improved economies of scale due to larger air handling units and more efficient ductwork. One of the best ways to uncover GMP issues in an existing facility is to plot the existing hygiene zones on a plan. The extent to which it is disjointed and unorganized represents a potential for GMP issues to exist. Such conditions are usually also representative of inefficient air systems, excessive material handling, and gowning problems. If such challenges are ignored and not corrected, the facility will increasingly become at risk of being identified by the regulating agencies as needing correction.

Incremental changes that occur in isolation can reduce the effectiveness of the entire facility. A change in one area can lead to bottlenecks, crossing of flows, or other inefficient and unproductive operational results. These are wasteful of time and manpower, all of which results in higher operating costs. Incremental changes also encourage expedient solutions that respond narrowly to the immediate business goal and discourage full consideration of the larger impacts to the facility now and in the future. It is necessary to have a larger game plan to avoid succumbing to these natural tendencies.

THE BUSINESS CASE FOR LEGACY FACILITIES

Why bother to preserve a legacy facility? In a global economy, surely there are alternatives to maintaining an old and outdated facility. By building new, however, there is much to be lost. Regardless of the current condition, by definition, legacy facilities have had a history of success. As such, established facilities incorporate attributes that can make them attractive to maintain as a vital part of a company's current and future supply chain.

The first and most obvious reason to maintain an existing, aging facility is the capital investment already in the physical plant. Over the years, a significant amount of money and time have gone into establishing and maintaining a site. Expenditures in the physical plant include the structure, foundation, and building enclosure; utility feeds both to the site and into the building; and to the extent they can be reused, the internal utilities and services. In addition, there are usually numerous support functions already in place, such as warehouse, office, cafeteria, and quality assurance and quality control (QA/QC) laboratories that can continue to be leveraged. To replace such a facility means the previous investment disappears in its entirety.

A less obvious advantage of a legacy facility is the knowledge embodied in the staff. Developing, sharing, and effectively using organizational knowledge is no small endeavor and impacts product quality, as acknowledged by the International Conference of Harmonisation (ICH) Q10, "Pharmaceutical Quality System." A tremendous amount of information is generated in establishing the critical process parameters and quality attributes of each product. While a formal system to gather, distribute, and utilize this information is important, the human factor cannot be undervalued, especially when dealing with existing products and processes. It is the existing staff that is the storehouse of this institutional knowledge. In addition, instilled in experienced staff is the company ethos and the industry's culture of quality. Staff knowledge and experience, if completely eradicated, are not easily or quickly replaced. Recruiting and training new personnel takes a significant amount of time and money.

The previous examples illustrate monetary and operational losses that occur when an existing facility is taken out of service. But the financial losses do not end there. Before a new facility can produce product, design, construction, and validation must occur. This takes a prolonged period of time that is measured in years. By itself, the design and construction of a new facility is a multiyear effort. Commissioning and validation extend that timeline even further. And at the end of this long road, regulatory approval is not guaranteed. The financial commitment for a company is huge, easily taking hundreds of millions of dollars. The extended time required to design, build, and validate a new facility, as well as hire and train personnel, is a monumental undertaking. In contrast, working with an existing facility will save time and represents a substantial savings.

The potential loss of a facility should give a company pause. There is much to be lost in terms of investment, infrastructure, institutional knowledge, and skilled personnel. The closing of an existing facility is disruptive and should only be undertaken if a significant benefit is realized. Yet, in spite of the natural advantages of any particular legacy facility, such a plant must also fit into the larger strategy of the company's entire global supply chain. But a strong and healthy facility, even if it is old, will invariably attract new products and will make a decision to close that site hard to justify. In this way, a plant's long-term sustainability can be ensured.

THE MASTER PLAN

As outlined in the preceding sections, there are numerous tendencies and pressures for existing facilities to become outmoded. An additional tendency is the natural inclination for people to opt for expedient solutions, which is to say prioritizing facility modifications that address the narrow needs and concerns of the immediate without maintaining a view toward long-term sustainable value for the plant. It is tempting to choose the expedient because it can appear to be the easiest to implement, the least disruptive, perhaps the least amount of work, and often the least first cost. However, focusing only on the expedient can lead to existing deficiencies being exacerbated, especially those related to material handling and personnel circulation. In other words, yielding to the expedient can create greater problems over time. It is in a facility's long-term interest to do more than just what it already does well. It needs to strive to stay vital within the larger context of the global organization and its supply chain. This means that a broader perspective must be used when making changes to the facility.

To be sustainable into the future, it is necessary to be strategic. Being strategic means having a set of goals and priorities, a considered policy, what is often referred to as a *vision*. It is necessary to continually ask: Where should the facility be in 5–10 years? What are the trends in the industry? What are the trends within the corporation? And ultimately, how can the facility position itself for a stronger future? Again, it is not enough to just do what a facility already does well. To not structure facility decisions strategically can result in options becoming limited and future opportunities lost. This in turn can only reduce a facility's value to its parent company.

The solution then is to create a strategic plan for the facility, what is commonly called a facility master plan. The goal of the master plan is to create a program, based on careful planning, that ensures the realization of the site's full value now and into the future. There are numerous functional components typically required for a manufacturing facility. These include the production area itself, but also all of the functions that support the manufacturing. These support functions typically include warehouse, QA/QC laboratory, office space, mechanical equipment, and personnel amenities such as cafeteria and gym. All of these need to be addressed in the master plan.

In developing a master plan, it is necessary to take a few common steps that can be enumerated simply as follows:

1. Define the issues (problem) and desired outcome.
2. Generate alternatives.
3. Evaluate the alternatives.
4. Formalize the final solution.

DEFINE THE ISSUES

The first step in any master planning process is to define the issues that need to be addressed. However, this is not always as easy as it may sound. Defining the issues requires the collection and processing of information. Correctly identifying information that is pertinent to fostering quality decisions is a critical first step. Sometimes planning personnel are overwhelmed by the accumulated detail and "can't see the forest for the trees." Alternately, if bad information is processed, you can end up with a situation described in a more contemporary phrase: "garbage in, garbage out." In addition, to overcome the tendency to view problems only in established and accustomed ways, it is important to not rely exclusively upon solutions that have worked before. It is the process of master planning that provides a disciplined approach that goes beyond existing assumptions and helps identify the real constraints and opportunities of a site. Gathering and processing data in this systematic way allows you to prevail against those natural but counterproductive tendencies.

Gather Data

The first step in defining the issues for a master plan is to gather the pertinent data. This information will serve as the basis for understanding and evaluating the existing constraints and opportunities of the site. Attention needs to be given at this stage to ensure that the information is complete and accurate. Required data that should be gathered include, at a minimum, the items shown in Table 3.1.

TABLE 3.1
Data

	Data Required	Evaluation Function
1	Corporate guidelines	Use as an evaluation tool of existing facility. Use in the development of appropriate alternatives.
2	International GMPs with which the facility will align	Use as an evaluation tool of existing facility. Use in the development of appropriate alternatives.
3	Processes and equipment available at the site	Determine process strengths and weaknesses. Identify processes that the supply chain depends on from this site.
4	Process capacity available at the site	Number of doses per year allows comparison of capacity to current usage and forms a basis for considering future options.
5	Process flow diagrams for all product types	Evaluate flows, gain a deeper understanding of process capacity, and identify opportunities for improvement.
6	Relationships with other sites in the supply chain	Understand how site fits within the supply chain. Determine any existing gaps in the supply chain, especially if this site can easily fill or reinforce those missing needs.
7	Current manufacturing schedule and volume projections	Where is the demand coming from? Where will it be in the future? In terms of process capacity, identify the likely growth areas.
8	Current marketing projections	Where is the demand coming from? Where will it be in the future? In terms of process capacity, identify the likely growth areas.
9	Known concerns or deficiencies	Known noncompliance issues need to be integrated into any action plan and may prove to be the driver for change.
10	Current flows of material, equipment, personnel, and waste	Identify crossings, backtracking, and anything that is in violation of unidirectional flow. Prioritize the most likely conditions that cause mix-up or cross-contamination.
11	Current hygiene zones	Identify inefficient grouping of HVAC or energy-intensive areas that force continued entry, exit, and reentry.
12	Container strategy	What form of containers are used and at what stages of process? Will changing container strategy improve staging, washing, or material handling?
13	Material handling strategy	Manual or hand charge, bin, vacuum convey, and gravity feed? Gain a deeper understanding of movement through the facility. Need for mezzanines and platforms?
14	Washing strategy	Manual or automated washers, and for what components, bins, and parts? Centralized or multiple locations? How does this integrate with the hygiene strategy?
15	Pallet strategy	Facility pallets vs. wood pallets. Transfer requirements and locations? Wash requirements and locations?
16	Warehouse capacity	How does the warehouse relate to current manufacturing, and how will it change with changes in production?
17	Lab capacity	How does capacity of the QA/QC lab relate to current manufacturing, and how will it change with changes in production?
18	Office capacity	How do office needs relate to current manufacturing, and how will they change with changes in production?

Analyze the Data

Defining the issues requires that first you gather the information necessary. However, until the information is processed, it is only raw data. To be meaningful and effective, the information gathered needs to be processed. It is through evaluation and synthesis that insight and understanding are developed.

There are a few essential issues that must be identified during this process. In the broadest sense, you need to ascertain the strengths and weaknesses of the facility and the potential opportunities, especially for growth. The existing process capabilities need to be evaluated and the strengths and weaknesses determined. Establishing the known areas of product growth and areas for potential new products is critical in determining how the site can play a role. Any processes on site that are unique within the larger corporate supply chain are important to identify. Gaps in the existing supply chain that the site can easily fill or reinforce are obvious opportunities that should be considered. Of particular note, all known compliance issues and concerns must be addressed as part of this effort. This will include crossing of material, personnel, and waste flows and backtracking due to nonsequential unit operations or other movements that are in violation of unidirectional flow. The conditions with the greatest potential to cause mix-ups and cross-contamination need to be prioritized.

Synthesize the Data

After the data have been evaluated and the important issues identified, the information needs to be organized into a coherent set of ideas that can be categorized and documented. The first of these is to formally write out the strengths, weaknesses, and opportunities of the facility. Utilizing a traditional strengths, weaknesses, opportunities, and threats (SWOT) matrix will structure the information in a manner that brings focus to the effort. A SWOT matrix is a traditional planning tool that allows a structured presentation of the items identified. The list of SWOT issues then become the objectives that need to be addressed as the master plan is developed.

Based on the established objectives, the next step is to set specific goals that need to be achieved by the master plan. These are the overarching issues that the master plan must address. The goals should be both short and long term. They need to address the shortcomings that have been identified, as well as being in alignment with the targeted GMPs and corporate standards. These goals represent a kind of ideal facility that becomes a guide to achieving the required outcome. The goals should be given a ranking of importance. This prioritization will establish the most important things needing to be accomplished, and thus make clear what the "must-haves" for the facility are.

The analysis, as described, will lead to an understanding of the site's deficiencies. These can include compliance, quality, safety, productivity, and health issues. They will relate to both the processes and the physical plant. Further, the analysis will provide an appreciation of the larger supply chain and how to leverage the facility's current standing, including potential opportunities that can be exploited. From this, the desired outcomes should begin to take shape. Later, it will be necessary to return to this information to create the criteria needed to evaluate the master plan options.

GENERATE ALTERNATIVES

With the knowledge obtained through defining the issues, it is possible to begin developing a master plan. However, an ideal strategic plan does not just appear fully developed. Creating a value-laden and realistic plan requires that different approaches be explored. This is a classic example of brainstorming where the goal is to identify multiple options that can be compared and evaluated. At this point, the maxim "quantity breeds quality" should be pursued. The rationale is that the more ideas generated, the greater the chance of overcoming established biases and producing a thorough, effective, and perhaps innovative solution.

The manufacturing processes are, of necessity, realized in physical form, in both equipment and spatial layout. Conversely, the placement of equipment within the building dictates numerous details of the process. There are many process and operational features, such as manpower requirements, that are influenced by the plan arrangement. Creating building plans that illustrate the alternatives is powerful because they make information visible. This form of visualization allows comparison and evaluation of spatial relationships, movement through the facility, and operational and work activities. Because the spatial relationship of equipment and activities is integral to how the processes are actually executed, developing a facility plan is a critical part of the master plan process.

Developing different plan options allows different questions and nuances to be investigated. Visually comparing the variations in plan is a robust evaluation technique and will lead to further questions and ideas. One critical feature of GMPs is the avoidance of mix-ups and cross-contamination through the appropriate personnel, material, and waste flows. Developing a plan is necessary to evaluate these essential flows. In addition, developing space plans makes it possible for initial costs to be assigned and brought into consideration. At the least, these initial costs will provide rough order of magnitude numbers that permit a relative ranking of the options.

EVALUATE ALTERNATIVES

Once the alternative plans are generated, evaluating and testing against a set of criteria needs to occur. The evaluation process follows a simple but familiar pattern:

1. Establish the evaluation criteria.
2. Test how each alternative fulfills the criteria.
3. Select the best option.

Establishing the evaluation criteria grows naturally out of the earlier data synthesis effort. The conclusion of that earlier activity should provide an understanding of the needs and desires for the site. Naturally supplementing this is all the information and knowledge that has been accumulated during the process. From this, a final list of criteria for the site needs to be agreed upon. Do not be afraid to add criteria that have not been identified previously. Consistency is less important than having the most appropriate criteria. Criteria examples might include staffing and cost considerations, the reduction of operational waste and redundancy, the improvement in facility compliance in terms of both international cGMPs and corporate standards, and enhanced productivity. In addition, the must-haves should be identified, as well as the "nice to have." This exercise alone will be instructive and will challenge some established assumptions. The resulting criteria should then be ranked to create a prioritized list indicating those items that are of greater and lesser importance.

With the evaluation criteria set, the alternatives can now be tested. Testing needs to be a thorough process that looks at every criterion and determines how well each alternative meets that standard. At this first stage, it is possible to divide the alternatives into those that address the must-haves and those that do not. Those that do not include must-haves can be eliminated outright. In this manner, the quantity of options tested can be paired down to a manageable number and thereby realize a significant savings in time and effort.

To test the remaining alternatives, it is best to use a methodology that brings discipline and structure to the process. There are numerous tools available for such an evaluation. Two we discuss here are a RAG analysis and a Kepner–Tregoe (K–T) analysis. These are two well-known business management tools used for decision making.

TABLE 3.2

Example of RAG Analysis

Evaluation Criteria	Alternative A	Alternative B
Uninterrupted operations	Red	Green
Material flow	Green	Amber
Gowning	Green	Green
Personnel flows	Amber	Green
Low operations cost	Green	Amber

Note: Black and white for this production. This analysis is normally done in color.

A RAG analysis is a simple, quick, yet powerful rating tool. RAG is an acronym for red, amber, and green. The colors, similar to those found in a traffic light, are indicators that are used to visually highlight the status of each evaluation criterion. A matrix is created with all the options listed on one axis and the evaluation criteria listed on the opposing axis. Within an option, each of the criteria is given either a red, amber, or green status. Red represents a negative correspondence between the master plan option and the criterion. Amber represents a minimal, neutral, or possible correspondence, and green represents a positive correspondence (Table 3.2).

The power of this method comes from the ability to easily visualize the relative strengths and weaknesses of each option due to the color coding. The options that are the least responsive to the evaluation criteria can be easy to identify. However, options that do not have strong differences become harder to choose between. To evaluate these options, a more rigorous tool may be necessary. One that uses a numerical rating system will often be successful in amplifying the distinctions between options.

There are several methods available. A K–T analysis is one of the most rigorous tools. It is a sophisticated procedure that not only prioritizes criteria but also considers weighting of those criteria. It is a structured method of decision making that is highly respected in business management.

To undertake a K–T analysis, first list the evaluation criteria. Assign each criterion a numerical value that represents its importance on a scale of 1–10, with 10 being the most important. Assess the alternatives against each of the criteria and rate the alternative's ability to meet that criterion, again, on a scale of 1–10, with 10 being the best. Then, multiply the importance of the criterion by the ability of the alternative to meet that criterion. This will result in a weighted score that reflects the priorities identified. Repeat this with each alternative and compare the totals (Table 3.3).

TABLE 3.3

Example of K–T Analysis

Evaluation Criteria	Importance Ranking	Alternative A Ability to Meet Criteria	Score	Alternative B Ability to Meet Criteria	Score
Uninterrupted operations	10	5	50	9	90
Material flow	9	8	72	7	63
Gowning	7	8	56	8	56
Personnel flows	8	7	56	8	64
Low operations cost	6	9	54	6	36
Total			288		309

It may be surprising what is revealed during this effort. Often the process causes reevaluation of the evaluation criteria itself, as well as their relative importance. This can result in a new deeper consensus regarding the needs of the facility and the importance of each criterion. In addition, it is not unusual that in the process a hybrid solution is identified. This option should be embraced, developed, and tested as rigorously as the previous alternatives. Another interesting occurrence is how many times cost starts as a less valued driver, but in the end becomes a top criterion. Do not be frustrated by this; it is a natural occurrence and should be considered appropriate. Without the bias of money, the other criteria can be more fully considered for their own merits. Once these "operational" issues are understood, it is only natural that monetary value also be factored into the evaluation.

Select an Alternative (The Master Plan)

The evaluation process naturally leads to two or three alternatives that balance the issues of a particular facility and seem reasonable. At this point, the top choices should be further scrutinized. This examination should include developing a greater level of detail, getting a deeper understanding of the costs, and again vetting the alternatives with the stakeholders with costs in mind. Actively challenging the options should also be pursued, exploring the potential problems and negative consequences that may have been overlooked previously.

This is perhaps less a selection process than a validation process. The evaluation effort is where alternatives that merit selection become apparent. At this later stage, it is appropriate to confirm the assumptions, the priorities, and the perceived constraints of the previous evaluation process, as well as to acquire buy-in from the stakeholders. This thorough process will overcome biases, preconceived notions, and create a well-balanced vision for the future.

In the end, the goal is not to make the choice that is perfect or has no defects, but to make the best choice. The perfect plan is usually not possible, especially in an existing facility. However, a plan that balances the many factors involved and that creates opportunity as well as additional value for the facility is realistic. The objective is to position the facility to meet the needs of the company and allow for modifications to keep up with current and future advancements. Needless to say, cost is always a factor. The master plan, however, does not need to be executed in a single initiative. A single large expenditure of money is probably the exception. A master plan is not an all-or-nothing proposition. Instead, a legacy facility master plan can serve as a framework within which work is executed over a period of time. As new opportunities for projects arise, the master plan should provide a structure within which the new work can be leveraged to achieve and maintain the long-term vision.

Create a Master Plan Document

The final crucial step in the master planning process is to consolidate the results of your efforts into a single written document. Collecting and organizing your work will bring clarity and transparency, solidifying the master plan into an actionable blueprint. Creating a formal document allows clear characterization of the conditions, circumstances, and priorities that went into the planning process, and it becomes a permanent reference guide for future decisions. In addition, a master plan document is a powerful communication tool that can be used to inform and educate a host of interested parties, including upper management. This can be especially helpful when developing budgets. Maintaining a sustainable future for your facility will be easier with a master plan serving as a foundation to achieve the goals and objectives identified. As the opportunities arise, the master plan should be consulted and execution of facility upgrades made to reinforce and fulfill the vision in the plan (Table 3.4).

TABLE 3.4

Example of Master Plan Table of Contents

1 **INTRODUCTION**
   1.1   Executive Summary
   1.2   Master Planning Objectives

2 **KEY SITE FEATURES**
   2.1   Site History
   2.2   Building Functions and Footprints
   2.3   Overall Site Constraints and Potential for Expansion
   2.4   Production Scenarios
   2.5   Utilities
   2.6   Warehousing Capacity Utilization
   2.7   QC/QA Operations
   2.8   Environmental
   2.9   Head Count
   2.10 Space Planning
         2.10.1   Administrative Offices
         2.10.2   Parking Spaces
         2.10.3   Cafeteria
         2.10.4   Conference Rooms
         2.10.5   Data Center

3 **EQUIPMENT OBSOLESCENCE**
   3.1   Existing Criticality
   3.2   Replacement Plan

4 **FUTURE VISION AND BUSINESS PLAN**
   4.1   Volumes Forecast and Transfer In/Out Projects
   4.2   Work Center's Capacity Utilization
   4.3   Production Scenarios
   4.4   Storage Scenario and Warehousing Requirements
   4.5   Lab Scenario
   4.6   Utilities and Energy
   4.7   Environmental
   4.8   Infrastructure and Personnel Facilities
   4.9   Automation and PPI

5 **MASTER PLAN**
   5.1   Selection Criteria
   5.2   Selected Plan Key Features
   5.3   Comparison against Key Business Drivers and Key Site Issues
   5.4   Equipment Layout
   5.5   Personnel and Material Flows
   5.6   Environmental and Hygiene Zoning
   5.7   Master Schedule and Key Dates
   5.8   Indicative Project Costs

6 **CONCLUSIONS AND RECOMMENDATIONS**
   6.1   Conclusions
   6.2   Key Recommendations

IMPLICATIONS FOR PERFORMANCE

It is the nature of a manufacturing plant that once built, the decisions that led to its form are fixed. Construction always reflects the era in which it was built. Buildings are the crystallization of a set of ideas and choices made at a specific time. But while a facility may be physically frozen at its completion, the pharmaceutical industry is not static; it continues to develop and adjust. Over the course of years, many changes occur. Paramount among them are technology and GMPs. The following quote from the FDA webpage titled "Facts About Current Good Manufacturing Practices (cGMPs)" makes this clear:

> The "c" in cGMP stands for "current," requiring companies to use technologies and systems that are up-to-date in order to comply with the regulations. Systems and equipment that may have been "top-of-the-line" to prevent contamination, mix-ups, and errors 10 or 20 years ago may be less than adequate by today's standards.

The implication of this statement is that "current" can potentially be considered to go in cycles of 10–20 years. While this is in no way a definitive timeline, it is a recognition of how change and evolution are constant, especially when it comes to technology.

An illustration of change in the industry can be found in the emphasis that regulatory agencies are placing on pursuit of science and risk-based approaches to drug production. One aspect of this is process automation technology (PAT), which has been embraced by the industry only since the FDA released guidance in 2004. Being a key factor in continuous manufacturing, the acceptance of PAT is helping to drive the development in the pharmaceutical industry of continuous manufacturing, which has been commonplace in many other industries for decades. Of course, you cannot stop the development of new therapies such as those being fostered by advancements in biotechnology and gene therapy. As therapies mature, the increased competition that comes from generics and biosimilars is another agent of change. Many of these factors did not exist, nor were they significant factors, in the industry 25 years ago.

It is easy to see that change is a constant presence in the industry. The corollary is that existing facilities, given their inherent condition of stasis, must be careful not to outlive their usefulness. To ensure a long and sustainable existence, a facility must embrace change. This must be done in a way that ensures constant renewal and future vitality. It requires a special effort focused on more than just doing what is already being done well. It takes a determination to overcome the established groupthink inherent in any preexisting operation and the nearsightedness that comes by focusing only on day-to-day operational details. The master planning process is a disciplined way to push beyond these natural obstacles. It methodically and systematically enables strategic planning for the long term. The process described in this chapter will arm facility personnel with a wealth of knowledge about the condition of their facility, the current state of the industry, and the facility's place within the larger corporate supply chain. This alone is a worthwhile endeavor that can return benefits for the site. However, the master plan goes further and creates a vision of what the facility can be and, more importantly, a blueprint on how to get there.

A master plan, however, should not be viewed as an inflexible and static tool that is not subject to change. Instead, a master plan should be seen as a framework that establishes the broad outlines for change and an instrument that can facilitate sound decisions when the opportunity arises. A master plan sets a general direction within which the specifics of its execution can be accomplished in a number of ways and even modified when particular needs are identified. It needs to be a living document subject to change, modification, and updating. With all that said, in the end, the most important aspect of a master plan is the action that is implemented as a result of the plan.

PROJECT MANAGEMENT ISSUES

Once a master plan is in place, there are options in how it can be executed. The first obvious approach is to upgrade the facility all at once. Ultimately, this would be the least cost because today's dollars are always less expensive than tomorrow's. But an extensive facility upgrade will be a significant capital cost, and it will not be lightly considered by management. Justification and return on investment will need to be clear. This may not be a hard case to make if there are significant compliance issues that have been uncovered either internally or by a regulatory agency. However, part of the position of this chapter is that a master plan should be used to prevent exactly this sort of a situation from arising in the first place.

An alternative approach is to use the master plan as a framework for future implementation. In this instance, as facility needs and projects are identified, the master plan serves as a vehicle to enable fast implementation and squeeze the most value from each undertaking. This approach does not require a lot of detail in the master plan but allows the evolution of specifics. In addition, it allows the cost to be integrated into projects that are mandated by other requirements, such as marketing and management demands. In terms of keeping a facility from falling behind, this is a strategy that all facilities should embrace. It is key to maintaining quality over the long haul. Once you understand that all facilities, once built, are slowing going out of date, it becomes imperative to find ways to stay ahead of the curve. A master plan should be viewed as a vision of the future that provides guidance for accomplishing that intention.

Is master planning worth the effort? When master planning is being considered, there are some typical objections that arise. Perhaps the most common rationalization is that things are too much in flux to be able to plan. As we all know from our own experience, planning is often ignored because it is not driven by necessity or urgency. We also know from experience that planning is a critical part of any endeavor. Albert Einstein is quoted as having said, "If I had an hour to solve a problem, I'd spend 55 minutes thinking about the problem and 5 minutes thinking about solutions." Taking the time to plan is critical to setting a course that leads to success. When the excuse given is too much fluidity, people are usually overwhelmed by the details. Focusing only on details causes one to lose sight of the larger issues and considerations. To overcome this resistance, it is necessary to break down the effort into smaller manageable tasks. The master planning process provides a structure and approach that enables a sequential accumulation of data and progressive development from the larger scale to the small. In this model, details are not the first consideration, but rather the result of the goals, drivers, and information gathered during the progress of the master plan.

Also implicit in this argument is the notion that a plan is too rigid to ever be of practical value to the site. However, as we have seen, a master plan needs to be strategic. Thomas Edison said, "Good fortune is what happens when opportunity meets with planning." When opportunity occurs, having a plan in place allows the most value to be realized. If a new product or technology is obtained, the site needs to execute it in a way that not only realizes the potential of that opportunity, but also reinforces the current portfolio, not closing the door on future opportunities. At its best, when done well, a master plan will reveal more potential for the site as each project is executed.

When a master plan is strategic, the specifics of the execution do not need to be handled exactly as originally intended. If the vision and structure of a master plan are maintained, even while the particulars of the implementation change, then value is not lost. Dwight D. Eisenhower, the 34th president of the United States and supreme commander of the Allied Forces in Europe during the Second World War, once said, "In preparing for battle I have always found that plans are useless, but planning is indispensable." The knowledge acquired from the planning process is invaluable. It informs all subsequent actions, increasing the likelihood of sound judgments and favorable outcomes. In addition, with a facility master plan, a strategic framework is created within which the practical actions of implementation can be easily modified and executed.

Another common excuse is the perceived financial cost of developing a master plan. The value of any plan is knowing where you are and where you are going. If your goals are clearly defined by the master plan, then resources can be quickly and efficiently deployed. Such knowledgeable and decisive action uses resources efficiently, reduces risk, and increases speed to market. If good decisions are invaluable in a successful business, then you can't afford not to plan. The real cost for establishing a master plan is the time for in-house staff plus any consultants that are hired.

For in-house staff, it is both the time spent on the effort and the time taken away from other responsibilities. In a lean organization, this can be difficult to manage. However, this alleged distraction has to be weighed against the delays and wasted effort that will occur if you are not prepared when an important opportunity or need arises.

A master plan increases the present value of the site by clearly delineating the potential that can be realized in the future. The document that results becomes a powerful communication tool that can be used internally and externally to clarify and solidify a facility's standing within a corporation's global supply chain. It can provide a basis for persuading senior management of the value of the site and to win new products. These are critical considerations that are necessary to engage in in order to maintain a site's competitive position within the organization.

TRENDS AND FUTURE DEVELOPMENTS

Today the pharmaceutical industry is experiencing numerous forces that are driving change in it. For a long time, the high cost of medical care and the desire to control costs have been a provocative and significant discussion within the industry. A partial response to this dilemma is found in the trend toward drug production based on a science and risk-based approach that is intended to drive innovation and efficiency. The FDA states its position in its final report of September 2004, "Pharmaceutical cGMPs for the 21st Century—A Risk-Based Approach":

> Using a scientific framework to find ways of mitigating risk while facilitating continuous improvement and innovation in pharmaceutical manufacturing is a key public health objective.

Two practical illustrations of this drive for science and risk-based drug production are seen in the advancement of PAT and quality by design (QbD). With global regulatory agencies encouraging innovation and continuous improvement in drug manufacturing, change is ensured for the design and construction of both new and existing facilities.

Consolidation in the pharmaceutical industry is also a force that continues in the industry. According to Bloomberg in a web post headlined "Consolidation Efforts Transform the Pharmaceutical Industry," in 1988 there were 42 members of the industry lobbying group Pharmaceutical Research and Manufacturers of America. In early 2014, of these 42 members, only 11 remained. Consolidation leaves companies with facilities that were inherited from previous owners and their value and place within a company's supply chain need to be reviewed and determined. As discussed earlier, a master plan lays out the current capacity and future potential of a facility, and can be a great asset in communicating a facility's value to its parent company.

Another significant development is the reorientation toward biologic therapies, what is referred to in the media as the biotech revolution. The potential of these new technologies is so significant that virtually every company is working to establish a presence in the field. How do older facilities that were built for established, traditional technologies respond, and what role should they play in the future? With the maturing of single-use technologies, will it become common for traditional pharmaceutical facilities to be converted to biological facilities centered on cell culture? These are intriguing questions.

An even newer trend is continuous processing. This is a technology that, after years of discussion and speculation, is showing signs of maturating to a point where it may finally find industry-wide implementation. When considering the future processing potential of a legacy facility, the role of continuous processing certainly needs to be investigated.

With today's complex, extended global supply chains, every facility must find its niche within its parent company's strategic portfolio. These trends and others continue to develop, and their impact on facility design is yet to be fully understood. They are both threats and opportunities. Smart money makes lemonade out of lemons. The discussion in this chapter illustrates the importance of a master plan in finding a facility's full potential and ensuring a vital and sustainable future.

SPECIAL DISCUSSION

Renovations of legacy facilities are problems of design in the same vein found in new construction. In both cases, many of the same principles and strategies must be utilized. However, in renovations you have the added problem of untangling the existing conditions and outdated technologies that were installed years earlier. In addition, it is usually necessary to maintain an existing facility in operation while making changes. In contrast, new construction is much more straightforward in that everything is new and does not need to take into account the relics from a previous time. Decisions are not hampered by existing conditions; there are no processes to maintain in operation or operating personnel to disrupt. The renovation of an existing facility is a complex undertaking. Besides all the requirements that need to be understood when designing a new facility, it is also necessary to identify and respond to the existing constraints. There are assumptions and preconceived notions embedded in an existing operation that often make understanding the value of change difficult. Existing facilities must be able to look past these limitations and find the opportunities and security that change can bring. With a useful life of approximately 20–30 years, it is not possible, every generation, to replace all of a company's existing facilities. Therefore, coming to terms with existing facilities and finding their best current value is a practical necessity.

FURTHER DISCUSSION

The following questions are intended to help prompt further discussion.

1. Should legacy facilities be abandoned for new facilities?
2. At what point are legacy facilities not worth revitalizing?
3. Can a legacy facility stay vital without a master plan?
4. Does a global supply chain improve or reduce the need to maintain legacy facilities?
5. Should continuous processing, biotechnology, and other new technologies be located only in new facilities?

ABOUT THE AUTHOR

Eric Bohn is a licensed architect with more than 35 years of experience in designing and building facilities for corporate and institutional clients. For the last 20 years, he has focused on the pharmaceutical and biotechnology industry, bringing his broad range of construction experience to these technologically intensive facilities. His designs include renovations and additions to existing facilities across the nation, as well as internationally. His master planning efforts have helped numerous clients understand the potential of their legacy facilities, as well as bring them back into compliance with current Good Manufacturing Practices. In 2011, his architectural design work was recognized when the Merck Global Clinical Supply Facility won the ISPE Facility of the Year Award for Integration. Eric is a long-standing member of ISPE and has lectured on design issues for his local chapter, as well as at the annual meeting. In addition, he is the author of numerous articles for industry publications, including *Pharmaceutical Engineering* and *Pharmaceutical Technology*. Mr. Bohn is a partner with JacobsWyper Architects, an architectural firm located in Philadelphia, Pennsylvania, that specializes in the design of facilities for pharmaceutical research and manufacturing.

RECOMMENDED READINGS

Ainsworth D, Planning and Designing a Pharmaceutical Facility: A Process Designer's View, PharmaTech, Iselin, NJ, September 1, 2005, http://www.pharmtech.com/planning-and-designing-pharmaceutical-facility-process-designers-view.

Bohn B, Master Planning the Legacy: Meeting Good Manufacturing Practices While Using Existing Pharmaceutical Manufacturing Facilities, *Pharmaceutical Engineering*, November/December 2013.

International Society for Pharmaceutical Engineering, *Baseline® Pharmaceutical Engineering Guides for New and Renovated Facilities*, Vol. 2: *Oral Solid Dosage Forms*, 2nd ed., International Society for Pharmaceutical Engineering, Tampa, FL, 2009.

International Society for Pharmaceutical Engineering, *Baseline® Pharmaceutical Engineering Guides for New and Renovated Facilities*, Vol. 3: *Sterile Manufacturing Facilities*, International Society for Pharmaceutical Engineering, Tampa, FL, 2011.

International Society for Pharmaceutical Engineering, *Baseline® Pharmaceutical Engineering Guides for New and Renovated Facilities*, Vol. 6: *Biopharmaceuticals*, International Society for Pharmaceutical Engineering, Tampa, FL, 2013.

Pena WM, *Problem Seeking: An Architectural Programming Primer*, 5th ed., Wiley, Hoboken, NJ, 2012.

U.S. Food and Drug Administration, Pharmaceutical cGMPs for the 21st Century: A Risk-Based Approach, Final Report, U.S. Food and Drug Administration, Silver Spring, MD, September 2004.

REFERENCE

1. William J. Curran, Governmental Regulation of the Use of Human Subjects in Medical Research: The Approach of Two Federal Agencies, *Daedalus*, 98(2), pp. 1–542, 1969.

4 Architectural Design Issues

Terry Jacobs

CONTENTS

INTRODUCTION

The architect is the unique integrator of the process flows, equipment, personnel flows, and mechanical systems into a building. The purpose of this chapter is to assist the reader in understanding how the architectural process works and what the key architectural concepts are in incorporating current Good Manufacturing Practices (cGMPs) into the design of pharmaceutical manufacturing facilities.

The architect must clearly understand the people, product, and process flows of the facility, as well as the manufacturing goals, to make the two-dimensional flow diagrams into a three-dimensional building that works efficiently, meets cGMPs, creates a positive workplace for the employees, and results in an efficient manufacturing facility whose output is a regulated product (Figure 4.1).

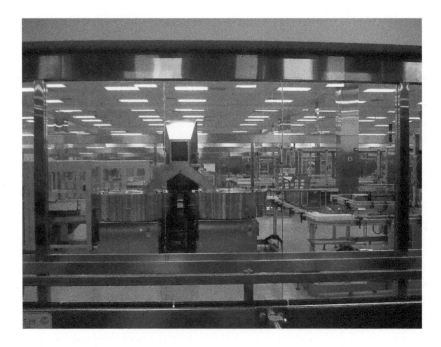

FIGURE 4.1   Current GMP packaging line.

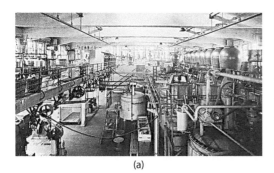
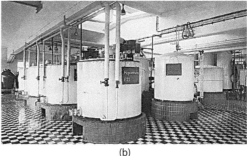

(a)   (b)

FIGURE 4.2   Legacy facilities.

The history of pharmaceutical manufacturing facility design has been one of the increasing compliance requirements from the U.S. Food and Drug Administration (FDA) and international regulators, as well as increasing complexity and integration of the process and mechanical systems into the facility. Pharmaceutical design has been slow to adopt new methods from other industries because of the time and risk required to validate new methods with the regulatory bodies. Changes are occurring in the pharmaceutical industry: the cost of goods has become an important factor, and there are new global standards with a trend toward lean manufacturing.

> Right now, manufacturing experts from the 1950s would easily recognize the pharmaceutical manufacturing process of today. It is predicted that manufacturing will change in the next 25 years as current manufacturing practices are abandoned in favor of cleaner, flexible more efficient continuous manufacturing. (Dr. Janice Woodcock, American Association of Pharmaceutical Scientists [AAPS], Annual Meeting, October 2011)

Many older legacy facilities have grown over time, resulting in a confusing mixture of small rooms with inadequate circulation and space (Figure 4.2). When renovating a facility, functionality, aesthetics, and building codes all present challenges.

Pharmaceutical facilities have traditionally been designed around batch processes, as opposed to continuous manufacturing (see Chapter 10 for a description of batch and continuous processing). The definition of a batch is "a specific quantity of a drug or other material ... [that] is intended to have uniform character and quality, within specified limits, and is produced according to a single manufacturing order during the same cycle of manufacture" [1]. A pharmaceutical facility manufactures in discrete batches, which may vary in size and length of the batch run. This requirement suggests a facility of rooms where batches are made, rather than a linear, assembly line–type facility. Traditionally, batch processing has been the norm, but a current trend is toward the design of continuous manufacturing facilities (Figure 4.3).

The advantages of continuous manufacturing are that it is an integrated process with fewer steps, minimal manual handling, increased efficiency, and shorter processing time. Architecturally, it results in smaller facilities, a more flexible operation, and smaller space requirements (or footprint). Another trend, which is discussed in more detail in Chapter 16, is sustainability; sustainable designs should also be integrated into the design process.

KEY CONCEPTS AND PRINCIPLES

UNDERSTANDING cGMPs

The main types of cGMP pharmaceutical manufacturing facilities include oral solid dosage (OSD) facilities, liquid and cream facilities, sterile facilities, active pharmaceutical

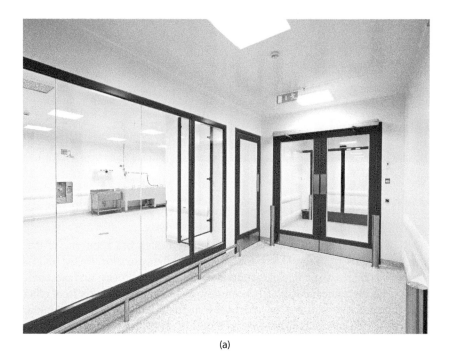

(a)

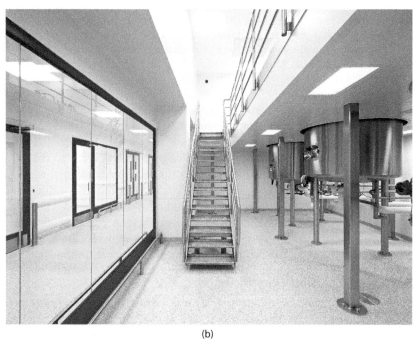

(b)

FIGURE 4.3 Current facilities with an open design and substantial glass and clean finishes. (Courtesy of Daldrop + Dr.Ing.Huber GmbH + Co.KG, Neckartailfingen, Germany.)

ingredient (API) bulk facilities, biopharmaceutical manufacturing facilities, and medical device facilities. In this section, key concepts common to the architectural design for all facility types are discussed. The design of these facilities is governed in the United States by the FDA and in other countries by their regulatory agencies. In the United States, this is referred to as cGMP. An understanding of cGMP requirements is critical to facility design. The following excerpt from the FDA illustrates the general guidelines, which are not prescriptive; that is, they will not give you a formula with which to comply.

> The cGMP requirements were established to be flexible to allow each manufacturer to decide individually how to best implement the necessary controls by using scientifically sound design, processing methods, and testing procedures. The flexibility in these regulations allows companies to use modern technologies and innovative approaches to achieve higher quality through continual improvement. Accordingly, the "c" in cGMP stands for "current," requiring companies to use technologies and systems that are up-to-date to comply with the regulations. Systems and equipment that may have been "top-of-the-line" to prevent contamination, mix-ups, and errors 10 or 20 years ago may be less than adequate by today's standards [2].

Because these regulations are written in general terms and not prescriptive terms, designers must interpret them and demonstrate that they meet the intent of the regulations.

Table 4.1 is an excerpt from the Code of Federal Regulations (CFR), Part 211, which covers the cGMPs for the design and construction of finished pharmaceutical buildings and facilities [3].

TABLE 4.1
cGMPs for Finished Pharmaceuticals

Title 21: Food and Drugs

Chapter I: Food and Drug Administration, Department of Health and Human Services

Subchapter C: Drugs, general

Part 211: Current Good Manufacturing Practice for Finished Pharmaceuticals

Subpart C: Buildings and Facilities

Sec. 211.42: Design and Construction Features

(a) Any building or buildings used in the manufacture, processing, packing, or holding of a drug product shall be of suitable size, construction and location to facilitate cleaning, maintenance, and proper operations.

(b) Any such building shall have adequate space for the orderly placement of equipment and materials to prevent mix-ups between different components, drug product containers, closures, labeling, in-process materials, or drug products, and to prevent contamination. The flow of components, drug product containers, closures, labeling, in-process materials, and drug products through the building or buildings shall be designed to prevent contamination.

(c) Operations shall be performed within specifically defined areas of adequate size. There shall be separate or defined areas or such other control systems for the firm's operations as are necessary to prevent contamination or mix-ups during the course of the following procedures:

(1) Receipt, identification, storage, and withholding from use of components, drug product containers, closures, and labeling, pending the appropriate sampling, testing, or examination by the quality control unit before release for manufacturing or packaging;

(2) Holding rejected components, drug product containers, closures, and labeling before disposition;

(3) Storage of released components, drug product containers, closures, and labeling;

(4) Storage of in-process materials;

(5) Manufacturing and processing operations;

(6) Packaging and labeling operations;

(7) Quarantine storage before release of drug products;

(8) Storage of drug products after release;

(9) Control and laboratory operations;

(10) Aseptic processing, which includes as appropriate:

(i) Floors, walls, and ceilings of smooth, hard surfaces that are easily cleanable.

Source: Code of Federal Regulations, Title 21.

HYGIENIC ZONES

The International Society for Pharmaceutical Engineering (ISPE) has written Baseline Guides for the design of OSD facilities, sterile facilities, API and bulk facilities, and biopharmaceutical manufacturing facilities, which have become reference guidelines for the industry [4–7]. Each facility type has both common and unique aspects from an architectural perspective, even though the processes to manufacture the products differ. The role of the process architect is to understand the unique aspects of the manufacturing process in the design. The ISPE Baseline Guides have established general levels of protection for facilities, or hygienic zoning of facilities, which relate to where the product is exposed, where it is packaged, and where it is stored in its final form. This is an important concept to understand, because the highest risk is where the product is exposed; the risk lessens when the product is packaged and when it is in its final shipping form. Pharmaceutical companies and other regulatory agencies also have complex and potentially conflicting guidelines and standards to address issues that may need to be evaluated.

It is necessary to establish hygienic zones for product protection. The zones have different air classifications, finishes, and gowning requirements. Table 4.2 outlines nomenclature used when creating hygienic zones commonly used in the industry.

TABLE 4.2
Product Protection and Segregation Approaches

ISPE Level			Description	
1	Black	Tertiary	There is minimal risk for product or product contact surface exposure. Raw materials and packaging components are in their received packaging. Final product is fully contained and protected by its completed shipping packaging. Typically within these areas, environmental conditions, which may include temperature, humidity, and air filtration quality, will be specified. Level 1 areas may include warehouse, shipping/receiving, palletizing, pallet wash, and equipment maintenance.	To provide control and accountability of product (chain of custody)
2	Gray	Secondary	There is risk for product or product contact surface exposure due to deviations (accidental product exposure). There may only be an initial layer of protection (e.g., bottle, blister pack, and pouch) separating the product from the room environment (e.g., secondary packaging, corridors adjacent to areas with exposed product, and transition spaces into level 2). Typically within these areas, environmental conditions, which may include temperature, humidity, and air filtration quality, will be specified.	Contain product if accidentally released to mitigate the risk of migration and cross-contamination with rest of facility. As a transition to or protection of white zones
3	White	Primary	Exposed product is present in these spaces, such as formulation, primary packaging, sampling, dispensing, production wash, clean storage, and transition spaces into level 3. Typically within these areas, environmental conditions, which may include temperature, humidity, and air filtration quality, will be specified and validated.	To protect product (quality)
Spaces outside the cGMP manufacturing areas			There is no product present. These areas are physically separated from cGMP manufacturing areas. These are typically support functions (e.g., offices, laboratories, and break rooms) for the facility.	Support of the manufacturing operation

CLASSIFIED AND NONCLASSIFIED SPACE

A classified space is an "area where HVAC systems are specifically designed to reduce airborne contaminants below a specified level as defined in ISO 14644-1…. And both temperature and relative humidity are controlled more tightly than in the ambient environment." These areas must be performance verified and qualified [8]. Classified space is also an area with airborne viable and nonviable particle contamination controlled within preset limits. A clean room is designated by ISO 14644-1 volume units (in operation) or European Commission (EC) grades A, B, C, and D (at rest and in operation). For pharmaceutical manufacture, a classified space implies ongoing environmental monitoring.

A controlled nonclassified (CNC) room environment is where closed processes and their immediate support systems may be located. The CNC space is cleanable, access controlled, and served with filtered ventilation air; procedural controls and personnel garment upgrades may be applied at the owner's discretion. In the biopharmaceutical industry, CNC has replaced the term *gray space* [8].

UNDERSTANDING PRODUCT, PEOPLE, MATERIAL, EQUIPMENT, AND WASTE

The key to designing a pharmaceutical manufacturing facility is to understand the flows of the product, people, material, equipment, and waste in the facilities. In Chapter 1, the facility drivers were discussed; that is, a certain output is required for the facility in terms of product. "Product and material flow provides the foundation for detailed facility design" [8]. The first task for the designers is to understand the basic flows in the facility. This is referred to as a block flow diagram (BFD) (Figure 4.4).

Block Flow Diagrams

A Block Flow Diagrams (BFD) is a simplified version of a process flow diagram (PFD). In the early development of a facility, BFDs serve as the critical transfer of process flow information to the designer. They are the earliest diagrams produced during programming and are distinct from true PFDs, which are used in equipment development. BFDs outline each unit operation within a given process in logical, direct, and sequential order. They also identify intermediate steps between unit operations (i.e., work in progress) and should follow a process from beginning to end, devoid of any relationship to a building or space. A separate BFD should be produced for each product within a facility, and even for each separate processes that may be required for a single product.

These diagrams are essential in identifying the total number of unit operations (or other process steps), which require physical space within the facility, acting as a key programming tool.

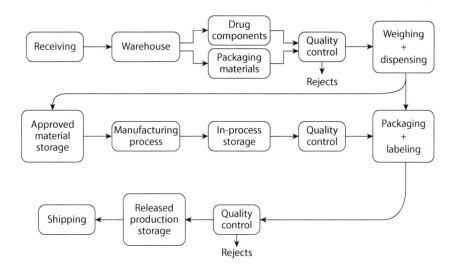

FIGURE 4.4 Block flow diagram.

In addition, they identify critical adjacencies between unit operations and allow the opportunity to discover efficiencies in layout, which will minimize movements and potential for mix-up. Throughout the design process, designers must refer to BFDs to ensure that facility design is in service to the ultimate driver—the production process.

Process Flow Diagrams

A PFD is a diagram commonly used in chemical and process engineering to indicate the general flow of plant processes and equipment. The PFD displays the relationship between major equipment of a plant facility; it does not show minor details, such as piping details and designations. The process engineer creates the PFD, which shows greater detail than the BFD. Different facility types, such as OSD facilities, sterile facilities, biopharmaceutical facilities, and API facilities, have different BFDs. The process architect needs to understand the BFD before proceeding with the design.

Airlocks

Airlocks are a physical solution to segregate and separate different functional areas and control airflow and pressurization. They may have manual or automated interlocked doors. Airlocks are generally used to separate areas of different area classifications. They may act as a "bubble," where the airlock has positive pressure relative to internal and external spaces, or as a "cascade," where doors are interlocked so that one door has to close before the other door is opened (Figure 4.5).

LEAN MANUFACTURING

Lean manufacturing or lean production, often simply referred to as lean, is a systematic method for the elimination of waste (muda) within a manufacturing system. Lean also takes into account waste created through overburden (muri) and waste created through unevenness in workloads (mura). The architect must work with the lean manufacturing engineer to ensure that the layouts developed support the goals in terms of overall flow and detailed flows within the rooms. Lean is discussed further in Chapter 17.

FACILITY FLEXIBILITY

Does the facility produce a single product with no flexibility? In a single-product facility, foreign contamination is the primary concern. In a facility with multiple products in dedicated equipment, contamination between areas of the facility is a concern. If the facility has multiple products in multiuse equipment, contamination is the principal concern.

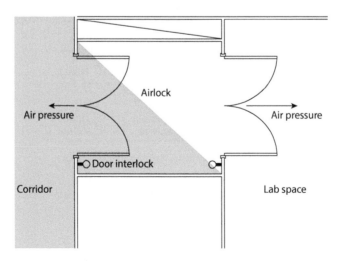

FIGURE 4.5 Airlock.

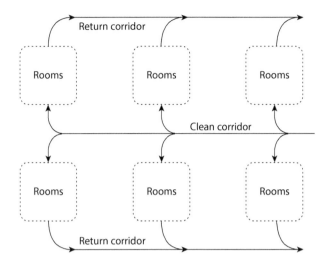

FIGURE 4.6 Unidirectional flow.

UNIDIRECTIONAL FLOW

Unidirectional flow occurs when the flow of people, material, and equipment goes in one direction and does not cross back on itself. This flow pattern is used when cross-contamination is a major risk, such as in vaccine, sterile, and biologic facilities. There is discussion in the industry about which products and material flows need to be unidirectional. In unidirectional facilities, separate "clean" and "dirty" corridors or areas are often used. Using clean and dirty terminology is not recommended, as clean and dirty corridors increase the gross square footage of the facility, which increases the cost; however, it may have functional benefits. The designer and owner need to weigh their options before making a decision. The goal is to demonstrate control of the product (Figure 4.6).

This may be a solution that works best for a facility, but it is not a requirement. The requirement is to prevent product mix-up, which may also be done procedurally. One may address these issues through air control and operating procedures. The design philosophy may be, however, that the facility design is a better place to ensure that this design goal is met. This is discussed in more detail in Chapter 7. Again, if cross-contamination is a risk, unidirectional flow is the preferred solution. This approach uses the physical design to ensure that mix-ups are less likely to occur.

There is increasing use of potent and cytotoxic materials in manufacturing. The layout of potent compound facilities is discussed in Chapter 14. Potent compounds, which require minimizing the chance of cross-contamination in the layout of the facility, are defined as an API or drug substance typically with an occupational exposure limit of less than 20 $\mu g/m^3/8$ h. Figure 4.7 illustrates a potent compound suite design with separate gowning and de-gowning, and a material and equipment airlock.

FUNCTIONAL PHARMACEUTICAL MANUFACTURING AREAS

From the BFD, there are certain areas that are generally common to all pharmaceutical manufacturing facilities. The discussions that follow are the generic areas typical in a pharmaceutical facility. Each has its own design considerations, as well as HVAC, plumbing, electrical, and finish requirements.

SHIPPING AND RECEIVING AREAS

Shipping and receiving areas are where incoming materials for the facility are received, and outgoing materials are shipped. These areas are generally black areas because there is no product exposure.

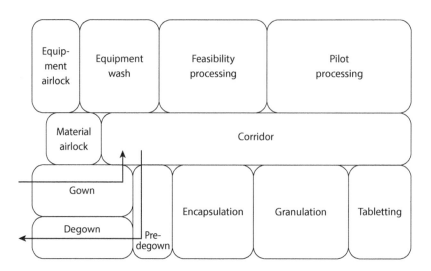

FIGURE 4.7   Potent compound suite.

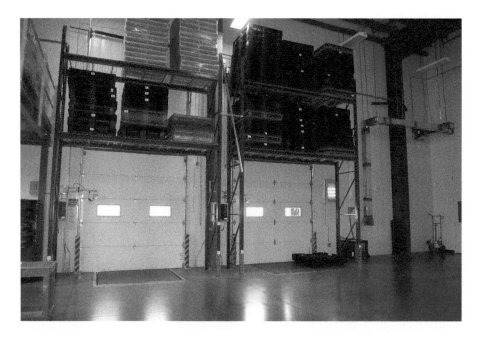

FIGURE 4.8   Receiving area.

Separate shipping and receiving areas should be provided to prevent mix-ups between incoming and outgoing goods. These areas are also generally separated by high-speed, roll-up doors from the general warehouse area as a buffer to the outside (Figure 4.8).

The components of the design of a shipping and receiving area include the number of loading docks required, whether the trucks should be visible from the street, the provision of security to the facility, and people using the loading dock. It is common to include a trucker's toilet in the area, so that there is no breech of the facility by outside people. Adequate space should be provided in the layout for the number of pallets required. This can be tested by actually laying out the pallets in the plan.

PALLET TRANSFER

Current facility design requirements do not allow wood pallets into the facility. The wood pallets are kept in the shipping and receiving area, and product is transferred to new plastic pallets that are dedicated to the facility. The purpose of the pallet transfer is to eliminate the possibility of contaminated pallets entering the facility. In addition, a pallet washer is needed to clean the pallets that have been used in the plant (Figures 4.9 and 4.10).

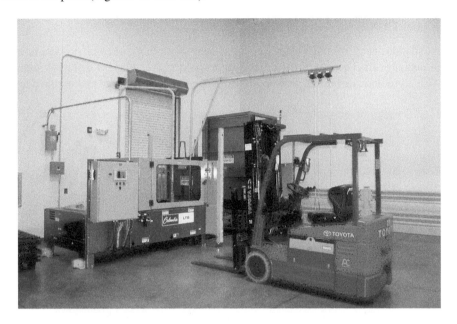

FIGURE 4.9 Pallet transfer.

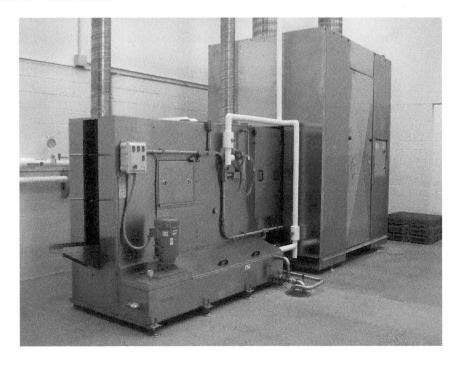

FIGURE 4.10 Pallet washer.

SAMPLE RECEIVING AND TESTING AREAS

Sample receiving and testing area is located through the shipping area doors into the warehouse area; it tests the raw materials as well as the packaging components that will be used in manufacturing the final drug. It is important to note that the areas where the sample is exposed for testing will be "white" areas with appropriate gowning and access requirements. These areas require two airlocks to separate them from the "black" area.

WEIGHING AND DISPENSING AREAS

Weighing and dispensing areas are where the raw materials for batch or batch processing are staged for the production run. These will differ in design and nomenclature for different facility types. Figure 4.11 is a prefabricated down-flow booth where the product is opened and weighed into drums.

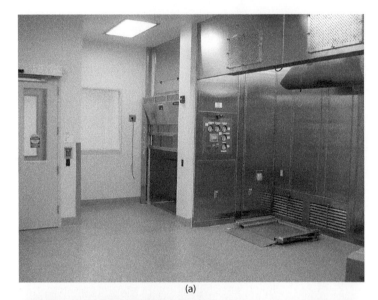

(a)

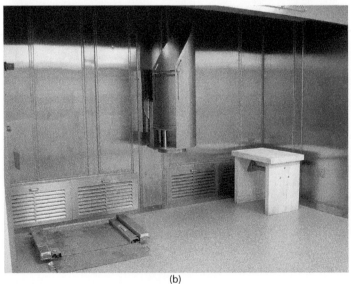

(b)

FIGURE 4.11   Two views of prefabricated weigh booths.

WAREHOUSES

Warehouse areas are generally "black areas," but usually have environmental controls (Figure 4.12).

As mentioned previously, there may be products that require special storage conditions, such as temperature and humidity control, as well as regulated products, such as narcotics that require a vault designed to Drug Enforcement Administration (DEA) standards [9]. It is key to design a facility that controls materials and prevents mix-ups [1]. Quarantine of raw materials and packaging components is required before the product is released after testing. This may be done by creating a physically delineated space or by use of computer control for the location of pallet spaces throughout the warehouse where the materials are in quarantine.

WAREHOUSE LAYOUTS

The size and capacity of the warehouse are driven by the number of pallet spaces that are required for storage of all materials. A pallet, made of fiberglass or metal (i.e., stainless steel or aluminum), is typically 40 in. wide and 48 in. deep. The pallet is the base component of the storage system (Figure 4.13).

A key concept to consider is the space required for upper and lower sprinkler heads in the rack, which must be located so they are not sheared off when pallet racks are installed. The height of the building may also impact whether in-rack sprinklers are required. The architect should coordinate

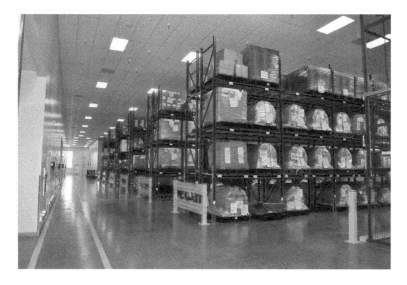

FIGURE 4.12   Warehouse facility.

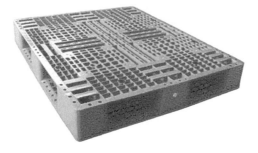

FIGURE 4.13   Typical pallet. (Courtesy of PNG Logistics, Lititz, PA.)

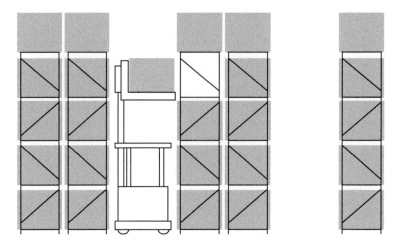

FIGURE 4.14   Narrow-aisle warehouse.

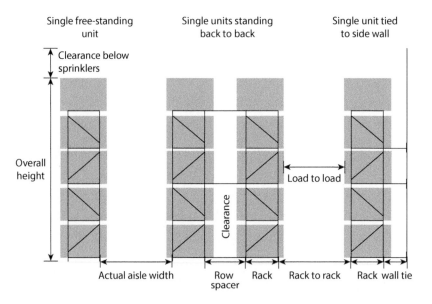

FIGURE 4.15   Basic rack configurations.

the sprinkler and ductwork with future racking plans to ensure that clear heights are maintained. Some facilities accomplish this through the architectural design, which dedicates certain physical areas using partitions, wire mesh, or coding and tracking of materials. Physical design options can be as simple as outlines on the floor or mesh partitions.

Another key concept to understand is the racking system and the aisle widths required when laying out a warehouse; to do this, the architect must be aware of the following typical warehouse configurations: (1) standard aisle, (2) narrow aisle, (3) wire guided, (4) robotic, and (5) flow rack. The aisles in a standard-aisle warehouse are typically about 12 ft, the aisles in a narrow-aisle warehouse are typically about 9 ft, and the aisles in a very narrow-aisle warehouse can be as little as 6 ft wide (Figures 4.14 and 4.15).

From the aisle widths and spacing of the pallets, a planning module may be established to create a structural grid. The height of the warehouse will be determined by forklift capabilities. It is important to be aware that the building height may be limited by the local zoning codes; there must also be an understanding about clearances for sprinklers from the top of pallets as per the insurance carrier and National Fire Protection Association (NFPA). The following codes should be considered: (1) NFPA 230: "Standard for the Fire Protection of Storage," (2) NFPA 30: "Flammable and Combustible Liquids Code," and (3) NFPA 13: "Installation of Sprinkler Systems."

WAREHOUSE STAGING AREAS

A staging area is a space where drums, pallets, and materials can be staged. It is important that these are not left in corridors, because it implies that there is not adequate space in the facility and can increase the risk of mix-ups. It is important to create a design layout of staging areas (Figure 4.16) and anticipate the number of pallets, drums, and so forth, that may be in the area to allow adequate space. The architect must draw the anticipated materials that will be staged.

MANUFACTURING OPERATIONS

The manufacturing room or area requirements are driven by the selection of the process equipment that is required to manufacture the product and the space needed for maintenance of the process equipment. The layout of the room is determined by the size of the equipment. The rooms then become the building blocks for the facilities. The process equipment must be laid out in the room, with associated staging and personnel space requirements, as well as all utility and access space for maintenance. Manufacturing operations may also be organized vertically, depending on the equipment (this is more common in continuous manufacturing facilities).

PACKAGING OPERATIONS

The packaging area is where the product in its final form is packaged for distribution. There are two types of packaging areas, primary and secondary packaging. Key concepts include the following: (1) understanding the packaging line philosophy, (2) providing adequate staging for materials and finished product, (3) providing visual connection between the packaging line, and (4) providing adequate storage space for packaging materials.

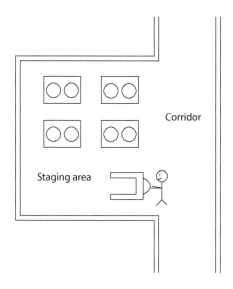

FIGURE 4.16   Staging area.

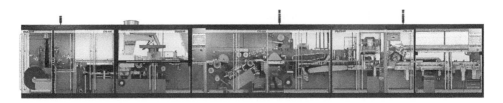

FIGURE 4.17   Blister line. (Courtesy of IMA Pharma, Leominster, MA.)

Primary Packaging Area

This is an area where the product may be exposed. In a packaging line, part of equipment may have exposed product, or product may be isolated within the line design. A packaging line is shown in Figure 4.17 (see also Figure 4.18).

Secondary Packaging Area

This is an area where the product is not exposed, as it is in its packaged form (e.g., vial or bottle), but it still needs to be packaged for shipment. These areas are generally open areas, where secondary packaging may occur in an automated form or by hand, depending on the scale of the facility. Architectural layouts need to consider the space required for each line and the space required for the cartons of packaging materials and the finished goods, which should be physically separate. The packaging lines are designed to minimize mix-up and confusion of batches, with full or half-height partitions. There is also a trend to separate the primary packaging area from the secondary packaging area, using a physical barrier or an enclosure around the section of the packaging line that has exposed product.

It is architecturally important to keep these areas as open as possible. This can be achieved by using partitions with glass to the ceiling and by creating views to the outside if possible.

Adjacent to the packaging areas are labeling rooms. Labeling rooms are where labels are stored and prepared for the packaging lines; these rooms should be secured.

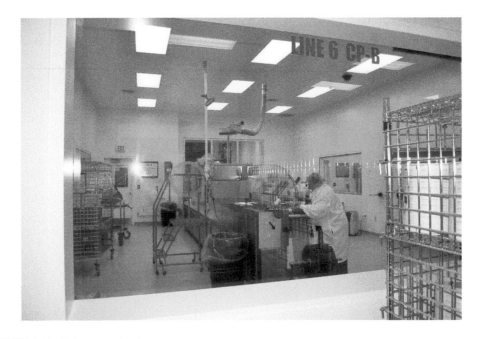

FIGURE 4.18   Primary packaging.

Locker Rooms, Gowning Rooms, and Changing Rooms

Locker rooms are designed to accommodate the needs of the employees and the "gown philosophy" of the facility (Figure 4.19). There may be several levels of gowning in a facility. Employees should progress from factory change to clean change in a logical progression. A changing or locker room is the one that supports the changing for employees. The architectural design of the area can reinforce the garment and changing philosophy of the facility, with step-over benches and a clear and logical progression. It is recommended that a bubble diagram of the gowning procedures be created to allow the physical design to follow. The gowning level and philosophy should be based on the risk to the product as well as to the employee.

There may be a changing area between the level 1 area (black) and then from the level 2 areas (gray) to the level 3 areas (white). The cGMP areas have the strictest gowning requirements. Gowning may be required to protect the product, the operator, or the environment [8]. The design of a gowning area for potent compounds or sterile facilities differs from that of an OSD facility. There is generally a de-gowning area in these facilities, as well as areas for decontamination. Gowning is also required for laboratory areas, where safety glasses and lab coats are required. To prevent cross-contamination, procedures must be established as to where personnel may go, such as toilet rooms, cafeteria, and break areas. Current trends are to have de-gowning or overgowning when employees leave the cGMP area to go to the cafeteria or toilet rooms.

Quality Control Laboratory

The quality control laboratory should be located in a central area, easily accessible to the plant, but also accessible to the laboratory personnel from the main entrance. A typical laboratory layout needs to allow for multiple high-performance liquid chromatography (HPLC) units, which are benchtop testing equipment. Unlike research laboratories, the design layout is unlikely to change dramatically from month to month, as the procedures are established. The design of support laboratories is discussed in Chapter 17.

DESIGN PROCESS

There are several critical and generally recognized phases in the design of a pharmaceutical facility. This section discusses the general descriptions of the activities that occur in these phases of the project. Figure 4.20 shows an overview of the design process.

The design phases generally organize the design from problem seeking to problem solving, followed by construction, commissioning, and validation. It is critical to include the commissioning and validation teams as part of the early design team.

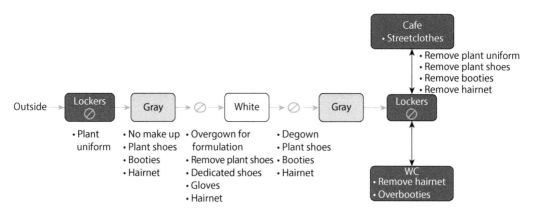

FIGURE 4.19 Employee gowning bubble diagram.

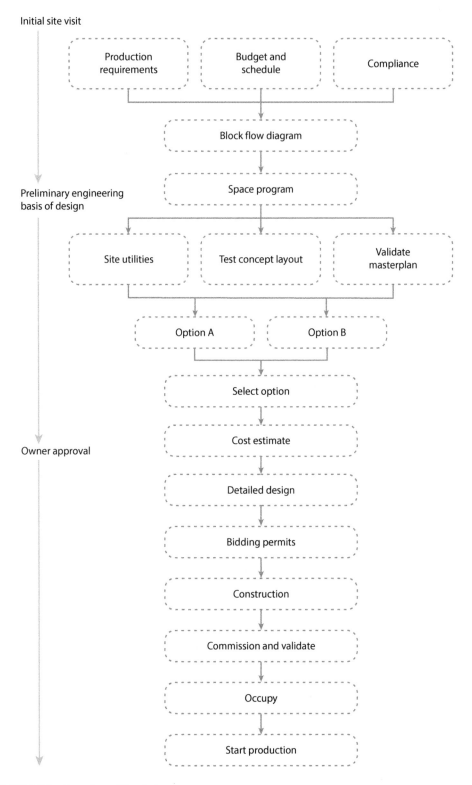

FIGURE 4.20 Overview of the design process.

PROGRAMMING PHASE

The programming phase is the problem-seeking phase. During this phase, the design criteria for the facility, not the design solutions, need to be defined. The process engineer creates a general BFD as well as more detailed PFDs of the manufacturing process. Based on the product forecast, the process engineer defines the manufacturing process and equipment needs to meet the production forecasts, as well as the associated storage requirements.

Based on the BFD, a space program is created, which is a list of the spaces and requirements for each space in the facility, including the sizes, number of each type of space, finishes, and sometimes predictions for future expansions. Interviewing the facility users by functional department to determine their needs to meet the facility output creates a functional space program.

Typical Space Program

The space program may be customized to add spaces to capture other requirements. An equipment layout is required to understand adequately the actual space required for the equipment and process (Figure 4.21). The space program is calculated in terms of net square feet (NSF), which is the space inside the rooms, and does not include space taken up by interior walls or services (Figure 4.22).

Measurement of gross square feet (GFS) is generally the total square footage of the building to the exterior wall. There are different definitions that vary slightly (see Building Owners and Management Association [BOMA]), but the general idea is the same. It is important to understand the differences in these diagrams (Figure 4.23).

The ratio of net square feet to gross square feet (NSF/GSF) equals the building efficiency. This is a useful tool when you are trying to determine how big your facility is from your space program. The space program in Table 4.3 shows a summary of the key areas.

When you have established the GSF of your building, you can apply a range of costs per functional area and begin to understand what the construction costs of the facility may be.

Room Criteria Cards

For the architect, the next step in the programming phase is to create room cards (also referred to as lab cards or room criteria sheets), which are defined as room layouts for each important functional

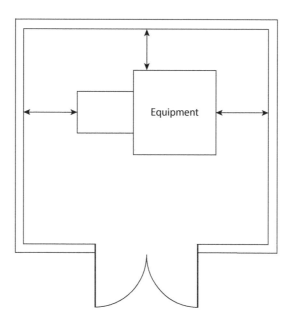

FIGURE 4.21 Equipment layout determines room size.

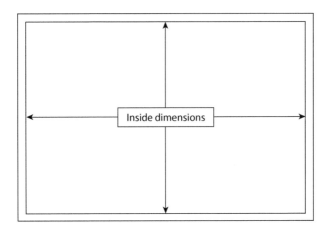

FIGURE 4.22 Measurement of net square feet.

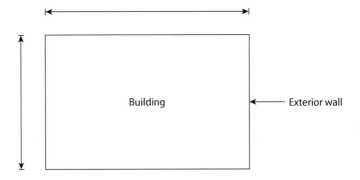

FIGURE 4.23 Measurement of gross square feet.

TABLE 4.3
Space Program

Space or Area	NSF	Less Efficient (%)	Middle (%)	More Efficient (%)	Range of GSF Less Efficient GSF	Middle GSF	More Efficient GSF
Warehouse	30,000	80	85	90	37,500	35,294	33,333
Shipping receiving	5,000	65	75	80	7,692	6,667	6,250
Manufacturing	40,000	50	55	60	80,000	72,727	66,667
Packaging	20,000	55	60	65	36,364	33,333	30,769
Quality control laboratory	5,000	50	55	60	10,000	9,091	8,333
Office support	15,000	55	60	65	27,273	25,000	23,077
Total NSF	115,000						
Total facility size (GSF)					198,829	182,112	168,429

Note: Conclusion: The facility of 115,000 NSF may range in size from 168,429 to 198,829 GSF before you test layout.

area and contain all of the important data about room finishes, ceiling heights, equipment layout, and all mechanical, electrical, and plumbing (MEP) requirements. This is done before the actual facility design is started. A typical room card format is illustrated in Figure 4.24. The room card is critical in the design of pharmaceutical manufacturing facilities because it captures all the users' needs and the engineering criteria at a very early date.

COMPLIANCE ISSUES

It is important to understand the regulated codes that are required to permit and construct a pharmaceutical manufacturing facility. The following sections cover the general descriptions and key concepts of which the reader should be aware.

Zoning Codes

Zoning and building codes impact the form, design, layout, and construction of a pharmaceutical facility. The zoning codes should be viewed as the "macro codes." The zoning codes cover the allowable use, amount of site coverage, building height, and parking requirements. Key concepts are discussed below.

> **Allowable use.** Each zoning code has zoned its township's land use into areas for different uses, such as residential, commercial, manufacturing, and research and development (R&D). In evaluating a site, the first issue to determine is if the manufacturing use that is proposed is actually permitted by the zoning code.
>
> **Height and area limitations.** The zoning codes determine the area and height limitations on the site. While this may be determined through a variety of methods, it is typically determined by the building footprint, and the total coverage of building and parking. The height limitations are important when determining the total height of the building, particularly if penthouses and other appurtenances are allowed. Some height restrictions vary from the setback toward the center of the plant site.
>
> **Hazardous materials.** Many zoning codes have language that references the codes use for storage and other functions of hazardous materials. It is important not to overlook these sections of the codes.

Building Codes

The building codes regulate the physical characteristics of the project. The primary purpose of building codes is to govern life and safety issues in construction. Chapter 13 fully covers this area, but there are several key areas that affect the design and layout of the facility. Most municipalities have adopted national codes, but they may have local supplements, which take precedence.

The use groups define the area limitations and construction type, depending on use. The following areas are typical use groups in a facility: (1) B: business for office and laboratory areas, (2) F: manufacturing, (3) S: storage and warehouse, and (4) H: 1–5 for hazardous materials. The use group also determines the height of the building, number of stories, and area allowed for each construction type; for example, type 1 construction is noncombustible protected, and type 2 is protected and unprotected. The construction type selected dictates aspects of how the building is constructed. The more fire protection that is used, the larger the area that is allowed to be built. The construction costs must be balanced with the type of construction. Hazardous areas are determined by the amount of hazardous materials present, and if there is a chance of deflagration.

Industrial Insurance Carrier Guidelines

The insurance carriers of every facility (e.g., Factory Mutual) have requirements for the facility. These requirements should be reviewed with the insurance carrier involved in the project. The carrier will provide comments on key design criteria, and this feedback must be incorporated into the design.

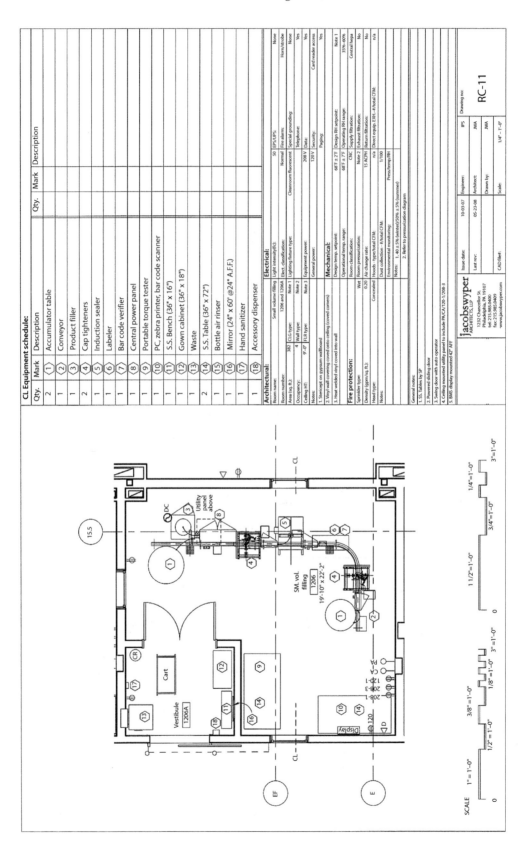

FIGURE 4.24 Typical lab card.

DESIGNING THE FACILITY

The programming phase has determined the project requirements for the equipment and the flow of people, product, and materials. The building and zoning codes have determined general area and size requirements. The architectural designer now organizes the facility into two- and three-dimensional layouts and tests the criteria based on the program. Several steps can be generally described, as discussed below.

Establish a Planning and Structural Module

This model may work with various functional areas of the facility. It is important to create a structural grid that will work for all areas of the facility, if possible (Figure 4.25). Special attention should be paid to very large pieces of equipment with large space requirements. The grid must work with the layout, but attention should also be paid to the most efficient structural grid in terms of tons of steel per square foot.

Functional Space Components

From the facility PFD and BFD, the functional space requirements may be drawn in a general manner to allow the designer to understand the physical size of these areas. For instance, the warehouse areas typically require a much larger footprint than the manufacturing areas. Figure 4.26 shows the approximate relative square footages of the functional areas.

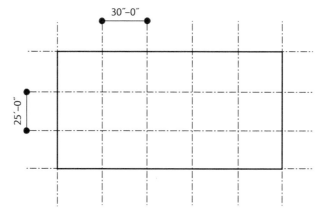

FIGURE 4.25 Structural grid example.

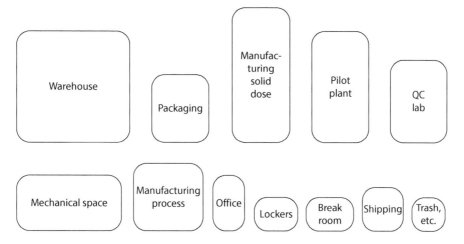

FIGURE 4.26 Functional space components.

It is important to also look at the vertical organization of the facility, in blocks that represent approximate sizes (Figure 4.27); then it is important to understand the relationships and adjacencies of these components and to have an overall concept of the flows within the building.

Mechanical Distribution Requirements

The mechanical distribution requirements for the facility, which must be determined in concert with the MEP engineer, are another key element that must be understood. The integration and allowance of adequate space for the MEP systems is critical in the design to allow for modification in the future. There are several possible locations for the MEP equipment, as illustrated in Figure 4.28. Roof-mounted equipment has the lowest cost but is functional. A penthouse is defined as an enclosed space on the roof, or partially below the roof of the building, where your mechanical equipment is enclosed. Having the equipment enclosed in a penthouse makes maintenance easier, as it provides protection from weather. Ground-mounted exterior HVAC units cost less but are hard to manage.

In addition to the equipment on the roof, penthouse level, or ground, MEP requires space within the building, which can be provided in an interstitial space or walkable ceiling level (Figure 4.29). An interstitial floor is a mechanical access floor completely above the manufacturing area and allows access from above. Walkable ceilings allow walking on all the ceilings above manufacturing areas and allow access from above.

Circulation and Future Growth

After understanding the BFD, PFD, and mechanical concepts, the designer creates concepts for circulation and growth of the facility. The designer must understand the gowning process and how it impacts the space requirements. The design also has to consider the hygienic zones of white, gray, and black and whether the facility must have unidirectional flow or is able to have two-way flow.

Following the general PFD, the functional areas must be organized to test the adjacencies and product flow. Figure 4.30 is a bubble diagram that tests the block area requirements and circulation.

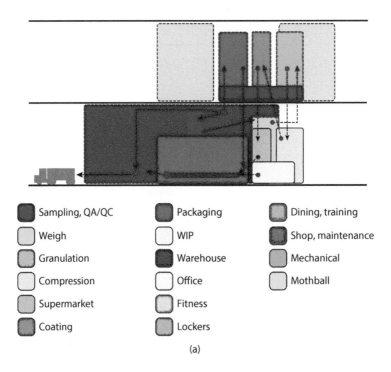

Sampling, QA/QC   Packaging   Dining, training

Weigh   WIP   Shop, maintenance

Granulation   Warehouse   Mechanical

Compression   Office   Mothball

Supermarket   Fitness

Coating   Lockers

(a)

FIGURE 4.27   (a) Vertical organization of the facility.   *(Continued)*

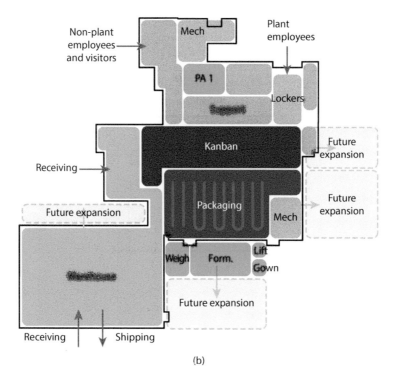

Non-plant employees and visitors

Mech

Plant employees

PA 1

Lockers

Support

Kanban

Future expansion

Receiving

Packaging

Future expansion

Future expansion

Mech

Weigh

Form.

Lift

Gown

Warehouse

Future expansion

Receiving

Shipping

(b)

FIGURE 4.27 (Continued) (b) Manufacturing facility layout diagram.

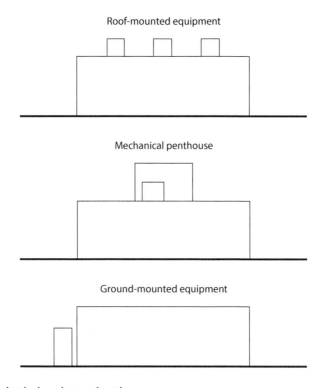

Roof-mounted equipment

Mechanical penthouse

Ground-mounted equipment

FIGURE 4.28 Mechanical equipment locations.

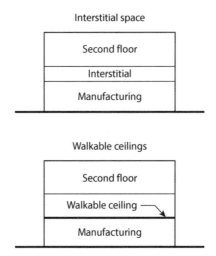

FIGURE 4.29   Interstitial space and walkable ceilings.

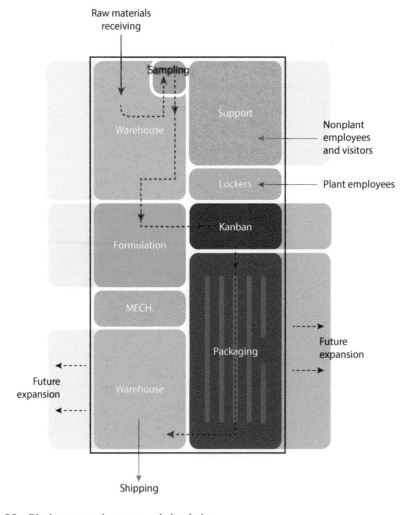

FIGURE 4.30   Block area requirements and circulation.

From this diagram, the designer should be able to test the ability to expand, as well as consider how areas would be renovated in the future. The designer should locate the break rooms on outside walls and establish circulation. The program can be "test-fit" into the facility. The test fit is the initial layout of rooms and staging areas, based on the approved program, and shows how the spaces fit. The floor plan and building section can now be tested against the criteria established during the programming phase, to confirm if the product flow and process flow work and if mechanical concepts have been established for the facility successfully. It is important that the MEP engineering designers develop mechanical concepts and the spaces they require at this early phase. They must determine the amount of space required for the air handling units (AHUs), compressed air systems, water systems, and electrical systems. The engineer should create schematic layouts of the equipment early, so that adequate space is provided, and a construction concept is established including those spaces.

Facility Image

In the end, the architect creates a building that has a presence and an image to portray to the public, customers, and employees. This will be a place where people come to work every day; thus, the facility should convey in the spaces outside the manufacturing area a sense of design that uplifts the employees by providing natural light and views.

Design reflects an attitude toward the process. The facility is making a product that improves people's lives; the facility should convey that with care toward design details, from the quality of the entrance and lobby to the offices, break rooms, lockers, and conference areas. These details can convey the respect and value the company has for its employees as well as its products.

The image of the facility, both from the exterior and interior, needs to be discussed at the earliest phase. The cost of the building's exterior needs to be identified so that the designer can present options. Manufacturing facilities should present a clean and crisp exterior that reflects the clean nature of the operation. This may be achieved with a variety of materials from metal panels to brick or other masonry to create an exterior that may be part of a campus or a stand-alone building (Figure 4.31).

Design Details and Material Finishes

The detailing and material finish selection in the design of pharmaceutical manufacturing facilities are critical to the final building success. There are no specifically FDA-approved materials; rather, there are materials that have become the current standards. There has been a trend toward using

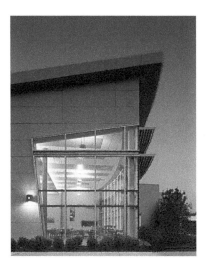

FIGURE 4.31 Photo of manufacturing facility in Newark, Delaware. (Courtesy of JacobsWyper Architects, LLP, Philadelphia, PA.)

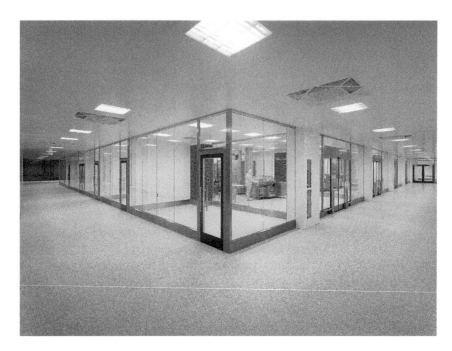

FIGURE 4.32   Floor-to-ceiling glass. (Courtesy of Daldrop + Dr.Ing.Huber, GmbH + Co.KG, Neckartailfingen, Germany.)

much more floor-to-ceiling glass (Figure 4.32). Glass is cleanable and opens up both the manufacturing and office areas. There is also a trend toward increased use of modular wall systems, as these systems have improved greatly in recent years.

Selection of finishes for pharmaceutical facilities must include the following considerations (as listed in the ISPE Baseline Guide on OSD facilities [4]): (1) durability, (2) cleanability, (3) functionality, (4) sustainability, (5) maintainability, and (6) cost-effectiveness. The finishes selected should also be based on the functional areas of the facility. There are industry and company guidelines that have established suggested levels of finishes for different functional areas. The purpose of these is to help prevent the escalation in costs of facilities in trying to anticipate what may be approved and accepted. This may be used as a base reference to select materials appropriate to the facility's needs and budgets. Table 4.4 is a matrix of finishes recommended for different functional areas.

Detailing of Pharmaceutical Facilities

Architectural details must be designed where dissimilar materials meet. Since these details are what is ultimately visible, it is important to spend time and attention in developing them. There are no FDA-approved details; however, details have been developed that help meet the goals of cleanability, durability, maintainability, and cost. Some typical details that are used in pharmaceutical facilities are discussed below.

There is a trend toward using high-impact drywall in facilities; however, it is important to know when a room will be washed down with a hose or when it will be wiped down. A wall that must withstand a hose needs to be made of different materials than a wall that will be wiped down; and is also more expensive. Details of interior door and window frames can be seen in Figures 4.33 and 4.34. Base details and a wall bumper detail follow in Figures 4.35 through 4.37.

There are many manufacturers who make modular wall systems that have different finish levels and provide doors, windows, and walkable ceilings. With these systems, the walls, ceilings, windows, doors, and all connections between them are provided as one system that works together to form cleanable rooms with walls as little as 2 in. thick.

TABLE 4.4
Finishes Recommended for Different Areas in a Facility

Area	Walls	Floors	Base	Ceiling	Details
Shipping area	CMU or gypsum wall or equivalent. Area needs to withstand abuse. Epoxy paint on walls not required.	Conc. with sealer or painted at minimum. Area needs to withstand forklift traffic.*	Vinyl base is adequate.	Ceiling is not required but a 2 × 4 lay-in ceiling with standard acoustical tile is recommended and acceptable.	Roll-up exterior doors. Dock levels. Bollard to protect covers. Thin coatings on concrete floors are not recommended.
Warehouse	CMU with block filler and semigloss paint. Gypsum wall above traffic areas.	Conc. with sealer or painted at minimum. Area needs to withstand forklift traffic.*	Vinyl base is adequate.	Ceiling not required but may want to consider for cGMP warehouse. Requirements for air conditioning and humidity control.	Coordinate sprinklers, ductwork, and lighting. Coordinate clearance from sprinkler heads to the top of pallets. Unless a floor coating is a troweled or broadcast epoxy, sealed concrete is recommended.
Packaging area	Impact-resistant gypsum wall with epoxy paint. Modular walls.	Vinyl composition tile (VCT) is acceptable. Seamless vinyl can be used. Epoxy.	Vinyl base or base compatible with the floor system.	2 × 4 acoustical ceiling. Where product is exposed, clean room tiles or gypsum ceilings.	Use glass walls between packaging areas to create openness. Ensure foot candles are adequate. Ceiling height in proportion to the space.
Manufacturing area	CMU with epoxy paint: plaster. Impact-resistant drywall with epoxy paint. Prefabricated metal wall panels. Seamless vinyl. Generally smooth finish.	Epoxy terrazzo. Broadcast epoxy. Seamless vinyl.	Epoxy terrazzo. Broadcast epoxy. Seamless vinyl. Flush detailing for sterile areas.	Vinyl-coated gypsum panels in ceiling grid. For sterile facility, flush ceiling (drywall or metal) is used.	Cove details are used on floor, wall, and ceiling intersections for sterile facilities (nice to have for OSD facility but not required). Test flows for moisture in slabs for any epoxy floors. Floor to ceiling glass.

Note: CMU, concrete masonry unit.

* If more than sealing is done to the concrete, a material that can withstand forklift traffic needs to be selected.

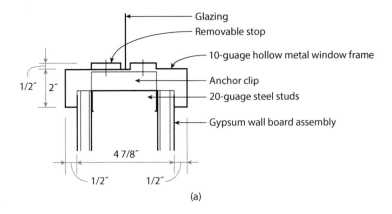

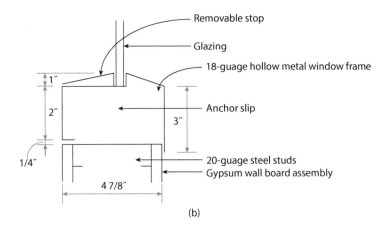

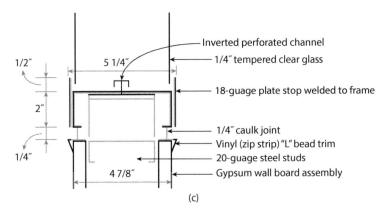

FIGURE 4.33 cGMP and non-cGMP window frames. (a) Standard window frame detail, (b) sloping sill, single-glazed window frame detail, and (c) flush, double-glazed window frame detail.

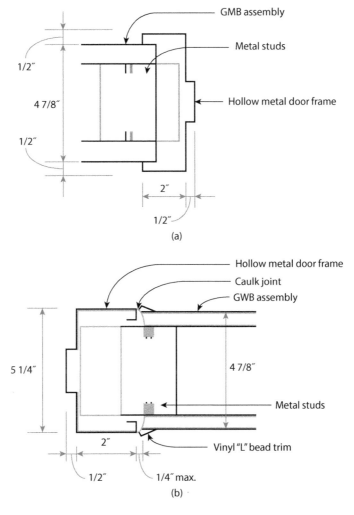

FIGURE 4.34 cGMP and non-cGMP door frames. (a) (Non-cGMP) standard door frame and (b) cGMP door frame. *Note:* The standard door frame has a small ledge.

Design Opportunities

The following are several key concepts in the design of a pharmaceutical manufacturing facility:

- Interior glass windows can be used in manufacturing spaces for visual control and safety, as well as aesthetics to provide visual openness in the facility (Figure 4.38).
- Natural light can be introduced into the facility in the packaging lines and, where possible, in break rooms.
- Color and floor patterns can be made in main corridors for way finding and differential functional areas.
- Well-designed and detailed amenity areas can be provided, such as break rooms, locker rooms, and cafeterias.
- Color and patterns can be used in floor materials, such as vinyl tile.
- The use of walkable ceilings and interstitial spaces helps create flexibility for mechanical modification and service.
- Crisp, modern building facades, which reflect a well-designed building, can be created.

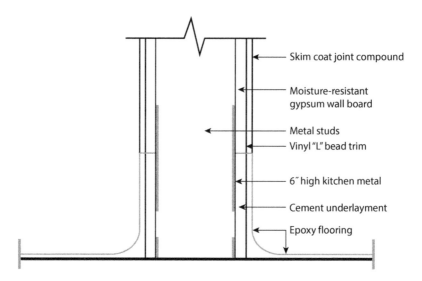

FIGURE 4.35 Flush base detail with epoxy flooring. Achieving a flush base detail is difficult with drywall. This detail is more typically used for sterile facilities.

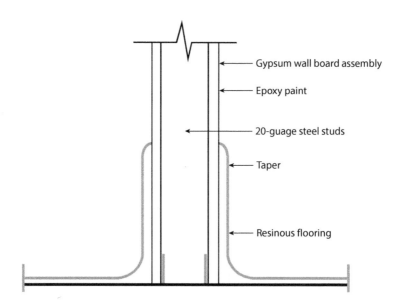

FIGURE 4.36 Semi–flush base detail. This detail is less difficult to construct and leaves a very small ledge where the epoxy meets the way.

Good cGMP design features include (1) clear layouts, (2) appropriate detailing and finishes, (3) adequate room sizes and staging areas, and (4) regulated presentation drawings that illustrate flows for people, product, and equipment.

Flexibility involves the ability to (1) adapt to different uses, (2) bring new services to the rooms, (3) easily clean, and (4) make modifications. Good architecture includes (1) clear organization, (2) natural light, (3) sustainability, (4) well-designed public spaces, and (5) the integration of the site and the building.

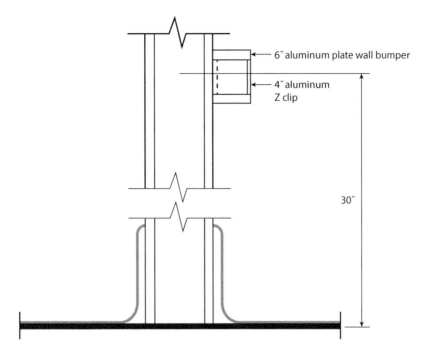

FIGURE 4.37 Wall bumper detail. Wall bumpers are critical to maintaining the walls in good condition from impact from carts and equipment, and so forth.

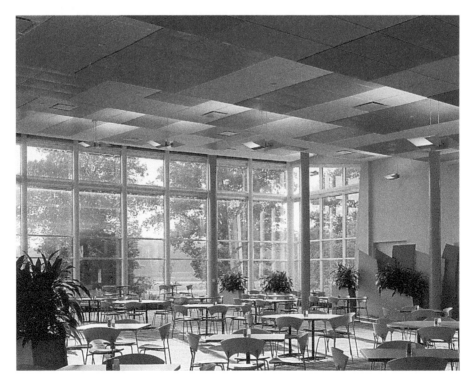

FIGURE 4.38 Use of glass and ceiling height in break area.

SUSTAINABLE DESIGN AND LEED BUILDING CERTIFICATION

Facilities today are designed around sustainable design principles, which minimize the use of natural resources in the design, construction, and maintenance of buildings. The goals are to minimize the energy uses of buildings and use materials that are renewable and sustainable. Leadership in Energy and Environmental Design (LEED) is a program sponsored by the U.S. Green Building Council (USGBC) that awards points for meeting these criteria. Major corporations are embracing these goals, and local municipalities are requiring them. Sustainability is discussed in Chapter 16. Many pharmaceutical manufacturing facilities have been LEED certified.

PREPROJECT FDA REVIEW

A recent trend has been to have a predesign completion review of the facility plans by the FDA. The architectural review can show the circulation for people, equipment, and product and demonstrate the hierarchy of finishes by using colored block plans. It will also show the approach for MEP system design and the overall compliance approach.

SECURITY

Post–September 11 concerns have brought security to the forefront. Security design starts with the site layout of a facility, with access to the site via a guard booth and a secure perimeter. There has been an increase in the use of card access to most areas of the facility. Possible contamination of critical facilities by terrorists should be considered in the design for critical products, such as vaccines.

RISK-BASED DESIGN

Risk-based design means there is a much earlier evaluation of risks and how the physical design is impacted. Risk assessments are described in Chapter 7.

BUILDING INFORMATION MODELING

There is a continuing trend of using building information modeling (BIM) for both the architects and engineers and increasingly the subcontractors for the integration of shop drawings and coordination and conflict resolution in the field. BIM tools allow for the comprehensive visualization of a proposed building, in which all elements are created and placed in three-dimensional space. The architect and consultants are able to link into a common model, which greatly streamlines documentation and aids in the effective coordination of equipment and infrastructure (Figure 4.39).

PROJECT MANAGEMENT

Manufacturing facilities are process-driven project types. Therefore, the design team is typically led by the engineer, so that the architect builds the facility around the process requirements. Three standard types of project delivery are shown in Table 4.5, with variations for pharmaceutical manufacturing facilities.

SUMMARY

The architect designs a pharmaceutical manufacturing facility around the process, and engineering systems are required to support the process. Attention to detailing of utility panels, functional flows, and personnel needs creates a facility that is efficient, safe, and attractive and an environment that is a good place to work. When these problems are solved, the building design needs to reflect the quality of the work being done, and architecture that contributes to the site and sense of place.

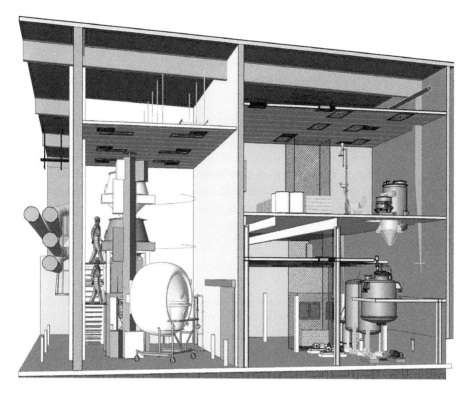

FIGURE 4.39 BIM model.

TABLE 4.5
Three Types of Project Delivery

Type	Comments
1. Design, bid, build, commission, and validate	• Takes longest • Possibly lowest price • Adversarial
2. CM	• CM on board early
a. With guaranteed price (at risk)	• Faster
b. Target budget (not at risk)	• Less adversarial
Design/build[a]: signing contract for design and construction	• Faster • As competitive as CM • Single point

Note: CM, construction management.
[a] Also referred to as engineering procurement and construction (EPC).

FURTHER DISCUSSION

1. Does the FDA dictate exactly how to design a facility?
2. Is the design process different for a sterile versus an OSD facility?
3. Is good design more expensive?
4. Does the FDA have a list of approved materials?
5. How do international codes affect design and compliance?

ABOUT THE AUTHOR

Terry Jacobs is a principal with JacobsWyper Architects, an architectural, planning, and interior design firm founded in 1981 in Philadelphia, Pennsylvania. The firm's practice focuses in part on large, complex projects for corporate and educational clients, including research laboratories and manufacturing facilities for the biotech, pharmaceutical, and research universities—many delivered using design build. Mr. Jacobs's extensive experience with pharmaceutical projects led him to coedit the first edition of *Good Design Practices for GMP Pharmaceutical Facilities* in 2005, and the second edition in 2015. Jacobs was an adjunct professor at both Temple University and Drexel University and a visiting critic at the University of Pennsylvania, all in Philadelphia. He has won design awards from the American Institute of Architects and the Pennsylvania Society of Architects. Jacobs earned his BA from Dartmouth College and his master's in architecture from the University of Pennsylvania. He was chairman of ISPE's Continuous Advancement Subcommittee and was president of the Delaware Valley Chapter of ISPE. He has been a course leader and speaker at numerous IPSE courses, and a member of the ISPE since 1981.

REFERENCES

1. U.S. Food and Drug Administration, Center for Drug Evaluation and Research, 21 Code of Federal Regulations, Parts 210 and 211, Current Good Manufacturing Practice for Manufacturing, Processing, Packing, or Holding of Drugs, U.S. Food and Drug Administration, Silver Spring, MD, http://www.fda.gov/cder/dmpq/cgmpregs.htm.
2. U.S. Food and Drug Administration, Facts About the Current Good Manufacturing Practices (CGMPs), U.S. Food and Drug Administration, Silver Spring, MD, http://www.fda.gov/Drugs/DevelopmentApprovalProcess/Manufacturing/ucm169105.htm.
3. Code of Federal Regulations, Title 21.
4. International Society for Pharmaceutical Engineering, *Baseline® Pharmaceutical Engineering Guides for New and Renovated Facilities*, Vol. 2: *Oral Solid Dosage Forms*, 2nd ed., International Society for Pharmaceutical Engineering, Tampa, FL, 2009.
5. International Society for Pharmaceutical Engineering, *Baseline® Pharmaceutical Engineering Guides for New and Renovated Facilities*, Vol. 1: Active Pharmaceutical Ingredients—Revision to Bulk Pharmaceutical Chemicals, 2nd ed., International Society for Pharmaceutical Engineering, Tampa, FL, 2007.
6. International Society for Pharmaceutical Engineering, *Baseline® Pharmaceutical Engineering Guides for New and Renovated Facilities*, Vol. 3: *Sterile Manufacturing Facilities*, International Society for Pharmaceutical Engineering, Tampa, FL, 2011.
7. International Society for Pharmaceutical Engineering, *Pharmaceutical Facilities*, ISPE Baseline Guide, OSD facilities, 2nd edition, International Society for Pharmaceutical Engineering, Tampa, FL.
8. Cole G, *Pharmaceutical Production Facilities: Design and Applications*, 2nd ed., CRC Press, Boca Raton, FL.
9. U.S. Department of Justice, http://www.deadiversion.usdoj.gov/21cfr/21usc/index.html.

5 Facility Utility Systems

Jack C. Chu, Leonid Shnayder, and Joe Maida

CONTENTS

INTRODUCTION

Under the Food, Drug, and Cosmetic Act, a drug is deemed to be adulterated unless the methods used in its manufacture (processing, packaging, holding, and the facilities and controls utilized) conform to current Good Manufacturing Practices (cGMPs). These require the drug to meet the safety requirements of the act, contain the proper strength and identity, and meet the quality and purity characteristics that it is represented to have. A properly designed and constructed manufacturing facility supports these practices.

The critical quality attributes (CQAs) and critical process parameters (CPPs) must be satisfied by the facility and utility system design and implementation. Professionals from architecture, engineering, and construction management must offer solutions for their portion of the design and installation challenge. Facility and utility design and construction work must be integrated into a complete and operational facility to facilitate the operations of production and maintenance, the company culture, and their quality systems.

This chapter presents pharmaceutical manufacturing utility system design criteria, and installation considerations, as well as critical utility system design concepts applicable to pharmaceutical manufacturing facilities design and construction.

PRODUCTION FACILITY AND UTILITY SYSTEMS DESIGN MUST FOLLOW GMP PRACTICE

Facility utility systems design and installation disciplines have a direct impact on the performance of manufacturing process systems and utility systems. In addition, the facility utility systems will have the greatest impact on the quality and consistency of the drug products, the safety of production personnel, and environmental compliance initiatives. Further, the facility utility systems design and installation can make up as much as 40% of the "brick-and-mortar" capital cost of a pharmaceutical manufacturing facility; the cost of proper maintenance programs could be 10% of the overall production budget.

KEY CONCEPTS

The facility utility systems discussed in this chapter are primarily mechanical systems that include heating, ventilation, and air conditioning (HVAC) systems and associated controls: electrical, plumbing, process piping and instrumentation and control systems, and fire protection systems.

EXECUTIVE SUMMARY

INTEGRATED APPROACH TO EXISTING FACILITIES' RENOVATION AND UPGRADE

In general, new facilities are built as supplemental to, or phased replacements for, existing production facilities. Most existing facilities have their own unique identities and established operation flows that cannot be disrupted by construction of the new facility. An integral part of programming and designing these projects is the development of phasing strategies that deal not only with construction activities and equipment movement but also with issues of safety and the prevention of product contamination or adulteration during facility construction and operation changeover periods. Design professionals must understand that some existing operational utility systems may not be designed with recognizable logic. Therefore, expediency, rather than flexibility and appropriateness, often dictates the layout of connection to existing utility systems; the possibility of future expansion is seldom a design determinant. A complete survey of these existing systems by a multidisciplinary architectural and engineering team is essential to orderly planning and integration. The project scope of work, and phasing of design and construction, will be based on the results of a thorough survey and the understanding of current and future production process flow, material flow, and personnel flow concepts.

UTILITY COMPONENTS, EQUIPMENT, AND SYSTEMS SURFACE FINISHES

Of all the architectural systems in a pharmaceutical manufacturing facility, the interior finishes are most uniquely identified with this specific building type. Particularly in the process areas, finishes are selected for their durability, resistance to cracking and microbial growth, and cleanability. Exposed engineering system components, and terminal equipment must also be selected to support these criteria to maintain facility integrity. For example, the exposed sheet metal vent ductwork will be made of stainless steel, type 304 or 316L, all electrical and instrumentation wiring will be concealed in the conduits, a metal jacket is required for all insulated piping, and so forth.

UTILITY SYSTEMS' OPERATIONAL RELIABILITY

Risk-based asset management (RBAM) must be performed for all facility utility systems to identify probable failure modes and operational reliabilities. Asset risk evaluation and assessment focus on the system-based approach. Components' risk assessment will be done by a preestablished preventive maintenance (PM) program. An engineering solution will be presented to production management based on the system risk identifying evaluation and mitigation processes. The following utility risk management strategies are commonly recommended:

Business continuity: Assets will continue their functionality as originally intended. This requires establishment of a maintenance and operational plan to minimize asset malfunctioning and eliminate critical single-point failures, for example, predictive maintenance (PdM), PM, and corrective maintenance (CM) programs.

Equipment redundancy: An alternative asset will be available to perform the same function as each existing asset. This requires a redundant asset or equipment in place for backup, for example, an online standby fan or pump unit.

Contingency plan: A disaster recovery plan will be provided to manage potential asset or equipment failure. Backup procedures to restore the normal operational condition are required, for example, automatically switching the power supply from a failed centralized supply line to a localized power source.

Minimize impact: Processes to minimize the impact due to the asset or equipment failure will be preestablished. Provide localized utility systems in addition to the centralized utility system, or multiple localized critical utility assets and equipment to support critical processes, for example, a local water-for-injection (WFI) system add-on to the centralized WFI distribution system, or multiple freezers with 35% spare capacity for backup to a failed freezer.

The cost of such strategies for asset redundancy or availability must be thoroughly assessed and justified based on the critical nature of the operations and the risks and consequences of failure. A cost-and-benefit model can be used for such assessments and will include the following primary factors:

- Drug product quality and GMP compliance requirements, which could have an impact on patient safety, for example, cross-contamination and microbial problems
- Production safety, for example, equipment safety and operator safety
- Business impact, for example, environmental compliance and product recall

CLEANABILITY, MAINTAINABILITY, AND SERVICEABILITY

The utility system's reliability requirements can be achieved by good engineering design practice, achievable construction deliverables, and a reliable maintenance program. Each utility system should be reviewed for maintainability by subject matter experts (SMEs), the group that will be responsible for operating and maintaining the system. Furthermore, utility system components should be located in a position where routine PM or CM can easily be performed with minimal impact to normal operations. Scheduled system shutdowns for service, in-line testing, and sampling methods should be carefully designed to minimize interruptions to production operations.

COMMISSIONING AND QUALIFICATION

Commissioning is required for all utility systems and equipment prior to putting in service, for example, HVAC, chiller system, domestic water system, and electrical distribution system. In general, validation (qualification) may not be required for the utility system unless it is classified as a critical utility system or equipment that has a direct impact on drug product quality and safety, for example, HVAC, WFI system, clean-in-place and steam-in-place (CIP/SIP) system, and compressed gas system. Reverification at a preestablished frequency will be required if the material produced by the utility system will be part of the drug, for example, WFI water and clean steam.

Commissioning, as defined in the American Society of Heating, Refrigerating and Air-Conditioning Engineer (ASHRAE) guideline, is

> the process of ensuring that systems are designed, installed, functionally tested, and capable of being operated and maintained to perform in conformity with the design intent … commissioning begins with planning and includes design, construction, start-up, acceptance and training, and can be applied throughout the life of the building.

The qualification process is a documented program that provides a high degree of assurance that a specific process, method, or system will consistently produce a result that meets predetermined acceptance criteria. See Chapter 7 for more discussion of commissioning and qualification.

MECHANICAL, ELECTRICAL, PIPING, AND INSTRUMENTATION CONTROL SYSTEMS

OVERVIEW

The primary objective for the design of production facility utility systems is to ensure that products manufactured using these systems are fit for use. Specifications and the CQAs of production should be understood in order to determine CPPs.

In general, facility-related mechanical systems include the following functional outputs:

- Heat transfer (both process and facility), for example, glycol chillers and heat exchangers
- Space temperature, humidity, and pressurization controls, for example, HVAC and building automation system (BAS)
- Space cleanliness and air filtration for space particle control: International Organization for Standardization (ISO) classification and high-efficiency particulate air (HEPA) filtration
- Provision of water and gases for product and process requirements: Domestic water and water softener
- Wastewater drainage and disposal of wastes

Utility systems are designed to accommodate facility and processes requirements that are determined primarily by the products manufactured, the processes utilized, established machinery and user criteria, and operational and maintenance factors and economic and scheduling requirements. Some specific requirements depend on whether the utility system or equipment comes in contact with product. The following sections discuss the various mechanical services, including HVAC systems, process and piping systems, and fire protection systems, and how these relate to the process requirements outlined elsewhere in this text.

HEATING, VENTILATION, AND AIR CONDITIONING SYSTEMS

The HVAC disciplines play a critical role in the manufacture of pharmaceutical products. The Food and Drug Administration (FDA), through current Good Manufacturing Practices and guidelines, has set strict facility requirements for the manufacturing environment that the HVAC systems support.

System Design Criteria

For people's comfort, ASHRAE standard 55, "Thermal Environmental Conditions for Human Occupancy"; ASHRAE standard 62.1, "Ventilation for Acceptable Indoor Air Quality" (Reference 3, Appendix 5); and ISO standard 7730 should be followed. If operators are wearing protective suits such as Tyvek suits, full-face respirators, or full-body suits with breathing air equipment, then lower space temperatures than those defined by ASHRAE may be required to provide operator comfort. For process and product controls, product may dictate the operating or process environment conditions. Many products can be hygroscopic or temperature sensitive during the manufacturing process. All of these conditions should be defined prior to selecting and sizing the HVAC system.

While regulations change over time and vary across countries, the major principles of regulation and guidance impacting HVAC design, installation, qualification, and maintenance in pharmaceutical manufacturing facilities are generally consistent. A few key principles are listed below:

Process contamination control and cross-contamination control: Control of pharmaceutical dust (from processing), air filtration, once-through air or recirculation air, space pressurization, and control of contaminants from personnel, and so forth
Production facility environmental control of critical parameters: Temperature, humidity control, pressurization, and filtration
HVAC system risk assessment: By processing zone, product or process specific, qualitative or quantitative

Contamination Control Criteria

The production environment where the drug is processed must be appropriately designed, constructed, and maintained. At every stage of processing, products and materials must be protected from microbial and other contamination. In oral products, the most serious potential contamination may be the contamination of one drug by another. Regulations predominantly suggest that the dissemination of pharmaceutical dust, including active product, must be controlled. This requirement for control of pharmaceutical dust includes minimizing the escape of dust from the process and the control of fugitive dust within the room.

Many common practices have been recognized by pharmaceutical professionals: In cases where dust is generated (e.g., during sampling, weighing, mixing, and processing operations, and packaging of dry products), specific provisions should be taken to avoid cross-contamination. When working with dry materials and products, special precautions should be taken to prevent the generation and dissemination of dust. This applies particularly to the handling of highly active or sensitizing material. Contamination of a starting material or a product by another material or product must be avoided. The risk of accidental cross-contamination arises from the uncontrolled release of dust, gases, vapors, sprays, and so forth, from active substances. Dust control systems for the removal of dust should be close to source of the contaminant.

Control of pharmaceutical dust in the ambient environment is the reason that regulations typically require "minimizing the risk of contamination caused by recirculation or re-entry of untreated or insufficiently treated air" (EudraLex Vol. 4 5.19 and Agência Nacional de Vigilância Sanitária [ANVISA]). This regulatory requirement is often used as the justification for using 100% exhausted systems without recirculation. However, regulatory agencies do recommend conducting an evaluation of cross-contamination potential in lieu of a ban on recirculation of air in multiproduct facilities. "A Quality Risk Management process, which includes a potency and toxicological evaluation, should be used to assess and control the cross-contamination risks presented by the products manufactured" (EMA *EU Guidelines for Good Manufacturing Practice for Medicinal products for Human and Veterinary Use*. Part 1. Chapter 5: Production).

In production areas, a risk evaluation plan should be established for the production facility and utility systems, production equipment, and manufacturing process systems. The production facility risk assessment should include weighing and dispensing, solution preparation, mixing and granulation, drying, tableting and encapsulation, tablet coating, and other processes. Risk analysis will determine whether a once-through air system or a filtered return air system is appropriate for a specific application. A risk-based approach to determining critical parameters is suggested by most regulations. The list of parameters that may be judged as critical can be broad. For instance, the following citation from WHO TRS 937, Annex 2 suggests a long list of parameters that may need to be qualified in an oral solid dosage (OSD) facility's HVAC design:

#8.2.17 for a pharmaceutical facility, based on a risk assessment, some of the typical HVAC system parameters and functions that may be qualified can include:

- temperature
- relative humidity
- supply air quantities for all diffusers
- return air or exhaust air quantities
- room air change rates
- room pressures (pressure differentials)
- room airflow patterns
- unidirectional flow velocities
- containment system velocities
- HEPA filter penetration parameters
- particle counts in the room air
- room clean-up rates
- microbiological air and surface counts where appropriate
- operation of de-dusting
- warning/alarm systems where applicable

Environmental Control Criteria

Although cGMP regulations establish the requirements for classified environments for bio and sterile manufacturing environments, most regulations do not require a classified environment for oral dosage manufacturing. However, this does not mean that OSD manufacturing environments are uncontrolled; rather, it suggests that oral drug manufacturing should be managed and well understood, though the cleanliness requirements are less than those for sterile products. The traditional approach to meeting control expectations was to "design to class 100,000 (ISO 8) but not certified" or "controlled but not classified space." This approach has been successful, but it does not offer a means of verifying that the intended goal has been reached. There is a growing regulatory expectation that facilities will be tested and qualified to an objective standard. For oral dosage facilities, the consensus appears to be that class 100,000 (ISO 8) in the "at-rest" state—equivalent to EU grade D—is a suitable background environment. As an example, the following is a citation from WHO TRS 937, Annex 2:

HVAC systems and components
    Note: The required degree of air cleanliness in most OSD manufacturing facilities can normally be achieved without the use of high-efficiency particulate air (HEPA) filters, provided the air is not recirculated. Many open product zones of OSD form facilities are capable of meeting ISO 14644-1 Class 8, "at-rest" condition, measured against particle sizes of 0.5 µm and 5 µm, but cleanliness may not be classified as such by manufacturers.

A rough comparison of the ISO and Federal Standard 209E is shown in Table 5.1.
Table 5.1 does not reflect the complexity of the ISO clean room standards. These should be considered thoroughly before embarking on a clean room design.
Specific facility and process criteria are defined in the following sections.

Temperature and Relative Humidity

Production facility temperature and relative humidity controls are critical to both process and production personnel. United States Pharmacopoeia (USP) excursion limits for finished product storage are 59°F–86°F (15°C–30°C) with a controlled room temperature (CRT) working environment

TABLE 5.1
ISO and U.S. Federal Standard 209E

ISO (Standard)	EU Grade	U.S. Federal Standard 209E (Reference Only)	Common Application in Pharm Industry	Recommended Air Change per Hour
1		—	NA	NA
2		—	NA	NA
3		1	NA	NA
4		10	NA	NA
5	A	100	Bio/vac/sterile operations	600
6	B	1,000	Bio/vac/sterile operations	35
7	C	10,000	Bio/vac/sterile/pharm operations	25
8	D	100,000	Bio/vac/sterile/pharm operations	15

Note: NA, not applicable.

of 68°F–77°F (20°C–25°C) with a maximum mean kinetic temperature (MKT) of 77°F (25°C). However, individual products may require a more stringently controlled environment.

Product temperature monitoring may be performed as an alternative to room temperature monitoring. Room temperature can be monitored by return or exhaust duct-mounted sensors or wall-mounted sensors that relay information to the BAS or separate sensors connected to an independent environmental monitoring system (EMS). Typically, a relatively tight control range is specified (i.e., 68°F–72°F), with an excursion alert occurring when a wider range is exceeded (i.e., 65°F–75°F), and a further excursion alarm occurring when a maximum range is exceeded (62°F–78°F). All values must be well inside the USP excursion limits.

Allowable space and system control tolerances must also be identified, as well as the impact of these tolerance requirements on the systems design. Proper outdoor ambient design conditions must be determined in order to select the air conditioning equipment. If outdoor conditions are chosen too conservatively, the equipment will be oversized, costing more than required and requiring more energy for operation. Conversely, if the selection does take variation of ambient conditions into consideration, the facility or process conditions may not be met under certain circumstances. An assessment must be made of the possible risks of not meeting space or process condition requirements and the effects on productivity.

Air Cleanliness
The level of acceptable airborne contamination within the space must be identified, whether required for product quality or employee safety. Environmental cleanliness is determined by several factors, including the quality and quantity of air introduced into the space, the effectiveness of air distribution through the space, and the effectiveness of the removal of the air contaminants. Removal of the contaminant as close to its source as possible is always the most effective method of contamination control—whether it is central filtration at an air handling unit before supply to the facility or dust collection at a point source of contamination within a space.

Clean room design takes contamination control to its highest level. Federal Standard 209 historically was the document governing clean room design. This standard has been replaced by the ISO 14644 and 14698 global clean room standards. Cleanliness is categorized by cleanliness classes, which are qualified by the quantity of 0.5 micron or larger particles per cubic foot of air within a specific area. Standard categories of cleanliness used in the pharmaceutical industry are ISO 5, 7, and 8 (Classes 100, 10,000, and 100,000 per U.S. Federal Standard 209E, which was replaced by the ISO standard). See Table 5.1.

Pressurization and Air Change Rates

Where airborne contamination, cross-contamination, or potent or hazardous material containment is a concern, one tool for control of airborne particulates is control of the differential pressure or direction of airflow between spaces with the following common practices:

- Bio and sterile operations: 15.0 Pa (0.06 in. of water column (WC))
- OSD operation: Between 5.0 Pa (0.02 in. WC) and 12.5 Pa (0.05 in. WC)

The velocity and direction of airflow between spaces should be satisfactory to reduce the transfer of airborne particulates or vapor. While there is not a numerical value for pressurization required in regulation, many current guidance documents suggest a mass airflow velocity of 100–200 fpm to control light dusts moving across a work area. Generally, smoke tests and Baulin Tubes may be used as evidence of the establishment of directional airflow between work areas. The air changes per hour method has been practically applied for engineering design and HVAC equipment specification. Common practice demonstrates the effectiveness of the proper air changes per hour (ACH) for various production facilities. See Table 5.1 for reference.

In many cases, the cleanliness of the production facility can be achieved by employing space temperature and relative humidity controls, airflow pattern and space pressurization controls, and air filtration and air system configuration controls, and controlling the air changes per hour within the space.

Other Considerations

The relative pressurization of the space will be determined primarily by the requirements of the product, but also by characteristics of the product that may adversely affect personnel. Space containment and isolation techniques can protect the product, the operator, or both. Where product contamination control is required, the space relative pressurization must be designed to ensure that the movement of exfiltrated air is from the clean to the less clean areas. In some cases dealing with hazardous products (e.g., high-potency compounds), this relative pressurization and the resultant air movement are reversed to contain the hazard and protect personnel. In these cases, product contamination can be controlled by the use of special laminar flow hoods or personal isolation suits, or positive and negative pressurization utilizing airlocks. Some operations may require flexibility for either positive or negative pressurization, depending on the application. A pressure differential of at least 0.05 in. water gauge with all doors closed is preferable between spaces with a pressure differential requirement. See Chapter 14 for more discussion on this topic.

Careful attention must be paid to the incoming air quality. This can be specific to the area in which the facility has been constructed, such as an agrarian or industrial area. An industrial area may have more corrosive or chemical-laden air, while an agrarian area may have a higher level of seasonal airborne particulate and bioburden. These issues must be carefully considered when selecting filtration systems so as to minimize the possibility of product contamination.

Most often, however, building intake reentrainment of its own effluent is the greater problem. Careful consideration must be made as to the impacts of building exhaust and relief systems, loading docks, and other incidences of vehicle exhaust and electrical generator exhaust. Analysis must be made of the building's impact on itself and other surrounding buildings, and their impact on the subject building. Potential future building activities should also be considered. Rooftop activity safety should also be analyzed, and a safe rooftop environment should be provided for routine maintenance activities.

Noise Considerations

Given the overriding concerns for durability and cleanability in process spaces, little can be done to dampen the acoustic qualities of finished surfaces. By definition, a cleanable space has smooth, hard finishes with simple geometries that reflect rather than absorb sound. This makes the control of noise contributed by utility systems critical in these spaces. Sound attenuation can be added to supply and exhaust air systems. Dust collection inlets tend to be the greatest contributor to space noise. Attention to design parameters can minimize the sound radiated from these inlets.

Manufacturing facilities also tend to utilize large process and utility equipment that can radiate noise to the outdoor environment. Local ordinances and the neighboring community may require that noise generated by this equipment be minimized. Methods of enclosure and the specification of sound attenuation devices can significantly reduce noise transmitted outside of the facility.

Cost Considerations

Pharmaceutical manufacturing facilities and processes are extremely costly to design, construct, and operate. When designing a facility and process, careful consideration must be given to the initial construction cost, balanced against life cycle operating costs. Careful analysis must be made of all of the components of the facility or process design. A cost-cutting measure taken during the initial capital expenditure may sometimes result in huge operating costs from years of inefficient operation. Conversely, a complex, capitally cost-intensive project can take too long to build and commission, which may affect the speed to market the product, and ultimately production and sales.

HEATING SYSTEMS

Heating of facility and process systems is generally accomplished utilizing steam or hot water as the heat source. There may also be intermediate methods of heat transfer utilizing a secondary steam or heating hot water system. Heating can also be provided by electric means, which is easily controlled but is expensive to operate and therefore not widespread. Heating systems for process equipment steam-in-place (SIP) for equipment sanitation are not covered in this chapter.

Heating of primary air at the central air handling unit is generally accomplished using hot water or low-pressure steam. Incoming ventilation air on high outside air volume systems in colder climates is generally heated utilizing low-pressure steam or a separate hot water system with a concentration of propylene glycol sufficient to prevent water system freezing (Figure 5.1).

It is preferred that heat required in a jacketed heat exchange process such as a kettle that has one level of product containment (the kettle wall) be provided by a non-plant source. This may be accomplished by using a secondary heat source such as an independent water or steam system utilizing plant steam as the primary heat source. This prevents plant system contamination in case of a boundary wall failure.

COOLING SYSTEMS

Cooling of facility and process systems is generally accomplished utilizing chilled water, condenser water, or direct refrigerant expansion (DX) as the heat sink. In isolated cases, a water and antifreeze solution or other heat exchange fluid may be utilized, generally without a phase change. There may also be an intermediate method of heat transfer utilizing a secondary chilled water system in concert with the plant systems outlined above. Primary chilled and condenser water is usually generated by a central cooling system. It is then distributed throughout the facility to points of use that include cooling coils, heat exchangers, and jacketed heat exchange processes. Piping for these plant water systems is generally welded or screwed black steel. Mechanical coupling systems are also utilized.

Plant chilled water is generally produced utilizing water-cooled or air-cooled chillers. Chilled water supply temperatures are usually in the range of 40°F–45°F and are determined by the requirements of the cooled medium, generally air.

Condenser water cools the condenser side of the chiller and is of a higher temperature. Condenser water supply temperatures are usually in the range of 85°F–95°F in the summer. Nonsummer condenser water supply temperatures can generally be maintained at lower temperatures. Water is

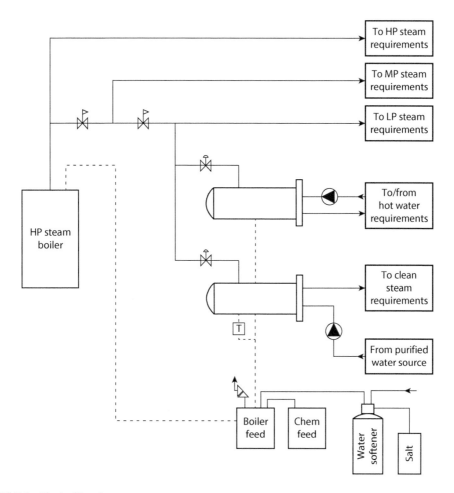

FIGURE 5.1 Typical heating system.

typically cooled by open cooling towers or closed-circuit coolers. Open towers utilize outside air to cool the water directly. Closed-circuit coolers circulate the water through tubing in the tower that is air cooled and sprinkled with water. Condenser water can also be used to cool processes besides chiller condensers. These include cooling of purified water processes, refrigerated processes, and jacketed processes. If the process does not require the lower temperatures of chilled water, condenser water can be a cost-effective solution, as it does not require the additional energy of the mechanical refrigeration process.

Cooling of space or process supply air is generally accomplished at the central air handling unit. Incoming ventilation air on high outside air volume systems may require additional dehumidification that the chilled water system cannot achieve (see the "Dehumidification Systems" section below). Terminal cooling is often required when an area with lower environmental temperature or humidity levels is served by a central system designed for maintaining higher temperatures and relative humidity (Figure 5.2).

HUMIDIFICATION SYSTEMS

In most cases, air supplied to the space or process will require moisture to be added to maintain relative humidity conditions. Moisture is generally provided utilizing steam injection and, in some cases, water atomized by utilizing compressed air. In the cGMP environment, the moisture added

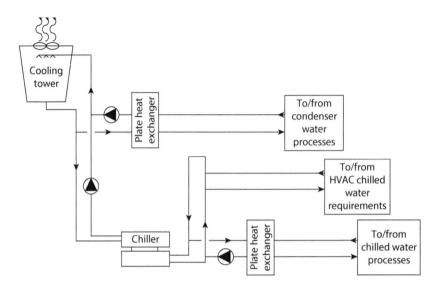

FIGURE 5.2 Typical cooling system.

must not be a source of contamination. Its source is therefore generally purified water that is then atomized or converted to clean steam. These humidifiers are typically constructed of stainless steel.

Dehumidification Systems

In cases of high latent loads from processes or high quantities of outside ventilation air, the building cooling system must be designed for the higher dehumidification requirements. Several moisture removal methods are available. These include low-temperature latent cooling used in concert with reheating, solid and liquid desiccant drying systems, and the injection of sterile, dry compressed air into the airstream. In all cases, room or process air can be treated centrally or locally. All methods must consider minimization of product contamination.

Supply Air Handling Systems

An air system has the greatest influence over the environment within the space or process that it serves. It assists in determining the temperature, moisture level, and cleanliness of that environment. It also assists in the relative pressurization of the space or process.

Space Supply Air Handling Systems

Supply air systems are divided into four specific components: prime movers, distribution, terminal control equipment, and terminal distribution equipment.

Prime movers on the supply air system are generally enclosed in an air handling unit comprising several components. The device that drives the air is a fan. The largest consideration for supply air fans in this industry is generally capacity control and turndown capability to accurately match the requirements of the supply air system. Coils are used to transfer heat into or out of the airstream. As described in the heating and cooling discussions above, many different heat transfer fluids may be used for heating and cooling.

Humidification devices are often placed inside of the air handling unit, but can also be installed within the ductwork outside of the unit, saving unit casing cost. Primary concerns in their specification are the moisture source and vapor trail, which are both potential contributors of biological and chemical contamination.

Air systems tend to be noisy. Contributors are primarily fans, dampers, and terminal air control boxes. Sound attenuation devices are often placed in or near the air handling unit to decrease the radiated noise of the fan. Attention must be paid to the type of attenuator, which could be a source of particulates and microbial contamination.

Filters are generally the first and last devices in the pharmaceutical manufacturing air handling unit. Intake prefilters protect the unit components from dirt and contamination. Final filters at the unit discharge protect the system and ultimately the space and process. Terminal filters are also often specified. See discussion below on terminal distribution equipment (Figure 5.3).

Distribution is generally sheet metal ductwork, although it can be piping or other materials. The greatest consideration is often the material. Galvanized sheet steel is most often used, but it is difficult to sanitize. If the ductwork material is open to product or product space or must be frequently decontaminated, it is often specified as stainless steel. Another important consideration is accessibility, both inside and outside for cleaning and testing. Other considerations for the ductwork design are the size of the ductwork and leakage rate.

Terminal control equipment includes air volume control boxes, terminal heating and cooling coils, terminal humidification, and sound attenuation. Air volume control boxes control the air quantity delivered to the space, and in concert with other supply, return and exhaust boxes within the space and adjacent spaces control space relative pressurization. Terminal cooling coils provide for space subcooling and dehumidification. Terminal heating coils are provided for reheat of space air to support dehumidification and room temperature control. Accessibility for maintenance is the primary concern for these devices. Terminal humidifiers may be used if needed to provide additional moisture to the processing spaces. As with central humidifiers, the primary concern is potential contamination from the moisture source or carryover. Terminal sound attenuation masks the noise from terminal boxes, and as with central attenuators, proper selection of the attenuator type is important to limit potential contamination from particulates and microbial growth.

Terminal distribution equipment includes diffusers, registers, grilles, and terminal filtration. Diffusers, registers, and grilles introduce air into a space. Proper application of the different types of devices is critical to maintain effective distribution. The airflow direction into the space is important. Unidirectional diffusers are often specified instead of aspirating type to provide, in concert with the exhaust terminal device, a "sweeping" effect in the room to more effectively remove particulate from the space. Another important consideration is device cleanability within the space. The device must not be a source of contamination. Terminal filtration is applied most often where space cleanliness is paramount. While this application of filtration can protect the space and product from contaminants within the air system, it can also protect the air system from product or contaminants within the space in case of system failure. Important considerations for the selection and placement of terminal filtration are its location, change-out requirements, and accessibility for testing.

Other important design considerations are as follows: The supply air system, more than any other system, controls the space temperature and relative humidity. Utilizing cooling and heating coils and methods of humidification and dehumidification, all within the supply airstream, each space is controlled to maintain the required conditions.

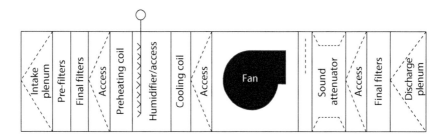

FIGURE 5.3 Typical air handling unit configuration.

In order to achieve specific cleanliness classifications, clean, HEPA filtered air is provided to the space. HEPA filtration is generally 99.97% or 99.997% effective on particles 0.3 microns or larger as measured by the dioctyl phthalate (DOP) method. DOP is a particulate matter that measures 0.3 microns in diameter or larger and is used in the testing of HEPA filter material (Figure 5.4).

Air is often terminally filtered to avoid contamination through ductwork. If the room is clean, the air is clean, and the space is positively pressurized, the only source of contamination to the product and process is from personnel or materials brought into the environment. By increasing the amount of clean air provided to the space, the density of contaminants is reduced by dilution. Many articles and papers have been published discussing the association between cleanliness class and the amount of clean air that must be delivered to the space.

The density of contaminants is also affected by the physical relationship of the source to the product, as well as the airflow patterns around them. A unidirectional or laminar flow of air should be provided with a minimum velocity of 90 fpm at the aseptic critical zone (or any ISO 5 area). Also, placing a source of contamination upstream of the product area must be avoided.

A means of avoiding local contamination and providing for a higher level of cleanliness at the critical area is to supply air at the point of use (e.g., directly over a filling line) in an enclosed or semienclosed environment. Semienclosed environments include laminar flow hoods or curtained laminar flow modules. Totally enclosed environments are completely enclosed stationary or portable equipment that house the critical procedure and sometimes the entire process in a controlled microenvironment. The popularity of these technologies is growing in sterile products manufacturing.

The U.S. FDA cGMP regulations for finished pharmaceuticals concerning HVAC systems are general. The proposed regulations dealing with large-volume parenterals, however, are more rigorous.

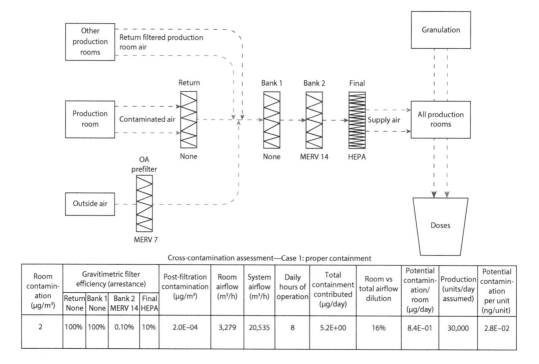

Cross-contamination assessment—Case 1: proper containment

Room contamination (µg/m³)	Gravimetric filter efficiency (arrestance)				Post-filtration contamination (µg/m³)	Room airflow (m³/h)	System airflow (m³/h)	Daily hours of operation	Total containment contributed (µg/day)	Room vs total airflow dilution	Potential contamination/ room (µg/day)	Production (units/day assumed)	Potential contamination per unit (ng/unit)
	Return None	Bank 1 None	Bank 2 MERV 14	Final HEPA									
2	100%	100%	0.10%	10%	2.0E−04	3,279	20,535	8	5.2E+00	16%	8.4E−01	30,000	2.8E−02

FIGURE 5.4 HVAC system configurations and filtration.

PROCESS SUPPLY AIR HANDLING SYSTEMS

Air can be utilized directly in the manufacturing process in various ways. It can be used to draw off dust and solvent fumes; it can be used to dry a granulation as in a fluid bed dryer or tray dryer; it can also be used to dry a tablet coating as it is applied, as in a film or sugar coating pan. Process exhausted air and its treatment is discussed later in the "Process Exhaust Air Systems" section.

The process supply airstream characteristics determine the environment within the process. These include temperature, relative humidity, and cleanliness. The process supply air temperature and relative humidity are solely determined by the product and process requirements. Air can be dehumidified, cooled, heated, and humidified, as required. Cleanliness is also determined by the product and process requirements. Because the air comes in contact with open product, it is often filtered through a HEPA filtration system.

Process air is generally provided to each process by an individual air handling unit, which may include a supply air fan, dehumidification, cooling coils, heating coils, clean steam humidifier, and final filtration, as required. Some processes utilize a powerful exhaust fan that precludes the need for a supply fan. Dehumidification, humidification, heating, and cooling can be applied as needed. Final filtration of the supply air is usually mandatory.

Cross-contamination prevention is a regulatory requirement. Process air handling systems should not be common to each other without positive separation systems (reliable fan operation, backdraft dampers, air control dampers, etc.). It is better to avoid the possibility of a problem by utilizing completely individual systems. The distance between the air handling unit components and the process is generally critical. Equipment and control reaction times and maintainability and accessibility will govern the location of support equipment relative to the process.

EXHAUST AND RETURN AIR SYSTEMS

Exhaust systems can have a great influence over the environment within the space or process that they serve. They evacuate contaminated air to be filtered or processed in some other manner and return it to the supply air unit or the atmosphere. They also assist in the relative pressurization of the space or process and can aid in the removal of unwanted heat and moisture from within a space or process.

SPACE EXHAUST AIR SYSTEMS

Several different types of exhaust air systems can serve each space. The general room air exhaust or return air system normally aids in maintaining pressurization, temperature, and relative humidity of the space, as well as the dilution of airborne contaminants to maintain cleanliness or a nonhazardous environment. Other exhaust systems, including dust collection and local scavenging systems for solvents, and so forth, remove air with more concentrated contaminants, generally at the source. This can include vapor, fume, or particulate contamination or even excess heat. Terminal capture device design is extremely important, as the more effective a collection device is, the more contaminant it removes from the source and the less air it uses.

Generally, room air that is difficult to treat for contaminants or from which it is impractical to remove excess heat before reuse in the space is exhausted to the outdoors. Regulations may require, however, that the air be treated before being released to the environment. If there is manageable contaminant and heat content, the air is generally returned to the space after processing (filtering) and cooling and dehumidification. This treatment may take the form of filtration or vapor or fume removal.

It is important to note that manifolded systems tend to have lower concentrations due to system dilution from unused points. Diluted airstreams are safer but tend to make contaminant removal more difficult and expensive.

A major consideration in particulate transport systems is the transport velocity. Low velocity will cause particulates to drop out of the airstream. High velocity will cause high distribution pressures and require more energy for transport. This concept is especially important in dynamic operation of manifolded systems. The potential for static electricity generated by the particulate movement must also be carefully considered, primarily from a safety standpoint. Distribution systems must be properly grounded to prevent discharge. Cleanability is also an important consideration, primarily in material selection and provision of access into the distribution system.

PROCESS EXHAUST AIR SYSTEMS

Air supplied to an open product process cannot be returned and must be exhausted. Process exhaust may have particulate, solvents, or other vapors or fumes. These, of course, may require treatment before release to the environment. See the "Exhaust Air Filtration," "Dust Collection," and "Vapor and Fume Handling and Treatment" sections below for discussion of exhaust processing methods. See the "Exhaust System Safety" section for discussion of explosion isolation, venting, and containment.

CONTAMINANT CHARACTERIZATION AND HANDLING

Space and process contaminants can include unwanted particulate, vapor, fume, or biological. These can be a nuisance or a hazard to product quality and personnel health and safety from a chemical or biological standpoint. The handling of the contaminants must be carefully considered, including the removal from the space or process and the support of dilution within the space or process, the collection and handling of the contaminants or contaminated air, and the treatment of this effluent. Table 5.2 generalizes primary treatment techniques and their application.

EXHAUST AIR FILTRATION

Particulate-laden air is treated with filtration to remove the contaminant to an acceptable level. The efficiency of the filtration system is measured by the percentage of particulate above a given size that is removed from the airstream that it is serving. Filter efficiencies generally range from 20% to 99.999% (these are called HEPA filters). Filtration can be done in stages of efficiencies to provide the appropriate overall effectiveness. For example, suppose that a high degree of filtration efficiency is required, say 95%, for a reasonably dusty environment, such as a coating process. Ninety-five percent efficient filters alone would continually overload in a short period of time and would require extremely frequent and costly replacement. A staged filter system, utilizing 35% and 60% prefilters and 95% final filters, would provide a much more effective system and require less expensive filter replacements.

Where the level of particulate in the airstream is extremely high or when unacceptable levels of fumes or toxic chemicals are present, alternate methods of removal must be employed. Careful consideration to filter change-out and potential exposure to filtered contents must be made when selecting filtration systems. Methods for removal of filter media are available to minimize or eliminate open handling of contaminated filters.

TABLE 5.2
Mechanical Approach to Waste Material Treatment

Technology/Contaminant	Particulate	Organic Vapor	Inorganic Vapor	Biological
Particulate filtration	X			X
Carbon bed filtration		X		
Wet scrubbing	X		X	X
Incineration		X		X
Adsorption		X		
Absorption		X		
Condensation		X		

DUST COLLECTION

Extremely high levels of particulate require larger filter surface areas and a means of collecting the particulate buildup from the filtration material. A dust collector is essentially a plenum. Particulate, which has been conveyed to the collector at high duct transport velocities, settles in the comparably lower velocity of the plenum. The particulate is then collected outside of the plenum, either via gravity to a container below or, in the case of larger installations, by a method of material conveyance, such as belt or screw conveyor.

Filters are generally located within the dust collector to capture the finer, more buoyant material. These filters are usually bags or cartridges. The downstream side of the filters is pulsated either mechanically or by utilizing a blast of compressed air to shake loose material collecting on the filter media. High-efficiency final filters may also be included, depending on overall system filtration efficiency requirements. As with exhaust system filtration described above, careful consideration to duct collector media change-out and potential exposure to collected contents must be made when selecting dust collectors.

Filtration is not always required, however. In the case of the cyclone separator, a high efficiency of particulate removal can be attained with a correct configuration, without the requirement for downstream filtration.

VAPOR AND FUME HANDLING AND TREATMENT

If the air exhausted from a process contains airborne toxic or otherwise harmful chemicals, it is probable that the Clean Air Act will require these materials to be removed from the air before release into the environment. These chemicals include organic and inorganic vapors and particulate. Organic vapors and particulate are most often found in the pharmaceutical manufacturing environment. Particulate filtering is discussed in the "Dust Collection" section above. Organic vapors can be dealt with in several ways. These include incineration, adsorption, condensation, and absorption.

Incineration converts organic vapors to carbon dioxide, water, and other elements using combustion. When these vapors are present in low concentration, a supporting fuel such as natural gas may be required to assist in burning the vapors.

Adsorption is the process by which organic substances are retained on a granulated surface. Some of these include activated carbon, silica gel, and alumina. Activated carbon is most effective and efficient.

Absorption is the process by which contaminants are transferred from a gas stream to a liquid stream. Some of these include water, caustic soda, and low-volatility hydrocarbons.

Condensation is the process by which the airstream is cooled or pressurized to the point of condensation of the organic compound to be removed. The condensate can either be recovered and purified for further use or disposed of in an approved manner.

Process effluent that requires particulate and vapor or fume treatment can be staged such that particulate is removed utilizing filtration, and then fumes or vapors are treated utilizing one of the methods outlined above.

EXHAUST SYSTEM SAFETY

In many processes, volatile materials are used. These materials may be flammable solvents, dusts or powders, or a combination of the two. In order for an explosion hazard to exist, a heat source, a fuel source, and an oxidizer are needed in sufficient quantities.

Explosions are classified as deflagration or detonation. A deflagration is an ignition and burning with a flame front. A detonation, which can be extremely violent, is a deflagration whose flame front velocity has exceeded the speed of sound. It is critical that a deflagration be contained and controlled and not allowed to become a detonation.

There are several control methods, including containment, isolation, venting, and arresting. These can be used separately or in combination with one another, depending on the size and volatility of the process. In smaller, less volatile processes, the equipment or distribution may be able to withstand an explosion. Generally, upon ignition sensing, the process must be isolated from other systems utilizing high-speed explosion dampers so that the equipment will contain the explosion. In larger and more volatile processes, the equipment cannot withstand the full force of the explosion and the process must be vented. In these systems, upon ignition sensing, the process will be isolated from other systems and, as the resulting pressure rises in the process, a vent will release to the outdoors and the explosion will be vented. In all cases, the reaction times of these systems are measured in fractions of a second and their selection is extremely critical.

Arresting is a process of removing the heat from the flame front. Arresting devices, placed in the airstream, are extremely efficient heat dissipaters. When a flame front passes through an arrestor, the heat is removed, even as the fuel and oxidizer are present.

To help avoid explosions, the system must be completely grounded to prevent buildup of static electricity, and devices and equipment should be spark-proof or purged with an inert gas.

MECHANICAL SYSTEM INSTRUMENTATION AND CONTROL

Similar to other pharmaceutical facilities, manufacturing facilities rely on BASs for coordinated control of the building mechanical and electrical systems. These may also be referred to as building management systems (BMSs) or facility management systems (FMSs). The BAS is separate from process control systems associated with manufacturing process equipment. The modern BAS consists of a network of direct digital control (DDC) controllers or control panels. These DDC panels are distributed controllers interfaced to their associated building systems through inputs and outputs. Examples of inputs are space temperature and relative humidity, airflow, room differential pressure, and valve and damper position indication. Examples of outputs are a fan start command, variable-frequency drive (VFD) speed control, and valve or damper modulation. Inputs come from instrumentation such as temperature sensors and valve limit switches. Outputs go to control devices such as starters, variable-speed drives, and automatic control valves.

The BAS is programmed to execute a sequence of operations for each building system to maintain building conditions within design parameters and operate the equipment efficiently and reliably. In order to achieve the required reliability, sequences of operation must include different operating scenarios, as well as planned failure modes. These include system operation upon the loss of building electric power and failure of major components or equipment devices. While each DDC controller operates in a stand-alone fashion, the controllers are networked together for coordinated operation and response to changes in conditions.

In addition to direct inputs and outputs through instrumentation and controls, other building systems and equipment are often integrated with the BAS through network communication interfaces. Chillers, variable-speed drives, and lighting control panelboards are examples of intelligent building equipment with self-contained microprocessor controls that commonly interface with the BAS. There are many available methods for interface. These include "open protocols" established by standard organizations or manufacturers' associations, older standard serial communication schemes, and proprietary interfaces developed by individual BAS manufacturers and third-party software vendors. The specifications for the intelligent building equipment and the specifications for the BAS must both indicate requirements for the network interface and require coordination of the communication interface between the equipment supplier and the BAS supplier.

The BAS may also monitor critical equipment such as freezers, refrigerators, and controlled environment rooms that support the manufacturing process. These monitoring functions may also be provided through a separate independent system. These functions need to be established early in the design process so that BAS panels are located where required and with adequate capacity to accommodate the full range of requirements.

The BAS can also aid in PM by automatically generating maintenance work orders on a scheduled or run-time basis. BASs can be interfaced with fire and security alarm systems to provide comprehensive monitoring and reporting capabilities. All of these capabilities can be provided on a single-building basis or for an entire building complex or campus.

Control of space conditions within established parameters is important to product quality, so these conditions must be monitored and archived as part of manufacturing records. Many BAS suppliers have developed reliable and secure data archiving software that is designed and qualified to meet industry guidelines for electronic record keeping. The need for this level of qualification must be determined during design and included in the system specifications. Often this application will require a more stringent level of quality control and documentation, including validation of the BAS or a portion of the BAS. Validation requirements for the BAS must be considered during design and addressed in the facility validation plan. Because validation increases the cost of BAS, it is sometimes appropriate to segregate the BAS into discrete segments for building system control and general monitoring and for monitoring and archiving of critical space conditions. With this approach, the more stringent quality control and documentation requirements associated with validation may be applied only to the segment of the system monitoring critical conditions.

Important design considerations include the implementation of well-thought-out sequences and consideration of dynamic turndown and system diversity. Accuracy must be carefully considered in the selection of components. Accuracy costs money, and selection can easily reach a point of diminishing returns. Carefully written failure sequences can lead to capital savings due to not purchasing redundancy and backup generation while minimizing productivity losses. Maintenance is an especially important consideration when it comes to instrumentation. Devices must be periodically calibrated according to an established plan.

PROCESS AND PIPING SYSTEMS

The process and piping systems, including plumbing, gases, true process systems, and fire protection, provide a critical role in the manufacture of pharmaceutical products. The FDA, through the current Good Manufacturing Practices and guidelines, has set strict facility requirements for the process and piping systems.

WATER SYSTEMS

Potable Water System

Potable water system supplied by the local authority to the building or site is generally referred to as domestic cold water. The facility domestic cold water is the base for all other water types required by the processes. The domestic cold water quality may be increased before any use in the facility by filtering, softening, or chlorinating. The potable water must be supplied under continuous positive pressure in a plumbing system free of defects that could contribute contamination to the water and therefore to any drug product. The base water quality must be potable as defined by the Environmental Protection Agency's Primary Drinking Water Regulations set forth in 40 CFR 141.

Domestic cold water is generally used for the following purposes:

- General nonpurified water usage, including toilet rooms, equipment wash (not including final rinse), and water fountains
- Source water for the domestic hot water system
- Source water for the purified water systems
- Makeup water for HVAC water systems

It is permissible for potable domestic cold water to be used for cleaning and initial rinse of drug product contact surfaces, such as containers, closures, and equipment, if it is considered to be potable water, meets the Public Health Service drinking water standards, has been subjected to a process such as chlorination for microbial control, and contains no more than 50 microorganisms per 100 ml. To prevent contamination of potable water from systems or processes, an air gap (in the case of an open filling operation) or a backflow preventer must be employed. This prevents contaminants (including product) from infiltrating water supply systems. Often, the prevention device is placed centrally in the system, thereby creating separate potable and nonpotable water systems, thus avoiding the requirement for multiple devices that need frequent inspection and maintenance.

Domestic Hot Water

The domestic hot water system utilizes domestic cold water as a source. Water is heated generally by steam or electric resistance and stored for use. Domestic hot water is generally circulated throughout the facility so that hot water is readily available without waiting for warm-up. Domestic hot water is used for ordinary facility usages such as toilet rooms and equipment wash (not including final rinse). Other hot water requirements are satisfied by heating the purified water. As with the domestic cold water system, a cross-contamination prevention device may be placed centrally in the hot water system, providing separate potable and nonpotable hot water distribution systems.

Purified and Process Water Systems

Purified water for process and cleaning needs is normally produced from domestic cold water. There are many grades of purified water, such as reverse osmosis (RO) water (purified by RO), deionized (DI) water, USP purified water, and WFI. Selection of the appropriate water grade is based on the requirements of process where the water is used. See Chapter 6 for further discussion on this topic.

DRAINAGE SYSTEMS

Drainage systems remove effluent from spaces, systems, or processes. Generally, the drainage system type, construction materials, and segregation and treatment requirements are dictated by the effluent involved, whether it is product-laden water, final rinse water, toilet room effluent, mechanical system drainage, solvent, acid, or caustic. In all cases, backflow considerations are critical. Different drainage system types are discussed in the following sections.

Sanitary Waste Systems

A separate sanitary waste drainage and vent system is provided to convey waste from toilets, lavatories, nonprocess service sinks, and floor drains. Sanitary drainage is connected to the site sanitary sewer system generally without treatment. Any other materials or product that may present a hazard or environmental problem in the sewer system must be conveyed by a separate waste and vent system.

Laboratory Waste Systems

A separate laboratory waste drainage and vent system is often provided in cases where acids or bases used in laboratory processes must be sampled and potentially neutralized before disposal into the sanitary waste system. A batch or continuous neutralization system may be utilized.

Process Waste Systems

A separate process waste drainage and vent system is often provided in cases where products used in the manufacturing process must either be contained separately or treated before disposal into the sanitary waste system. If they are contained, they are usually removed by tanker truck and disposed of off-site. Because the process drainage may be potentially hazardous and poses a potential environmental contamination threat, the drain system must either be protected (e.g., by using a double-wall piping system) or installed in a location that is easily monitored (e.g., exposed service corridors).

Hazardous Material Waste and Retention

Separate hazardous waste drainage systems are provided in cases where hazardous materials such as solvents, toxins, radioactive materials, and concentrated chemicals must be contained. Generally, these systems are limited in distribution and highly contained. They can either be local, such as in-lab safety containers, or larger, such as of a solvent spill retention system in a dispensing area.

Storm Drainage Systems

A separate storm drainage system is provided to drain rainwater from all roof and area drains. This system is generally not combined with any other drainage systems. Precautions must be taken to ensure that contaminated fluids cannot flow into the storm drainage system.

General loading dock apron area drains can connect to the site storm drainage system and are typically provided with inline sand and oil interceptors. In case of potentially hazardous material spills, a valve is generally provided in the drainage system to isolate the affected drainage area.

PLUMBING FIXTURES AND SPECIALTIES

Washing Facilities and Gowning Areas

The FDA requires that adequate washing facilities be provided for personnel, including hot and cold water, soap or detergent, air dryers or single-service towels, and clean toilet facilities easily accessible from working areas. Gowning areas are also required and must be equipped with surgical-type hand-washing facilities and warm-air hand-drying equipment. Other fixtures must be provided to meet specific facility requirements and those of the local building codes and standards.

Gas Systems

Many types of gases are utilized in the manufacturing process. The most prevalent of these include compressed air used in the process and controls, breathing air for hazardous environments, nitrogen, vacuum, vacuum cleaning, natural gas, propane, and other process systems. All gases used in manufacturing and processing operations, including the sterilization process, should be sterile filtered at points of use to meet the requirements of the specific area. Any gases to be used at the filling line or microbiological testing area must also be sterile filtered.

The integrity of all sterilizing air filters must be verified upon installation and maintained throughout use. A written testing program adequate to monitor integrity of filters must be established and followed. Results are recorded and maintained.

Compressed Air

In general, compressed air should be supplied by an oil-free-type compressor and must be free of oil and oil vapor unless vented directly to a noncontrolled environment area. It should also be dehumidified to prevent condensation of water vapor (generally to around −40°F dew point). Centrally distributed compressed air is generally provided at 100 to 125 psig, and the pressure is reduced at the use points as required.

Breathing Air

Breathing air is generally provided for use by personnel working in hazardous environments. It can be provided centrally through a breathing air distribution system or at the local level with backpack-type breathing air units worn by each person. Personal units are more cumbersome but less expensive than a central system. In either case, the system must be designed to work with the delivery device employed by the user. Air must be purified to meet Occupational Safety and Health Administration (OSHA) grade D breathing air requirements. System reliability must be provided in the design with redundancy or storage to provide for escape time in case of equipment failure.

Nitrogen

Nitrogen is an inert gas generally utilized in the pharmaceutical laboratory and manufacturing environments primarily for the purging of electrical equipment in volatile or explosive environments. If nitrogen is utilized extensively throughout the facility, a central distribution system will generally be provided. Nitrogen, however, can also be provided locally utilizing small individual bottles or generators. In the central system, nitrogen may be distributed at 100–125 psig with pressure regulation as required. Laboratory nitrogen is generally provided at lower pressures (40–90 psig).

Vacuum

Vacuum is utilized throughout pharmaceutical laboratory and manufacturing facilities. A great deal of vacuum is utilized in encapsulation and tablet compression areas. Vacuum is generally generated at between 20 and 25 in. Hg and provided at between 15 and 20 in. Hg at the inlet. Once again, process and equipment requirements will dictate pressures and quantities.

Natural Gas and Propane

Natural gas and propane are sometimes required in the pharmaceutical laboratory environment and for such processes as maintaining solvent oxidization and heating hot water and generating steam. Gas is generally distributed to laboratory outlets at 5 to 10 in. WC.

FIRE PROTECTION SYSTEMS

This section describes, in general terms, the various automatic fire suppression and protection systems and their application in pharmaceutical manufacturing facilities. Pharmaceutical manufacturing facilities are typically provided with automatic fire suppression and protection systems throughout. The provision of specific suppression and protection throughout the facility might be the consequence of a strict code requirement, a trade-off for increased allowable building area or height, or simply good fire safety and life safety design practice.

DESIGN CODES AND STANDARDS

Fire protection systems are designed and installed in accordance with locally adopted building codes and National Fire Protection Association (NFPA) standards. Insurance underwriter's requirements and guidelines (FM, IRI, Kemper, CIGNA, etc.) may also be incorporated as applicable.

SPRINKLER SYSTEMS

Wet sprinkler system: A sprinkler system with automatic sprinkler heads attached to a piping system containing water and connected to a water supply so that water discharges immediately from sprinkler heads that are opened directly by heat from a fire.

Dry-pipe sprinkler system: A sprinkler system using automatic sprinklers attached to a piping system containing air or nitrogen under pressure, which, when released during the opening of the sprinkler heads, permits the water pressure to open a dry-pipe valve, which allows water to flow into the piping system and out of the opened sprinkler heads.

Preaction sprinkler system: A sprinkler system using automatic sprinklers attached to a piping system containing air that may or may not be under pressure, with a supplemental detection system (smoke, heat, or flame detectors) installed in the same areas as the sprinklers. Actuation of the detection system opens a valve that permits water to flow into the sprinkler piping system and be discharged from any sprinkler heads that may be open. Preaction systems can operate in one of three ways. Single-interlock systems admit water to the sprinkler piping upon operation of detection devices. Noninterlock systems admit water to the sprinkler piping upon operation of detection devices or automatic sprinklers.

Double-interlock systems admit water to sprinkler piping upon operation of both detection devices and automatic sprinklers.

Deluge sprinkler system: A sprinkler system using open sprinkler heads attached to a piping system connected to a water supply through a valve that is opened by the operation of a detection system (smoke, heat, flame detectors, etc.) installed in the same areas as the sprinklers. When the valve opens, water flows into the piping system and discharges from all attached sprinkler heads.

Antifreeze sprinkler system: A wet-pipe sprinkler system using automatic sprinkler heads attached to a piping system containing an antifreeze solution and connected to a water supply. The antifreeze solution is discharged, followed by water, immediately upon operation of sprinkler heads opened directly by heat from a fire.

Foam-water sprinkler system: A special system of piping connected to a source of foam concentrate and a water supply and equipped with appropriate discharge devices for extinguishing agent discharge and for distribution over the area to be protected. The piping system is connected to the water supply through a control valve that is usually actuated by operation of automatic detection equipment (smoke, heat, flame detectors, etc.) installed in the same areas as the sprinklers. When this valve opens, water flows into the piping system, foam concentrate is injected into the water, and the resulting foam solution discharging through the discharge devices generates and distributes foam. Upon exhaustion of the foam concentrate supply, water discharge will follow the foam and continue until the system is shut off manually.

Foam-water spray system: A special system of piping connected to a source of foam concentrate and to a water supply and equipped with foam-water spray nozzles for extinguishing agent discharge (foam and water sequentially, in that order or in reverse order) and for distribution over the area to be protected. System operation arrangements parallel those for foam-water sprinkler systems, as described previously.

Closed-head foam-water sprinkler system: A sprinkler system with standard automatic sprinklers attached to a piping system containing air, water, or foam solution up to the closed-head sprinklers and which discharges foam or water directly onto the fire after the operation of a sprinkler. These systems can also be dry-pipe or preaction-type systems.

STANDPIPES

Standpipes are designed and installed in accordance with locally adopted building codes and NFPA standards. Typically, standpipes are required if the floor level of the highest story is more than 30 ft above the lowest level of fire department vehicle access or the floor level of the lowest story is located more than 30 ft below the highest level of fire department vehicle access. Standpipes are also typically required if any portion of the building floor area is more than 400 ft of travel from the nearest point of fire department vehicle access.

The installation of standpipes and hose stations may be desired independent of code requirement, especially if there is an on-site emergency response organization trained to respond to fire emergencies.

FIRE WATER SOURCE AND CONVEYANCE

The water supply for automatic fire suppression and protection is provided in accordance with the locally adopted building code and NFPA standards. If an adequate supply of water is not available from a public source, an on-site source of water will need to be provided. If the source of water has inadequate pressure to provide the required sprinkler protection, a fire pump (electric or diesel) will also need to be provided. The decision as to whether the pump is electric or diesel will need to be made based on the availability of electricity, reliability issues, underwriter requirements, maintenance issues, and cost.

GENERAL DESIGN REQUIREMENTS

The building will typically be provided with one or a combination of systems to provide automatic fire suppression and protection throughout the building. Suppressing agents other than those mentioned above, such as CO_2, dry chemical, foam, and halon alternatives, can be used to address specific hazards, but not as a suppression agent throughout the entire facility.

In general the first choice for automatic fire suppression is a wet-pipe sprinkler system. This most common type of system provides the quickest actuating, most reliable, and least expensive type of suppression for most applications. Wet-type sprinkler systems are generally used throughout most of the facility.

Protection of spaces for storage, handling, and dispensing of flammable and combustible liquids is a prime candidate for low-expansion foam-water sprinkler systems such as closed-head foam-water sprinkler systems, due to containment requirements in the event of fire and subsequent sprinkler discharge or flammable or combustible liquid discharge. High-expansion foam and dry chemical systems are also applicable to these spaces.

In areas that are susceptible to water damage or where contamination is a concern, the use of preaction sprinkler systems is appropriate. These spaces may include computer rooms, high-voltage electrical rooms, telecommunications rooms, sterile areas, containment areas, and other GMP spaces. At a minimum, a single-interlock preaction system can be provided. Where the accidental or unnecessary discharge of water is a concern, a double-interlock preaction system can be provided.

Dry-pipe valve systems are appropriate for use in unheated spaces such as remote detached buildings, warehouses, outside loading docks, combustible concealed spaces, and parking garages. Antifreeze sprinkler systems are also appropriate for unheated spaces but are typically limited for applications requiring 20 sprinkler heads or less, such as small loading dock areas or vestibules. Caution must be taken with the application of these systems to support local water company requirements with regard to cross-connection control (backflow prevention) due to the addition of antifreeze to the sprinkler system.

CONTROL AND MONITORING

Water flow detection sensors and alarms are typically provided for each floor, zone, or specific hazard space and are monitored by the building fire alarm system. Each floor or zone is equipped with electrically supervised water supply control valves that are also monitored by the building fire alarm system. Other conditions, such as fire detection and loss of air pressure, are monitored for preaction, dry, and deluge-type systems.

PORTABLE FIRE EXTINGUISHERS

Portable fire extinguishers are provided to suit the type of hazard and are provided in accordance with locally adopted building codes and NFPA 10, "Portable Fire Extinguishers." Extinguishers are typically of the dry chemical multipurpose ABC type, but can be water, CO_2, or other substance, depending on the occupancy and hazard involved.

ELECTRICAL AND POWER DISTRIBUTION SYSTEMS

ELECTRICAL SYSTEM DESIGN CONSIDERATIONS FOR FACILITY RENOVATION OR NEW CONSTRUCTION

Understanding the following is essential when designing electrical systems for a pharmaceutical manufacturing facility:

- Electrical utility and services characteristics when selecting a site for a pharmaceutical manufacturing plant.

- Normal and emergency electrical power distribution systems within the manufacturing plant.
- Electrical distribution and utilization equipment, such as transformers, motor controllers, lighting, industrial control panels, light fixtures and motors that are commonly installed in the manufacturing plant.
- Requirements and recommendations within the United States for installation, maintenance and operation of electrical equipment for hazardous areas and for the risk assessments associated with potential arc flash and shock hazards.
- The requirements of the production facility and critical processes, such as the product's specifications and its CQAs. In some instances, the facility should be equipped with a special lighting system due to the drug material's sensitivity to light.
- Electrical power and control equipment and components must be selected properly based on legally adopted building codes and published industrial standards. This is especially true for installations in clean rooms and production areas.
- Electrical Codes and Standards. Table 5.3 lists some of the codes and standards that provide the minimum requirements and guidelines for the design of electrical installations within the pharmaceutical plant and facility in the United States and countries in the European Union (EU). Other countries have similar codes and standards. Although there are similarities between the codes and standards utilized in the United States, plants designed using U.S. codes and standards are not acceptable in the EU, and vice versa.

POWER DISTRIBUTION OVERVIEW

Electrical power distribution circuits installed within pharmaceutical plants should deliver reliable electrical power. Electric power is reliable when the power supply at the point of utilization is at the proper voltage, is clean with minimal noise (harmonics), and is derived from an adequately sized power distribution system that has selectivity.

The frequency of power system failures is inversely proportional to the power system reliability. Power system failures are caused by either an electrical fault or the loss of utility power. Reliability is greatly enhanced with the installation of on-site backup power supply systems, which include uninterruptible power supplies (UPSs) and emergency generators. Upon the loss of normal power, the backup power systems must provide emergency power for a defined period of time for critical or essential loads and for legally required loads, such as egress lighting and exit signs. In addition to the minimum periods of time for operation that are defined by building codes, the operating times for the delivery of emergency power has to consider the effect of the power interruption on the process, including the completion of a batch process or bringing the process to a point where the quality of the product will not be jeopardized.

Advances in power electronic technologies, which are nonlinear loads, will continue to enhance the cGMP process and other systems within manufacturing plants. Nonlinear loads include VFDs, uninterruptable power supplies, electronic ballasts in lighting fixtures, light-emitting diode (LED) lighting power supplies, and other devices that creates a direct current (DC) power source, including

TABLE 5.3
Minimum Electrical Design Requirements for Electrical Installation

Codes and Standards	United States	EU
Installation	NFPA 70 (NEC®)	IEC 60364
Electrical machinery	NFPA 79	IEC 60204
Equipment and material	Underwriter's Laboratory (UL)	CE and ATEX

personal computer power supplies. The high-frequency on and off switching action of these devices create nonlinear distortion, which causes noise on the electrical power distribution system feeding the nonlinear loads. This noise is commonly referred to as harmonics. Harmonics can never be eliminated, but can be attenuated and must be considered in the design of electrical power circuits for pharmaceutical equipment. Excessive harmonics can be destructive and can interfere with the operation of the process instrumentation.

The voltages shown in Table 5.4 are commonly specified for manufacturing equipment based on the electrical power available from the public utility at the location of the plant site.

In urban areas where the electrical infrastructure is substantial, the utility circuit is a more reliable source of electric power than on-site power generation. The reliability of the utility power circuit or circuits at the site where a pharmaceutical plant or facility might be constructed should be a consideration in the site selection. Utility circuits that run on pole lines next to busy highways are much less reliable than utility circuits that are not subjected to vehicular traffic accidents. Because of harmonics, pharmaceutical plant services should always have a dedicated utility or plant-owned transformer. The transformer is integral to or ahead of its incoming electrical service to the pharmaceutical plant. Neighboring facilities that could be connected to the same utility transformer will have harmonics, possibly including the most destructive third harmonic. The third harmonic and other triplet harmonic currents will not pass through a two-winding, delta–wye or wye–wye, three-phase transformer. Non-triplet harmonic currents and voltages, the 5th, 7th, 11th, 13th, 17th, 19th, etc., will pass through the transformer but will be attenuated by the impedance within the transformer's windings.

When selecting a location to construct a new pharmaceutical plant, the "stiffness" of the utility's power distribution system must also be considered. Stiffer power systems produce high short-circuit power and are better in absorbing the harmonics created by nonlinear loads within the pharmaceutical plant. Systems that can produce high short-circuit power will, however, require overcurrent protective devices with higher short-circuit ratings, resulting in higher initial costs.

A power distribution system that is properly designed will include overcurrent and overload protection equipment that provides selectivity. Selectivity is "a general term describing the inter-related performance of relays and breakers, and other protective devices; complete selectivity being obtained when a minimum amount of equipment is removed from service for isolation of a fault or other abnormality."[*] In other words, when complete selectivity exist, only the faulted (short-circuit or overloaded) portion of an electrical distribution system will be disconnected, allowing the remaining portions of the electrical system to continue to operate properly. The term *selectivity* also can refer to a system's ability to transfer to an alternate power source when power is lost from the normal source.

TABLE 5.4
Common Voltages

North America (60 Hz)	Europe and Singapore (50 Hz)
120 V, 1 phase, 3 wire	230 V, 1 phase, 3 wire
208 V, 1 phase, 3 wire	400 V, 1 phase, 3 wire
240 V, 1 phase, 3 wire	400 V, 3 phase, 4 wire
208/120 V, 3 phase, 5 wire	400/230 V, 3 phase, 5 wire
240 V, 3 phase, 4 wire	
277 V, 1 phase, 3 wire	
480 V, 1 phase, 3 wire	
480 V, 3 phase, 4 wire	
480/277 V, 3 phase, 5 wire	

---

[*] Institute of Electrical and Electronics Engineers (IEEE) Standard C37.100-1992.

Normal Power

Normal electrical power is the electricity that is normally provided by the electric utility and is available at the process and other equipment within the pharmaceutical plant. It is delivered to the equipment through the plant's normal electrical power distribution system.

Normal power sources must be within the allowable voltage tolerances for the manufacturing equipment. The design of power sources and power distribution systems must consider voltage drop across conductors and transformer taps, while also considering the amount of nonlinear loads and the risk of an arc flash hazard event. Transformers need to have primary or secondary winding taps that can be adjusted to account for the voltage drop. Good design limits the voltage drop across feeders to 2% and across branch circuits to 3%. Distributing electric power at a higher voltage than the utilization load voltage is typically the preferred approach. Using 480 V feeders with local 208/120V transformers reduces problems with voltage drop, reduces the short circuit levels at 120/208V utilization equipment and reduces the risks of electrical hazards when the equipment is maintained.

Emergency Power

Emergency power distribution system circuits that carry emergency power for life safety systems must be reliable and comply with adopted building codes. Typically, emergency egress lighting levels of 1 foot candle are required in the United States and 1 lux in the EU. Emergency egress lighting is required along the floor along the path of egress from the building upon the loss of normal power. Exit signs and fire alarms are additional examples of life safety loads. Emergency power may also be provided for optional manufacturing processes and manufacturing equipment. Defining the emergency power requirements and selecting the power sources are important steps in the design of electrical power systems within the plant.

Emergency power sources can be storage batteries, on-site electrical synchronous power generator sets, two separate utility services when the utility circuits are deemed extremely reliable, UPSs, or unit equipment (DC battery-powered light fixtures that illuminate DC lamps on the loss of alternating current [AC] normal power). Unit equipment and light fixtures used for emergency lighting must be selected and located so that the loss of an individual lighting element (lamp) cannot leave an area entirely in the dark.

Emergency power for life safety systems, when required, must be available seamlessly or within an acceptably short period of time (e.g., within 10 s) as defined by applicable codes and standards. Emergency power for optional loads needs to be available based on the process or HVAC requirements (typically within 60 s). Diesel engine generator sets can be used with automatic transfer switches (ATSs) to meet the 10 s requirement, whereas natural gas engine sets will typically take too long to come up to speed. Another consideration is the possible requirement for having the fuel on site. This requirement may change in certain localities as the reliability of the natural gas supply continues to increase.

Reliability

Reliable electrical power systems deliver continuous electricity to loads at their utilization voltage. When designing an electrical power distribution system for the manufacturing plant, each load should be evaluated as to its relative need for reliable power compared to other loads within the plant. The fewer electrical circuits and electrical components there are between the power sources and the load, the more reliable the power system is for the load. This is the reason building codes require that the number of feeders within the manufacturing plant between the service and the elevator branch circuit be kept to a minimum.

The reliability of the electrical power distribution system directly affects the production and other operation of the manufacturing plant. The plant's electrical power distribution system should be designed based on a projected number of failures per year and the time it takes to repair these failures. Electrical power distribution systems should be kept as simple as possible.

POWER DISTRIBUTION SYSTEMS

Power distribution systems are composed of components that include

- Utility-owned or plant-owned service transformers that are typically provided in a pad-mounted, weatherproof enclosure and installed outdoors.
  - Utility-owned transformers typically use mineral oil and should be located as far away from the building as possible, never near windows and doors. These need to be installed per the utility company requirements and are protected by utility-owned overcurrent and short-circuit protective devices, often fuses. Mineral oil transformers may explode when they catch fire.
  - Plant-owned transformers will require medium-voltage (>1,000 V) plant-owned overcurrent and short-circuit protective equipment, typically either a medium-voltage fused load break switch or a medium-voltage circuit breaker with protective relays. Plant-owned transformers can be located indoors or outdoors and can use mineral oil and other liquids or be dry, having cast coil construction. In order to comply with insurance company requirements, ester-based fluids such as EnviroTemp®, which is not harmful to the environment and is less flammable then mineral oil, have been used. Even though the cost of the EnviroTemp liquid filled transformers may be higher, money can be saved by eliminating the need for separation, containment, barriers, and deluge sprinkler systems.
- Low-voltage (1,000 V) utility service or services that deliver power to the pharmaceutical plant or facility start at the secondary terminals of the service transformers. Electrical power may be supplied to the plant or facility by one or more utility services dependent on the total demand or load or as required by code. In the United States, the National Electric Code (NEC®) requires a separate electric service for electric fire pumps for the plant's sprinkler system. Each service which can consist of more than one set of service entrance conductors must terminate on the line side of no more than six adjacent service disconnecting switches that have overcurrent protection. Overcurrent protection can be provided by fusible switch or circuit breaker. The fuse or circuit breaker will provide overload protection for the service entrance conductors and short-circuit and overload protection for the feeder on the load side of the protective device. For services and feeders with voltage above 150 V to ground but not exceeding 600 V phase to phase, the service-fused disconnect switches and circuit breakers rated at 1,000 A and higher must also have ground fault protection (GFP) when installed in the United States. Because ground fault protection can result in nuisance tripping, the size of the service's fused disconnect switches and circuit breakers should be considered when designing the service distribution equipment with the intent of increasing reliability while maintaining selectivity.
- Feeders are used to distribute power between the service disconnecting switches or circuit breakers and the panelboards, sometimes referred to as load centers, and motor control centers that have short-circuit and overload protective devices (fuses or circuit breakers) located throughout the plant. Transformers, which have a primary feeder and a secondary feeder, are part of the power distribution system.
- Branch circuits include short-circuit and overload protective devices in the panelboards or motor control centers and the conductors that connect utilization equipment and motors to the power distribution system.
- In addition to overcurrent and short-circuit protection, consideration should be given to providing undervoltage protection and surge protection on the feeders and the service. This is especially true for power systems that have motor starters that do have solid state overload relays with single phase protection.

MOTOR CONTROL CONSIDERATIONS

- All motors require control, short-circuit protection, and overload protection.
  - Manual motor starters consist of an on and off switch with a thermal overload device. Short-circuit protection is provided by the circuit breaker or fuse protecting the branch circuit to the motor starter. Building codes provide the criteria for selecting and sizing the motor disconnect switch, the short-circuit protection, and the overload protection. Some small motors can have integral overload protection and do not require an external overload device.
  - Combination automatic starter use an electrically operated contactor, which is specifically sized for the motor's full load current, a separate short-circuit device and a separate overload device to protect the motor. The contactors come in various forms, including full-voltage nonreversing; reversing, which switches two-phase conductors to reverse the direction of the motor's rotation; and reduced voltage. The short-circuit device can be a fuse, a thermal magnetic circuit breaker, or a magnetic-only circuit breaker that is referred to as a motor circuit protector. The size and selection of overload and short-circuit protection are defined within building codes.
  - VFDs, which are being used more than ever before, replace the electro-mechanical motor starters. VFDs have many benefits, including their ability to soft start, run loads at optimum speeds, and even know when a pharmaceutical batch is blended based on the change of viscosity. VFDs also have an excellent power factor. VFDs have to be selected based on their application. The same VFD will have a different horsepower rating for constant torque loads versus variable torque loads. VFDs can include overload protection for the motor when the overload protection that is integral to the VFD meets the requirements of the building codes. Short-circuit protection can be provided by a fuse or thermal magnetic circuit breaker, not by a motor circuit protector, which is sized to protect the VFD.
  - Solid-state overload relays normally provide single-phase protection and GFP, whereas thermal elements, although less expensive, do not.
  - The use of capacitors for motor power factor correction or to reduce the sizes of power distribution equipment, as was commonly done for many years, should be avoided. Nonlinear loads, such as VFDs and UPSs, create harmonics on the power system that could create a high resonant short circuit at specific frequencies within the capacitor. The high currents will cause heating and can blow current-limiting fuses protecting the capacitors. Capacitors cannot be connected to the load side of VFDs.
- Appliances, such as heaters, ovens, and anything that is not a motor, which plug into or are connected to electrical outlets within the electrical power distribution system, are protected by the branch circuits' fuses and circuit breakers.

ENERGY CONSERVATION

Energy conservation codes have been adopted by states and local governments within the United States. One of the code requirements is the ability to turn off half of the light fixtures within a space that is not equipped with occupancy sensors. In addition to code requirements, the plant operating costs can be reduced through conservation efforts such as: the use of high-efficiency motors (when the load on the motor is 60% or more of its nameplate rating); the use of dry transformers rated at 80°C rise versus 150°C rise; the use of LED lighting fixtures, which will not only reduce electrical loads, will also reduce the heat load in the space; and the use of VFDs for variable torque loads, such as fans within air handling units.

GROUNDING

Incorrect power system and equipment grounding is the most common cause of problems and outages within manufacturing plants. These are not failures in the power system but are failures in the design and installation of the power systems. Because of the requirement to install GFP on 1,000 A and larger feeders, entire sections of the plant could lose power for a relatively small fault when the GFP device trips instead of the small circuit breaker feeding the branch circuit where the ground fault occurred.

Building a pharmaceutical plant and not performing power systems studies during its design versus after the construction documents are issued is foolish and will lead to design-related failures. Having proper and complete one-line diagrams, which identify the grounding of transformers, generators, and ATSs, along with the complete time–current characteristic (TCC) coordination curve, is essential during the design and not afterwards.

There are two types of electrical grounds:

- System grounds, which connect the neutral or common conductor of a grounded power system to earth. With the exception of outdoor service transformers, the neutral conductor is grounded at the service disconnect switch only. The size of the grounding electrode conductor and the types and numbers of grounding electrodes, which include ground rods, are defined by building codes. Except for autotransformers, a new power distribution system is separately derived on the secondary of every transformer, and the transformer secondary neutral conductor must be grounded at one point only, either ahead of or at the first overcurrent fuse or circuit breaker on the secondary of the transformer.
- Equipment or earth grounds, which include metal raceways and non-current-carrying copper conductors run with the current-carrying conductors, are bonded together to ground at many points within a power distribution system. These serve as the path for return ground fault currents to the transformer and are essential to the proper operation of short-circuit devices.

Grounding systems should be commissioned after installation. Measurements of grounding data will be stored in the engineering files and are not generally verified periodically. Usually grounding measurements are repeated only on as-needed bases, if there are reasons for retesting. Visual review of bonding should be included in the PM procedures.

HAZARDOUS AREAS

Classified areas, as the term relates to electrical installations within pharmaceutical plants, may include areas surrounding equipment where flammable and combustible liquids or combustible dusts are processed, transmitted, handled, or stored. Hazardous area analyses are performed to determine if areas are classified or non-classified, the boundaries of the classified areas, and level of the hazard within each defined boundary.

Hazardous area analysis for flammable and combustible liquids considers the containment media, the ventilation within the area, the temperature, the volume and pressure of a combustible substance, and the characteristics of the combustible substance for locations where combustible substances are handled, stored, or transported. Where a process uses open flames, the areas are not classified. Hazardous area analysis for combustible dust considers the quantity of dust, the natural and mechanical ventilation, and housekeeping practices.

In the United States, at a minimum, the following standards are used for hazardous area analysis:

- NFPA 497, "Recommended Practice for the Classification of Flammable Liquids, Gases or Vapors and of Hazardous (Classified) Locations for Electrical Installations in Chemical Process Areas"

- NFPA 499, "Recommended Practice for the Classification of Combustible Dusts and of Hazardous (Classified) Locations for Electrical Installations in Chemical Process Areas"
- NFPA 70, "National Electrical Code®" (NEC®) Articles 500, 501, 502, and 503 are used for installations in hazardous areas that are classified using the class/division system. NEC® Article 505 is used for installations in hazardous areas that are classified using the class/zone system. One system must be selected, and areas classified under one system cannot overlap into areas classified under the other system. Areas cannot be classified under both systems, and there are restrictions on where these areas can be next to each other.

In Europe, ATEX Directive 99/92/EC (Reference 8, Appendix 5) defines three zones for gases, mists, or vapors (Zone 0, Zone 1, and Zone 2) and three zones for dusts (Zone 20, Zone 21, and Zone 22). These zones require equipment of Category 1 for Zones 0 and 20 (very high level of safety), Category 2 for Zones 1 and 21 (high level of safety), or Category 3 for Zones 3 and 22 (normal level of safety).

Electrical circuits and components that are installed within hazardous areas might be installed within explosion-proof enclosures where the heat generated by an explosion within the enclosure caused by an electric spark is eliminated before leaving the enclosure, or within air-purged enclosures, which will not allow the volatile vapors or dust to enter the enclosure. The requirements for purged enclosures can be found in other NFPA and International Electrotechnical Commission (IEC) standards.

Low-energy circuits such as thermocouples that are commonly used for instrumentation may be classified as intrinsically safe circuits and can be installed using general wiring methods. NEC® Article 504 provides the minimum installation requirements for these circuits.

HAZARD ASSESSMENT

Power system equipment that is installed in accordance with applicable codes and maintained in accordance with the manufacturers' and testing agencies' requirements, and when applicable, within closed cabinets or boxes, does not present hazards to people or the facility. When cabinets are opened or the equipment is being interacted with in a manner other than normal operation of the equipment, electrical hazards can exist. Empirical formulas that can predict the incident energy, which is the energy on a surface released by sustained electrical arcs have been developed and published for electrical power circuits. These formulas and associated methods are included within, or incorporated by reference into, safety standards for the purpose of warning workers of the potential arc flash hazards. Understanding how to reduce the potential arc flash hazards, through both design and the use of arc energy reduction devices, is now a fundamental part of the design of electrical power circuits. Not performing arc flash analysis during the design of a power distribution will reduce the reliability of the power distribution system for all but the simple power distribution systems and must be considered when installing electrical equipment within clean rooms or process areas within the pharmaceutical facility.

PREVENTIVE MAINTENANCE AND CLEANABILITY

Electrical circuits and components should be inspected on a periodic basis and should have an annual comprehensive PM program. NFPA 70B, which is not a legally adopted building code, provides guidance for electrical maintenance requirements. In Europe, the periodic inspection is defined by local regulations and may not require annual activities.

All electrical devices should be rated by the manufacturer and will function to meet the requirements of the processes and environmental conditions where the equipment is installed. Periodic inspections and maintenance activities will be developed to ensure the integrity of electrical systems.

PM procedures performed within clean rooms and production areas are most frequently related to inspecting and cleaning electrical devices. The housekeeping of electrical equipment always has many levels, starting with surface wiping and ending with contact cleaning. It is important to keep electrical devices clean and in good operational condition. Electrical failures can disable a significant part of the plant and may be even the entire plant operation.

Electrical equipment within clean rooms and production areas must be specified to be cleanable and, in some cases, able to be washed down. Equipment that does not meet these requirements not only violates the adopted building code but also jeopardizes the integrity of the pharmaceutical products. Standards for specifying equipment for various levels of exposure to water, duct, and so forth are published in both the United States and EU and must be followed to comply with the building codes.

PROCESS EQUIPMENT AND MACHINERY

Standards that should be followed for the electrical design and installation of electrical power and control systems for pharmaceutical processes and equipment include NFPA 79, "Electrical Standard for Industrial Machinery," in the United States and IEC 60204, "Safety of Machinery—Electrical Equipment of Machines—Part 1: General Requirements," in the EU.

FURTHER DISCUSSION

1. Describe the components and function of a typical heating system.
2. Describe the components and function of a typical cooling system.
3. Describe each of the different types of sprinkler system contained in this chapter. List the benefits and drawbacks of each system.

ABOUT THE AUTHORS

Jack C. Chu has more than 30 years of pharmaceutical experience in both engineering and productions, including facilities, critical utilities, process systems, automation systems, and manufacturing operations. His experience includes R&D operations, safety assessment, pilot plants, and pharm-biomanufacturing. His focus is on vaccine manufacturing process and engineering. Jack has worked more than 20 years for Merck & Co., Inc. in various positions and responsibilities. He is a frequent speaker for various pharm conferences and technical programs and holds professional engineer licenses in many states; he has been a member of the International Society for Pharmaceutical Engineering (ISPE) since 1997. He is the chairperson for developing the ISPE Baseline Guide *Oral Solid Dosage Forms* in 1998, the second edition in 2009, and the third edition in 2015. Jack is the coauthor of *Good Design Practice, GMP Facility*, Second Edition (2015) and *Facilities and Support Systems Optimization—GMP Compliance, Productivity, and Quality*. Jack lectures on pharmaceutical manufacturing engineering in the graduate study program at Stevens Institute of Technology, Hoboken, New Jersey.

Leonid Shnayder is an industry professor in the pharmaceutical manufacturing and engineering program at Stevens Institute of Technology, Hoboken, New Jersey. He came to Stevens after a 30-year career in the industry, where he worked as both a process engineer and a research scientist on a wide variety of projects. His areas of expertise include finished pharmaceutical manufacturing, biotechnological processes, and clean-in-place and clean process utilities (pure steam, water-for-injection, USP purified water, etc.). He was responsible for the process design of biotech facilities for Amgen, Wyeth, and ImClone, and finished pharmaceutical facilities for Merck, Boehringer Ingelheim, Wyeth-Lederle, and others. Prior to that, he worked as a research scientist in process development with a national pharmaceutical company in Russia, where he was involved in the development and optimization of various fermentation processes, including biosynthesis of penicillin, oxytetracycline, and other antibiotics.

Joe Maida is an entrepreneur and engineer. After obtaining a BS and an MS in electrical engineering from Drexel University, Philadelphia, Pennsylvania, and 4 of his 18 current project engineering licenses, Joseph, with the help and support of his wife, Nancy, left his job with Day and Zimmermann, Inc. and started Maida Engineering, Inc. Since 1978, as president of Maida Engineering, Joseph has personally or administratively overseen many of the numerous large and small projects in various markets and a number of disciplines performed by his company. Joseph's technical skills and knowledge have evolved from performing engineering on relatively simple to very complex projects. Some of his personal projects, which were completed during the last 10 years, include the replacement of the motors, drives, lubrication systems, and controls for two helicopter blade 4,050 hp dynamic balancing towers; the replacement of an existing wind tunnel's AC wound rotor and DC motors with a 18,000 hp synchronous motor and a 22,000 hp, 36-pulse VFD; the engineering and design of a 6 MW, 13.2 kV mission-critical electrical power generation and distribution system for the Philadelphia Veterans Medical Center; the conceptual design and code analyses and preparation of the functional specifications for the replacement of the motor, drives, and controls for the tram systems within the St. Louis Gateway Arch; the installation of 5 MW standby power distribution system and priority load management control system for a pharmaceutical R&D campus; a new cement plant's 34.5 kV and 4,160 V, 20 MVA power distribution system; a hazardous area analysis for areas containing fossil fuel dust; numerous power system studies, including load flow, voltage drop, short circuit, equipment evaluation, TCC coordination, motor starting, harmonics, and arc flash analyses; the remodeling of numerous commercial kitchens; the power distribution and control of new outdoor and indoor lighting; a new command center; the study for upgrading a large data center's standby and interruptible power supplies; the installations of new services, feeders, and branch circuits for pharmaceutical, fiberglass, and cement plants and commercial buildings, HVAC and mechanical equipment and renovations to buildings; and the Mechanical, Electrical and Piping (MEP) design for a 120-apartment university student resident complex. Joseph is a member of the National Society of Professional Engineers (NSPE), Purdue Society of Professional Engineers (PSPE), Institute of Electrical and Electronics Engineers (IEEE), and Practicing Institute of Engineers (PIE), through which he reviews and approves courses and activities for professional engineering credit hours of the State of New York.

6 High-Purity Water

Gary V. Zoccolante

CONTENTS

INTRODUCTION

The importance of process water to a pharmaceutical manufacturing facility cannot be overstated. Production of water used for drug manufacturing is a great challenge in every aspect of design, implementation, and maintenance. Water is the most widely used material in pharmaceutical manufacturing and is often the most costly. The percentage of water in finished products varies from zero to greater than 90%. A greater volume of water is used in cleaning and rinsing processes than in formulation in most facilities. Regardless of the water volume used in the actual drug, formulation of all pharmaceutical water is subject to current Good Manufacturing Practices (cGMPs) even when the water does not remain in the finished product.

Water treatment systems are often investigated in great depth by U.S. Department of Health and Human Services Food and Drug Administration (FDA) inspectors. Poor design and inadequate maintenance of water systems have led to countless FDA 483 citations, warning letters, and in certain cases, recalls of pharmaceutical products.

Optimization of pharmaceutical water systems is a risk management exercise that requires extensive utilization of good engineering practice (GEP). The design team must make decisions regarding water quality, method of generation and distribution, sanitization method, instrumentation and control, data acquisition, and other design details. Construction and maintenance specifications are all based on the impact of the consequences of water system success or failure. Optimization is a delicate balance of acceptable risk and available financial resources. Pharmaceutical companies are under intense pressure to reduce costs while maintaining maximum product safety with minimal patient risk. Competence in pharmaceutical water requires knowledge of pharmacopeial requirements, GMPs, GEP, chemistry, microbial control, sanitization strategies, many unit processes, generation options, storage and distribution options, and commissioning and qualification requirements.

This chapter provides readers with information in all of these areas that can be utilized in conjunction with the recommended related reading to be able to produce a conceptual design for a pharmaceutical water system. Practical options are provided for the generation and distribution of pharmaceutical water so that the reader can know what has been done in existing facilities. Advantages and disadvantages are presented to aid in the selection of desirable configurations.

EXECUTIVE SUMMARY

Sound water system design requires knowledge of both external and internal quality requirements. External requirements are set by pharmacopeial groups worldwide. Internal requirements are typically set by quality groups and often exceed external requirements. Pharmacopeial groups set the therapeutic drug standards for a country or region, as well as standards for drug ingredients. Water standards are set by these pharmacopeial groups. Required water quality and methods of manufacture often vary with different regulatory groups. The required water quality is determined by use and product destination. Use can be for product manufacturing, active ingredient production, cleaning, medical device manufacturing, ophthalmics, topicals, consumer products, and many other applications. The water design team must properly specify the correct water quality. The products and product destinations must be defined to understand what regulatory requirements must be met. Parenteral products require a minimum of water for injection (WFI) quality. Oral dosages require a minimum of purified water (PW) quality.

Inspection agencies such as the U.S. FDA work in conjunction with pharmacopeial groups to enforce regulations and set requirements for GMPs. GMPs are rarely specific regarding water and must be interpreted to be properly applied. Groups such as the FDA are likely to find more issues with water system GMP compliance than with water quality compliance.

All water systems must comply with GMPs, and system design is a risk assessment exercise. The variation in system design and cost is extreme, as risk aversion and company standards vary significantly. Pharmaceutical companies assess many factors, including product dosage form, water use, destination, and product name recognition. Large cost discrepancies occur from differences in materials of construction, instruments and control, sanitization methods, documentation, testing, and many other factors.

System maintenance is critical to proper operation. Regulatory agencies frequently monitor maintenance, standard operating procedures (SOPs), operator training, record keeping, and other related factors. In many cases, soundly designed systems have been cited by regulators for improper maintenance and poor operator compliance with SOPs.

Systems usually comprise generation equipment and storage and distribution equipment. Water quality requirements must be met at both locations, and proper sanitization of both system segments is critical. Sanitization of generation equipment is either chemical or thermal, and distribution sanitization is chemical, heat, or ozone. The sanitizer choice impacts cost, microbial control effectiveness, and system uptime availability. Selection of sanitization methods for generation and distribution is one of the most important decisions that water system designers must make. The decisions significantly impact microbial control, risk, and costs. Both capital cost and operating cost are affected.

Pharmaceutical companies have historically produced WFI by distillation. Distillation has historically been a required method in all countries complying with the European Pharmacopoeia. Recently the European Pharmacopoeia Commission posted a press release regarding adoption of a revision of its monograph for Water for Injections (0169). "Up to now, the production of Water for Injections (WFI) had been limited to distillation only. The revision allows for production of WFI by a purification process equivalent to distillation such as reverse osmosis, coupled with appropriate techniques. The revised monograph will be published in the Ph. Eur. Supplement 9.1 and will become effective in April 2017." This revision aligns the EP WFI requirements closely with the USP and JP WFI requirements and will likely increase the implementation of robust membrane based alternative systems in the future. Distillation will certainly remain in operation in many facilities and be implemented in many new facilities, but the overwhelming domination of distillation for WFI will likely change significantly. Many other locales, including the United States, allow alternative methods of production, but if a product is manufactured for worldwide distribution, distillation must be used until the EP WFI revision becomes effective in April 2017. PW can be produced by any method. Chemically regenerated ion exchange (IX) units dominated PW production decades ago, as membrane-based production was new and unproven. Membrane-based production is dominant now, as most companies try to minimize chemical discharge. Chemical discharge is also eliminated with use of off-site regenerated IX systems.

GOOD MANUFACTURING PRACTICES

One of the most significant issues in water system design and operation is that although the GMP requirements are well documented in writing, they are very general and subject to continually tightening interpretation as cGMPs. The FDA establishes cGMP requirements beyond those that are documented in legal compendia, but rarely publishes written guidelines with any level of detailed engineering guidance.

Most of the GMP requirements for water are derived from broad statements in 21 CFR 211. These general statements relate to the requirement for water used in production or cleaning processes to not "alter the safety, identity, strength, quality or purity of the drug product." The statements directly open all water system unit operations, contact surfaces of equipment and piping, installation, and maintenance to FDA scrutiny. All materials must be proven to be compatible with the product and process and must not contribute objectionable contaminants.

Additional 21 CFR 211 GMP requirements for verification of proper cleaning and sanitization procedures mandate written records and procedures for these steps. All rinse and cleaning water qualities must be proven to be appropriate.

Most of the engineering details that are considered to be cGMP requirements have evolved over decades of system development since the birth of the concept of GMP manufacturing. Several key concepts of cGMP production of water have been adopted from the long considered, but never adopted "Good Manufacturing Practices for Large Volume Parenterals," 21 CFR 212. This legislation was proposed in 1976 and finally removed from consideration in 1994. Although the "GMPs for LVPs" document was never approved, many concepts proposed in the document have become commonplace in pharmaceutical systems. Some of these concepts include storage tank vent filters, minimal piping dead legs, sloped and fully drainable distribution systems, flushed pump seals, double-tube sheet heat exchangers, and elimination of use point filters. These concepts and others will be discussed in more detail in pharmaceutical water system design section.

Due to the perceived ambiguity of cGMP regulations, great disparity exists in both individual and corporate views regarding what constitutes a cGMP-compliant water system. System costs may vary by more than an order of magnitude from company to company, with all groups believing that each system is optimized for cGMP construction and good design practice. The proper materials of construction, surface finishes, level and accuracy of instrumentation, automation level, data acquisition and trending, sanitization methods, system and component draining, use of microbially retentive filters, and many other factors are open to interpretation. The decisions made by the design team in these areas of design and construction have great impact in capital cost, operating costs, and risk management. The team may solicit input from consultants' vendors and construction contractors to help in completion of the design specifications. Significant capital and operating cost savings are available to those who properly interpret the cGMP requirements and do not overdesign the system.

PHARMACOPEIA GROUPS

It is important to understand the roles of the FDA and the U.S. Pharmacopeial Convention (USPC). The USPC is a private not-for-profit organization established to promote public health. The USPC works closely with the FDA and the pharmaceutical industry to establish authoritative drug standards. These standards are enforceable by the FDA. More than 4,700 standards monographs are published in the United States Pharmacopeia (USP) and National Formulary (NF). The monographs for water used in pharmaceutical manufacturing for products used in the United States are published in the USP.

Other pharmacopeial regulations, such as the requirements of the European Pharmacopoeia (PhEur), the Society of Japanese Pharmacopoeia (JP), and the Chinese Pharmacopoeia (CP), may need to be considered in the water system design and water quality testing for products that are exported from the United States. The ultimate destination of drug products or drug substances determines the regulatory requirements that must be satisfied.

WATER QUALITY REQUIREMENTS

The types of water defined in the pharmacopeial monographs, such as PW and WFI, are known as compendial waters. Other quality waters used in manufacturing, not defined by USP or other recognized compendia, are known as noncompendial waters. Noncompendial waters can be used in many applications, such as production of many active pharmaceutical ingredients (APIs) and in many cleaning and rinsing steps.

Noncompendial waters are not necessarily lower quality than compendial waters. Noncompendial waters range from water that is only required to meet the U.S. Environmental Protection Agency (EPA)

National Primary Drinking Water Requirements (NPDWRs) to water that is specified to exceed the requirements for WFI. Noncompendial water systems are not necessarily less tested, maintained, or validated than compendial waters, and are subject to the same cGMP requirements.

The water quality specification required for manufacturing is a function of several factors. Where will the product be shipped? If production is for the United States only, the water specification will be principally based on USP requirements. Shipment to Europe will require compliance with PhEur requirements, and shipment to China will require compliance with CP requirements. Many other countries utilize USP, PhEur, CP, or JP regulations or have their own requirements. In addition to pharmacopeial requirements, water specifications reflect product and process requirements and corporate views toward FDA and cGMP regulations.

Microbial control methods for water systems frequently impact the total cost of water production more than attainment of the chemical attributes of water outlined in USP and other appropriate compendia. The chemical attributes of compendial water listed in the monographs of the governing pharmacopeial groups are generally easily met with a properly designed and maintained system.

The microbial requirements are not stated in the USP monographs, as of this writing, but the maximum action levels are documented in the USP 38 general information chapter <1231> and have been defined by the FDA in the 1993 FDA "Guide for Inspections of High-Purity Water Systems." Although the chemical quality of water must be met consistently at points of use, proper microbial control is the focus of many FDA inspections.

SAMPLING

A sampling and testing plan must be developed for every pharmaceutical water system. This is a cGMP requirement, certainly GEP, and necessary for monitoring system operation and control. It is important to design sampling points into the unit processes to be able to monitor each process for validation, normal operation, and troubleshooting. Test protocols and frequency must be established for each unit process, as well as every use point.

Samples for quality control purposes, as opposed to process control purposes, must be collected in an appropriate manner. As an example, use point samples for hose connections must be collected from actual production hoses using the same flush cycle used in production to prove proper water quality. Regulators do not require sample collection to be done in an unsafe manner, but expect sampling to be done as close to the use point as practical.

Unit process tests should be based on the expected unit performance (e.g., effluent chlorine level for an activated carbon unit employed for dechlorination). Use point testing must be sufficient to prove compliance with both chemical and microbial requirements. Most of the chemical requirements may be proven with online or laboratory conductivity and total organic carbon (TOC) monitoring from a single distribution system sample location. Periodic use point testing is required to verify the single-loop sample location.

A single distribution loop sample for microbial performance is not acceptable. Each use point must be tested at a sufficient frequency to prove that the system is in microbial control. The 1993 FDA "Guide for Inspections of High-Purity Water Systems" suggests microbial testing for a minimum of at least one use point per day, and that all use points are tested at least once weekly. Several recent industry guides have suggested that use point microbial tests can be conducted at reduced frequencies relative to the FDA guide text.

VALIDATION, VERIFICATION, AND QUALIFICATION

It is accepted that all pharmaceutical water systems will be validated or qualified. *Validation* was the term used for decades for the completion of test and inspection protocols to prove that the system was appropriate for the intended purpose. Other terms, such as *verification* and *qualification*, are also used today for this process. Verification and qualification are often used in risk-based qualification of systems. Validation is used for the purpose of the following discussion. The validation plan must be completed to some degree prior to specification of the water system. All equipment suppliers, contractors, commissioning agents, and other implementation parties must be aware of the requirements for documentation, automation life cycle, commissioning and validation overlap, and many other factors to ensure a successful validation. Critical information, such as proper life cycle methodology, instrument certifications, material certifications, weld documentation, and so forth, often cannot be created after the fact if the requirements were not known prior to manufacturing and installation. The most successful validations generally occur when the validation group has been involved throughout the project design phase.

Many groups, including the FDA, International Society for Pharmaceutical Engineering (ISPE), American Society for Testing and Materials (ASTM), and International Conference for Harmonisation (ICH), have promoted a change to a risk-based qualification process. The process of system qualification may be referred to as validation, qualification, or verification, dependent upon company preference and process. The ISPE *Baseline Pharmaceutical Engineering Guide*, Volume 5, *Commissioning and Qualification*, provides a practical approach to traditional system qualification. The ISPE *Good Practice Guide: Approaches to Commissioning and Qualification of Pharmaceutical Water and Steam Systems* and ASTM E2500 provide guidance on risk-based qualification. See Chapter 7 for further discussion.

RELATED READING

The ISPE Baseline Guide *Water and Steam Systems* (Volume 4, Second Edition) provides an excellent overview of all aspects of pharmaceutical water. ISPE *Approaches to Commissioning and Qualification of Pharmaceutical Water and Steam Systems* provides insight into risk-based and traditional qualification methods. The 1993 FDA "Guide to Inspections of High-Purity Water Systems" provides readers with insight into areas that inspectors may pursue.

MONOGRAPH REQUIREMENTS

USP 38 (as of this writing) includes monographs for seven types of pharmaceutical water. Three types of bulk water are defined, as well as five types of packaged waters. The three bulk waters are USP purified water (PW), USP water for injection (WFI), and USP water for hemodialysis. The packaged waters are bacteriostatic WFI, sterile water for inhalation, sterile WFI, sterile water for irrigation, and sterile PW.

Most pharmaceutical products are manufactured with either PW or WFI. PW and WFI have the same chemical purity requirements. The monographs require that the water purity is proven by conductivity and TOC. The conductivity requirement using USP <645> can be met with online testing (Stage 1) or in laboratory testing (Stages 1, 2, or 3). The Stage 1 conductivity test requires measurement of conductivity and water temperature. The conductivity limit varies from 0.6 μS/cm at 0°C to 3.1 μS/cm at 100°C. Intermediate values include 1.3 μS/cm at 25°C and 2.7 μS/cm at 80°C.

Stage 1 conductivity requirements can be reliably attained with a variety of system configurations using common water purification processes. Most pharmaceutical water systems are designed to meet Stage 1 conductivity to take advantage of online testing to provide significant data for trending and minimize laboratory testing. Point-of-use testing generally requires laboratory analysis. Pharmaceutical water that does not meet the Stage 1 conductivity limit can be laboratory tested to meet the Stage 2 or 3 limits.

The TOC test is a limit response test with a theoretical limit of 500 ppb. The test is designed to accommodate virtually any TOC analyzer that meets the USP suitability requirements. Most manufacturers go beyond the pass–fail 500 ppb response test and record and trend values well below the 500 ppb limit. The FDA has been promoting process analytical technology (PAT) for pharmaceutical manufacturing. PAT requires online or at-line instrumentation with recording and trending of critical aspects of systems. Alert and action levels are much closer to normal operating levels than prior periods and well below specification limits. Online TOC and conductivity testing are encouraged with PAT thinking.

The microbial limits for USP PW are not defined in the legally binding monograph. The general information chapter <1231>, "Water for Pharmaceutical Purposes," states that a maximum of 100 colony-forming units (cfu) per milliliter may be used as an action level, and this is also stated in the 1993 FDA "Guide to Inspections of High-Purity Water Systems." The requirements of this general information section are not legally binding, but the FDA has stated publicly on many occasions that this is the maximum level acceptable for USP PW. The actual action level may be much lower than the maximum action level of 100 cfu per ml and is determined by the manufacturer (subject to FDA approval) as a function of product, process, and system performance. Some products and processes require an absence of certain objectionable species, such as *Pseudomonas aeruginosa*, as well as a low total viable plate count.

WFI has the same chemical requirements as PW and has a limit of 0.25 endotoxin units (EU) per milliliter. The microbial level for WFI is also absent from the monograph but is stated to be a maximum action level of 10 cfu/100 ml in USP Chapter <1231>. This is in agreement with FDA views.

The USP 38 PW monograph states, "Purified water is water obtained by a suitable process." This essentially leaves the process selection open to all technologies. The USP 38 WFI monograph states, "Water for injection is water purified by distillation or a purification process that is equivalent or superior to distillation in the removal of chemicals and microorganisms." Several prior volumes of USP limited WFI production to distillation or reverse osmosis (RO).

Distillation currently produces more than 99% of USP WFI. Other processes, such as a combination of RO, deionization (DI), and ultrafiltration, have a significant history of production of WFI quality water for rinsing, API production, and other uses as well as WFI where allowed.

WATER QUALITY SELECTION

The water quality or qualities selected for the pharmaceutical process must be consistent with the final product requirements. The final rinse water must be the same quality as the water used in manufacturing. Oral products must use a minimum of USP PW for manufacturing, and PW is normally used as final rinse water. Since the method of manufacture for PW is not stated by USP, there is little advantage to use of noncompendial water for final rinse water where PW is acceptable.

Parenteral products must use a minimum water quality of USP WFI for manufacturing, and WFI is used in most plants for final rinse water. It is acceptable to use WFI quality noncompendial water for final rinse in parenteral processes if practical. Production of noncompendial WFI quality water may or may not be less expensive than WFI.

The ISPE Baseline Guide *Water and Steam Systems* recommendations are shown in the water quality decision tree in Figure 6.1. Expanded views for laboratory, manufacturing, and cleaning are also shown (Figure 6.2).

The water quality requirements for API and bulk pharmaceutical chemicals (BPCs) are complex. The minimum water permitted in API or BPC manufacturing is water meeting the U.S. EPA NPDWRs or equivalent. APIs use a wide range of waters for manufacturing, initial rinses, and final rinses up to and including WFI. The ISPE Baseline Guide *Water and Steam Systems* water quality recommendations for API manufacturing are shown in Figures 6.3 and 6.4.

The FDA may expect WFI to be used in certain inhalation products depending on use. Water quality exceeding USP PW or WFI requirements may be required for some products, such as intrathecals. A large-volume parenteral product may have to be produced with water with endotoxin limits well below WFI limits, dependent upon the expected patient weight and dosage volume. The manufacturer is required to determine the appropriate water quality.

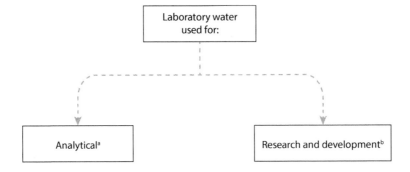

ᵃSome analytical methods require USP compendial waters.
ᵇIf both cGMP and non-cGMP operations follow the cGMP path.

FIGURE 6.1   Laboratory water.

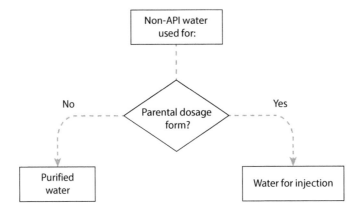

FIGURE 6.2   Water for manufacture.

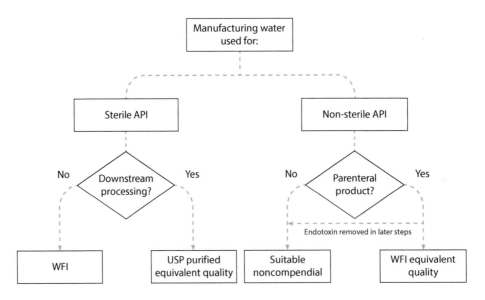

FIGURE 6.3   API process water decision tree—minimum water quality.

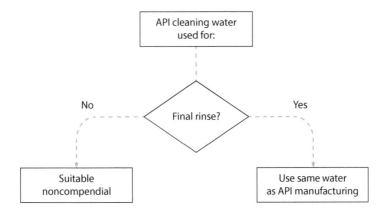

FIGURE 6.4 API cleaning water decision tree.

FOREIGN PHARMACOPEIAL REQUIREMENTS

European Pharmacopoeia 8 has monographs for PW and WFI, as well as a third bulk water, highly PW. The EP 8 PW requirements are similar in many respects to USP 38 PW as of this writing. The chemical purity is defined by TOC and conductivity, but also by a traditional pass–fail test for nitrates.

EP 8 requires WFI to be produced by distillation without exception until April 2017 when the new language that is similar to USP WFI language becomes effective. The chemical requirements are the same as for EP 8 PW, with the exception that the conductivity limit at 20°C is 1.1 µS/cm. The microbial requirements are the same as for USP WFI. The EP 8 endotoxin requirements are the same as those in USP, although the units are expressed as IU/ml rather than EU/ml. The Japanese Pharmacopoeia allows for membrane-based WFI systems. The Chinese Pharmacopoeia is similar to EP 8 in requiring distillation for WFI production.

DESIGN AND COST FACTORS

The capital and operating costs for pharmaceutical water systems can vary significantly as a function of the processes and materials of construction selected. WFI systems has fewer acceptable options for generation, storage, and distribution than PW systems. The microbiological requirements are much tighter for WFI than for PW, and WFI is generally utilized for the most critical pharmaceutical applications. Most WFI systems utilize distillation, are similar in construction, and tend to favor conservative approaches to system design, as detailed in this chapter.

The selection of an appropriate sanitization method for generation, storage, and distribution equipment can impact capital and operating costs significantly. Thermally sanitizable systems generally have higher capital costs due to a greater content of stainless steel components but usually require considerably less labor for sanitization and have less downtime. Thermal sanitization is easier to automate and validate and typically allows attainment of lower microbial levels.

Chemically sanitized equipment has been proven to be acceptable in many applications and may have a lower capital cost, but generally requires more labor to prepare chemicals, verify attainment of proper chemical level during sanitization, and prove proper removal of residual chemical in rinse steps. Implementation of chemical sanitization is not driven by superior performance, but rather by capital cost. Hot water sanitizable equipment is generally higher in capital cost, but lower in operating cost, as sanitization is typically automated where chemical sanitization is labor-intensive.

Future needs and system expansion should be considered at the time of system design. Some unit processes may be practically expanded with a reasonable capital investment, while others are extremely difficult to expand without additional space, equipment, and controls. RO units that are designed for expansion may have increased capacity within the original dimensions through addition of pressure vessels and membranes. Column-based processes such as softeners and activated carbon units are generally impractical to expand without additional unit implementation. Low-cost processes such as softeners are often best oversized initially to allow for anticipated expanded flows in the future. Expansion may be practical from a mechanical perspective, but it may not be practical when production and qualification are considered. Downtime for expansion work and qualification must be considered.

Determine System Capacity Requirements

One of the most critical and difficult steps in the programming of a water system is determination of the optimum generation and storage and distribution system sizing. Optimization requires accurate information regarding individual use point demand and the total manufacturing cycle. Users must provide data regarding flow, pressure, and temperature for each use point over a daily and weekly schedule. At times, this information is estimated prior to confirmation of the production cycle. The water usage chart in Figure 6.5 is an example of projected water consumption on an hourly basis. These data can be used in conjunction with a generation production rate, tank size, and tank makeup levels, as shown in the storage-tank-level chart in Figure 6.6. This exercise predicts tank levels throughout the day to project sufficient or insufficient levels over the operating day. If an insufficient tank level is indicated, changes must be made. Generation output can be increased, tank volume can be increased, or peak draw volumes can be reduced.

All parties involved must resist the tendency to overestimate consumption, or the system may be significantly oversized. Significant system oversizing wastes capital, can lead to microbial issues during operation, and can needlessly increase wastewater generation. Future needs should be considered during system design. Systems can often be designed to run at low flows initially and to be operated at higher flows later, as production needs increase. GEP minimizes capital expenditure without incurring unacceptable risk.

Determining the Optimum Generation System

Good design practice can be applied in the selection of the pharmaceutical water generation system process and equipment specification. Generation system selection should be based on accurate source water information, proper water quality specifications, life cycle cost analysis, sanitization methods, reliability, maintenance requirements, and several other possible factors.

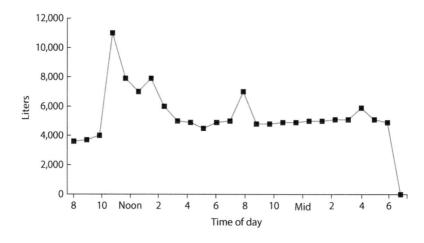

FIGURE 6.5   Water usage chart.

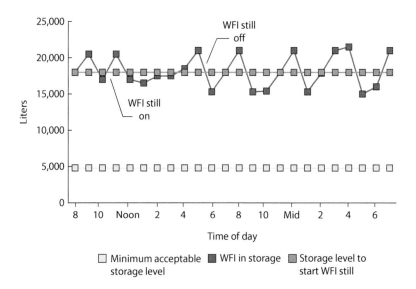

FIGURE 6.6 Tank-level chart.

PHARMACEUTICAL WATER SYSTEM DESIGN

Pharmaceutical facilities may utilize a single grade or multiple grades of water. The water requirements may include the compendial grades of USP WFI or PW or various noncompendial grades. The first decision to make is whether a single grade of water is the best regulatory and economic choice, or multiple grades provide more logical operation. A higher grade of water, such as USP WFI, can also serve as a lower grade, such as USP PW. USP PW, of course, cannot be used as USP WFI. The cost to produce USP WFI may be higher than the cost to produce USP PW, so significant analysis is usually required to optimize system design.

Consider a facility that requires both USP WFI and USP PW. The facility could be best served by production of WFI only to serve both WFI and PW if several factors exist. If the WFI quantity required significantly exceeds the PW requirement, if all or most of the water is used hot (>65°C), and if the WFI and PW use are reasonably congruent, a single WFI system with hot storage is probably the best choice. If the PW requirement is greater than the WFI requirement, the PW is used at ambient temperature, the WFI and PW use points are reasonably divergent, heating and cooling resources are limited or expensive, and separate systems to produce and distribute WFI and PW are probably more logical.

After the choice of single or multiple water systems is made, the systems must be optimized for generation method and storage and distribution method chosen. Generation systems will generally comprise several of the pretreatment, final treatment, and polishing components discussed later in this chapter.

USP Purified Water and Water for Injection Generation Systems

Proper design of USP water systems requires consideration of many factors. Major factors include USP specifications, cGMP requirements, feed water quality, required system availability, raw water cost, plant wastewater discharge limits and costs, labor availability, outside service availability and competence, chemical handling, utility availability, and cost and designs with prior successful history. Previously successful system designs should always be weighed against other viable options unless the prior system design is obsolete or not cGMP.

The ISPE Baseline Water and Steam Guide Committee, after meetings with FDA personnel, determined that the specified water quality for pharmaceutical use must be met at the outlet of the generation system, as well as at the use points. Although some water quality parameters (particularly microbial levels in hot or ozonated storage systems) may improve in storage, the water quality should not fail as generated and depend on improvement in storage to comply with the quality specifications.

System configurations based on RO, IX, and distillation will be reviewed. Each of these systems is discussed in detail later in this chapter. Distillation-based systems have an extensive history of production of both USP WFI and PW. The alternate designs have been primarily utilized for PW production, with a few WFI applications. All designs will be assessed for the capacity to produce both compendial waters.

Most high-volume USP PW systems utilize RO as the primary purification process, with varying additional polishing processes. A technology map shows the most common options for the basic RO-based USP PW systems (Figure 6.7). The number of process steps implemented is usually a function of feed water quality, finished water quality specification, and risk assessment. The addition of an appropriate final endotoxin and microbial reduction process allows production of WFI quality water if the process is proven to be equal or superior to distillation.

The first pretreatment purification step is primary filtration for reduction of coarse suspended solids. Multimedia filtration is selected when labor must be minimized or the expected suspended solids level is low. Disposable cartridge or bag filters minimize capital cost and are a good choice for low suspended solids or low-flow applications.

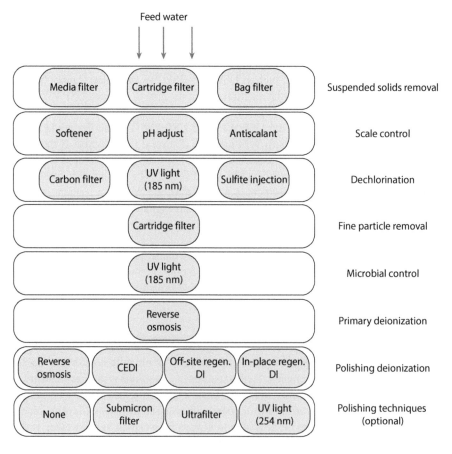

FIGURE 6.7 Reverse osmosis technology map. (Courtesy of Evoqua Water Technologies LCC, Warrendale, PA.)

Scale control is the next pretreatment step. Softening for hardness removal is by far the most popular choice. Addition of antiscalant chemicals is a lower capital cost option. This option is not used in nearly as many applications as softening but is popular where discharge of softener regeneration brine is an issue. Reduction of pH is also used in a small number of systems. The scale control through reduction of pH is very effective, but the negative consequences of carbon dioxide generation limit use of this low capital cost option.

Disinfectant removal is accomplished through implementation of activated carbon, sodium sulfite injection, or ultraviolet (UV) light. Activated carbon may be the highest capital cost option when thermal carbon sanitization is included. Activated carbon is used in a majority of systems when all flow rates are considered because the activated carbon requires little operator attention and can remove any municipal level of chlorine or chloramines. Sodium sulfite injection is the lowest cost option. Dechlorination is effective, but the application rate must be carefully controlled to avoid RO fouling or membrane oxidation. UV light can also be very effective. The sizing of UV light must take peak chlorine or chloramine levels into account.

Final particulate removal prior to RO is accomplished with disposable cartridge filtration. The optimum filter rating is often determined in service. The filter particulate retention and cost must be balanced against RO cleaning frequency and downtime for the application.

The final pretreatment option is microbial reduction through application of UV light. Many companies prefer to place UV light units downstream of activated carbon units to reduce the effluent microorganisms.

The primary treatment process of RO reduces the inorganic, organic, and microbial contaminants to or near USP PW requirements. USP PW TOC and microbial levels are very likely to be met in the RO product water. The conductivity requirement is generally not met after a single pass through RO, and further polishing is typically implemented.

A second pass of RO is a popular option at this point in the system for feed to multiple-effect (ME) stills and USP PW production (and in some cases, USP WFI). The still feed option is popular, as chloride, silica, and conductivity requirements are often met. Some systems also meet the USP PW conductivity limits out of the second RO pass. The product water meets Stage 1 conductivity requirements in some applications and Stage 2 or 3 in others. This design is excellent for low TOC and microbial levels.

Most USP PW systems utilizing RO as the primary process implement an IX process to ensure consistent attainment of USP conductivity with variation in feed water and RO performance. All of the IX, also known as deionization (DI), combinations with RO allow consistent production of USP PW.

Automatic in-place regenerated mixed-bed deionizers (DIs) provide process control but require chemical handling. Off-site regenerated IX units allow conductivity attainment at minimal capital cost. Some internal process control is lost, as outside service is required. The final IX option is CEDI. This option is popular when chemical handling is undesirable and off-site regenerated resin is not cost-effective or does not meet quality assurance requirements.

Many RO/DI-based systems incorporate one or both of the optional post-IX polishing options shown in the RO system technology map. UV light bacteria reduction follows a majority of IX units in systems where microbial control is desired. This process is not implemented when resin regeneration or hot water sanitization provides sufficient microbial control.

Microbially retentive filters with ratings of 0.02–0.45 μm are often implemented to produce extremely low bacteria levels in RO/DI water. These filters allow consistent attainment of low total plate count levels and are very useful where indicator organism limits, such as no *Pseudomonas aeruginosa*, no *Burkholderia cepacia*, or no Gram negatives, exist.

The final option shown in Figure 6.7 is ultrafiltration. This option can provide the endotoxin and microbial control necessary to produce WFI water. Ultrafiltration modules are available in polymeric and ceramic construction. Both membrane types have extensive history in the production of WFI quality water. Some ultrafiltration membranes can be run continuously hot at 80°C or higher for self-sanitizing operation. Systems using the many RO and IX options in the RO system technology map are in great use because they provide consistent USP PW with minimal chemical consumption and are often the lowest evaluated life cycle cost.

Primary filtration may or may not be required to protect other pretreatment components, such as softeners and activated carbon units. The choice of no filtration, multimedia filter, or disposable filter is based on the same logic as the RO-based systems.

Almost all distillation pretreatment systems utilize softening for scale control of the still directly, or to protect a pretreatment RO unit, if implemented, from scale. The use of just softeners as the only scale control is more common for vapor compression (VC) stills than for ME stills. Softening of still feed water can provide adequate protection against hardness-based salt scale but does not eliminate silica scale if sufficient feed water silica is present to make silica scale an issue. The softening can also be accomplished with nanofiltration rather than regenerable softeners.

All stills need protection from chlorine corrosion if feed water disinfectants are present. Activated carbon is currently the most popular choice. Sodium sulfite injection and UV light are used in a relatively small population of distillation feed water systems. The tolerance for feed water free chlorine is generally even lower for stills than most RO units. Either process can require extremely expensive repair when feed chlorine is not reduced to extremely low levels in accordance with the manufacturer's recommendations.

A disposable cartridge filter typically follows media-based pretreatment processes such as activated carbon and softening units. The cartridge removal rating can be relatively coarse and is usually in the 5- to 10-micron range.

The most critical choice in still pretreatment system design is whether to implement inorganic solids reduction. This decision has significant capital cost, operating cost, and maintenance and reliability consequences. The still selection must be made simultaneously to optimize the system. The still feed water requirements for conductivity, silica, hardness, chloride, and other factors must be known.

Some VC still installations operate successfully without RO or IX processes upstream. Still blowdown is generally significantly higher than the rate for RO or DI feed. Others implement RO, IX, or RO/IX upstream to meet requirements for either silica or product water conductivity guarantees, or simply to minimize maintenance and maximize reliability.

Most ME installations incorporate a minimum of RO as feed water inorganic level control. ME stills typically limit chloride, silica, and feed conductivity as a minimum. Single-pass RO can meet these requirements on relatively low total dissolved solid (TDS) waters. Product-staged, or two-pass, RO is very popular on higher TDS waters to meet the feed requirements. RO and any one of the IX processes are often combined to produce ME feed water with minimal inorganic, organic, microbial, or endotoxin contaminants. A final filter for retention of resin fines may be used after the final IX process.

IX system process selection may be based on in-place regenerated or off-site regenerated resin. The first process step is coarse suspended solids reduction, and the selection of multimedia filtration or a disposable filter is determined, as in the cases of RO or distillation-based systems.

Dechlorination typically follows filtration, and the complete removal of chlorine or chloramines is not as critical as pretreatment to RO or stills. The IX resins used in most pharmaceutical systems are tolerant of low levels of chlorine. Activated carbon is the most common selection, as the carbon media can also provide some protection against anion resin organic fouling if the carbon is sized and maintained correctly. UV light is an excellent choice since total dechlorination is not critical and the UV light can provide microbial control.

Some IX-based systems employ anion resin organic scavenging units on high TOC feed waters. These units can provide more consistent and greater TOC reduction than activated carbon on many feed water supplies. This unit process can help to meet the final USP TOC requirement, as well as to protect the IX anion resin from organic fouling.

Coarse cartridge filtration is frequently employed before IX units if multimedia, carbon, or organic scavenging units are upstream. These filters would serve little purpose if no media beds are implemented upstream.

The primary IX process for conductivity attainment may be mixed-bed DI, separate-bed DI, or both. Mixed-bed DI can meet the USP conductivity requirement on almost any EPA qualified feed source. Separate-bed DI units may be implemented upstream for in-place regenerated systems to take advantage of the simpler separate-bed regeneration procedure for the bulk of regenerations. Separate-bed units may be employed in off-site regenerated systems if the economics are favorable.

Countercurrent regenerated separate-bed DI units can meet the USP conductivity limits without mixed-bed polishing on many feed waters. The final reason to consider separate-bed DI units is the superior microbial control impact of the pH shifts through the resin beds.

Most systems utilizing IX resin use filtration downstream of resin beds. Filtration rating ranges from coarse (5–10 μm) for resin fine retention to 0.1 μm or tighter for microbial retention. The operating cost of microbial retentive filters may be high on high colloidal content feed waters.

UV light units are also common downstream of DI units for microbial control. The necessity is based on microbial limits and other microbial control methods, as in RO/DI system design.

All of the DI options discussed have been utilized successfully in hundreds or thousands of applications. The greatest risk in DI systems that do not utilize RO upstream is failure to meet the USP TOC requirement if the feed water is high in TOC. Several DI systems have successfully utilized ultrafiltration or organic scavenging units to compensate for no RO membrane on difficult water supplies.

All IX resins can contribute high TOC levels when first placed in service. This TOC contribution can cause failure of the USP TOC requirement. Special resins that have been through a TOC extraction process can be implemented to eliminate the problem. These resins should be used when new resin is used in off-site regenerated units. New regenerable units can use these resins or go through several exhaustion and regeneration cycles of standard resins to provide low TOC levels.

The most significant advantages of DI-based systems are potential low capital cost if no chemicals are used or if chemical handling and neutralization equipment exist, higher water recovery than RO-based systems if RO wastewater is not reused, and excellent flow rate flexibility.

The principal disadvantages are chemical handling for in-place regenerated systems and process control issues for off-site regenerated systems. Operating costs can be high or low as a function of feed water source, resin regeneration cost, and water consumption.

PRETREATMENT

Most pharmaceutical water systems include pretreatment equipment, primary (or final) treatment equipment, and sometimes polishing equipment. Typically, polishing technologies are not used downstream of distillation. Pretreatment equipment selection must be made after selection of the primary treatment equipment. Pretreatment equipment must be properly selected to protect the final treatment equipment and, in some cases, to meet the final water quality requirements.

Pretreatment equipment typically is implemented to control scale, fouling, and oxidation of final treatment equipment. Scale, or precipitation, occurs when the solubility of sparingly soluble salts is exceeded in the concentrate streams of RO and distillation units. Scale is commonly controlled with several process options. The options are briefly discussed below. More information is available in the ISPE Baseline Guide *Water and Steam Systems* and other pharmaceutical water system design books.

Scale Control

The most common form of scale control is the use of water softeners upstream of stills and RO units. Water softeners utilize cation exchange resin in the sodium form to remove divalent cations such as calcium, magnesium, barium, and strontium. The most common forms of scale in RO units and stills are calcium carbonate, calcium sulfate, calcium fluoride, barium sulfate, strontium sulfate, and silica. Softeners cannot control silica scale, but they can prevent formation of the other forms of scale through the removal of calcium from the feed water in exchange for sodium. Sodium salts are highly soluble. Softeners operate on a batch basis and are regenerated with a sodium chloride brine solution. The method of brine introduction and brine volume can be optimized to reduce operating cost.

Softener construction varies broadly. Vessel construction is typically fiberglass-reinforced plastic (FRP), lined carbon steel, or stainless steel. Piping materials are typically polyvinyl chloride (PVC), copper, or stainless steel. Multiport valve units are used, as well as individual valves. All of these designs are proven in thousands of applications.

Instrumentation commonly includes a flow monitor to measure service and backwash flows and inlet and outlet pressure gauges. Hardness monitors can be used on the effluent to detect the breakthrough of hardness and can be used to initiate regeneration of the softeners.

Antiscalant and antifoulant chemicals can also be used to control scale and fouling in RO units. Several antiscalant chemicals are very effective in inorganic scale control, including all of the calcium salts previously mentioned and various silica compounds. These chemicals also have antifoulant properties and can be very useful in minimizing particulate fouling. The antifoulant properties limit deposition of inorganic and organic particulates and colloids. The capital cost of antiscalant systems is generally significantly less than the capital cost of water softeners. The operating cost may be higher or lower, depending upon feed water quality.

Antiscalant chemicals have been successfully utilized in RO feed water applications for decades, but some issues must be addressed. The application rate of the antiscalant chemical must be correctly projected and adjusted. Underapplication of the chemical may result in significant scaling of the RO or distillation equipment, and overapplication may lead to significant membrane fouling requiring frequent cleaning.

Adjustment of feed water pH can also be utilized to minimize scale in RO systems. Lowering of the pH increases the solubility of most sparingly soluble salts. Lowering of pH converts some bicarbonate to carbon dioxide that is not removed by RO. The system design must address this carbon dioxide, or an alternate scale control method must be implemented.

Fouling Control

Pretreatment equipment is often included to minimize fouling in RO primary treatment systems. Fouling is a mechanical coating of membranes rather than a chemical precipitation such as scale. Fouling occurs from common feed water contaminants such as silt, dissolved organics, colloids, heavy metals, and microorganisms. Different pretreatment processes are utilized for the different foulants.

Silt, colloids, and other types of particulate are generally controlled through different methods of filtration. Large particulate or suspended solids are typically minimized through pretreatment steps such as multimedia filtration, disposable cartridge filtration, nanofiltration, and ultrafiltration, or through a clarification or flocculation process.

The most common particulate fouling control is use of a multimedia filter as the first component of the pharmaceutical water system. Multimedia filters are pressure filters generally employing three active layers of media filtration in a pressure vessel utilized in a downward service flow. The active layers vary but are most commonly anthracite, followed by a layer of sand, with a final filtration layer of fine garnet. Multimedia filters can generally filter down to the 7- to 10-micron range, although not on an absolute basis.

Multimedia filters are sized as a function of the pretreatment requirement and the feed water quality. Multimedia filters are generally sized larger to provide better filtration ahead of RO systems than they would be for either distillation units or demineralizers. The flow rate of multimedia filters upstream of RO units is generally in the range of 5–8 gpm/ft^2 of filter surface area, with a maximum of 10 gpm/ft^2 for continuous duty. When multiple filters are used, the instantaneous velocity through the filter will obviously increase when one of the filters is out of service in a backwash or maintenance mode. It is not an issue to increase the velocity through the remaining filters in service for the brief period of filter backwash and rinse. A multimedia filter media bed is shown in Figure 6.8.

The most common alternative to multimedia filtration is an inexpensive disposable cartridge filter or bag filter. These filters reduce the capital cost, reduce the generation of wastewater, but generally increase operating cost. Manual labor is required to change the cartridges or bags, and the media replacement cost can be significant in some applications. Disposable cartridge filters and bag filters are available in a very wide range of materials, filtration ratings, and costs. Disposable cartridge filters and bag filters can filter just as effectively as multimedia filters, or better as a function of the disposable filter micron rating. In cases of high flow and high suspended solids, multimedia filters are generally the better choice since they are typically automatically backwashed and necessitate very little labor.

Organic fouling reduction is not always included in RO pretreatment. When organic fouling reduction is included, it is generally an organic scavenger, activated carbon filtration, or ultrafiltration.

Organic scavengers utilize specially selected anion resins in a pressure vessel configuration very similar to that of water softeners. The anion resin selected has the ability to remove a wide variety of dissolved organics from feed water and have the organics eluted from the resin during a regeneration process.

Activated carbon has been used in several applications for organic reduction, as well as dechlorination. The reduction of organics varies greatly with time in service, application, and feed water properties. The reduction of organics through use of activated carbon may range from only a few percent to as high as perhaps 80%. It is difficult to predict the effectiveness of organic reduction with activated carbon without pilot testing.

Pretreatment systems must also address the issue of microbial fouling of final treatment equipment. Microbial fouling is an issue in membrane systems, such as RO and ultrafiltration, and also

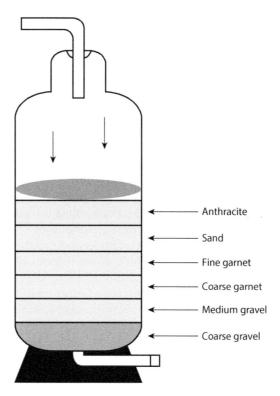

FIGURE 6.8 Multimedia depth filtration. (Courtesy of Evoqua Water Technologies LCC, Warrendale, PA.)

in media processes, such as multimedia filters, disposable cartridge filters, softeners, and activated carbon units.

Microbial fouling can be effectively controlled through the presence of residual chlorine in the feed water to many processes. Some processes, such as multimedia filters, disposable cartridge filters, and softeners, as examples, generally tolerate levels of chlorine that are high enough to control microbial growth and low enough to not cause significant media oxidation.

Other processes, such as RO, ultrafiltration, or microfiltration units, frequently incorporate membranes or media that are not chlorine tolerant. Residual feed water chlorine is not a viable option in this case. Microbial fouling control methods in these cases often include the use of UV light upstream of the process in order to moderate the microbial level in the process feed water, frequent sanitization with hot water at temperatures of 80°C or higher, or frequent chemical sanitization with a range of oxidizing and nonoxidizing biocides.

UV light has been utilized for decades to control microorganism growth in water systems. The UV light spectrum includes several wavelengths that are effective in minimizing the replication of microorganisms in the water stream. UV units typically incorporate UV lamps that are housed inside of quartz sleeves that allow penetration of UV light into the water stream.

The microbial control of UV units is based on UV radiation penetration of the cell wall of the microorganisms. UV light is absorbed by DNA.* The absorption of UV energy inhibits the ability of the microorganisms to replicate. UV units are commonly referred to as sterilizers, but this is generally inaccurate since, while UV units typically provide a significant reduction in microbial counts from the influent stream to the effluent stream, they are not expected to sterilize the process stream.

Oxidation Control

Another critical part of pretreatment systems is the implementation of a process to remove feed water disinfectants from the process stream. Most municipal feed waters utilize chlorine or chloramines for bacterial control. Many private supply systems utilize injection of chlorine for the same microbial control purpose. The chlorine or chloramines damage many pretreatment and final treatment components. Ammonia can be a by-product of dechloramination, and the system must be designed to remove the ammonia or USP conductivity limits may not be met.

Distillation units and RO units employing the widely used thin-film composite membranes are subject to extreme damage from chlorine compounds. Most distillation units are only rated up to 0.02 ppm free chlorine, and most manufacturers recommend that nondetectable levels should be present. Manufacturers of thin-film composite RO membranes have various rating systems for chlorine tolerance. Most are rated in chlorine parts per million–hours of contact, but none of the manufacturers provide any membrane warranty if oxidation of the membrane is present. The reality is that chlorine should be at nondetectable levels ahead of all distillation and thin-film composite RO systems for the most reliable operation.

Dechlorination or dechloramination is accomplished in most pharmaceutical systems through implementation of activated carbon, injection of sodium sulfite compounds, or use of UV light. All of these processes have significant advantages and disadvantages.

Activated carbon was by far the most widely used dechlorination process until recent years. Activated carbon is still used in approximately 80% of new systems that are implemented in the pharmaceutical industry. Activated carbon is capable of removing chlorine or chloramine to virtually nondetectable levels, preparing the effluent water for further purification in the final treatment processes. The activated carbon process is relatively passive and typically does not require significant operator attention other than the sanitization process.

The principal issue with activated carbon use is the potential effluent microbial level. Activated carbon units can provide an ideal environment for microbial growth. This issue is well managed with regular sanitization with clean steam or hot water at 80°C or higher. Steam is very effective,

---

* Soli et al. *Credit to ISPE Baseline Guide Volume 4: Water and Steam Systems, Second Edition*, 2011.

but the carbon unit must be well designed to avoid channeling of steam through the carbon bed. The channeling could leave unsanitized cold areas.

Hot water is more easily distributed to provide complete heating of the carbon unit, and plant steam can be utilized as the heating source. Both hot water and steam can effectively control microbial levels in carbon units.

Activated carbon is generally provided on either a deep bed column basis, where the carbon remains in service for generally a minimum of 6 months to a maximum of approximately 2 years, or on a disposable basis, where the carbon may be changed as frequently as every 2 weeks. Both methods of carbon implementation have been widely used with success in pharmaceutical systems.

Activated carbon units are normally provided with inlet and outlet pressure gauges and flow instrumentation to ensure appropriate backwash flow rates. Thermally sanitized activated carbon units are typically provided with temperature indication to ensure that appropriate temperatures are reached for the thermal sanitization procedure. A thermally sanitizable carbon unit is shown in Figure 6.9.

The use of sodium sulfite compounds (sodium sulfite, sodium bisulfite, or sodium metabisulfite) has increased significantly in recent years. Injection of sodium sulfite compounds for dechlorination or dechloramination is almost always the lowest capital cost alternative for this process.

Sodium sulfite injection can be very effective for the removal of chlorine or chloramines (combined chlorine). The application rate varies with the compound utilized. Applying sodium sulfite at the correct rate is one of the issues in use of this technology for dechlorination. Sodium sulfite

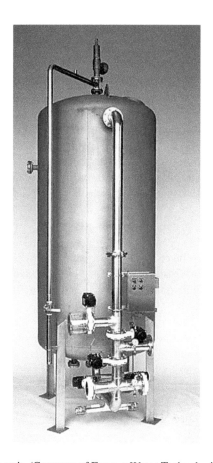

FIGURE 6.9   Activated carbon unit. (Courtesy of Evoqua Water Technologies LCC, Warrendale, PA.)

systems must address feed water chlorine or chloramine spikes, as complete removal is required without excessive overapplication of sulfite.

Underapplication of sodium sulfite can lead to residual chlorine or chloramines and therefore may result in oxidation of downstream equipment. Overapplication of sodium sulfite can lead to rapid fouling of RO units.

Instrumentation of sodium sulfite injection systems varies. Instrumentation to measure free chlorine or combined chlorine should be incorporated to ensure proper performance of the system. Oxidation and reduction potential (ORP) monitors are commonly used for this purpose with mixed success. Monitors to directly measure free chlorine or combined chlorine have also been used and have been successfully combined with feed-forward control technology.

The newest alternative method for dechlorination in pharmaceutical water systems is use of UV light. Low-pressure and medium-pressure units can be effectively utilized, as is the case for microbial control. Extremely high-intensity levels are required for quantitative reduction of free or combined chlorine. The range of UV light energy can vary from 10 times the energy required for microbial control to as high as 150 times the energy required for germicidal control.

Many factors are considered when sizing UV units for dechlorination or dechloramination. These factors include the disinfectant utilized, range of concentration of disinfectant in the feed water, water temperature, feed water TOC level, and UV unit that is to be utilized. UV light is very effective in reduction of free or combined chlorine levels, but significant energy must be applied to reduce typical feed water levels to nondetectable levels.

The greatest advantage of UV dechlorination is that no microbial risk exists, as is the case with both sodium sulfite injection and activated carbon dechlorination. The massive doses of ultraviolet light applied are lethal to feed water microbial levels. The capital cost is generally higher than sodium sulfite injection, but lower than or equal to thermally sanitized activated carbon units.

The principal disadvantage of ultraviolet light dechlorination is that the attainment of chlorine levels below the limit of detection is quite difficult without significant UV light energy levels being employed. The effectiveness of UV dechlorination is a direct function of the feed water disinfectant level and the UV energy level applied. Significant increases in feed water disinfectant level, such as those encountered when coliform microorganisms are detected in municipal feed water, may present a challenge to UV light dechlorination. Sodium sulfite injection can be used as a supplemental dechlorination method when peak chlorine levels are encountered.

Significant advantages and disadvantages exist with all of the common methods of pharmaceutical water system dechlorination. A great debate exists regarding the most effective method of dechlorination, but all of the technologies have been employed successfully in the industry.

Primary (Final) Treatment

Water systems may incorporate one or more final treatment processes. The most commonly implemented primary treatment processes for USP PW and WFI production are RO, IX, and distillation. These processes may be used individually or in various combinations.

Reverse Osmosis

RO is a process utilizing a semipermeable membrane capable of removing dissolved organic and inorganic contaminants from water. Water can permeate through the membrane, while other substances, such as salts, acids, bases, colloids, bacteria, and bacterial endotoxins, are quantitatively rejected and concentrated in a waste stream. RO can reject up to 99.5% of the inorganic salts that comprise the largest contaminant group of raw feed water. Rejection of organics, microorganisms, and endotoxins can also be handled. The only feed water contaminant group that is not effectively rejected by RO is dissolved gases.

Many water purification processes are operated on a batch basis. Contaminants are removed in a process and collected on the process media. The contaminants are then removed in a regeneration or backwash procedure and the removal or regeneration is repeated. RO is a continuous pressure-driven process that depends on cross-flow contaminant removal into the waste or concentrate stream for effective operation.

The recovery (percent of feed water that becomes purified product water) of RO systems is typically about 75%. The recovery can range from as low as 25% to levels approaching 90%. The significant wastewater generated from the RO process is a significant concern in many facilities. Higher recovery rates reduce wastewater but can lead to more frequent RO cleaning requirements and lower product water quality. More complex designs can maintain high product water quality, high recovery, and low-frequency membrane cleaning. Lower recovery rates improve product water quality and process reliability but can increase water consumption unless the RO wastewater is utilized elsewhere. RO wastewater can often be utilized in cooling tower makeup or other applications, and then RO can be a very efficient process from a standpoint of water conservation.

The output of an RO array of membrane modules is a function of the applied transmembrane pressure (feed pressure minus product pressure) and the feed temperature. The product water output of a fixed-membrane area increases with an increase of pressure or temperature. If low-cost heat is available, it may be wise to heat the feed water in cold water applications to somewhere in the range of 50°F–70°F. This reduces the feed pump pressure and energy requirement. Low-cost heat is generally not available, and in most cases, the lowest-energy-cost application of RO is to use low-temperature feed water from the source with higher applied membrane driving pressures. System optimization requires an analysis of the best temperature–pressure combination.

Most pharmaceutical RO units incorporate membranes utilizing thin-film composite membrane construction. Thin-film composite membranes are degraded rapidly in the presence of chlorine at municipal drinking water levels. The dechlorination of the feed water does allow the opportunity for some bacterial growth to occur, and sanitization methods must be taken into account. All RO units can be configured to be compatible with a range of chemical sanitization agents. Many units are supplied with RO membrane modules that allow hundreds of sanitization cycles with water at 80°C. The hot water sanitization is extremely effective in microbial control but does not generally eliminate the need for periodic membrane chemical cleaning. Hot water sanitization is typically significantly more effective than chemical sanitization.

RO can be successfully implemented in pharmaceutical systems in several ways. The most common application of RO in pharmaceutical water systems is utilization of RO upstream of an IX process to produce USP PW. The combination of RO and IX easily exceeds the requirements for conductivity, TOC, and microbiology when properly applied. RO units can be implemented upstream of off-site regenerated IX units to reduce the cost of resin replacement. RO is frequently utilized upstream of CEDI units to provide appropriate feed water quality. RO units are also utilized upstream of regenerable deionizers to reduce regenerant acid and caustic consumption. All of these combinations of RO and IX technologies reliably produce USP PW and can be designed to meet even higher noncompendial standards.

RO is also used to pretreat the feed water to a polishing RO unit. These systems are known as product-staged or two-pass RO and are generally capable of producing water that meets the requirements of the USP PW for TOC and conductivity. Some installations produce water that meets the USP Stage 1 conductivity level, allowing online measurement, while others produce water that passes the Stage 2 or 3 laboratory tests.

RO is commonly implemented as part of a pretreatment system for still feed. RO units alone, or with IX, produce feed water meeting the still requirements for chloride, silica, and other contaminants. The reduction of endotoxin in the still feed stream ensures extremely low endotoxin levels in the distillate. An RO unit is shown in Figure 6.10 (see also Figure 6.11).

Microbial levels in the RO product water can be an issue. RO can control product water microbial levels to meet WFI requirements (less than 10 cfu/100 ml) when properly designed and maintained. Most RO applications do not require microbial levels even approaching WFI requirements. The product water microbial levels from most RO units meet USP PW specifications.

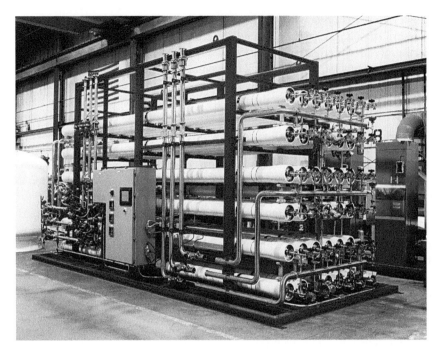

FIGURE 6.10   Reverse osmosis. (Courtesy of Evoqua Water Technologies LCC, Warrendale, PA.)

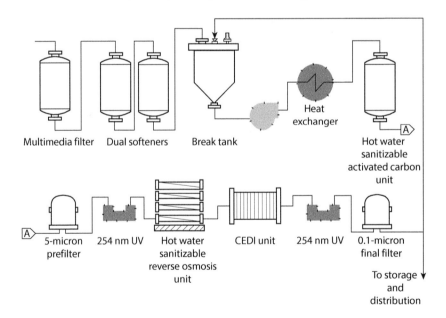

FIGURE 6.11   Reverse osmosis–continuous deionization system. (Courtesy of Evoqua Water Technologies LCC, Warrendale, PA.)

High RO product water microbial levels generally occur as a result of poor sanitization proce-dures, infrequent sanitization, or poor pretreatment design and maintenance. RO membranes are now available for continuous operation at 80°C. This operation is self-sanitizing and allows RO to consistently meet the WFI microbial requirement of less than 10 cfu/ml.

The common RO pretreatment processes have been reviewed in the Pretreatment section.

RO is widely used for final treatment in pharmaceutical water because the process removes a wide variety of contaminants with minimal chemical consumption and reasonable energy costs. The process is reliable when the pretreatment and RO systems are properly designed and maintained. The membrane barrier protects the finished water from contamination under normal and most peak feed water contamination conditions.

Ion Exchange

IX is incorporated in many USP PW systems, WFI systems, and noncompendial systems. The common IX processes are off-site regenerated IX, in-place regenerated IX, and CEDI. All of the processes incorporate cation exchange resin for cation removal and anion exchange resin for anion removal. The processes have similarities in performance but can differ significantly in capital cost, operating cost, chemical consumption, wastewater generation, maintenance requirements, microbial control, and outside service requirements.

Microbial control varies greatly in IX technologies. Some are tolerant of sanitization and some are not. Hot water sanitization and frequent chemical regeneration have been successfully implemented in pharmaceutical water systems.

Off-site and in-place IX resins are the same materials. The difference is simply that off-site regeneration transfers the regeneration process to outside service companies. In-place regeneration requires pharmaceutical companies to implement chemical storage, chemical handling, and neutralization equipment to perform resin regeneration. The off-site versus in-place regeneration decision is based on consideration of capital cost, operating cost, chemical handling, process control, and other factors. Off-site regenerated resin systems are generally much lower in capital cost than in-place regenerated systems, as significant chemical handling equipment and piping are eliminated. The outside services of a resin regenerator are required unless new resin is purchased for each exchange. Most systems use regenerated resin, but many pharmaceutical companies do purchase new resin for each exchange because they feel that quality control is improved. Many quality resin regeneration companies exist, but all should be periodically audited to ensure that the resin regeneration process is accomplished in a GMP manner.

Off-site regenerated IX resin systems can be the only final treatment utilized to produce USP PW, or may follow RO to remove the ionic contaminants that have passed through the RO process. IX can remove ionized contaminants to virtually immeasurable levels. The decision to utilize IX alone or use RO upstream of IX is generally based on cost and technical considerations.

IX units can reduce feed water TOC, but not necessarily to USP levels on all water supplies. RO may be implemented upstream of IX units to ensure consistent USP TOC attainment. IX systems without RO pretreatment reliably produce USP PW in many installations where the feed water TOC levels are not too high.

Since RO typically removes greater than 98% of feed water ionized solids, the throughput of downstream IX units is increased substantially. When RO is implemented upstream of off-site regenerated IX units, the payback is fast in most cases. If TOC attainment is not an issue, the decision to utilize RO pretreatment is usually based on whether the additional capital cost of RO equipment is offset in a reasonable time by reduced resin regeneration costs.

All IX systems (no RO) are generally limited to relatively low daily makeup volume on relatively low TDS feed waters. Polishing components such as UV light microbial reduction units, disposable cartridge filters, and even ultrafilters are commonly placed downstream of the IX units. The disposable cartridge filters may be rated in the range of 5-micron removal for resin fines or may be as tight as 0.1 micron absolute for microbial retention.

High makeup volume systems more commonly use CEDI or in-place regenerated IX units for the IX polishing process. Systems implementing pretreatment and in-place regenerated IX (but no RO) were the dominant USP PW generation system design for decades until about 1990. At that time, RO-based systems began to claim a majority of new large-volume systems. Large-volume, in-place regenerated IX systems are rare in new applications, as most companies wish to reduce chemical consumption and utilize membrane technology or distillation. Most systems that use in-place regenerated ion units also utilize UV and filtration devices downstream for control of microbial levels and resin fines (particulates). The cost of microbially retentive filters downstream of IX units can be excessive on high colloidal-level feed waters when RO is not employed upstream.

The final IX process that is commonly used in pharmaceutical water production is CEDI. The CEDI devices are able to remove ionizable contaminants from water without the requirement for chemical regeneration. CEDI units use IX membranes, IX resin, and direct current (DC) electrical potential to transport ionized species from a feed stream into a concentrate stream. Some of the IX resin in the unit are continuously regenerated with H^+ and OH^- that are created from splitting of a minor portion of the feed water stream.

Almost all CEDI units are placed downstream of RO. The RO unit upstream improves the feed water quality to a level suitable for feed to CEDI. The RO unit also minimizes the conductivity level of the RO product stream, making the removal of the remaining ionized contaminants by CEDI practical. CEDI feed water must be relatively low in hardness, organics, silica, suspended solids, and TDSs, and free of oxidizing agents for reliable operation.

CEDI units typically exhibit bacteriostatic or bactericidal effects within the resin–IX membrane module. The electric field and water-splitting by-products provide this microbial control. This can significantly retard microbial growth within the resin–membrane matrix. This effect does not extend into piping areas outside of the electric field, so periodic sanitization is still required. Some units can be chemically sanitized or sanitized with hot water up to 80°C, while others can only be chemically sanitized.

The posttreatment considerations for CEDI are similar to those for other IX processes. Many systems use UV light downstream for additional microbial control. Some systems also use postfiltration for particle control or additional microbial control. Some systems rely on hot water sanitization microbial control and use no posttreatment.

All of the IX processes are well proven in thousands of applications. All are frequently combined with RO to easily exceed all USP PW attributes. All of the processes have been utilized successfully in the production of USP WFI and many grades of noncompendial water.

Distillation

Distillation is one of the oldest water purification processes and has an extensive history in the production of pharmaceutical water. Distillation is the predominant process worldwide for production of WFI and is also used to produce PW and noncompendial waters. As stated earlier, distillation is the only process allowed by EuPhr for production of WFI. Distillation utilizes the phase change from liquid to vapor and removal of entrained liquid droplets to purify water. This process can, with appropriate pretreatment, reduce feed levels of ionized solids, suspended solids, organics, certain gases, microorganisms, and endotoxins to meet USP WFI and PW requirements.

The basic process requires energy, in the form of steam or electricity, to evaporate feed water, disengage entrained water droplets, and condense the vapor to form pure water. The evaporator and droplet disengagement features differ between manufacturers and basic still types. The dominant still types are ME and VC. Both are capable of cGMP production of WFI and PW. These types differ in energy consumption, pretreatment requirements, cooling water requirements, and maintenance needs.

ME stills incorporate more than one evaporator in order to recover the latent and sensible heat from pure vapor for reuse (and an increase in operating efficiency). The number of evaporators, or effects, may be as few as 2 or as many as 10. Standard units generally incorporate from three to eight effects. The feed water is evaporated in the first evaporator. The vapor produced in the first effect becomes the heating medium in the second effect. The first effect pure vapor is condensed in the second effect heating section and eventually travels to the condenser for final cooling and recovery as pure distillate. The pure vapor generated in each effect is utilized as the heating medium in the next effect throughout the ME still. The pure vapor from the last effect goes directly to the condenser. ME stills also use multiple heat exchangers to recover energy from condensate, blowdown, and interstage condensate to improve efficiency.

The multiple effects are utilized for efficiency, and the water is only evaporated once, not multiple times. The distillate quality is the same as from a single-effect still. A common myth is that distillate from a three-effect still, as an example, is triple distilled.

An increase in the number of effects increases the capital cost of the still for a fixed output and reduces the operating cost through reduction of heating steam and cooling water. Economic optimization requires a balance of capital cost increase against a reasonable payback period.

Since a temperature differential between heating medium and feed water must exist in each effect, an increase in number of effects is usually accompanied by an increase in the first effect heating steam temperature. ME stills operate at higher temperatures than VC stills. The feed water quality requirements are generally higher for ME stills than VC to minimize evaporator scale. The specifications vary with manufacturer and blowdown rates, but most ME pretreatment systems significantly reduce silica, chloride, hardness, TDSs, and oxidizing disinfectants to low levels. Many ME pretreatment systems incorporate either product-staged RO or RO and IX to provide extremely reliable ME still operation.

ME stills share the vast majority of the still marketplace with VC. Some prefer ME distillation because they believe that the minimum number of moving parts in ME stills is a maintenance advantage. As stated previously, the water quality produced by the various still types is usually not a significant consideration. The final distillate quality from any well-designed still meets WFI or PW requirements with proper feed water. The distillate conductivity is often more a function of feed water quality than still design.

VC stills also recover latent heat from previously evaporated pure vapor for efficiency purposes. Feed water is evaporated on a surface of a tubular heat exchanger in an evaporator section. The heat source is most commonly steam but can be electric in smaller units. The pure vapor is drawn into a compressor, and in the compression cycle the pressure and temperature of the pure vapor are increased. The higher-temperature pure vapor exits the compressor and enters a heat exchange unit in the evaporator, where the latent heat is transferred to feed water and more pure vapor is produced. The condensed pure vapor loses sensible heat in an additional exchanger or exchangers and a classical condenser with cooling water is not required.

VC stills are generally regarded as the most efficient still option. These stills are used in most very high-volume applications and can be found in multiple units in some facilities producing several hundred gallons per minute of distillate. VC stills can produce very small distillate volumes also and compete with ME stills across a broad spectrum of flows.

The required pretreatment systems upstream of VC stills vary greatly with feed water quality, corporate standard designs, and personal preferences. VC stills have an upper limit on silica in the evaporator. Feed water silica level may necessitate IX or RO as pretreatment for reliable operation and minimum blowdown. When silica is not a factor, many VC installations use simple pretreatment systems that may include particle filtration, softening, and dechlorination. Many facilities prefer this simple pretreatment scheme, while many others believe that still reliability is increased and maintenance decreased through implementation of RO or IX as VC pretreatment. The 1993 FDA "Guide to Inspections of High-Purity Water Systems" suggests consideration of membrane pretreatment upstream of stills to ensure attainment of low product water endotoxin levels. The guide documents multiple-still endotoxin failures with required retrofit of membrane systems upstream.

The presence of chloramines in still feed water can cause pretreatment changes for ME or VC stills. Stills cannot remove ammonia, and ammonium will be converted to ammonia in a hot distillation process. The presence of even a small amount of ammonium in the distillate can cause a significant increase in distillate conductivity. The still pretreatment system must be capable of ammonia removal when ammonia is present in the feed water or ammonia is generated in other process steps.

STORAGE AND DISTRIBUTION SYSTEMS

PROCESS CONSIDERATIONS

The design requirements for storage and distribution systems vary with the water quality specifications, generation system quality, and risk assessment. The storage and distribution system must maintain the water quality within the specified quality limits. Deterioration of quality is acceptable as long as the quality attributes do not fall out of specification.

The USP WFI monograph requires the system be designed to "protect [WFI] from microbial contamination." The FDA expectation for maximum WFI microbial level is 10 cfu/100 ml. This requires a conservative storage and distribution system design. The FDA expectation for PW is a maximum of 100 cfu/ml. This is three logs higher than the WFI specification and allows consideration of some designs that are not practical for WFI.

Almost all WFI distribution loops are constructed of sanitary 316L or 316 stainless steel tubing, fittings, and valves. The 316L or low-carbon material is required for welded assemblies for proper welding. These systems use orbitally welded joints where possible and use sanitary triclamp joints for mechanical connections. Most piping is pitched to allow for complete drainage for steam sanitization (if utilized) or maintenance.

This construction is considered by most to be cGMP and is one of the cGMP common practices to come from the previously discussed GMPs for LVPs. Most companies utilize this construction unless technical considerations favor alternate construction.

A few WFI distribution systems are constructed with polyvinylidene difluoride (PVDF) plastic piping because the products cannot be made with the metal levels in WFI that arise from contact with stainless steel. Some companies favor PVDF because passivation initially and periodically is not required as with stainless steel systems. There is an industry trend to move away from frequent scheduled passivation of stainless steel systems (such as annually) to following a scientific basis for passivation. Implemented methods of determination for passivation include visual inspection, water testing for heavy metals, implementation of a rouge monitor, and filtration testing for metal particulate.

PVDF piping can be operated at 80°C continuously with continuous piping support and expansion loops. PVDF can be intermittently sanitized with low-pressure steam or hot water. Hot water is sufficient and presents less of a risk of exceeding the rated temperature than steam. The PVDF piping costs are often similar to 316L stainless steel piping when the stainless steel is properly specified.

Almost all WFI systems are operated at continuous high temperature (>65°C) or intermittently high temperature. Few variations exist, and since almost all WFI systems are sanitary 316L stainless steel construction, most WFI systems are quite similar in design. The differences exist in instrumentation, surface finish, and other details.

Most PW storage and distribution systems are variations of a few basic designs. Water can be stored at continuous high temperature (>65°C), ambient with intermittent hot water sanitization, ambient with continuous or intermittent ozone, and ambient with periodic chemical sanitization or cold (generally <10°C) with periodic sanitization. When water is stored at continuous high temperature, it may be distributed at high temperature or ambient temperature.

CONTINUOUS HOT STORAGE

A typical continuous hot storage and hot distribution system is shown in Figure 6.12. The water may be used hot or may require some method of heat exchange if colder temperatures are required. The continuous hot system is self-sanitizing, and microbial problems are virtually always external to the sanitary system. Poor hose practices, airborne contamination, poor sampling practices, or other factors may contribute to unacceptable use point microbial counts, but poor counts from the sanitary system are unlikely.

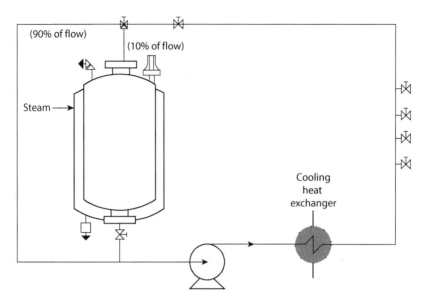

FIGURE 6.12 Hot storage, self-contained distribution. (Courtesy of Evoqua Water Technologies LCC, Warrendale, PA.)

A continuous hot system is generally considered to be the most conservative, lowest-risk storage system design. The capital cost is relatively high, as almost all hot systems are constructed from 316L stainless steel sanitary components and require insulation. Continuous hot system operating costs may not be high if all of the water is used hot for manufacturing. This situation is ideal for continuous hot operation.

Most facilities require cooled water for manufacturing, and the energy costs for heating and cooling may be significant. A very significant percentage of the pharmaceutical industry is willing to incur these energy costs for the low-risk system operation.

Use point heat exchangers for cooling or cooled subloops are commonly employed where hot water is not suitable for manufacturing. The ISPE Baseline Guide *Water and Steam Systems* provides guidance regarding use point heat exchanger implementation options. The guide also illustrates the energy-efficient implementation of self-contained cooled subloops off of hot storage tanks. The key point is to recirculate all or most of the cooled water back to the subloop, rather than constantly reheating all of the unused cooled water for return to the hot tank. A system flow schematic is shown in Figure 6.12.

OZONATED STORAGE

An excellent alternative to continuous hot storage with cooled water for usage is continuously ozonated storage, as shown in Figure 6.13. The continuous application of ozone ensures low microbial counts in storage, and the ozonated water in storage can be used to periodically sanitize the distribution system. Ozone can destroy most microorganisms (those not embedded in biofilm) in seconds of contact time, is easily removed from manufacturing water with UV light, and has been successfully documented in many installations. Microorganisms embedded in biofilm necessitate significantly longer ozone contact time for destruction.

Pharmaceutical companies must demonstrate that ozone has been completely removed from water for manufacturing. Residual ozone in USP PW or WFI utilized in manufacturing would violate the monograph prohibition of "no added substances." Online monitors are typically utilized to prove the absence of ozone in distributed water. The residual ozone in water from

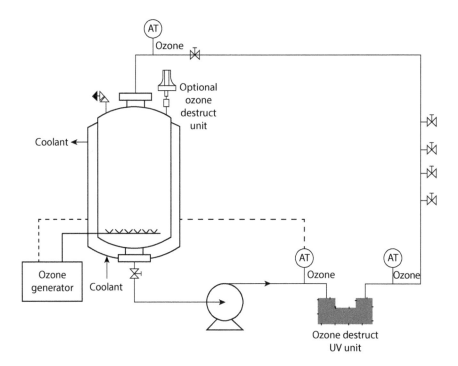

FIGURE 6.13 Storage and distribution. (Courtesy of Evoqua Water Technologies LCC, Warrendale, PA.)

storage is removed with in-line ultraviolet units downstream of the distribution pump. These UV units use approximately three times the energy, per gallon processed, as UV units sized for microbial control. Distribution system sanitization is easily automated and accomplished by shutting off the UV units when system sanitization is desired. The ozonated water from storage is allowed to enter the distribution system and sanitization is accomplished.

Continuous addition of ozone to stored water will cause an increase in conductivity. The increase may cause the conductivity to rise above the USP conductivity limit during lengthy periods of low or no water usage. This issue is eliminated or minimized through repurification of some of the stored water, use of appropriately low applied ozone levels, or purging of some stored water, resulting in the addition of low conductivity makeup water to storage.

Since ozone is an extremely strong oxidizing agent, material compatibility must be addressed in system design. Most ozonated systems use components constructed of 316L or 316 stainless steel. PVDF piping, fittings, and valves are also very compatible with ozone. Gaskets and other elastomers must be carefully selected.

The capital cost of most ozonated systems is similar to that of continuous hot systems. The capital cost of a small ozone-based system may be higher than that of an intermittent hot system, as the cost of an ozone generator, ozone mixing devices, instruments, and an UV light unit may exceed the cost of heating equipment and insulation. The capital cost of large hot water sanitizable systems may exceed the cost of ozonated systems if insulation costs are high. The operating cost of ozonated systems may be much lower than that of continuous hot systems if the makeup water is generated at ambient temperature and the water is used at ambient temperature.

AMBIENT STORAGE

Many systems utilize ambient temperature water storage without continuous or intermittent ozone. These systems rely on periodic hot water sanitization (80°C–121°C) or chemical sanitization.

Properly designed sanitary 316 stainless steel systems with daily hot sanitization are commonly used with great success in both WFI and PW applications. Many systems operate successfully with hot sanitization less frequently than daily, but the microbial risk increases.

Chemical sanitization is the least desirable of all sanitization options. Chemical sanitization is usually implemented as a result of budget limitations rather than technical superiority. Chemical sanitization is limited to PW applications and is typically used with plastic piping (polypropylene or PVC) to minimize capital costs.

Chemical sanitization is usually considerably more time consuming than thermal or ozone sanitization and less effective. The required contact time with organisms is greater, and other time factors apply. Each use point must be drained and tested to prove the presence of chemical during sanitization and the absence of chemical after rinsing. Higher microbial counts after sanitization may occur for a short period if the biofilm is disturbed, but not completely inactivated.

Plastic piping systems with chemical sanitization can be successfully implemented. This design is best utilized when the acceptable microbial counts at use points are relatively high. Frequent sanitization helps. A properly designed and maintained makeup system with tight microbial control also helps significantly.

DISTRIBUTION STORAGE TANK DESIGN CONSIDERATIONS

Distribution tank capacity optimization was reviewed earlier in this chapter. Other design specification considerations include material, surface finish, pressure rating, vacuum rating, temperature rating, access, fitting number and type, instrumentation, spray balls, vent filters, rupture disks, nitrogen blanketing, support, steam jacketing, and insulation.

TANK ATMOSPHERIC ISOLATION

Proper isolation of WFI or PW in storage is an absolute cGMP requirement. An appropriate hydrophobic, integrity testable, microbial retentive vent filter or nitrogen blanketing is acceptable. The filter, normally rated at 0.2 μm absolute or tighter, should be heat traced in hot applications to prevent filter plugging due to condensation. Proper integrity tests for vent filters prior to use and after use must be implemented.

Proper pressure and vacuum protection should be provided. A pressure rupture disk is often implemented. A vacuum rupture disk is usually implemented if the tank is not rated for full vacuum. Rupture disks can be equipped with an alarm function to notify operators of rupture and tank atmospheric exposure. Relief valves are utilized in lieu of rupture disks in some instances.

DISTRIBUTION PIPING DESIGN CONSIDERATIONS

The optimization of the distribution system configuration, tubing or pipe size, and flow rate or rates requires significant thought. The distribution system must be able to deliver the proper flow and pressure to all users under varying demands. The flow rate in each individual loop is generally at least 50% greater than the maximum instantaneous demand to allow proper pressure control and avoid water hammer incidents. The system must be maintained at a positive pressure, or system sanitization would be required if air is presumed to have entered the system.

The number of parallel loops is normally minimized for cost and control purposes. One serpentine loop is ideal for control, instrumentation, ease of balancing, and sometimes capital cost. Each individual loop length is ultimately constrained by pressure drop. Multiple loops are generally used in large systems to limit the pressure drop in each loop to ensure that water can be delivered to all users at the required pressure and flow. Each loop is normally individually instrumented to monitor proper flow, pressure, and temperature.

CONTINUOUS RECIRCULATING OR NONRECIRCULATING CONFIGURATION

Although many consider continuous recirculation of water a cGMP requirement, this is not true. Most systems due continuously recirculate at reasonable velocity in an attempt to minimize microbial attachment to piping surfaces. This is logical and somewhat effective, but not a regulatory requirement.

Nonrecirculating or "dead-end" systems can be validated and pass audit if continuous flow or proper flushing and sanitization procedures are implemented and documented. Some nonrecirculating systems have continuous usage and are dynamic at all points without having to bear the cost of return piping back to the tank. Other systems utilize timed flushes to drain or effective sanitization to demonstrate proper microbial control.

DEAD LEGS

Extreme attention is paid to piping layout to minimize dead legs in order to minimize microbial growth opportunity and meet cGMP expectations. The older interpretation of an acceptable dead leg meeting GMP guidelines was a maximum of six pipe diameters (using the branch diameter) measured from the centerline of the main run to the center of the branch isolation valve. The six-pipe-diameter dead leg "rule" was based on hot (nominal 80°C operating temperature) sanitary stainless steel tubing distribution systems. The current view of most companies is to minimize the dead leg to the smallest practical. Many companies strive to limit the dead leg to two pipe diameters (branch diameter) or fewer, measuring from the pipe wall of the main run to the center of the branch isolation valve. When plastic piping materials or ambient operating temperatures are utilized, the dead legs should be as close to zero as possible.

DISTRIBUTION PIPING VELOCITY

Water system design for decades has frequently considered water velocity, turbulence, and minimization of boundary layer in flow rate and pipe sizing. Strict, high-velocity limits were common. The theory was and often still is that the turbulence produced by high velocity will inhibit microbial attachment to piping surfaces and minimize biofilm formation. An absolute velocity or Reynolds number is not a cGMP requirement and is not completely effective in practice. No evidence exists to indicate that FDA inspectors seek a particular minimum water velocity.

Data indicate that microbial attachment can eventually occur at almost any velocity or Reynolds number (a common measure of turbulence). Biofilm control is best achieved through effective sanitization methods and continuous measures, such as high or low temperature, residual ozone, UV light, and filtration.

Water velocities as low as 2 ft/s have proven to be sufficient. From a practical point, extremely low continuous velocities are unlikely because this would require large pipe diameters at increased capital cost. Most systems utilize water velocities in the range of 3–10 ft/s to minimize pipe diameter and cost. Higher velocities would produce unacceptably high-pressure drops in long piping runs.

The most important consideration is to avoid designing for a high absolute minimum velocity under all possible operating conditions. This difficult constraint may result in small return lines, high pressure drop, and validation difficulties.

DISTRIBUTION PIPING MATERIAL

Although the term *distribution piping* is used in this text and is the common term for a water distribution network, tubing is more common than pipe in distribution systems. Stainless steel tubing (316L) is used in almost 100% of WFI systems. Sanitary stainless steel tubing for WFI distribution has a lengthy history of successful operation. Alternative designs should be based on technical considerations rather than economic considerations. Almost all new PW systems in large manufacturing facilities also use 316L stainless steel tubing construction.

Some manufacturing facilities use PVDF tubing, fittings, and valves to eliminate passivation but maintain the options for use of ozone or hot water sanitization. Polypropylene piping has also been implemented when chemical sanitization of distribution is the choice.

Pipe, rather than tubing, is utilized in some manufacturing and laboratory applications. The pipe is almost always plastic material and may be utilized for economic or technical considerations. The economic considerations may be considerable if PVC or polypropylene piping is utilized rather than 316L stainless steel tubing and fittings. A sanitary stainless steel tubing system is typically five to eight times the cost of a PVC system and two to four times the cost of a polypropylene piping system. New PVC systems are quite rare.

The piping or tubing material selection must be compatible with the continuous or intermittent sanitization method. Continuous hot or ozonated systems are restricted to stainless steel or PVDF. Polypropylene and PVC systems are typically chemically sanitized, although a small percentage use intermittent ozone sanitization. Polypropylene is not ozone compatible. Chemical, heat, or ozone compatibility should always be confirmed by the piping manufacturer.

The choice of distribution material and joining method is critical relative to the microbial limit specification. Almost any configuration can be properly maintained to meet the PW maximum allowable microbial action level of 100 cfu/ml. Lower levels and the absence of indicator organisms such as *Pseudomonas aeruginosa* or *Burkholderia cepacia* are more consistently achieved with sanitary stainless systems. Extremely low microbial levels can be achieved with piping, but continuous heat or ozone is recommended.

Plastic piping can contribute excessive organic extractible contaminants when usage is low and the piping is new. Some low-usage plastic systems require periodic purging of water from storage or use of TOC reduction UV units in recirculation to control TOC levels.

Joint Method

Stainless steel sanitary tubing system joints are automatically orbitally welded where possible, hand welded where necessary, and manually clamped in a sanitary manner for instrumentation and access. PVDF and polypropylene are joined with welded joints where possible and joined mechanically where necessary. Different weld methods are available and produce varying degrees of weld surface smoothness. Some joining methods for plastic piping actually produce smoother joints than stainless steel orbital welding. Smooth surfaces are desirable for the lowest microbial requirements. Smooth surfaces cannot completely inhibit microbial attachment, but the initial attachment can be delayed. A smooth surface is particularly important with intermittent chemical sanitization.

PVC systems use solvent welded joints for most joints and incorporate flanged and threaded mechanical joints. These joints are more likely to contribute to microbial issues than welded joints. PVC systems are generally used where low microbial levels are not required.

Surface Finish

Stainless steel tubing systems are normally specified for surface finish. WFI surfaces are normally in the range of 15–20 Ra in microinches. PW system stainless surfaces are normally in the range of 25–40 Ra in microinches. Surface finish is generally less critical where continuous sanitization with heat or ozone is implemented than in ambient nonozonated systems. Most self-sanitizing systems still use highly polished tubing regardless of the technical justification.

Plastic systems are not specified for surface finish. PVDF surfaces are typically smoother than the highest mechanical polish stainless steel surfaces. Polypropylene piping surfaces are also extremely smooth. PVC surfaces provide the most surface crevices in the common plastic piping materials.

TOTAL SYSTEM DRAINING

Systems incorporating steam sterilization or sanitization must be designed to facilitate complete draining prior to steaming and during steaming. These systems must also be designed to allow complete venting of air. Systems that use hot water, ozone, or chemical sanitization are frequently designed for complete draining, but it is not absolutely necessary. Flushing residual chemicals out of systems can be validated.

DISTRIBUTION SYSTEM POLISHING COMPONENTS

Ideally, the water quality specifications are met out of the generation system and no polish processes are required in distribution. Compendial water systems rarely need polishing in distribution. Laboratory systems meeting high-level laboratory water specifications often need polishing components in distribution to meet tight levels for conductivity, TOC, and microbial level. Continuous hot systems typically incorporate no additional purification processes in distribution. Ozonated systems implement UV light units for ozone removal, but typically use no other distribution processes.

Ambient nonozonated systems are the most likely to incorporate distribution polishing technologies. These processes may be used to improve or maintain conductivity, TOC, or microbial levels. IX processes may be incorporated where extremely low conductivity values are required. These conductivity values are generally well below USP allowable values. These extremely low conductivity requirements should be questioned and justified.

Implementation of the IX process generally involves UV light units or filters for microbial and particulate control. UV light units can provide adequate microbial control downstream of IX and are not a regulatory issue. Filters implemented for particle control downstream of IX are also not a regulatory issue.

Microbial retentive filters in distribution or at use points can be very effective, but generate significant cGMP debate. The only written prohibition of filters in distribution was in the previously discussed GMPs for LVPs. Since these requirements were never adopted, the use of microbial retentive filters is subject to interpretation.

Almost all, if not all, pharmaceutical companies ban the use of microbial retentive filters in WFI distribution because they believe that FDA acceptance is unlikely. FDA does not disallow in-line or use point filters if they are properly validated and maintained, but many firms do not do this properly. Use point filters can mask system microbial control problems. Proper microbial sampling should be done upstream and downstream of filters to ensure that the entire system is in proper microbial control.

Many companies also shun filter use in PW distribution for similar logic. Some companies use a single bulk filter after distribution IX units in PW applications. The effectiveness of microbial retentive filters has been proven for decades in pharmaceutical, microelectronics, chemical process, and other applications. The issue has nothing to do with effectiveness and is strictly a perceived regulatory issue. I have observed successful microbial retentive filter use in hundreds of properly designed and operated systems.

Many people believe that a single bulk filter, used as part of a total microbial control plan and properly maintained, is perfectly appropriate for pharmaceutical use in PW applications. Multiple use point filters are rarely necessary and are used extremely infrequently.

Some low-endotoxin noncompendial or PW systems utilize an ultrafiltration unit in distribution to ensure extremely low endotoxin levels. These units are similar to the units described earlier but are generally sanitary in construction. These systems typically produce water with endotoxin levels well below USP WFI requirements.

SUMMARY

Water is often the most expensive utility in pharmaceutical plants. Considerable capital and operating cost reductions can be realized through optimization of water quality specification, generation system design, storage and distribution system design, and proper maintenance. FDA is not an engineering agency and does not publish strict engineering guidelines. Many individuals have expressed a desire for greater FDA detailed engineering requirements. This is not likely to occur, and this provides an opportunity for companies to optimize water generation and distribution and prove that the system is appropriate for the application through proper validation.

TRENDS AND FUTURE DEVELOPMENTS

The pharmaceutical industry is moving to risk-based design and qualification of water systems. Risk-based design and qualification require greater process knowledge and enhanced system data generation. The concept is extremely sound and can lead to more consistent water quality attainment, increased uptime, and lower costs.

Pharmaceutical companies are placing greater value and emphasis on energy and water conservation. Technologies to accomplish this are available with reasonable return on investment analysis.

Cost containment is a trend in water, as in all other aspects of pharmaceutical manufacturing. This has led to greater acceptance of standard designs to reduce engineering costs and production time.

FURTHER DISCUSSION

1. What are the differences between water for injection (WFI) and purified water (PW)? What are the uses of each, and how are they produced?
2. What are the differences between compendial and noncompendial water? Is compendial water cleaner than noncompendial water?
3. Why is pretreatment necessary?
4. Describe a reverse osmosis–continuous deionization system.
5. Why is polishing sometimes necessary?

ABOUT THE AUTHOR

Gary V. Zoccolante is pharmaceutical technical director for Evoqua Water Technologies, a firm that provides water system equipment and services globally. Gary has more than 40 years of experience in the design, operation, and troubleshooting of pharmaceutical water systems. He has been involved in the development of equipment for pretreatment, reverse osmosis, deionization, ultrafiltration, and distillation. Gary was a committee member of five ISPE guides, including two baseline water and steam guides, two guides on commissioning and qualification of pharmaceutical water and steam systems, and a guide on ozone sanitization of pharmaceutical water systems. Gary developed the ISPE pharmaceutical water course and has presented the course to hundreds of pharmaceutical industry personnel, including FDA staff. Gary has chaired courses for many groups and presented for ISPE, Interphex, the American Institute of Chemical Engineers, the American Institute of Mechanical Engineers, Parenteral Drug Association, and many others. Gary has authored many papers and books on pharmaceutical water production, system operation, and qualification. He holds several patents for pharmaceutical water processes. Gary is a graduate of Northeastern University, Boston, Massachusetts, with a BS degree in mechanical engineering.

7 Commissioning, Qualification, and Validation

Christina Meyer Dell Cioppia

CONTENTS

INTRODUCTION

Within the past 30 years, the pharmaceutical industry's perception of and attitude towards validation has changed profoundly. Validation was historically viewed as a hindrance to progress and facility operation. It resulted in massive paperwork, project cost overruns, schedule delays, and operational burdens. Thirty years ago, activities related to validation generally were not even considered until well into the construction phase of a capital project. Times have changed, and now it would be unusual for a project to be initiated without considering the ultimate requirement to design, build, and hand over a validated facility. While facility designs for a validated facility are profoundly altered by the requirements of validation, project teams now recognize that most of the design elements are subject to intense scrutiny, justification, documentation, and verification. It is now standard practice to use the life cycle approach for the design, verification, validation, and operation of a facility since these are recognized as interdependent parts of a whole. The early phases of the life cycle set the stage for successful handover and operation in the future.

The word *validatability* has been coined to express those elements of the design that are subject to validation. Designs must be more than merely functional; they must be capable of meeting the preestablished requirements that regulatory agencies and industry standards have set for the validation of various systems. Project teams recognize that facility design and ultimate validation are intertwined. A well-structured team fosters communication and cooperation between the design, procurement, construction, quality, and validation teams.

EXECUTIVE SUMMARY

This chapter gives a brief history of what is broadly referred to as validation, but often means commissioning and qualification. This also includes an overview of the expectations of regulatory agencies and industry practices to deliver a validated facility and an overview of the evolution of validation from the 1970s to today. The concentration is on current Good Manufacturing Practice (cGMP) issues related to commissioning, qualification, and validation (CQV) during the design phase of a facility. This includes an overview of the role of the concepts quality by design (QbD) and good engineering practice (GEP) in the design process. This chapter focuses on the specific CQV activities associated with the three main phases of facility design: conceptual design, preliminary design, and detailed design.

HISTORY OF VALIDATION

Many legislative acts and regulations have been born out of tragic events that have killed or injured thousands of patients. Examples of such events are discussed below.

In 1937, sulfanilamide was used widely in tablet and powder form to treat streptococcal infections. There was a demand for the drug in liquid form, so it was dissolved in diethylene glycol and sold as Elixir Sulfanilamide, but it killed 107 people, many of whom were children. This dramatized the need to establish drug safety before marketing and was the impetus behind the passage of the Food, Drug, and Cosmetic (FDC) Act of 1938. The act required that new drugs show safety before being sold [1].

In 1941, nearly 300 deaths and injuries resulted from the use of sulfathiazole tablets, an antibiotic tainted with the sedative phenobarbital. In response, the Food and Drug Administration (FDA) drastically changed manufacturing and quality control requirements, which led to the development of cGMPs.

In 1952, nearly 180 cases of often deadly blood diseases were caused by the antibiotic chloramphenicol. Two years later, the FDA engaged the American Society of Hospital Pharmacists and the American Association of Medical Record Librarians, and later the American Medical Association, in a voluntary program of drug reaction reporting [1].

In 1962, thalidomide was sold as a treatment for anxiety and gastritis in Europe, and later to treat morning sickness in pregnant women. The drug was advertised by its manufacturer as being completely safe for everyone, including mother and child "even during pregnancy." By 1960, thalidomide was marketed in 46 countries (but not in the United States), with sales almost matching those of aspirin [2]. Unfortunately, more than 5,000 infants in Europe and more than 10,000 infants worldwide were born with phocomelia, a malformation of the limbs. Media reports on how Frances Kelsey, MD, an FDA medical officer, helped prevent approval and marketing of thalidomide in the United States stirred up great support for the FDA and stronger drug laws. This led to the passage of the Kefauver–Harris Amendments, which required drug makers to prove that their drug worked and was safe before the FDA could approve it for sale [1].

In 1982, after several deaths from cyanide-laced acetaminophen (Tylenol) capsules, the U.S. Congress passed the Federal Anti-Tampering Act in 1983, making it a crime to tamper with packaged consumer products [1].

To understand the history of and basis for validation, it is necessary to understand the history of drug products in the United States. In the early 1800s, the United States depended largely on Europe for pharmaceuticals, which made the United States a dumping ground for foreign adulterated and even banned drugs, with often tragic results. This concern led to the publication of the first United States Pharmacopeia (USP) in the 1820s. Yet, adulterated drugs continued to make their way into the U.S. market. Public outcry grew during the Mexican–American War of 1846, when, right or wrong, adulterated drugs were blamed for high-mortality rates among U.S. soldiers. This led to the signing of the Drug Importation Act of 1848, which prohibited the importation of adulterated drugs into the United States. The act was supposed to be enforced by government-appointed inspectors stationed at key points of entry into the United States. Sadly, the law was an abject failure.

In addition to the fact that inspectors were not always the best qualified for their duties, the act did not address the growing problem of adulterated domestic medicines [2].

The FDA began in 1862, when President Lincoln appointed a single chemist, Charles M. Wetherill, to serve in the Department of Agriculture. This marked the beginning of the Bureau of Chemistry, the predecessor of the FDA. The FDA's true roots as a consumer protection agency began in 1906 with the passage of the Pure Food and Drugs Act. The act prohibited interstate commerce in misbranded and adulterated food, drink, or drugs. The Meat Inspection Act was passed the same day after shocking disclosures of unsanitary conditions in meat packing plants [3]. Today, the FDA oversees most food products (other than meat and poultry), human and animal drugs, biologically derived therapeutic agents, medical devices, cosmetics, and animal feeds. In 2013, the FDA employed more than 14,000 full-time employees [4] with an operating budget of $4.5 billion [5].

Clearly, the FDA is involved in much more than inspecting drug manufacturers and writing 483 citations, a form issued by the FDA notifying a company of objectionable conditions, however, keeping the U.S. drug supply unadulterated is a major part of the FDA's efforts, of which validation is a key activity. Validation in the pharmaceutical industry appears to have its origins in the United States during the early 1970s. The term *process validation (PV)* was introduced to the pharmaceutical industry by Ted Byers and Bud Loftus of the FDA. The FDA's objective was to enhance the quality of sterile drugs produced in the United States in response to well-publicized sterility issues with parenterals. Since validation seemed to have been an outgrowth of a major regulatory crisis, firms that did not make parenteral products were clearly skeptical of what was perceived to be an FDA overreaction to a problem unique to sterile product manufacturers. Despite these misgivings, FDA pressure was such that validation activities for sterilization processes were underway at virtually all U.S. parenteral manufacturers by the middle of the decade. The definition of validation in the 1970s provided little clear guidance as to its real intent, nor could anyone have foreseen in that definition the substantial impact validation was to have on the industry eventually.

"Validation is the attaining and documentation of sufficient evidence to give reasonable assurance, given the state of science and the art of drug manufacturing, that the process under consideration does, and/or will do, what it purports to do" (Ted Byers, June 1980).

Within this context, the industry began its first validation efforts. The goals of industry during this early period were in reaction to the lack of clarity on what validation really was and what it was required to be in a compliant state. This led to doing everything conceivable (often meaning mountains of paperwork) to "satisfy the FDA" out of a fear of the consequences of noncompliance. The solution was to keep the FDA happy and keep the facilities operating. The initial area of activity within the industry was almost totally directed toward sterilization and aseptic processing.

As firms focused on sterilization validation programs, the FDA continued to make presentations in support of validation and an industry perspective began to evolve. It was clear that the FDA intended to emphasize validation and impose it beyond just sterilization. Validation had become a part of cGMP expectations throughout the parenteral industry. Soon, the FDA recognized the merits of validation for all types of processes.

By the end of the 1970s, validation was largely a regulatory exercise that remained isolated from the rest of the firm and was certainly not an area of high concern during the design phase of a project. In 1987, the FDA published its "Guideline on General Principles of Process Validation" [6]. While there was initial opposition to the guideline's tone, there was general consensus that validation was now a way of life for the pharmaceutical industry. Within the guideline, the FDA provided the following definition that clarified expectations:

"Process validation is a documented program which provides a high degree of assurance that a specific process will consistently produce a product meeting its predetermined specifications and quality attributes" [6].

The 1987 guidance, which was revised in 2011, specifically included active pharmaceutical ingredients: "This guidance outlines the general principles and approaches that the FDA considers to be appropriate elements of process validation for the manufacture of human and animal drug and biological products, including active pharmaceutical ingredients (API or drug substance), collectively referred to in this guidance as drugs or products. This guidance incorporates principles and approaches that all manufacturers can use in validating a manufacturing process" [6].

It is important to discuss the terms *qualification* and *validation*. While these terms are often used interchangeably, their meaning is quite different, often leading to confusion. Early on, *validation* became synonymous with the activities focused around protocols, data acquisition, and reports. Validation had myriad interpretations, depending on the audience. However, in the simplest terms, equipment and systems are commissioned and qualified, but processes are validated. In the context of a design guide, this chapter focuses mainly on commissioning and qualification.

Commissioning includes predelivery inspection (PDI), factory acceptance testing (FAT), site acceptance testing (SAT), and field commissioning. Qualification includes design, installation, operational, and performance qualification (PQ). These may be combined with commissioning or verification, but the focus is on equipment and systems; these activities are engineering activities. PQ is the final step before validation. Commissioning and qualification confirm and document that systems are "fit for purpose." Following these activities, processes can be validated.

Qualification was not a significant part of many programs when validation first became a required activity in the late 1970s. The focus of regulatory guidance was on PV, which was often referred to as process qualification. Aspects of equipment and system installation and functionality were only minimally addressed. It was recognized that to ensure the reliability and consistency of validated processes, the equipment must function in a reliable manner. Measurement and confirmation of system operation could serve as a predictor of its ability to provide acceptable results in a subsequent PV study. With this, the qualification of equipment and systems as a precursor to validation became a standard feature of a sound validation program.

Validation generally refers to PV and also includes other product/process-related activities, such as methods validation, cleaning validation, mixing studies, shipping validation, dirty hold-time studies, and clean hold-time studies. These activities are critical to compliance and arguably more important than qualification: if a process cannot be validated, it is not a viable process; however, if a system cannot be qualified, the process in it cannot be validated.

In the early 1990s, there was a lack of understanding on the part of industry as to what validation really entailed and how this could add value. At the same time, the fear of 483 citations resulted in an overkill approach to qualification and validation. While the cost of qualifying and validating a facility was viewed as excessive, this was far eclipsed by the cost of a bad inspection and not being first to market.

The evolution of CQV has been driven by a number of factors, including greater industry involvement in the development of industry standards and regulatory guidelines, a greater focus on process understanding in developing and executing validation programs, and a realization that validation is not an endpoint in the project life cycle. Validation is a continuum of activities that, if properly executed, will greatly ensure product quality and patient safety, streamline regulatory inspections, and offer the opportunity for process improvements.

QUALITY BY DESIGN

In 2002, the FDA announced the pharmaceutical cGMPs for the twenty-first century. The initiative was an attempt to integrate quality systems and risk management approaches into existing programs with the goal of encouraging industry to adopt modern and innovative manufacturing technologies. This was spurred by a number of factors and goals, including (1) the need to harmonize cGMP with other non-U.S. pharmaceutical regulatory systems and with the FDA's own medical device quality system regulations; (2) the need to make the development of innovative medical products more efficient, so that safe and effective therapies could reach patients sooner; (3) the need to stress the importance for manufacturers to use robust quality systems and appropriate process knowledge to aid in implementing process improvements; (4) the hope that effective quality systems would lower the risk of manufacturing issues, better control product quality and reproducibility, and result in shorter and fewer FDA inspections; and (5) the provision of the necessary framework for implementing Quality by Design (QbD), continual improvement, and risk management in the drug manufacturing process [7]. The overarching philosophy articulated in the FDA's quality systems approach is, "Quality should be built into the product, and testing alone cannot be relied on to ensure product quality" [7].

QbD means designing and developing a product and associated manufacturing processes to ensure that the product consistently attains a predefined quality at the end of the manufacturing process. An essential element of the life cycle approach to CQV is the concept of QbD, which has become a catch phrase that most organizations throw around freely; QbD needs to be implemented during the product development phase through a thorough understanding of the product. QbD provides for a proactive approach to pharmaceutical development through process knowledge. At the project level, this is accomplished by understanding critical quality attributes (CQAs) of the product. CQAs are the physical, chemical, biological, or microbiological properties or characteristics that should be within an appropriate limit, range, or distribution to ensure the desired product quality. CQAs are generally associated with the drug substance, excipients, intermediates (in-process materials), and drug product [8]. Following identification of the CQAs, associated critical process parameters (CPPs), which control CQAs, are identified. There should be CPPs associated with each CQA. The design effort and subsequent project phases, including construction, commissioning, qualification, and validation, can then focus on delivering a process and facility that consistently deliver products that achieve these CQAs.

The implementation of QbD is not something that can take place as an afterthought well into design. QbD concepts include a life cycle approach, which requires that CQV be considered early and throughout the project. Input often is not provided early due to budgetary constraints, lack of resources, or the belief that the early design phases are purely engineering functions that will be impeded by CQV and quality input. This often leads to increased project costs due to rework and schedule slippage.

The project team has a shared goal: everyone shares the desire to bring safe, effective, and often lifesaving products to market; to meet project budgets and schedules; and to deliver a facility that surpasses operational and quality needs, expectations, and requirements. The continuously conflicting constraints of schedule, budget, and quality exist on every project. There is no perfect design that incorporates all operational, schedule, budgetary, and regulatory requirements into an easily validated design. These areas generally become points of contention between different project disciplines. Finding a successful balance between them is what defines a successful project.

GOOD ENGINEERING PRACTICE

GEP is key to successful implementation of QbD on any project. ASTM E2500 defines GEP as "those established engineering methods and standards that are applied throughout the life cycle to deliver appropriate and effective solutions" [9]. Examples of GEP include project and design management, the use of registered professional engineers, document control, project controls, the use of preapproved engineering specifications and standards, structured and documented design reviews, and change control. For areas and systems that are critical to product quality, GEP is supplemented by enhanced documentation, inspection, and testing activities, including qualification and validation. GEP must be applied throughout the project life cycle to deliver cost-effective facilities that meet user quality, safety, environmental, and regulatory requirements.

PROJECT AND ENGINEERING CHANGE CONTROL

Project change control (PCC) refers to the planned and documented method for the review, evaluation, approval, and communication of project changes before handover of the project to the end user.

PCC is an essential element of GEP and critical to implementing QbD on any project. The purpose of PCC is to ensure that proposed changes are properly evaluated to control effects on schedule, budget, safety, system performance, user requirements, product quality, and compliance with applicable regulations. PCC is an engineering project function. Typically, the project manager is responsible for implementing PCC to ensure that (1) controls are in place to prevent changes from being made without notification of and approval by appropriate members of the project team, (2) changes are properly documented, (3) changes are properly reviewed and approved by appropriate team members, and (4) changes are communicated to appropriate members of the project team. The project team may include engineering, construction, commissioning, qualification, validation, quality, regulatory affairs, operations, maintenance, automation, and environmental health and safety (EHS), as well as system owners. Changes need to be properly closed out, with all impacts addressed, including changes to documents affected by the change.

PCC is critical to GEP; however, it can limit the progression of the project during the early project phases. During the conceptual and preliminary design phases, design of the facility is very fluid, and PCC during these early phases is not recommended. PCC is typically implemented at the completion of the preliminary design phase with issuance of "issued-for-design" (revision 1.0) documents.

PCC should not be confused with site change control or quality assurance change control. Site change control refers to the planned and documented method for review, approval, and documentation of changes to critical drawings and documents, following turnover of the project to the site system owners.

Quality assurance change control is critical to keeping systems and processes with a product quality impact in a compliant, validated state. During facility design, construction, and commissioning, changes are handled by project engineering, according to GEPs. Quality may not be routinely involved in the PCC process, since these changes are typically linked to the technical management of the project and engineering documents. However, the PCC system should allow for quality review and input into the change when the change affects a qualified or validated system, a cGMP critical document, such as user requirement specifications (URSs), or the approach to CQV (i.e., a schedule change that dictates a family approach to media-hold studies, where three media-hold studies might be conducted on the first bioreactor, with only one study conducted for each subsequent bioreactor).

PROJECT LIFE CYCLE METHODOLOGY AND CQV

The use of a life cycle methodology requires that CQV and quality considerations be raised early in the project. This proactive approach is critical to the handover of a compliant facility. It is also critical that appropriate resources, which are often in short supply, focus on areas that ultimately have an impact on product quality and patient safety. Using quality personnel to approve equipment specifications, building footprints, process calculations, and other engineering deliverables is not a wise use of their time and expertise; it is also often detrimental to schedule and budget. However, focusing these resources on high-level, product-impacting documents, including master plans, USRs, and cGMP design reviews, is certainly critical to the success of the project.

The following sections detail typical deliverables throughout the project life cycle that impact quality; these are not intended to be a comprehensive list of all deliverables through each project phase. Project phases are described in this chapter as the concept, preliminary, detailed design, execution, validation, and closeout phases. Other naming conventions are often used, such as the feasibility phase, project definition phase, basic engineering phase, or basis of design phase. Many companies have defined the specific phases and required deliverables in structured guidelines or standards. Depending on the project scope, size, schedule, and deliverables, these phases may be combined, and deliverables may fall into different phases than those presented here. Projects typically progress from one phase to the next after completion of defined "stage gates."

These stage gates must be completed before a formal decision is made to authorize progression to the next project phase. Often, these stage gates include critical deliverables, which form the foundation for later project deliverables, such as system URSs. The stage-gate approach to project phasing has become an industry-accepted practice. It has been shown to be effective in producing a quality driven design, where disciplined teams are careful to check the quality of deliverables at each gate. A formal project review should be conducted at the completion of each phase to review the status of the project, the deliverables completed during the phase, and the direction of the project against the initial project charter. Projects generally proceed to the next phase with open deliverables, with the exception of critical stage-gate items that are prerequisites for the next phase. Finally, it should be noted that the intent of the following sections is not to limit the input of CQV and quality representatives during the design phase of the project; the intent is to focus often limited resources in the areas most critical to product quality, licensing, and ultimately, patient safety.

CONCEPTUAL DESIGN PHASE

This phase begins soon after the manufacturers recognize the need for a new facility or renovation, and for large projects, it generally precedes approval of the capital appropriation request. Its purpose is to provide an initial definition of the project in terms of scope, cost, and schedule by evaluating and selecting high-level business and technical options that can achieve the business need and provide the basis for the initial confirmation of financial viability. This phase therefore generally begins with broad, high-level URS, in which the goals of the facility are described quantitatively and qualitatively.

Quantitative goals are numerical measures used to define the facility in physical terms relative to size, dimension, and layout. Quantitative goals are objective and easy to define. Qualitative goals are more subjective in nature. These include goals for compliance, such as a design that meets worldwide cGMP requirements, is highly automated, or is state of the art in terms of technology. Quality and CQV input at this stage of the project are highly recommended, since this will highlight areas where regulatory concerns may influence design. This stage of the project may take longer than expected, as management teams often challenge cost or schedule objectives, necessitating the development of other options to achieve agreement on scope, estimated cost, schedule, and functionality of the finished facility.

PROJECT AND ENGINEERING DELIVERABLES

Typical deliverables from the conceptual design phase that have a CQV impact are discussed below. These are mainly project and engineering deliverables except where noted. However, a number have a quality impact, and as such, review and approval of the items by the CQV and quality representatives are highly recommended.

User Requirements Brief

The user requirements brief is typically developed by the engineering and design team to provide a comprehensive overview of the project and key drivers, including overall business and technical objectives, scope, schedule, cost, and requirements for regulatory compliance. This sets the direction for the project and should be reviewed but not approved by the CQV and quality teams.

Block Flow Diagrams

Block flow diagrams (BFDs) show major steps in the manufacturing process. Incoming and outgoing flows are shown, with process items shown in blocks (rather than as equipment). These are precursors to the process flow diagrams (PFDs).

Process Flow Diagrams

These depict the process flow, including material and energy balances, with BFD blocks replaced by equipment. The PFDs are the precursors to piping and instrumentation diagrams (P&IDs).

Conceptual Equipment Arrangements or Layouts

These indicate the location of major equipment items in the facility and are a prerequisite to material, equipment, and personnel (MEP) diagrams. At this phase, room classifications may be shown on the classification diagrams or listed in tabular form for classified spaces. While these are engineering deliverables, these should be reviewed by quality.

Material, Equipment and Personnel Flow Diagrams

These Material, Equipment and Personnel (MEP) diagrams show the flow of material, equipment, personnel, and waste through the facility. MEP diagrams should accurately depict these flows from entry into the facility through exit. These will be refined in later phases; however, broad MEP philosophies should be established at this phase, including the following: (1) Is two-way flow acceptable in certain areas? (2) What areas need to be fully segregated? (3) Is batch-to-batch full segregation required? (4) Is temporal segregation acceptable? (5) Are combined personnel and material airlocks acceptable, or are combined entry and exit airlocks acceptable? (6) Is the flow of personnel from less clean to cleaner areas, with increased gowning requirements, incorporated into the design?

Often, MEP diagrams are accompanied by a narrative describing flows throughout the facility from entry through exit. Such descriptions are very beneficial in helping the entire project team understand gowning regimes and assumptions, airlock considerations, cross-flows, and potential areas of concern with the overall design. A meeting is also helpful if a facility design meeting is going to be scheduled with the regulatory agency (see the Regulatory Review Meeting section of this chapter). It is critical to review owner design guidelines and quality directives in the review of MEP diagrams. Often, these stipulate requirements that are more stringent than agency requirements.

LEVEL II SCHEDULE

The project schedule developed at this phase establishes overall project milestones and priorities. Input from CQV should ensure that enough time is included in the schedule for all CQV activities and precursors (e.g., system prerequisites, calibration, mechanical completion, developmental runs, engineering runs, water system PQ activities, environmental monitoring, process and cleaning validation, and retest).

MAINTENANCE OF AN INTEGRATED SCHEDULE

Maintaining an integrated schedule is critical to achieving the overall project schedule and ultimately cost objectives. Separate, independent schedules are of little, if any, value. The integrated schedule should include timelines for engineering, procurement, construction, start-up, commissioning, qualification, developmental runs, turnover, validation, and regulatory filing and approval, with increasing levels of detail provided as the project progresses.

SUPER SKID AND SKID MODULE PHILOSOPHY

This consists of an evaluation of the potential to modularize certain elements of the project for the purpose of ease, speed of construction, inspection, testing, and scheduling. While this is certainly an engineering deliverable, it is a critical item for the CQV team, since it will have an impact on the system identification listing, system impact assessments, and overall inspection and testing approach.

Concept Phase Estimate

At this phase, this is generally a ±20%–30% estimate, depending on the level of deliverable completion or company practice. For CQV-related activities, a factored, not a detailed estimate, is applied. Depending on company practice, project size, scope, and type of facility, the level of engineering required for this phase may be in the range of 5%–25% and could represent 1%–5% of the total installed cost of the project.

Regulatory Strategy Document

This identifies the agencies and governments with which the facility will be licensed, their governing codes, and the related submission and inspection strategies to be followed by the project. The CQV strategy document would then be aligned with the regulatory strategy.

CQV Strategy Document

This document describes the strategy and approach that will be taken for the CQV of the new facility and for maintaining the facility in a cGMP-compliant manner. The strategy document often points to the concepts that will be used for CQV activities throughout the project; for example, "The overall strategy outlined in this document employs the concepts outlined in the ASTM E2500, 'Standard Guide for Specification, Design, and Verification of Pharmaceutical and Biopharmaceutical Manufacturing Systems and Equipment' and the ISPE *Baseline Pharmaceutical Engineering Guide for New and Renovated Facilities*, Volume 5, *Commissioning and Qualification*" [9, 10]. This is a high-level document that does not describe specific systems and may sit over or under the site validation master plan (SVMP). A separate CQV strategy document is not always developed. Often, the elements of the CQV strategy document are included in the site CQV master plan or project-level master plans.

Critical Quality Attributes and Process Parameters

Process understanding is a basic tenet of the life cycle approach to CQV and product quality. This is the basis for facility design. Process understanding is critical to understanding the risks that may be present in the process and mitigating these risks in the design. Key to process understanding is an understanding of CQAs and CPPs. The International Conference on Harmonisation (ICH) Q8 definitions follow: (1) The CQAs are physical, chemical, biological, or microbiological properties or characteristics that should be within an appropriate limit, range, or distribution to ensure the desired product quality. (2) The CPPs are process parameters whose variability has an impact on CQAs, and therefore should be monitored or controlled to ensure the process produces the desired quality [8]. The CQAs are identified during product development, with the process then further developed by conducting multivariate experiments to consistently produce a product meeting CQAs. To consistently deliver a product meeting CQAs, it is critical to understand the impact of material attributes and process parameters on CQAs, and then identify, control, and monitor the sources of variability in materials and the process. With this, there should be CPPs associated with every CQA. Wherever feasible, the design should allow monitoring of CQAs. This can allow for process control strategies that provide process adjustment capabilities to ensure control of all critical attributes. The CQAs and CPPs should be incorporated into URSs, which are the basis for all subsequent activities related to facility design, commissioning, qualification, validation, and handover.

System-Level URSs

Ideally, system-level URSs would be available at the completion of the conceptual phase and include CQAs and CPPs. The purpose of the URS is to describe the system intent, in terms of high-level performance requirements, including those related to cGMPs. The URS documents are used to ensure that cGMP regulatory expectations, CQAs, CPPs, and owner quality directives are incorporated into the design. It is very important to note that user requirements are not synonymous with design requirements. User requirements should focus on what is needed, without describing how the requirements will be achieved. Design requirements may be more stringent than user requirements to ensure that additional safety factors are designed into the system. User requirements should never be more stringent than design requirements.

A decision should be made at the project level as to which systems will require separate URS documents. For systems that do not have a quality impact (e.g., plant utility systems) and simpler pieces of equipment (e.g., standard refrigerators, freezers, and incubators), URSs may be incorporated in equipment specifications. All requirements indicated in the URS should be verified during design reviews and later field verified during CQV as appropriate. Non-cGMP requirements (i.e., safety, maintenance, operability, and expandability) may or may not be included in URS documents, depending on project or owner procedures and guidelines.

Engineering typically interviews user groups to determine and document user requirements on a system-by-system basis. Sources of user requirements may include the following: (1) product license requirements for an approved product; the product license stipulates critical process criteria and ranges; (2) the CQAs and CPPs and ranges defined in technology transfer documents; (3) owner guidelines and procedures; often, owner procedures stipulate more stringent requirements than regulatory bodies, so it is critical that there is parity between URS and the most stringent requirements; (4) Guidance issued by regulatory agencies, such as the FDA and European Medicines Agency (EMA); (5) the USP and International Organization for Standardization (ISO) standards and ICH guidelines; and (6) material compatibility requirements.

When documenting the user requirements, it is important to avoid overspecifying; for example, the URS might include a requirement that vessel internals are thoroughly wetted by spray balls. However, the URS should not specify the number of spray balls or rotation requirements. Overspecification leads to overly stringent requirements that are often unnecessary. This often leads to schedule delays and cost overruns. Overly detailed URS documents that go beyond performance lead to excessive documentation. Design review or design qualification needs to verify each item, which typically leads to editing and reapproving URS documents under PCC procedures. This can have a tremendous impact on cost and schedule.

Avoid underspecifying with statements that are too vague. For example, statements such as "the system must meet cGMP requirements" do not specify a particular user requirement. "Nice to have" items should also be avoided, as these are convenience items that may be desirable but are not truly cGMP critical. These items are often the focus of value engineering and often removed from the design at a later date.

It is important to include ranges. User requirements should not stipulate set values or overly stringent acceptance criteria; rather, URSs should include an acceptable range of values for critical attributes and parameters.

In the author's opinion, URSs are among the most important deliverables of the project. The URS documents are the foundation of all subsequent design deliverables and field verification activities. They are also generally one of the key deliverables required at the stage gate to go from the concept to the preliminary phase. Unfortunately, these are often rushed because of schedule pressures, copied from previous projects, and not given the attention they deserve.

Concept Phase cGMP Design Review

The cGMP design review completed at this phase examines and documents applicable regulatory requirements (e.g., FDA, EMA, Canadian, and owner), as well as expectations for the overall facility. These regulatory requirements, as well as CQAs and CPPs, should be verified as being incorporated into user or system requirements and other available design documents during this initial review.

The design effort will not have progressed to allow for a review of each individual system. Rather, this review focuses on the overall facility and examines high-level arrangements and flows to ensure that a practical approach has been taken to ensure adherence to cGMP concepts, as well as agency and owner regulatory requirements and expectations. Key areas examined during this phase include (1) material receipt, quarantine, release, and reject; (2) MEP flow diagrams; (3) layout diagrams; (4) gowning regimes; (4) area classifications; (5) user requirements; (6) heating, ventilation, and air conditioning (HVAC) zoning diagrams; (7) airflow diagrams; (8) cGMP philosophies; and (9) automation philosophy.

The design review team should consist of key members of the project team, including project, engineering, automation, quality, validation, manufacturing personnel, EHS, and other subject matter experts (SMEs) as appropriate. At the completion of the cGMP design review, a report should be issued summarizing the areas examined, regulatory requirements and expectations, reference documents, decisions made, and potential risks.

PRELIMINARY DESIGN PHASE

The objective of this phase is to refine and converge technical options to identify a single project concept and develop this concept to generate issued-for-design documents. During this stage, technical documents from the concept phase are detailed, with additional deliverables developed in accordance with the deliverables list. Deliverables completed during this phase should be approved for design. Once documents are issued as revision 1.0 (or 0.0), PCC procedures should be put into place. Deliverables impacting CQV activities are described below.

PIPING AND INSTRUMENTATION DIAGRAMS

P&IDs depict all equipment, ancillary items, instrumentation and controls, piping, valves, equipment and instrument tags, fluid flows, tie-ins, and notes to give a detailed view of process, utility, and support systems. These are developed from PFDs. The P&IDs are purely engineering deliverables and need not be approved by CQV or quality. However, these drawings should be provided to the CQV team for review, since they are key reference drawings against which systems are compared during commissioning and qualification. The P&IDs should be reviewed against URS documents during design reviews, to ensure that CQV expectations are incorporated. This would include items such as sample valves, minimum distances, slopes, block and bleed valves on clean-in-place (CIP) circuits, and use point filters. Once P&IDs are approved, change management should be imposed to ensure that affected members of the design and CQV team are notified when a change is requested.

Basis of Design Documents

Basis of design (BOD) documents provide a description and the design criteria for key areas, including HVAC, process, automation, process, process utilities, plant utilities, electrical, and support areas. For example, the BOD for HVAC would describe temperature and relative humidity ranges, classifications, air-change rates, differential pressures, controls, automation, and the design basis. BOD documents with a cGMP impact (e.g., those for HVAC, process utilities, automation, and CIP) are often referenced in deliverables for GxP systems; however, these are purely engineering deliverables and should not require quality approval.

System Identification and Development of a Systems List

This is typically a CQV deliverable, with input from the project team, including system owners, engineering, and construction. This involves dividing the facility, project, or area into logical systems. A number of factors should be considered when developing the systems list, including skid or module philosophy, vendor or subcontractor scope, construction schedule, system owner, delayed installation of use point equipment, and the impact of the system on product quality.

Depending on the above, systems may be identified on a P&ID basis (i.e., each P&ID is a separate system), skid basis (i.e., all items within a skid are considered one system), vendor or subcontractor scope basis (i.e., purified water generation separate from storage and distribution), or a system impact basis (i.e., if there are very few quality-critical components within a particular system, include those components within the scope of a different quality-critical system). Systems should be numbered in accordance with a company standard nomenclature, and referenced throughout the project life cycle. To the fullest extent possible, the same system boundaries should be maintained during construction, commissioning, and qualification.

SYSTEM-LEVEL IMPACT ASSESSMENT

The process of completing an impact assessment was first formally presented in the ISPE Baseline Guide *Commissioning and Qualification* (2001). Although this was first presented over 15 years ago, before the launch of the FDA's pharmaceutical cGMPs for the twenty-first-century initiative and before more formal and detailed procedures for conducting risk assessments became popular, most companies still use some form of the system-level impact assessment as presented in the original ISPE Baseline Guide. The impact assessment process is used to determine which systems should be subject to qualification practices in addition to GEP. Using this approach, systems are classified according to the definitions below.

Direct-Impact System

A system that is expected to have a direct impact on product quality is designed and commissioned in line with GEP and subject to additional qualification practices. A system is defined as direct impact if it meets any of the following criteria: (1) it comes in contact with the product (e.g., air quality); (2) it provides an excipient or produces an ingredient or solvent (e.g., water for injection [WFI]); (3) it is used in cleaning or sterilizing (e.g., clean steam); (4) it provides status preservation (e.g., nitrogen); (5) it produces data that are used to accept or reject product (e.g., electronic batch record system or CPP chart recorder); or (6) it is a process control system (e.g., programmable logic controller or distributed control system) that may affect product quality, and there is no system for independent verification of control system performance in place [10].

Indirect-Impact System

An indirect-impact system is one that is not expected to have a direct impact on product quality, but typically will support a direct-impact system. Example include plant steam and chilled water. These systems are designed and commissioned following GEP, and not subject to qualification practices.

No-Impact System

A system that will not have any impact, either directly or indirectly, on product quality is a no-impact system. These systems are designed and commissioned following GEP.

The system-level impact assessment is a CQV deliverable that should be approved by quality.

System Boundary Definition

This is typically a CQV deliverable. After the systems are identified, system boundaries should be identified. This is generally performed using P&IDs. Attention should be given to system interfaces to ensure that all elements of the project are included within the scope of the systems and also to ensure that the same system elements are not included in more than one system scope.

Equipment Specifications

Equipment specifications for long lead items are generated during this phase. These are engineering deliverables that need not be approved by quality; however, specifications should incorporate all URS and system specific and include specific requirements for deliverables and activities to support qualification, such as requirements for documentation, inspection, testing, FAT, and SAT.

Turnover Package Matrices

These are detailed listings of documentation requirements from vendors, the facility designer, and construction. Turnover packages are compiled by system, with system boundaries and package contents defined in the turnover package matrix. Typically, three types of turnover packages are compiled, and the contents are often specified in company procedures: (1) vendor turnover packages (VTOPs), (2) engineering turnover packages (ETOPs), and (3) construction turnover packages (CTOPs).

Development of the matrices and compilation of the turnover packages are generally not CQV activities; however, a great deal of the documentation included in the packages is critical to the CQV effort. Missing or late documentation is one of the major contributors to construction and commissioning punch lists, as well as deviations and schedule delays during the qualification and validation phases. It is strongly recommended that the CQV team provide input into these matrices to ensure that items necessary to support CQV activities are included. It is further recommended that professional documentation management resources be used to expedite, manage, compile, and verify the turnover packages to provide the CQV team with timely and complete documentation.

Vendor Document Requirement Matrices

A vendor document requirement (VDR) is an attachment to equipment data sheets and specifications that details the documents that the vendor must provide to support operations, maintenance, FAT, SAT, construction, quality, and CQV. The detailed VDR listing also includes an indication of the quantities required for each document (e.g., original equipment manufacturer manuals), format required (i.e., electronic or hard copy), and date required (i.e., prior to FAT, prior to shipment, or with shipment).

To the fullest extent possible, VTOPs should be verified during pre-delivery inspections, FAT and vendor SAT. These should be placed under project document control. Applicable documents from the VTOP are verified as part of field commissioning and qualification activities.

Engineering Documentation Requirements

This matrix delineates engineering design, specification, and procurement documents that must be supplied by the engineering contractor. Documents are compiled into ETOPs. The engineering documentation requirements and associated ETOPs are generally compiled by the engineering firm responsible for the design and reviewed and approved by the system owner for completeness.

Construction Documentation Requirements

This matrix delineates data and documentation that support the construction and mechanical completion of the system. The construction documentation requirements are compiled by the construction manager and reviewed and approved by the system owner for completeness. Many of the items included in the CTOP are CQV critical and reviewed during the field execution phase.

Preliminary Phase cGMP Review and Design Qualification

A second cGMP review and design qualification is often conducted at the completion of the preliminary design phase to verify that product, process, license, regulatory, and owner quality directives are incorporated into the approved system-level URS.

Risk Assessments

ICH Q9, "Quality Risk Management," defines risk as "the combination of the probability of occurrence of harm and the severity of that harm" [11]. Achieving a shared understanding of the application of risk management among diverse stakeholders is often difficult. Each stakeholder tends to perceive different potential harms, place a different probability on the likelihood of that harm occurring, and attribute different severities to each harm. The risk assessment process attempts to minimize the subjectivity involved in assessing risks.

A risk assessment is a systematic approach for evaluating new systems or changes to existing systems to identify and prioritize potential risks and their impact. If done correctly, there are numerous advantages to conducting risk assessments, including assisting in the decision-making process and prioritizing efforts to address issues; identifying major quality and regulatory concerns before they become a problem; identifying safety issues, environmental issues, and operational flaws; and finalizing the CQV approach and determining validation requirements. Finally, and perhaps most importantly, the risk assessment process forces an understanding of the process and what might go wrong to validate the selection of the manufacturing process and confirm the appropriateness of the design. An overview of a typical quality risk management process is shown in Figure 7.1.

The risk assessment process consists of identification of potential risks, assessment of the likelihood of the risk and potential failure modes, and evaluation of the severity of the risk. The deliverables from the risk assessment may be quantitative (e.g., risk number and risk score) or qualitative (e.g., high, medium, or low).

After the risk is assessed, the next step is to mitigate the risk by removing it, reducing it, or accepting it. Risk mitigation must reduce the risk to an acceptable level. Ideally, the risk can be eliminated in the design; more often, the risk can be reduced or mitigated through the process control system or other design modifications. It is less desirable to control risk procedurally, particularly in new facilities. Alternatively, a decision may be made to accept the risk based on the overall risk classification.

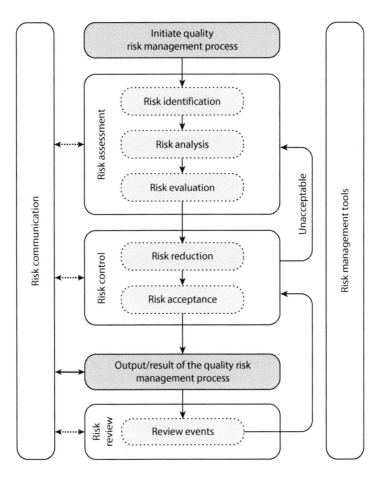

FIGURE 7.1 Risk management process. (From International Conference of Harmonisation, Guidance for Industry Q9: Quality Risk Management, International Conference of Harmonisation, Geneva, June 3, 2006. http://www.ich.org/fileadmin/Public_Web_Site/ICH_Products/Guidelines/Quality/Q9/Step4/Q9_Guideline.pdf)

Risk assessments are often conducted numerous times throughout the project design and are typically completed at the following milestones: (1) at the completion of the preliminary design phase, (2) during the detailed design phase, (3) before change on an existing system, (4) as the result of quality investigations or remediation, and (5) following an accident or recordable incident.

Finalize Templates and Review or Approval Process

It is critical that the templates to be used for all CQV deliverables and related items are defined before work begins on the actual deliverables. Significant detrimental effects on project schedule and budget can be avoided if formats are finalized during the early design phases. Since finalizing templates is not related to the design, templates can be finalized before the preliminary design phase; ideally these are defined by company procedure. In addition to defining the templates, the process for document flow, review, and approval must be finalized and communicated to the project team. A listing of all project-relevant standard operating procedures (SOPs) and guidelines (new and existing) should be made available during this phase.

Validation master plans (VMPs) have become a common practice for most capital projects. Most organization's quality directives stipulate that VMPs are a requirement, and often approval of the VMP is a project stage-gate deliverable. Although there is no regulatory requirement to complete a VMP, the VMP is an expectation. Annex 15 to the European Union (EU) Guide to GMP, "Qualification and Validation," states, "All validation activities should be planned. The key elements of a validation program should be clearly defined and documented in a VMP or equivalent documents" [12]. The term *VMP* is somewhat all-encompassing and, depending on the project phase, systems, and audience, has many different meetings. This chapter focuses on the project commissioning and qualification master plan (PCQMP), since this is most often a capital project deliverable. The hierarchy of VMPs is depicted in Figure 7.2.

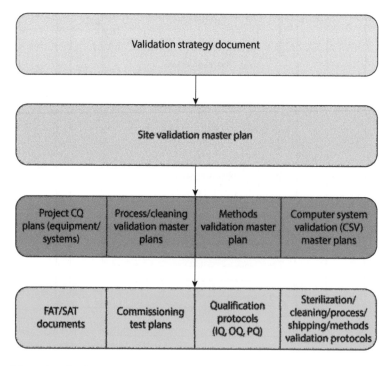

FIGURE 7.2 Hierarchy of validation master plans.

PROJECT PLANS

Site Validation Master Plan

Each site involved in manufacturing, distribution, or testing of drug products should have a SVMP to define the overall approach to commissioning, qualification, validation, and ongoing maintenance of the facility in a cGMP-compliant state. The SVMP should include details for managing the overall CQV program, including roles and responsibilities for initial CQV, risk assessments, design qualification, change control, document control, periodic review and revalidation, equipment- and system-specific inspection and testing activities with acceptance criteria, handling of deviations, and corrective actions. Individual project plans typically refer to the SVMP.

Project Commissioning and Qualification Master Plan

During the preliminary design phase of a project, the PCQMP should be developed. The PCQMP describes the scope of the project, responsibilities for project life cycle activities and deliverables that support commissioning and qualification, and the overall plan for operation of the project systems under cGMP requirements. The PCQMP should reference the SVMP.

The PCQMP should be a plan and not just a document to complete a stage gate or satisfy a quality directive or regulatory expectation. The plan should describe the facility, systems, specific instructions, deliverables, inspection and testing requirements, acceptance criteria, references, and responsibilities to hand over a compliant facility in accordance with regulatory and owner requirements. There is no standard format for PCQMPs, although several regulatory documents, such as Annex 15, give a listing of minimum expectations. A basic outline is provided in Table 7.1.

Computer System Validation Master Plans

Computerized systems are typically qualified using the system development life cycle methodology presented in the Good Automated Manufacturing Practice (GAMP) Guidelines 5 [13]. The level of validation depends on the complexity, uniqueness, and criticality of each system. GxP-regulated computerized systems include hardware, software, networks, interfaces, equipment, instruments, and procedures that create, modify, maintain, archive, retrieve, or distribute data used during the production of clinical and commercial product, testing, and distribution. Computer system VMPs are developed to describe the documentation, responsibilities, review, and testing requirements for each computer system throughout the project and validation life cycle. On a project level, a computer system validation master plan may be combined with the PCQMP; however, a separate document is often written.

Laboratory and Methods Validation Master Plan

This provides a description of the philosophy and strategy to support validation activities for laboratories and is typically developed by the quality control group. Test methods used for release, stability, in-process testing, and validation studies must be validated. Pharmacopoeial or compendial methods must be verified and documented prior to use to ensure that they can be correctly implemented. Microbiological methods, in all cases, require validation.

Process and Cleaning Validation Master Plan

Generally, a stand-alone process and cleaning validation master plan is developed. The process and cleaning plan describes the activities required to demonstrate that the new equipment and systems areas will be validated to meet cGMPs for cleaning and PV. As these activities are generally done in conjunction with each other, a combined process and cleaning validation master plan is generally developed, although separate plans may also be utilized.

TABLE 7.1

Contents of a Project Commissioning and Qualification Master Plan

Introduction	This gives an overview of the project scope, location, timing, and regulatory expectations (i.e., the facility will be designed to meet FDA, EMA, Japan, and owner regulatory requirements).
Purpose and scope	This describes the purpose of the plan (i.e., details the activities, responsibilities, procedures, and deliverables for completing CQV activities associated with the project), identifies the scope of the plan, and indicates exclusions from the plan. This may point to other owner VMPs (e.g., the site master plan) and other validation plans.
Responsibilities	High-level responsibilities for generation, execution, review, and support of the deliverables and activities delineated in the plan should be indicated for each functional area, such as the project manager, SMEs, manufacturing, metrology, facilities management/maintenance, automation, validation, quality control, quality assurance, and regulatory.
Facility/process description	A high-level overview should be provided. This should not be a repeat of the BOD documents, nor should this provide minute details that are subject to change. Rather, this should give an overview of major processing areas, critical utility systems, HVAC, automation, and support, with appropriate references to design documents.
System listing and CQV requirements	A table listing the equipment and systems included in the scope of the PCQMP, impact of each system, and CQV requirements for each should be included in the plan.
Overview of CQV deliverables	A high-level overview of each type of deliverable should be provided. This should reference the owner's specific SOPs and guidelines to be used in the execution of the project.
General and specific CQV activities acceptance criteria	Key acceptance criteria (i.e., general and specific) for the items listed in the systems listing should be provided. This would include general inspection and testing activities (typical for all systems), as well as system-specific testing and acceptance criteria. General items may include alarm and interlock testing, transfer testing, functional testing, and power-loss testing. Specific items would include inspection and testing activities unique to particular systems, such as environmental monitoring of classified spaces, media-hold studies for bioreactors, media fills for aseptic processing lines, empty and loaded chamber temperature mapping of autoclaves, and sampling of high-purity water systems.
Punch-list and deviation procedure	An overview of the procedure for identifying, documenting, and resolving punch-list items (i.e., nonconformances found before qualification) and deviations (i.e., nonconformances found during qualification/validation) should be provided, referencing a specific procedure for details.
SOP/guideline listing	A listing of all SOPs and guidelines to be used in the execution of the deliverables detailed in the PCQMP should be listed.
High-level schedule	It is the author's preference not to include a schedule since this is subject to change. The opposing view is that a schedule should be included since the PCQMP is an actual plan, and achieving a schedule is a major goal of the plan. Whatever the ultimate decision, if a schedule is included, it should be kept at a very high level to avoid excessive revisions to the VMP.
A responsible, accountable/ approval, conferred, and informed (RACI) matrix	A RACI matrix lists specific deliverables for each system, turnover packages, FAT, SAT, commissioning protocols, qualification protocols, and final reports. Additionally, the RACI matrix defines responsibilities for other activities that support the CQV effort, such as calibration, SOP development, developmental studies, engineering runs, sampling, sample analysis, environmental monitoring, and supply of consumables and test equipment. It is important to assign responsibility for each area to one functional group (and on a systems basis to one person). Assigning responsibility to more than one group leads to confusion and is equivalent to assigning responsibility to no one.
References	All references used in the development of the plan should be listed, with revisions and dates indicated.

Extractable and Leachable Testing Master Plan

This may be combined with the PV master plan; the key point is that this testing must be planned and completed. Extractability and leachability data are key elements of regulatory submissions, and with the increased use of disposable components, this cannot be overlooked. This testing must be built into the development schedule to ensure the availability of data.

Shipping Validation Master Plan

This plan describes the approach, studies, and acceptance criteria to validate the handling, storage, and shipping of products and intermediates.

Construction Quality Assurance Plans

It is recommended that the construction manager develops a construction quality assurance plan to describe the procedures that will be used to verify and document activities with a cGMP quality impact. Much of this documentation is compiled into the CTOP and used to support later commissioning and qualification activities. With this, it is critical that a plan be in place to verify and document these activities. Examples of construction quality assurance–related activities include (1) material receipt inspections and material control; (2) postconstruction cleaning; (3) materials of construction and lubricant verification; (4) welding procedures, welder qualifications, inspection and documentation, and weld maps; (5) as-built isometrics and P&IDs, (6) passivation, and electropolishing surface finishes; (7) calibration and loop checks; (8) pressure tests, cleaning, and flushing; (9) clean construction techniques; (10) training records; (11) SOPs; (12) leak testing; (13) spray ball coverage; (14) HVAC system testing and balancing; (15) SAT documentation (if within the scope of the construction manager); (16) integrity tests; and (17) punch-list documentation and closure.

REGULATORY REVIEW MEETING

In recent years, it has become quite common to request a pre-operational review meeting with the regulatory agency to review the facility design at the completion of the preliminary design phase or at the completion of detailed design and preconstruction. Scheduling a review meeting is strongly recommended, since this may reveal potential areas of concern in the design phase rather than in conjunction with an inspection. This also opens up dialogue with the agency, which can result in a more timely review and approval of the application. The application sponsor must submit a request to the agency for a preoperational review; the agency will not accept a request from the engineering company, construction manager, or any other subcontractors involved in the design.

Design review meeting requests typically occur at the completion of the concept phase, but more commonly occur at the completion of preliminary. This generally involves a review of the following key documents, which should be delivered to the agency in advance of the meeting: layouts; MEP diagrams; PFDs; classification, airflow, and zoning diagrams; master plans; listing of any elements of the design that may be unconventional; and the PCQMP.

Preconstruction design review occurs at the completion of detailed design and, in addition to the items above, may also involve a review of the more detailed design deliverables available at this phase, including P&IDs; clean utility systems; drainage systems; HVAC systems, including pressurization plans; control systems; and facility review, including gowning regimes, airlock philosophies, and monitoring of critical environmental factors.

A review meeting does not guarantee approval of the facility. It does, however, give the facility sponsor the opportunity to understand the agency's current opinion as to whether the facility would comply with cGMPs at the time of the review. In particular, if there are any aspects of the design that may "push the envelope" of current industry practice (e.g., the increased use of gray space rather than classified space), the meeting provides an excellent opportunity to receive the agency's opinion in regard to these areas.

ESTIMATES

At the completion of preliminary design, a definitive funding estimate is commonly developed. At this phase, this is generally a ±10%–20% estimate, depending on the level of deliverable completion. Depending on company practice, project size, scope, and type of facility, the level of engineering required for this phase may be in the range of 25%–40% and could represent 3%–10% of the ultimate project total installed cost. As this is typically a definitive estimate for funding purposes, detailed input is required from each discipline, including CQV.

DETAILED DESIGN PHASE

This phase of the project is the most intensive from a design perspective and involves the greatest engineering resource requirements. During this phase, drawings and specifications are prepared in sufficient detail to construct buildings, purchase and install equipment, commission and qualify equipment and systems, and validate the facility and process. Resource requirements to complete commissioning and qualification deliverables increase greatly during this phase, with the bulk of commissioning, qualification documents, and support documents written and approved.

COMMISSIONING AND QUALIFICATION APPROACHES

The traditional approach to equipment qualification is to perform commissioning on an informal basis to ensure that systems are mechanically complete and functional before qualification. With this approach, commissioning represents prequalification to ensure that suppliers and subcontractors have completed their respective work and to ensure that systems are ready for subsequent qualification.

Most organizations use a leveraged approach to commissioning and qualification, where activities completed during commissioning (e.g., FAT, SAT, and site commissioning) are leveraged to support qualification rather than repeated during qualification. This approach was first formalized in the ISPE Baseline Guide *Commissioning and Qualification* of 2001 [10]. This guide introduced the formal process of system-level impact assessments, component-level impact assessments, and leveraging commissioning to support qualification. Goals of this leveraged approach include (1) cost savings, by leveraging rather than repeating documentation and testing activities completed during earlier project phases; (2) schedule savings, by pulling back activities normally completed during qualification to the construction and commissioning phase; and (3) focusing often limited quality assurance resources by requiring enhanced documentation only for those systems with a direct impact on product quality, including additional documentation, testing, quality assurance change control, and quality assurance review and approval.

While there are numerous benefits in the ISPE Baseline Guide approach, using quality assurance change control during commissioning is very often problematic. Subjecting systems to quality assurance change control during FAT, SAT, and other commissioning activities essentially leads to commissioning turning into qualification. The flexibility offered during the commissioning phase to shakedown systems without quality assurance approval to make changes is lost. Additionally, the original Baseline Guide focused on equipment. With the release of ICH Q8 ("Pharmaceutical Development") and ICH Q9 ("Quality Risk Management"), the focus has become more on product and process understanding [8, 11].

ASTM E2500, "Standard Guide for Specification, Design, and Verification of Pharmaceutical and Biopharmaceutical Manufacturing Systems and Equipment," attempts to update the Baseline Guide [9]. Key concepts presented in the American Society for Testing and Materials (ASTM) guide include a focus on product and process understanding, an approach in line with concepts described in ICH Q8 and Q9; a focus on systems and processes being fit for their intended purpose; and an understanding of roles and responsibilities, maximizing the use of vendor and supplier data and applying GEP to support specification, design, and verification.

Key differences between the approach presented in the ISPE Baseline Guide and ASTM E2500 include melding of commissioning, installation qualification (IQ), and operational qualification (OQ) into one process referred to as verification; replacement of PQ with performance testing; the

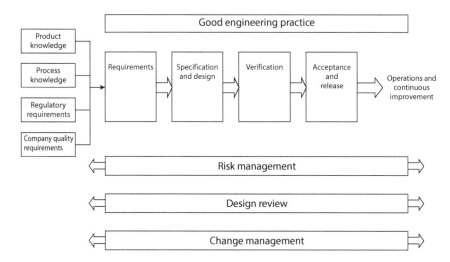

FIGURE 7.3 Specification, design, and verification process.

implementation of project or engineering change control through verification, with quality assurance change control beginning at performance testing; replacement of impact assessments (system level and component level) with repeated risk assessments; more of a reliance on vendors and SMEs for verification activities; and verification test plan management and approval by engineering, with performance testing management and approval by quality.

An overview of the specification, design, and verification process presented in ASTM E2500 is given in Figure 7.3.

There are numerous advantages to the approach presented in ASTM E2500, including forcing an early definition of needs, using the expertise of SMEs and vendors, focusing quality involvement in those areas that are critical to product quality, minimizing the duplication of effort between commissioning and qualification by replacing separate processes with one, using a pragmatic change control procedure, potential pulling back the schedule, and potentially saving money if fewer activities are duplicated.

Many organizations are using a hybrid CQV approach that melds successful concepts from ASTM E2500 with those from the ISPE Baseline Guide. This melded approach includes early definition of needs; functional and process-focused risk assessments; system-level impact assessments; use of the expertise of SMEs and vendors with active but focused quality involvement; use of engineering rather than quality change control through the commissioning phase; leveraging of commissioning to support qualification, rather than replacement of commissioning; and qualification with verification to allow for the use of existing quality systems and address concerns with regard to regulatory compliance. The following CQV-related deliverables are completed during the detailed design phase, using this hybrid approach.

VENDOR FAT AND SAT PROTOCOLS

Vendor-supplied FAT and SAT documents are typically submitted to the project team for pre-execution review and approval during the detailed design phase. Both FAT and SAT are considered commissioning activities, with the project team responsible for ensuring that FAT and SAT requirements are communicated to system vendors and subcontractors in equipment specifications and subcontractor bid documents.

The FAT/SAT documents are approved by engineering or project team members and generally not by quality. Vendor FAT documents should be evaluated by key project stakeholders to ensure

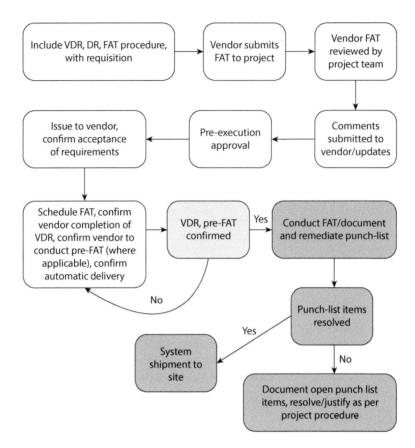

FIGURE 7.4 FAT process.

that requirements, as stipulated in equipment specifications, are included. The FAT documents should be evaluated to ensure that all documentation, inspection, and testing activities are properly captured. An overview of the FAT process is given in the flow diagram in Figure 7.4.

Inspection and testing activities completed during FAT and SAT may be used to support qualification activities, also called leveraging. If this testing is to be leveraged to support later activities, it is recommended that FAT documents (and SAT) be reviewed by CQV and potentially quality. If owner quality directives stipulate that these documents must be approved by CQV and if quality testing is to be leveraged, then, of course, this would be a project expectation. If FAT and SAT activities are leveraged and not repeated during site qualification, these must be documented according to cGMP documentation practices as follows: (1) Documents are revision controlled with acceptance criteria clearly indicated. (2) Results are clearly indicated, with a method of indicating "pass" or "fail" for results. (3) The signature of the person performing the test and the date of the test are clearly indicated on each data sheet. (4) Nonconformances and punch-list items include a method of recording and documenting the resolution of these items. (5) All handwritten entries are made using permanent ink at the time the activity takes place. (6) Corrections to entries in the FAT and SAT are made by striking through the incorrect entry with a single line and inserting the correct entry in such a way that the original entry remains legible.

DETAILED DESIGN REVIEW OR DESIGN QUALIFICATION

The design review or design qualification during this phase requires engineering, vendor, supplier, and subcontractor documentation to ensure that URS are achieved in the design. This design review is especially critical, since this is the final opportunity to make changes to the design to ensure that requirements are incorporated into the delivered system. Each of the requirements indicated in the URS should be verified during this review. Additionally, the design review often includes an indication of when the URS requirement will be verified during field execution of CQV activities.

DEVELOPMENT OF COMMISSIONING DOCUMENTS

The ISPE Baseline Guide *Commissioning and Qualification* defines commissioning as "a well planned, documented, and managed engineering approach to the start-up and turnover of facilities, systems, and equipment to the end-user that results in a safe and functional environment that meets established design requirements and stakeholder expectations" [10]. The term *commissioning* typically encompasses the following tasks: physical completion and inspection, setting to work, regulation and adjustment, and testing and performance testing.

All systems are commissioned, with the degree of formality and rigor based on the criticality (e.g., cGMP, EHS, and operational) and complexity of the system. For direct-impact systems, the commissioning effort (including inspection, FAT, and SAT) may assist qualification activities by providing testing and documentation necessary to support the qualification effort and ensuring that systems are ready for qualification before the qualification phase.

Regardless of the approach used for integrated CQV, it is critical to commission all systems before qualification. Moving directly from mechanical completion to qualification without first verifying that the system is properly installed, documented, and functioning is a sure path to endless deviations and massive schedule and budget overruns during the qualification phase.

For direct-impact systems, commissioning test plans resemble installation and operational qualification (IOQ) protocols. However, while IOQ documents focus on those items with a cGMP impact, commissioning protocols will include installation and functional verification of the entire system.

DEVELOPMENT AND APPROVAL OF QUALIFICATION PROTOCOLS

Qualification protocols include installation qualification (IQ), operational qualification (OQ), and performance qualification (PQ). During the detailed design phase, protocols should be generated and pre-execution approved. It is recommended that a combined IOQ, rather than separate IQ and OQ documents, be generated; this will minimize the number of documents generated and lead to scheduling and budget efficiencies.

Installation Qualification

An IQ is performed to verify that the system is built and installed in accordance with design specifications and applicable regulatory codes and guidelines. Note that much of IQ can be leveraged from earlier project phases (e.g., FAT, SAT, mechanical completion verification, and commissioning). The decision to leverage earlier project activities and the specific activities that will be leveraged should be detailed in the PCQMP and rationalized as part of the risk assessment process.

Operational Qualification

An OQ is performed to verify system operation within specified ranges of parameters, such as temperature, pressure, and flow. Execution of the OQ involves testing parameters that regulate the process and product quality; however, actual product is not used during OQ. Typical, non-system-specific OQ tests include verification of the proper operation of programmed sequences, controllers, indicators, recorders, pressure-hold studies, transfer verification, spray ball coverage testing, integrated functional checks, alarm and interlock testing, and power failure testing.

As with IQ, much of OQ can be leveraged from earlier project phases, provided prerequisites are met. For projects where commissioning is heavily leveraged, IOQ documents may serve largely as a documented audit of commissioning documentation to confirm that cGMP critical items and functions have been properly verified, tested, and documented. However, if extensive troubleshooting of systems is required during the commissioning phase, the decision to repeat commissioning testing activities may be recommended.

Performance Qualification

The PQ is not synonymous with PV, developmental runs, or engineering runs. PQ protocols are developed during the detailed design phase to verify that the pharmaceutical-grade utility, environment, equipment, or support system produces the required output. This output may be a product contact utility (e.g., clean compressed air and WFI), sterilization condition (e.g., autoclave), aseptic condition (e.g., media fills), or environment (e.g., HVAC system).

DEVELOPMENT OF SOPS

Development of SOPs for a new facility is a monumental task that is often overlooked until the field execution phase. Typical procedures needed for equipment and systems include operation, cleaning, preventive maintenance, and calibration. While SOPs are not CQV documents, these are needed to support the CQV effort. At a minimum, SOPs should be available in draft form at the start of operational testing. As the CQV effort proceeds, these can be updated to reflect more closely the proper operating methods for the equipment. Where feasible, SOP development should begin in the detailed design phase. For skidded systems, operational and maintenance SOPs will be based on vendor-supplied information. For stick-built systems, operational SOPs will be based largely on functional specifications and design documentation provided by the engineering project team.

PROJECT MANAGEMENT ISSUES

Having a validated process and licensed facility is the quintessential goal of any project. If all project objectives have been met, but the facility cannot be licensed, the project has been an abject failure. That being said, cost and schedule are incredibly important too. Key to successfully managing budget and schedule is to both understand and control the scope. All too often, basic project management principles are not applied to CQV, and the effort is treated as more of an art than a science. Endless "lessons learned" sessions have included detailed horror stories of projects that took years to qualify and validate, armies of consultants churning out volumes of documents, thousands of deviations, and endless change orders. To the extent that a company predefines its CQV practices, standards, documentation formats, and requirements procedurally and sets up a framework for the project team to apply, these risks can be minimized.

Using an established project control system to monitor schedule, performance, cost, and change for CQV activities is critical. This will allow for the identification of baseline cost, schedule, and progress to maximize project control, as well as the opportunity for continuous project improvement and corrective actions. The level of rigor associated with the project control system should be commensurate with the size, complexity, criticality, and risk associated with the project. However, for any CQV project, there must be a baseline understanding of and plan for control of schedule, cost, scope, and productivity.

SCHEDULE CONTROL

High-level project milestones should be established at the start of the project, with detail added at the system level as the project progresses. Ultimately, the CQV schedule must be integrated into the overall project schedule, taking into account all items included in the RACI matrix and all prerequisites. The CQV lead should provide input into the overall project schedule and work with the design team, construction manager, other subcontractors, system owners, and support functions to ensure that prerequisites are detailed in the schedule. Reports showing planned, actual, and forecast dates for each key deliverable should be issued on a regular basis.

In putting together the integrated schedule, it is critical to include prerequisites for each CQV deliverable. Before the execution of qualification field activities, the following activities must take place or specific items must be available to avoid excessive deviations: (1) Commissioning and qualification documents must be approved for execution. (2) Each system must be mechanically complete with critical punch-list items resolved. (3) Calibration and loop checks must be complete. (4) Turnover packages must be compiled with all GxP critical data included. (5) Shakedown and commissioning must be complete with critical punch-list items resolved. (6) Depending on the control system, separate automation qualification must be complete (prior to OQ). (7) Operational SOPs should be available (at a minimum in draft form). (8) Consumable items and test equipment must be available. (9) All prerequisite systems must be available. System dependencies should be built into the project schedule (e.g., before an autoclave can be qualified, clean steam, plant steam, compressed air, and electricity must be available).

It is very easy and sadly very common for the CQV schedule to slip into a state of chaos. Consider a capital project with 100 separate qualified systems, with each system having 8 separate deliverables for a total of 800 deliverables. Assume that all deliverables must be completed in 1 year. This translates to the generation, review, and approval of roughly 16 deliverables a week. Completion of each deliverable involves five steps; each deliverable needs to be written, issued for comment, reviewed and commented on by the approval signatories, updated, and issued for approval. If the schedule allows for 5 days for each step, then completion of each deliverable requires 25 days. Now assume two revision cycles on each deliverable, with a 6-day turnaround time on each step. It does not seem like much of a strain on the schedule; however, the completion of each deliverable now requires eight steps, 6 days per step, or 48 days—almost double the time originally budgeted in the schedule. Multiply this by 800 deliverables and the product is schedule chaos. The moral of this story is to: (1) Enforce the number of revision cycles. If given numerous opportunities to review a document, all opportunities will be used. (2) Enforce document turnaround times. This is difficult to do, and the responsibility ultimately falls on the project manager to instill a culture of urgency in the project team to review all deliverables within the allocated time. (3) Minimize the number of document approvers. Every approver of a deliverable has other responsibilities, most of which probably seem much more critical than reviewing and approving documents. Every approver is therefore a source of schedule delays. (4) Ensure adequate resources are available to review and approve all documents. If the project team includes only one quality representative working part-time on the project, this could pose a risk to the schedule. (5) Ensure all prerequisites are built into the integrated project schedule. A stand-alone CQV schedule that does not incorporate prerequisites is of little value.

PERFORMANCE MONITORING AND EARNED VALUE

Some form of performance monitoring should be implemented on any project. Simply assuming that everyone is busy so the work must be getting done is not the best gauge of project performance, nor will this control the budget or schedule. At the start of any fixed-scope CQV project, the earned value system for performance monitoring should be established. Earned value is determined by comparing the budget (in hours and dollars) to the actual hours and dollars expended. This comparison provides performance factors and a trend history. By analyzing trends, a performance factor for job completion can be forecast. Consider that same project discussed previously with 800 deliverables. The budget for each deliverable is 30 h, resulting in an overall deliverables budget of 24,000 h. Labor costs are $100 an hour, resulting in an overall deliverables budget of $2.4 million.

TABLE 7.2
Cost Overruns

Budget/earned hours per deliverables	30/30
Spent hours per deliverable	40
Productivity	earned/spent = 75%
Estimated hours to complete all deliverables	24,000/0.75 = 32,000
Estimated cost to complete all deliverables	$2,400,000/0.75 = $3,200,000
Projected overrun	$800,000 or 33%

Unfortunately, for a number of reasons, each deliverable is taking an additional 10 h to complete. In the scheme of things, an additional 10 h does not seem problematic. Everyone is still working at full speed and the work is getting done. However, as shown in Table 7.2, this results in 33% overrun of the project budget.

Ideally, earned hours will be equal to or greater than actual hours spent, and this is a reasonable expectation after an initial project learning curve. By regularly monitoring progress and productivity, using quantifiable methods, the health of the project can be quickly determined and appropriate corrective actions taken.

SCOPE AND CHANGE CONTROL

All projects experience changes that affect cost and schedule. These usually fall into the following categories: scope changes, schedule delays, additional document revisions, and field failures (punchlist, deviations, and unbudgeted retest). As with all areas of the project, effective scope and cost tracking offer the opportunity to evaluate planned and unplanned changes, investigate alternatives, and minimize the negative impact of change on both schedule and budget.

FUTURE DEVELOPMENTS

In 2014, the FDA approved 41 novel drugs, including Lynparza for the treatment of advanced ovarian cancer, Blincyto for the treatment of B-cell precursor acute lymphoblastic leukemia, Harvoni and Viekira Pak for the treatment of hepatitis C, and Zykadia to treat non–small cell lung cancer [14]. While these drugs treat vastly different illnesses, they do have one thing in common: all are examples of targeted drug therapies, often referred to as personalized medicines. Unlike conventional therapies, personalized medicines are tailored to the individual characteristics of each patient.

On July 9, 2012, the FDA's Safety and Innovation Act (FDASIA) was signed into law. One of the goals of FDASIA is to promote innovation to speed patient access to new products. Under FDASIA, new drugs may be given special designations to expedite development and agency review. This includes granting fast-track, breakthrough therapy, accelerated approval, and priority review designations. The goal of these designations is to expedite the development and review of new drugs with preliminary evidence indicating the drug may offer a substantial improvement over other available treatments for serious or life-threatening diseases, and especially for those that offer treatments where no other therapies are available. The ultimate goal is to bring these therapies to patients as soon as it can be concluded that the benefits justify the risks [15]. This has led to earlier patient access to new, often lifesaving therapies.

Many believe that targeted therapies will eventually replace more conventional therapies. These have the potential to offer hope to patients and their families battling illnesses where no other hope exists.

So what does this have to do with integrated facility design and integrated CQV? Safe, effective, available drugs have saved millions of lives and given greater quality of life to those suffering from illnesses that in the past were untreatable. Targeted therapies offer even greater promise to treat illnesses, while allowing patients a greater quality of life throughout treatment. Conventional facility designs, project execution approaches, and product delivery logistics need to adapt to different and often small-scale technologies used for targeted therapies. An individual batch may be a treatment for one individual patient or a small population with a rare disease, and the delivery of that batch may mean the difference between life and death for that patient or population. The need to deliver lifesaving therapies to market quickly in the context of small patient populations demands that new regulatory and licensing approaches be adopted by agencies, with consequent adaptation of design and validation methodologies by the industry. Pressure on designers and validators to complete projects in much less time will become even greater, whether for traditional pharmaceuticals or targeted therapies, due to the priority of the medical need and competitive pressures.

To meet the needs of this evolving trend, plant designs supporting these therapeutic solutions will evolve to include highly flexible, small-scale, and fully contained systems, with flexible automation and a preponderance of disposable components and contact parts. Such designs could be configured with different, prequalified unit operations in many different ways to suit the needs of the process, while minimizing some of the historical validation needs, such as cleaning via the use of disposables. Modular approaches to validation documentation may evolve to allow streamlined qualification testing of each new configuration before PV.

FURTHER DISCUSSION

1. What is the role of the FDA? Describe the relationship between the FDA and pharmaceutical companies.
2. What are commissioning and qualification?
3. What is change control?
4. What factors are important when developing user requirement specifications (URS)? What are common issues that arise?
5. How are targeted therapies changing the validation process?

ABOUT THE AUTHOR

Christina Meyer Dell Cioppia is senior vice president of validation and regulatory compliance with Amec Foster Wheeler (AFW), where she is responsible for CQV projects worldwide. Before joining AFW in 2003, Christina held various positions with Kvaerner Process for 14 years as a process engineer, CQV specialist, project manager, director, and ultimately vice president of validation. Christina has assisted biopharmaceutical, vaccine, pharmaceutical, and aseptic processing firms worldwide in the areas of commissioning, qualification, validation, design reviews, cGMP audits, program development, project management, training, remediation, and worldwide regulatory compliance. Christina holds her BS in biochemical engineering from Rutgers University, New Brunswick, NJ, and an MBA in industrial management from Fairleigh Dickinson University, Teaneck, NJ. She is a frequent industry speaker and contributing author to the *ISPE Baseline Guide: Commissioning and Qualification*.

REFERENCES

1. U.S. Food and Drug Administration, *A History of the FDA and Drug Regulation in the United States*, 1st ed. U.S. Food and Drug Administration, Silver Spring, MD, 2013.
2. Fintel B, Samaras AT, Edson C, The Thalidomide Tragedy: Lessons for Drug Safety and Regulation. Introduction to Food Regulation in the United States, *Helix Magazine*, July 28, 2009.
3. U.S. Food and Drug Administration, Milestones in Food and Drug Law History, U.S. Food and Drug Administration, Silver Spring, MD, May 14, 2009, http://www.fda.gov/AboutFDA/WhatWeDo/History/Milestones/default.htm.

4. U.S. Food and Drug Administration, Distribution of Full-Time Equivalent (FTE) Employment Program Level, U.S. Food and Drug Administration, Silver Spring, MD, http://www.fda.gov/downloads/AboutFDA/ReportsManualsForms/Reports/BudgetReports/UCM301553.pdf.

5. U.S. Food and Drug Administration, FY 2015 Operating Plan, 3, U.S. Food and Drug Administration, Silver Spring, MD (downloaded June 1, 2015), http://www.FDA.gov.

6. U.S. Food and Drug Administration, Guideline on General Principles of Process Validation, 4, 6, 1987, U.S. Food and Drug Administration, Silver Spring, MD, http://www.fda-consultant.com/provalid.html.

7. U.S. Food and Drug Administration, Quality Systems Approach to Pharmaceutical Current Good Manufacturing Practice Regulation, U.S. Food and Drug Administration, Silver Spring, MD, September 3, 2006, http://www.fda.gov/downloads/Drugs/GuidanceComplianceRegulatoryInformation/Guidances/UCM070337.pdf.

8. International Conference of Harmonisation, Guidance for Industry Q8 (R2): Pharmaceutical Development, International Conference of Harmonisation, Geneva, November 16, 2009, http://www.fda.gov/downloads/Drugs/GuidanceComplianceRegulatoryInformation/Guidances/UCM073507.pdf.

9. ASTM International, Standard Guide for Specification, Design, and Verification of Pharmaceutical and Biopharmaceutical Manufacturing Systems and Equipment, 2, ASTM International E2500-13, ASTM International, West Conshohocken, PA, November 1, 2013, http://www.astm.org/Standards/E2500.htm.

10. International Society for Pharmaceutical Engineering, *Baseline Pharmaceutical Engineering Guide: Pharmaceutical Engineering Guides for New and Renovated Facilities*, International Society for Pharmaceutical Engineering, Tampa, FL, 2002, pp. 29, 30, 51.

11. International Conference of Harmonisation, Guidance for Industry Q9: Quality Risk Management, International Conference of Harmonisation, Geneva, June 3, 2006, http://www.ich.org/fileadmin/Public_Web_Site/ICH_Products/Guidelines/Quality/Q9/Step4/Q9_Guideline.pdf.

12. European Commission, Final Version of Annex 15 to the EU Guide to Good Manufacturing Practice, European Commission, Brussels, July 4, 2001.

13. International Society for Pharmaceutical Engineering, *GAMP 5: A Risk-Based Approach to Compliant GxP Computerized Systems*, International Society for Pharmaceutical Engineering, Tampa, FL, 2008.

14. Woodcock J, FDA Continues to Lead in Precision Medicine, n.p., March 23, 2015, http://blogs.fda.gov/fdavoice/index.php/2015/03/fda-continues-to-lead-in-precision-medicine/.

15. U.S. Food and Drug Administration, Guidance for Industry: Expedited Programs for Serious Conditions—Drugs and Biologics, U.S. Food and Drug Administration, Silver Spring, MD, May 2014, http://www.fda.gov/downloads/Drugs/GuidanceComplianceRegulatoryInformation/Guidances/UCM358301.pdf.

16. Carleton F, Agalloco J, *Validation of Aseptic Pharmaceutical Processes*, M. Dekker, New York, 1986, p. 1.

8 Process Engineering

Art Meisch

CONTENTS

INTRODUCTION

ROLE OF PROCESS ENGINEERING IN THE PHARMACEUTICAL INDUSTRY

Process engineering forms the bridge between the underlying sciences of chemistry, biology, and pharmacology and manufacturing operations. The process engineer translates the basic science and technology of the process steps into a commercially feasible production process. This task includes scaling up unit operations and converting them into the sizing, specification, and selection of the production equipment systems. These systems must meet the required production capacity for the selected products, while simultaneously meeting the constraints of capital and operating costs. The process engineer must also consider current Good Manufacturing Practice (cGMP) regulations, safety, and environmental issues.

RELATIONSHIP OF PROCESS ENGINEERING TO OTHER DESIGN DISCIPLINES

Every aspect of the pharmaceutical manufacturing facility is focused on supporting the process operation and allowing it to function as intended. The design of these facilities is a team effort; typical teams are comprised of process; instrumentation and control system; mechanical, civil or structural, and electrical engineers; architects; manufacturing personnel; validation and quality operations personnel; and frequently, scientists and engineers from research and development. A key responsibility of the process engineer is to communicate the processing system's requirements to the other design team members so that they can design a facility that achieves the production objectives.

IMPACT OF cGMPs ON PROCESS ENGINEERING

The cGMPs require that the production processes manufacture products that consistently meet quality, efficacy, and stability requirements. A well-documented scientific basis for process operations ensures that when they are carried out under the documented conditions, the correct drug results.

   The process and the facility are designed to prevent both trace contamination and cross-contamination of the drug products. Typical sources of trace contamination are water used in production, equipment and piping systems, and environmental particulates. The responsibility of the process engineer is to specify and design process equipment and piping systems that will prevent contamination and can be easily cleaned, as well as to establish safe environmental conditions within the manufacturing facility to protect the product. The International Society of Pharmaceutical Engineering (ISPE) Baseline Pharmaceutical Guides provide an excellent resource for identifying and addressing cGMP issues.

EXECUTIVE SUMMARY

HISTORICAL PERSPECTIVES ON PROCESSING IN THE PHARMACEUTICAL INDUSTRY

Many of the earliest pharmaceutical chemicals were extracted by the individual user from natural substances (e.g., willow leaves and bark yielded molecules similar to those of acetylsalicylic acid or aspirin). Early manufacturing efforts also extracted pharmacologically active chemicals from plants and animal tissues. Digitalis, for example, is still extracted from plants commercially. Animals were used to produce some of the first vaccines and antibiotics; for example, cows were used to make the smallpox vaccine. Of course, the use of genetically engineered plants and animals, both multicellular and single cellular, is at the forefront of today's technology for both biologicals and even synthetic pharmaceuticals. Beginning in the late 1800s, chemists began to develop methods to produce naturally occurring chemicals synthetically. Aspirin, for example, was first synthetically manufactured in the 1800s from coal tar. The trend of using chemical reactions to manufacture pharmaceuticals grew throughout the 1900s, especially after World War II, to become the production method of choice for most active pharmaceutical ingredients (APIs). Fermentation has been used since the 1940s to produce antibiotics, and biotechnology has been used with increasing prevalence to produce more targeted molecules since the 1980s. Today, a combination of chemically produced "small molecules" attached to biologically produced "large molecules" is becoming common.

TYPICAL PROCESSING TECHNOLOGIES

Pharmaceuticals are chemicals with health effects that interact with living animals or humans. Production of pharmaceuticals depends on chemical synthesis, extraction from natural material, biological processing, or a combination of these processes. After the pharmaceutical chemicals are produced, they must be formulated for human use, which entails delivery targeted to a particular area of the body and absorption of the appropriate dose. The primary delivery methods include oral (i.e., solid or liquid), topical, inhalant, and injectable.

PHARMACEUTICAL PROCESSES

This section discusses the primary processes used in the production of pharmaceuticals. The dosage forms are discussed first, followed by a discussion of the processes used to manufacture the APIs found in the final dosage forms.

DOSAGE FORM PROCESSING

Drug products are administered in oral solid, oral liquid, topical, inhalant, and injectable forms. Oral solids comprise the largest volume of drug products. Below is a brief overview of the key processing steps and equipment used for each dosage form. For all, the starting point in the process is the API, produced by chemical synthesis or biological processing. Generally, dosage form processing focuses on bringing about physical, not chemical, changes.

Oral Solid Dosage Forms

The fundamental process steps in oral solid dosage forms include dispensing, granulation, drying, milling, blending, tableting, coating, encapsulation, and packaging (Figure 8.1).

Dispensing is the accurate weighing of the solid and liquid ingredients that constitute the dosage form; these include APIs, excipients, lubricants, disintegrants, and coatings. As corrosion is not a major concern, dosage form equipment is generally fabricated from 316L stainless steel. Containment of dust, however, is a major issue throughout solid dosage form processing, starting with the dispensing operation. High-potency APIs may be handled in isolators, downflow booths, or exhaust hoods; nonpotent materials are generally handled with exhaust hoods or downflow booths.

Once dispensed, the finely divided powders are granulated to form a larger particle (agglomerate) that contains a uniform concentration of all of the constituent solids. Granulations are often created with a liquid to aide in agglomeration, although for some products, dry granulation (without a liquid) is possible. This liquid may be United States Pharmacopoeia (USP) water, or it may be a flammable solvent, depending on the final product. Since most APIs dissolve in water, the amount of liquid used in granulation is very small and is added while the solids are blended. Granulations are performed in a wide range of equipment, including rotating blenders, agitated stationary blenders, and fluid-bed processors.

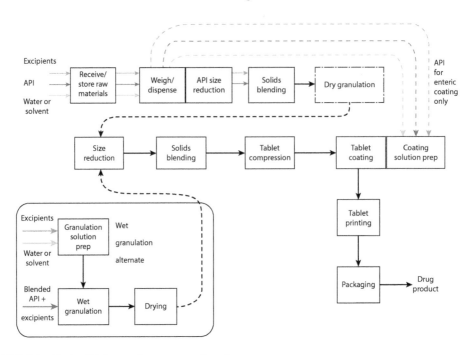

FIGURE 8.1   Oral solid dosage form process flowchart.

After a wet granulation is formed, the liquid must be removed by drying. If a fluid-bed processor or a jacketed blender is used, then drying is done in the same equipment. Tray- or truck-drying ovens are still used; however, they are becoming less popular because they require extensive manual handling and because potent materials are difficult to contain during processing. Microwave drying is used with highly potent compounds to provide contained drying as part of a high-shear granulator (see below).

The dried granulation is milled with limited energy input to produce a uniform particle size for tableting operations. There is a trend toward "single-pot processing" for potent compounds, in which granulation, drying, and milling are performed in a single integrated equipment train. After milling, the granulated materials are blended to develop a uniform concentration. Blending can take place in an intermediate bulk container (IBC) or in a fixed piece of equipment (e.g., a V-blender or twin-shell blender). The blended material is usually transported in an IBC to the tablet press, where the final tablet is formed. Tablet presses are very complicated machines that depend on uniform flow properties of the granulation to produce the uniform composition of tablets (Figures 8.2 and 8.3).

Often, many of the ingredients in the blend are included to allow the tablet press to perform its function consistently. Because of this complexity, small-volume products are sometimes produced as capsules, which simplifies the granulation steps. The tablet is usually coated, either in a coating pan or in a fluid-bed coater. Coating solutions can be aqueous or solvent based, with some tablets requiring more than one coating step. Some coatings (e.g., enteric coatings) contain a different API from the tablet itself to provide an initial pharmacological effect before the tablet disintegrates in the digestive tract. Coating solutions are prepared in jacketed, agitated tanks. The solution is usually heated slightly to promote dissolution of the solid ingredients and then cooled to room temperature before being added to the coater. Tablet coaters use large volumes of filtered, conditioned air to dry the coated tablets. Occasionally, when flammable solvents are used, nitrogen is used in place of air in the coating operation. Because of the large-volume requirements and process economics, the nitrogen is normally recycled after the solvents and dust particles are removed. In general, large, sophisticated

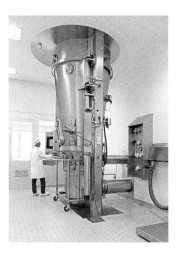

FIGURE 8.2   Fluid bed. (From Glatt Air Techniques, Inc.)

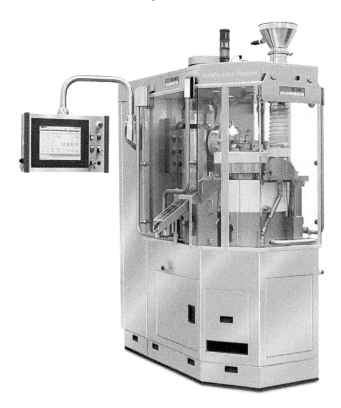

FIGURE 8.3   Tablet press. (From Korsch America, Inc.)

air (or nitrogen) handling systems are required to support each coating pan or fluid-bed unit. Coated tablets are printed with the manufacturer's product information and then packaged (Figure 8.4).

Liquid and Semisolid Dosage Forms

This broad category includes oral liquid, topical, inhalant, and injectable dosage forms. While there are significant differences in facility design for oral liquids and topicals compared to inhalants and

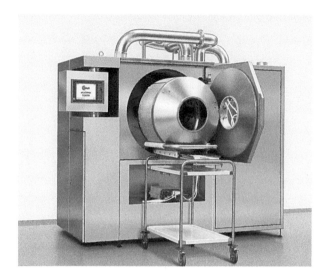

FIGURE 8.4   Coating pan. (From Glatt Air Techniques, Inc.)

injectables, the basic process unit operations are similar. Most of these product types start with dispensing and then proceed to a liquid-phase blending step, using a jacketed, agitated vessel. After the blending step, the product containers are filled and then packaged.

Since the API is normally a solid, the same dispensing issues exist as discussed above for oral solid dosage forms. For oral liquids, the API is usually blended in either ethanol, which is flammable, or USP purified water. Most oral liquids are blended at ambient temperature. Topical dosage forms range from low-viscosity liquids to moderate-viscosity lotions to high-viscosity creams and ointments. Lotions, creams, and ointments frequently are emulsions formed by intense agitation of two distinct liquid phases—one aqueous based and the other oil based. Each liquid phase is first prepared in separate jacketed, agitated vessels by dissolving the required solid ingredients in water or oil while heating (to aid dissolution). After each liquid phase is prepared, both the water and oil phases are combined, using intense agitation (a homogenizer) to disperse the phases and form a stable emulsion. Containers for highly viscous topicals are filled at elevated temperatures to improve flow during filling.

Injectables must be sterile, as they directly enter the body, bypassing the protection offered by the digestive tract. Therefore, while the actual process steps for injectables are relatively simple, those that ensure that the product is sterile and stable are not. The product, either liquid or solid, is usually filled into small glass or plastic containers. Since most injectables are water based, the processing starts by dissolving the API in water for injection (WFI). After this formulation is prepared, it is normally filtered through 0.2-micron filters to ensure sterility, before filling a vial, syringe, or other container. If the API can tolerate the heat, then the filled, stoppered containers are steam sterilized (terminal sterilization). Containers of injectable liquids that cannot be terminally sterilized must be filled under aseptic conditions. Many injectable products are then dried after filling, using a vacuum freeze-drying process called lyophilization. Vials and all items that come in contact with the sterile product must also be sterile. Chapter 11 provides further discussion on sterile facilities.

Inhalants, like injectables, bypass the digestive tract. They must have a low bioburden but may not need to be sterile. Inhalants require the means to provide a dose of a fixed, repeatable size (metered dose), as well as the means to propel the dose into the throat. Most commonly, a solution or a suspension of the API is prepared in a liquid, which is then placed into the dosage container and a propellant added to pressurize the container. When used with an engineered nozzle, this assembly provides consistent doses of the API. Processing starts with dispensing the API and any other ingredients, and then adding the API to a liquid to form a solution or a uniform suspension. If water is used, it is USP purified or, in some cases, WFI, to reduce the bioburden. After the blending step, the liquid is filtered prior to filling containers. The use of dry powder inhalants, rather than the liquid solution or suspension, has grown considerably over the past 15 years.

PROCESSING OF APIS

APIs are produced primarily by chemical synthesis, biological processing, or a combination of both. Extraction of natural materials, from either plants or animals, can be completed by one or both of these processes. The paragraph below describes chemical synthesis, and Chapter 12 provides a discussion of biological processing and the facilities in which it occurs (Figure 8.5).

Chemical synthesis describes a series of chemical reactions that produce the API; these chemical reactions are accompanied by a number of other unit operations, which separate and purify the final API. The primary chemical synthesis unit operations are reaction, heat transfer, extraction, distillation, evaporation, crystallization, filtration, drying, and size reduction. Most chemically derived APIs complete the initial reaction in a liquid phase in organic solvents; they are then solidified, separated from the solvent and other impurities by filtration, and finally dried under vacuum to remove the last traces of solvent. The dried API is then milled to reduce its particle size range for formulation into the final dosage form. Pharmaceutical plants that produce APIs require multiproduct, flexible equipment trains. A brief discussion of the unit operations and the equipment commonly used at these plants follows (Figures 8.6 and 8.7).

Reactions

Most reactions are liquid-phase batch reactions, carried out in a pressure vessel with an agitator and an external jacket. The final API frequently requires from 3 to 10 separate reaction steps, depending on the complexity of the API molecule and on the commercially available intermediate chemicals. Each of these reaction steps usually requires separation and some purification. The early steps also

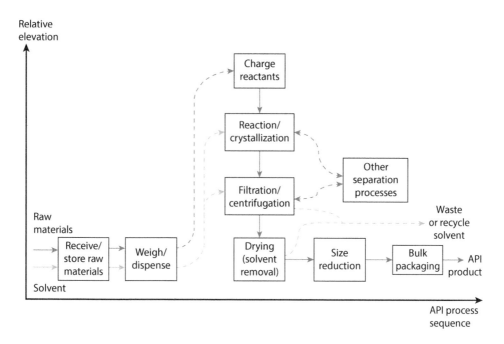

FIGURE 8.5 API process flowchart.

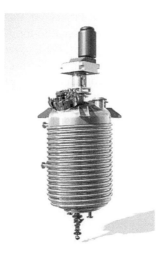

FIGURE 8.6   Reaction vessel. (From DeDietrich Process Systems, Inc.)

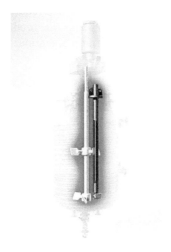

FIGURE 8.7   Reaction vessel. (Courtesy of DeDietrich Process Systems, Inc., Mountainside, NJ.)

generally require a greater volume of reaction materials, and therefore a larger reactor than later steps; for example, in these multistep processes, it is not uncommon for the first step to take place in a reactor four to five times the size of the final-step reactor. Typical reactor volumes used for production processes range from 500 to 5,000 gallons. Research and development reactors generally range from 5 to 500 gallons.

The reaction chemicals in API processes are frequently highly corrosive. The most common materials of construction for reactors are glass-lined steel and Hastelloy C, which are able to withstand high temperatures and resist corrosion. Associated equipment, piping, and product contact instruments must provide similar corrosion resistance. Piping materials include Teflon-lined steel, Hastelloy C, glass-lined steel, and armored glass, although the armored glass is less frequently used in production plants because of safety issues.

Reaction pressures are generally below 150 psig, except for some gas–liquid phase reactions, which can require up to 6,000 psig. Reaction vessels must also be capable of holding a full vacuum, to accommodate many operations that occur below atmospheric pressure to limit the temperature

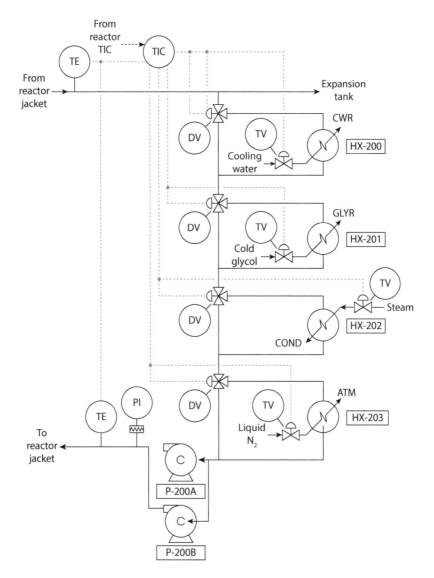

FIGURE 8.8   Schematic of heat transfer module. ATM, vent to atmosphere; COND, condensed steam; CWR, cooling water return; DV, automated diverting valve; GLYR, cold glycol return; HX-xxx, heat exchanger; N₂, nitrogen; P-xxxx, pump; PI, pressure indicator; TE, temperature sensing element; TIC, temperature controller; TV, automated temperature control valve.

exposure of the reaction product. Processing temperatures normally range from –20°C to +250°C, with some reactions occurring at as low as –70°C (Figure 8.8).

Heat Transfer

It is critical to control the reaction temperature, including the rate of temperature change. Heat transfer in batch API reactors is accomplished by using an external jacket (on the reactor) with heat transfer fluid flowing through the jacket. Unfortunately, there is an inverse relationship between the reactor volume and the relative reactor surface area; that is, the larger the reactor, the less relative heat transfer area there is available. This issue is especially critical in designing reactors for highly exothermic reactions. Design tools, such as internal heat transfer coils and external heat exchangers that increase heat transfer, are not available for pharmaceutical reactors because they create cleaning problems and do not comply with cGMP regulations. Therefore, the reactor size or the rate of reaction must be limited for highly exothermic reactions. The construction material of the reactor also impacts the rate of heat transfer through the reactor wall; for example, glass-lined reactors have heat transfer rates about one-half those of Hastelloy C reactors. Furthermore, because of the potential to degrade the reaction products thermally, the maximum temperature of the fluid in the jacket must be limited frequently. When using glass-lined reactors, care must be taken to limit the temperature gradient across the glass lining to prevent damage to the glass.

Reactor heat transfer systems most commonly use a single-jacket heat transfer fluid over the entire temperature range of –70°C to +250°C. This fluid is heated or cooled indirectly, using heat exchangers. In plants with fewer reactors (generally less than 15), it is more economical to use independent heat exchange modules for each reactor. These modules consist of a circulating pump and from two to four heat exchangers, using steam, cooling water, chilled water, chilled heat transfer fluids, and liquid nitrogen, to bring the jacket fluid to the desired temperature. In facilities with many reactors, it is more economical to provide a hot (around +250°C) and a cold (around –25°C) central system, which circulates the heat transfer fluid. In these facilities, each reactor has a jacket circulating pump and controls to bleed in the appropriate hot or cold central fluid to achieve the desired temperature. Temperatures below –25°C are achieved by the following: (1) closing off the reactor jacket loop from the central systems, (2) using a dedicated heat exchanger for each reactor jacket loop, and (3) using liquid nitrogen to reach jacket temperatures as low as –70°C. For temperatures below –25°C, it is important to recognize that carbon steel becomes too brittle to use for the jacket loop heat exchangers, pump, piping, and instruments; thus, stainless steel must be used for the reactor jacket and all of the reactor heat transfer system components. Depending on the corrosiveness of the reaction chemistry, either stainless steel or Hastelloy is used for the reactor.

Extraction

Extraction is the transfer of solute from one liquid phase to another immiscible liquid phase. This is often one of the first purification steps following a reaction. If there is sufficient volume available, extraction is carried out in the reaction vessel, by the addition of the second immiscible solvent to the reactor, followed by a period of agitation to disperse the two liquid phases. Agitation is then stopped, and the two phases are allowed to separate by gravity, based on their relative densities. The denser (lower) phase is then removed from the bottom of the vessel. Further processing is performed on the phase that is rich in the product solute. If the reactor does not have sufficient volume to perform the extraction, another agitated vessel is used, after transferring the entire batch from the reactor. Centrifugal extractors are used for liquid phases that share similar densities and are therefore difficult to separate by the force of gravity.

Distillation

Batch distillation is used in some reaction steps to remove an undesired reaction by-product. Distillation is normally performed in the reactor in conjunction with a distillation column above the reactor. Most distillations are performed in a vacuum to limit product temperatures and enhance the removal of the unwanted by-product. Some very large manufacturing facilities have central solvent recovery systems that use distillation to recover and purify solvents for reuse.

Evaporation and Crystallization

After the desired chemical product is produced in the reactor, it is usually solidified as small particles in a slurry to separate it from the reaction solvent, unreacted raw materials, and unwanted by-products, all of which remain in a liquid state. Solidification is accomplished by increasing the product concentration by heating and evaporating the solvent and by crystallizing the product by cooling. Evaporation and crystallization can occur in the batch reactor but frequently occur in a separate agitated, jacketed vessel that is located directly above the filtration device; this location minimizes the transfer distance of the slurry, thereby avoiding pipeline plugging problems and limiting any potential damage to the structure of the solid crystals (Figures 8.9 and 8.10).

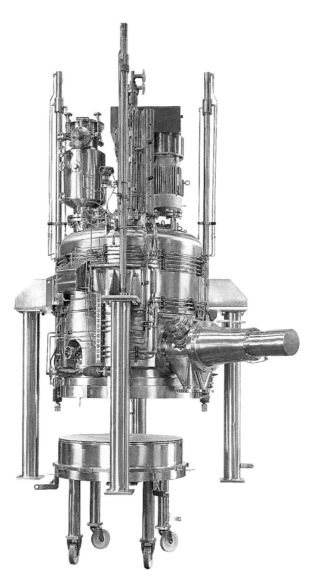

FIGURE 8.9 Pressure filter. (Courtesy of DeDietrich Process Systems, Inc., Mountainside, NJ.)

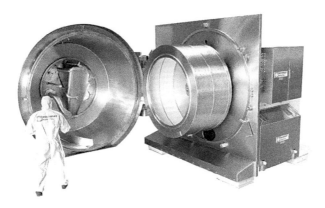

FIGURE 8.10 Centrifuge. (Courtesy of Robatel, Inc., Pittsfield, MA.)

Filtration

Once the slurry is formed with the solidified product, it is filtered to separate the solid product from the now undesired liquid-phase components. The product is collected on the filter, while the liquid is collected in tanks for reuse, recovery, or disposal. In all filtration operations, there is resistance to moving the liquid through the filter media, as well as the collected bed of solids. The two commonly used methods of overcoming this resistance are the use of pressure and the use of centrifugal force; therefore, the filtration equipment is a pressure filter or a filtering centrifuge. These items must be corrosion resistant, meaning that they must be constructed of Hastelloy or a similar metal, as fabricating the intricate parts with glass-lined metal is impractical.

When the bed (cake) of solids is formed on the filter media, it is usually washed with cold, pure solvent to displace dissolved impurities in the still wet cake. Usually the wash liquor is collected in separate tanks from the initial (mother) liquor from the first filtration. Depending on the process, it may be economical to take the mother liquor and subject it to another evaporation or crystallization step to solidify additional product, which can be recovered in another filtration step. The wash liquor is generally considered waste. The product cake discharged from the filter or centrifuge is then vacuum dried. Without drying, the product cake presents many handling problems. For a large-volume product, the filter or centrifuge feeds the discharged cake directly into the dryer by gravity. This arrangement eliminates most of the handling problems associated with the wet cakes. However, most production plants are multiproduct facilities, and the filters and dryers are decoupled to increase flexibility, unless they are designed for highly potent compounds. If the filters are decoupled from the dryers, then the cake is discharged to a lined drum or an IBC. These are then staged until the drying step is scheduled. Getting the wet cake out of these containers frequently requires manual intervention.

Drying

The purpose of the drying step is to remove any remaining solvent used during processing. To limit thermal degradation of the product, drying is performed in a vacuum to evaporate the solvent at reduced temperatures. Typical API drying temperatures are limited to +80°C. Production plant dryers are usually agitated, jacketed vessels, frequently fabricated of Hastelloy for corrosion resistance. Glass-lined rotating dryers are also used, although less and less frequently. Research and development facilities still use vacuum tray dryers, but because operator exposure is a major issue, they are seldom used in new production facilities. The dryer requires a heating medium for the jacket, a vacuum pump, a condenser, and a solvent collection tank for the solvent removed during the drying process. Heated water is the most common heat transfer fluid used in the dryer jacket. The dried product is cooled, discharged from the dryer, and then either milled or packed for shipment to the dosage form facility that will use the API (Figure 8.11).

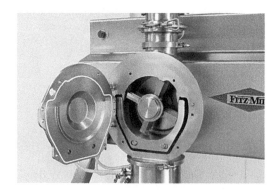

FIGURE 8.11   Mill. (Courtesy of Fitzpatrick Company, Elmhurst, IL.)

Size Reduction

The API must be milled to provide a uniform particle size before use in the final dosage form. Impact mills with an internal screen are the most commonly used mills, with air-classifying and air-swept mills becoming increasingly popular. When the product is dry during the milling operation, corrosion is not a concern, so the mill systems are fabricated of stainless steel. An impact mill with a screen is essentially a vertical flow-through device, with the mill outlet connected to the pack-out system to fill either lined drums or IBCs. Air-classifying mills and air-swept mills use the carrier gas (i.e., filtered, dried air or nitrogen) to either limit the size of a particle that can leave the mill or cause the solid particles to collide with each other to reduce their size further. These mills require a milled product collector to separate the solids from the carrier gas and accumulate the product.

INTERACTIONS WITH THE FACILITY AND SUPPORT SYSTEMS

PROCESS WATER

Dosage form operations usually require USP purified water for oral and topical products and WFI for injectables and some inhalants. Chemical synthesis may require USP purified water, depending on the specific step in the process; for example, final-step API processes almost always use USP purified water. However, early-step processes may simply use potable or deionized water. See Chapter 6 for a detailed discussion of this topic.

FACILITY ISSUES

Dosage Form Facilities

Dosage form facilities generally are not required to meet code requirements for hazardous buildings, except for limited areas that handle flammable liquids; therefore, there is considerably more layout flexibility than in buildings where chemical synthesis takes place. In dosage form facilities, the manufacturing equipment is frequently integrated with the building; for example, fluid-bed processors are installed through floors, and coating pans, autoclaves, and lyophilizers are installed through walls. The combination of cGMPs and the use of potent compounds requires the segregation of the individual process operations in separate rooms.

Flexible dosage form facilities for products that are not highly potent may also provide separate rooms for each process step, such as granulation rooms, milling rooms, tableting rooms, and coating pan rooms. With this layout, the facility provides isolation and product protection to satisfy cGMP regulations, while allowing a high degree of flexibility to run different batches or processes at the same time. Materials are moved from room to room as required by the processing step. In potent compound facilities, the trend is to include an integrated suite, containing granulation, drying, milling, and blending equipment with closed transfers between equipment. Tableting and coating are in separate rooms, using IBCs to transfer product. Coating does not require the same level of containment equipment as the other processes, as the potent active compound is contained by the tablet and its coating.

API Facilities

Buildings in which chemical synthesis takes place (to process APIs) must comply with code requirements for hazardous buildings because of the use of large quantities of flammable solvents. These building codes limit the size and height (i.e., the number of stories) and dictate how close they can be to other buildings on the site or to the property line. There are also strict limits on the maximum distance a person has to travel for egress. Hazardous buildings are required to use pressure-resistant walls and floors as well as pressure-relief panels. Furthermore, the process equipment is highly integrated with the building; for example, vessels, filters, and dryers are installed through floors, and centrifuges are installed through walls. The combination of cGMPs and the use of potent compounds requires the segregation of the individual process operations in separate rooms. All of the above-mentioned requirements make the layout of API facilities a challenge.

Typical layouts of flexible API facilities for products of normal potency provide reactor areas or rooms, filtration and centrifugation rooms, drying rooms, and milling rooms. A facility with this configuration provides isolation and product protection as mandated by cGMP regulations, while allowing a high degree of flexibility to run different processes at the same time. Products are moved from room to room as required by the processing step. Potent compound facilities often include an integrated suite containing reactors, filtration equipment, and drying equipment with closed transfers between equipment. These suites frequently make use of multiple floors to provide gravity flow from reactors to filtration and drying equipment. This approach reduces overall facility flexibility, since the suite and its equipment are dedicated to a single product during the operation, regardless of whether all of the equipment is used. The benefit of this approach is increased containment of the potent material.

PROJECT MANAGEMENT ISSUES

CAPITAL COSTS

To develop an accurate capital cost estimate for a pharmaceutical manufacturing facility, it is necessary to define explicitly the process equipment needs, the necessary support equipment, the utility equipment needs, and the building and site requirements. There is no true shortcut to obtain an accurate cost estimate. In very early project planning, historical square footage costs are often used. While the cost per square foot of a process facility normally falls within a reasonable range, depending on the type and scale of the process, it is difficult to quickly determine the square footage required. In order to develop a credible estimate of the space required, the process engineer must define the process equipment needed to meet the manufacturer's objectives, participate in discussions about equipment layouts, and estimate the utility requirements so that support systems can be sized and their layouts developed. This is a process that, depending on the scale and type of facility, cannot be done quickly.

PROJECT SCHEDULES

In most projects, the delivery of the process equipment to the construction site is on the critical path (i.e., limits the rate of completing the project) because of the long fabrication time of the equipment (from 5 to 15 months) and because the installation of the equipment is often integrated with the facility. To maintain the project schedule, the process engineer must size and specify the equipment quickly, so that contracts can be bid, vendors can be selected, vendor engineering can be performed, and the equipment can be fabricated.

In some cases, to save time, prefabricated modules that are immediately ready for installation can allow parallel construction of the facility and the process. However, because of the intense integration of the process equipment within API facilities, they are arguably the most complicated pharmaceutical manufacturing projects, often limiting the use of these fully prefabricated systems. The API facilities also need a large amount of process piping, so that most of the actual construction is expended at the plant site and inside the process building. Because of these constraints, typical schedules for large API projects can take 3–4 years from concept development to commissioning and qualification.

TRENDS AND FUTURE DEVELOPMENTS

CHANGES OVER THE PAST 10 YEARS

The biggest change over the past 10 years for all types of pharmaceutical processing has been the increased potency of the APIs. Before 2000, few products were highly potent, so existing processes and manufacturing facilities were not designed to handle these compounds; however, there have been extensive efforts to modify existing facilities for potent compound processing. In addition, new multifunctional processing equipment that improves containment and limits the number of transfers between equipment systems has become commercially available. This makes the design of a potent compound facility much more straightforward. However, the need for additional space has not changed, as potent compound handling requires more space around equipment and for containing waste (e.g., collected dusts), as well as more airlocks.

EXPECTED CHANGES IN THE NEXT 10 YEARS

Pharmaceutical processing has traditionally been done in discrete batches; however, in the past several years, continuous processing has been implemented for some products. This trend will no doubt continue over the next 10 years and become more widely used, in both API and dosage form production. Primary commercial application of continuous processing has been in dosage form manufacture. See Chapter 10 for information on continuous manufacturing.

SPECIAL DISCUSSION

CONTROL SYSTEMS

Dosage form facilities normally use an "island of automation" approach, with each equipment system having its own vendor-supplied control system. These individual control systems communicate with a plantwide supervisory system for overall coordination and batch data storage. These systems must meet the electronic batch record requirements of Title 21 of the Code of Federal Regulations (CFR), Part 11.

Facilities for API production usually integrate all process support systems into a plantwide control system. Control systems are based on either programmable logic controllers (PLCs) or distributed control computers with multiple operator interfaces that use graphic displays. The level of automation varies from facility to facility. Production facilities with well-established products and processes often program their full-batch recipes, including the automated addition of ingredients and process steps. Highly flexible facilities (e.g., contract manufacturing plants and pilot plants) usually do not program the entire batch recipe, but depend on operator input for the addition of ingredients, temperature, and pressure set points, for example. Some equipment systems include a vendor-provided PLC that interfaces with the plantwide control system. Examples of such equipment systems are centrifuges, agitated filters, filter–dryers, agitated dryers, and modular skid systems. Since production data are normally stored in the control system, they must meet the electronic batch record requirements of 21 CFR 11. See Chapter 7 for a detailed discussion on automation and control systems.

POTENT COMPOUND CONTAINMENT

The trend in the industry is toward the production of more highly potent compounds (i.e., APIs are limited to operator exposure levels below 100 $\mu g/m^3$ of room volume). Compounds with exposure limits below 1 $\mu g/m^3$ are increasingly common. Typical containment devices include isolators, split butterfly valves, downflow booths used with IBCs, double-lined fiber drums, disposable plastic containers, and disposable bags. Processes with potent compounds often carry out multiple process steps in each piece of equipment (e.g., a filter–dryer in place of a separate centrifuge or filter and a separate dryer). See Chapter 15 for information on exposure control for occupational and patient populations and Chapter 14 for a detailed discussion on containment issues and solutions.

It is important to consider the need for extra floor space and extra headroom around the containment devices when designing API facilities for potent compound handling. Potent compound facilities require more floor space for the same amount of equipment than a normal potency facility. Much of this additional floor space is occupied by airlocks to separate the potent compound areas within the facility; for example, a typical potent compound suite has three airlocks, which include a personnel gowning airlock, a decontamination or de-gowning airlock, and a material airlock.

Cleaning

Dosage Form Equipment

Clean-in-place (CIP) spray nozzles, using an aqueous detergent solution, are the typical cleaning method for dosage form equipment. The final rinse for this equipment normally uses USP purified water. Equipment for injectables and some inhalants is rinsed with WFI and then steam sterilized.

API Equipment

It is difficult to clean reactors and crystallizers using CIP spray nozzles and a cleaning solution, as hardened or sticky deposits are often well adhered to the vessel walls and agitator. Cleaning therefore involves "boiling-up" the vessel with organic solvents to dissolve these remnant process materials. The boil-up may be preceded by spraying an organic solvent into the vessel via spray nozzles, but extreme caution must be taken to ensure that the vessel is inert when spraying flammable solvents. Solvent cleaning is frequently followed by aqueous cleaning, using a detergent solution and a final water rinse. This final rinse may require USP purified water, depending on the use of the vessel. Filters and centrifuges may also be cleaned with solvents, followed by aqueous cleaning and rinsing. Mills are most commonly cleaned with aqueous solutions.

Environmental Health and Safety

Dosage Form Facilities

The primary environmental health and safety (EHS) issues in dosage form processing relate to the presence of combustible dusts, flammable organic solvents, and highly potent product materials. While combustible dusts present explosion hazards, the energy release is far less than when a flammable liquid explodes. Safety measures for combustible dusts include the use of 10-bar pressure-rated equipment to contain a dust explosion or the use of an explosion suppression system to limit the extent of a dust explosion. For flammable liquids and potent compounds, the precautions are similar to those used in chemical synthesis facilities. From an environmental standpoint, dust control devices are required for virtually every plant. Dosage form facilities that extensively use organic solvents generally use thermal oxidizers to remove the organic vapors from venting gas streams.

API Facilities

Chemical synthesis processes present numerous EHS issues because of the use of flammable organic solvents, toxic raw and intermediate materials, and highly potent product materials, and the potential for runaway chemical reactions. In addition, the use of high temperatures (+250°C or higher), extreme low temperatures (–70°C or lower), and an asphyxiant (nitrogen) makes it imperative that extreme caution be taken in the design and operation of API facilities.

Common health and safety measures in the design include closed processing to contain the hazardous materials, the use of nitrogen to provide an inert atmosphere inside the process equipment, an integrated control system with extensive safety interlocks to reduce the potential for human error, overpressure relief for process vessels coupled with catch tanks to contain releases, and pressure-resistant room walls and pressure-relief panels to direct explosive energy away from other rooms in the facility. As a secondary health precaution, operators use personal protective equipment in the event of a failure of the primary barrier between them and the hazardous materials.

Air emission control devices are required for all plants. These typically include a combination of scrubbers, low-temperature condensers, thermal oxidizers to remove organic vapors, and dust collectors to remove solid airborne particles. Organic liquid wastes are classified as hazardous wastes and are segregated from aqueous wastes for off-site disposal. At very large plants, organic liquid waste may be recycled for reuse in early-step processes, using a solvent recovery distillation system. Aqueous wastes may be fully treated on-site at very large plants, but more commonly are limited to pretreatment (pH adjustment) on-site followed by disposal to publicly owned treatment works. Solid waste is also generated, including process materials, as well as filter cloths, drum liners, disposable containers, and gowning materials. Since all of these may contain some process material, they are usually classified as hazardous waste and disposed off-site. See Chapter 15 for a more in-depth discussion on health and safety issues.

- *Active pharmaceutical ingredient (API)*. The API is the chemical entity that causes the pharmacological effect in the living body.
- *Bulk pharmaceutical chemical (BPC)*. An API or an intermediate chemical used in the manufacture of the API is a BPC.
- *Final dosage form*. This is the form in which the drug product delivers the API.
- *Oral dosage form*. This is a formulation of an API and other material (excipients) in a solid, liquid, suspension, or dissolvable form that is taken by mouth and provides the appropriate dose of the API.
- *Topicals*. These are formulations of an API and excipients that are applied to the skin.
- *Inhalants*. These are formulations of an API and excipients that are inhaled.
- *Injectables*. These are formulations of an API and excipients that are injected into the body, bypassing the digestive tract. Extra precautions must be taken to ensure the sterility of injectables. These are also called parenterals.
- *Excipient*. This is a nonactive ingredient in the dosage form that is used to provide a reasonably sized dose that can be readily handled and measured. Excipients are also used to bind materials together in a tablet, to stabilize a solution or suspension, or to provide a protective coating.

FURTHER DISCUSSION

1. Continuous processing has historically been applied to products that have a large volume demand and well-defined process parameters and controllability, so that slight variations in the process outcome over time can be maintained within well-defined product specifications. Discuss benefits and disadvantages of continuous processing in the biopharma industry. Consider technology issues (such as process development requirements and availability of commercially proven equipment), production issues (such as personnel staffing, reliability, maintenance, and materials supply, storage, and movement), cGMP issues (such as product quality, uniformity, and lot traceability), and facility issues (such as relative space requirements and configuration).
2. More than 90% of the drugs produced today are small molecules, produced via chemical synthesis. In addition, the majority of drugs are administered via oral solid dosage forms. However, the majority of drug patents applied for today are for large molecules, produced

via biological processes. Small molecules are generally very stable and can tolerate aggressive chemistry of the digestive tract. Large molecules are not very stable and easily become denatured in the digestive tract. Discuss the implications for the longer-range future of biopharmaceutical processing. Consider issues related to patient compliance and relative ease of taking the final drug product.

3. Conjugation of small molecules with monoclonal antibodies is becoming more widespread, particularly in cancer treatment. The therapeutic benefit is that the small-molecule active ingredient is delivered directly to the cancer cells. Discuss process options for this merger of bioprocessing and chemical synthesis for production of the antibody drug conjugate.

ABOUT THE AUTHOR

Art Meisch is a senior project director at CE&IC, Inc., an engineering/consulting firm specializing in the design of processes and facilities for the pharmaceutical and biotech industries. Art is a professional engineer with more than 42 years of experience in the planning, design, construction, commissioning, and validation of a variety of pharmaceutical projects, including sterile products, oral dosage forms, topicals, and active pharmaceutical ingredients derived by both biological and chemical processing. He holds a BS and MS in chemical engineering from Rensselaer Polytechnic Institute, Troy, New York, and an MBA from Rider University, Lawrenceville, New Jersey.

Art has led biopharma industry seminars on the following topics:

- Potent compound containment
- Process systems considerations
- cGMP issues related to utility systems
- Introduction to bulk pharmaceutical facilities: a review of the ISPE guide
- Containment in bulk pharmaceutical chemical pilot plants
- Methodology for determining BPC reactor capacity requirements

He has also authored the following biopharma industry publications:

- ISPE Baseline Guide *Active Pharmaceutical Ingredients*, 2nd ed., "Sterile Bulk" chapter.
- "BPC Pilot Plants: Bridges to the Future," *Pharmaceutical Engineering.*
- "Reflections on Documentation: A Plea for Practicality," *Journal of Validation Technology.*

FURTHER READING

International Society for Pharmaceutical Engineering, *Baseline® Pharmaceutical Engineering Guides for New and Renovated Facilities*, Vol. 1: *Active Pharmaceutical Ingredients*, 2nd ed., International Society for Pharmaceutical Engineering, Tampa, FL, 2007.

International Society for Pharmaceutical Engineering, *Baseline® Pharmaceutical Engineering Guides for New and Renovated Facilities*, Vol. 2: *Oral Solid Dosage Forms*, 2nd ed., International Society for Pharmaceutical Engineering, Tampa, FL, 2009.

International Society for Pharmaceutical Engineering, *Baseline® Pharmaceutical Engineering Guides for New and Renovated Facilities*, Vol. 3: *Sterile Product Manufacturing Facilities*, 2nd ed., International Society for Pharmaceutical Engineering, Tampa, FL, 2011.

International Society for Pharmaceutical Engineering, *Baseline® Pharmaceutical Engineering Guides for New and Renovated Facilities*, Vol. 4: *Water and Steam Systems*, 2nd ed., International Society for Pharmaceutical Engineering, Tampa, FL, 2011.

International Society for Pharmaceutical Engineering, *Baseline® Pharmaceutical Engineering Guides for New and Renovated Facilities*, Vol. 6: *Biopharmaceuticals*, 2nd ed., International Society for Pharmaceutical Engineering, Tampa, FL, 2013.

International Society for Pharmaceutical Engineering, *Baseline® Pharmaceutical Engineering Guides for New and Renovated Facilities*, Vol. 7: *Risk-Based Manufacture of Pharmaceutical Products*, International Society for Pharmaceutical Engineering, Tampa, FL, 2010.

International Society for Pharmaceutical Engineering, *ISPE Guide: Biopharmaceutical Process Development and Manufacturing*, International Society for Pharmaceutical Engineering, Tampa, FL, October 2013.

International Society for Pharmaceutical Engineering, *ISPE Guide: Science and Risk-Based Approach for the Delivery of Facilities, Systems, and Equipment*, International Society for Pharmaceutical Engineering, Tampa, FL, 2011.

International Society for Pharmaceutical Engineering, *Good Practice Guide: Process Gases*, International Society for Pharmaceutical Engineering, Tampa, FL, 2011.

International Society for Pharmaceutical Engineering, *Good Practice Guide: Technology Transfer*, 2nd ed., International Society for Pharmaceutical Engineering, Tampa, FL, 2014.

Edward J. Tannebaum, AIA and Samuel Halaby

CONTENTS

INTRODUCTION

This chapter provides an overview of the means and methods of today's manufacturing technology, the facilities that use these technologies, and the regulatory and environmental employee health and safety challenges that provide the context for ensuring quality. The focus of this chapter relates to the good design practices necessary to develop or upgrade oral solid dosage (OSD) manufacturing facilities.

MEETING INDUSTRY AND MARKET NEEDS

Industry and market needs have increasingly dictated the course of OSD manufacturing. Historically, OSD products date back to the seventeenth century in the United States. Until the 1920s, 80% of the medicines were compounded by pharmacists in liquid, powder, and tablet form. As a result of the health care needs of the military in World War I, high-technology medicines were necessary to treat injured soldiers and cure diseases among war-torn populaces, which became major health issues. The production of tablets of newly created drugs became a prominent industry in the United States. The common OSD products include tablets; hard- and soft-shell gelatin capsules; layered, coated, osmotic, extended-release tablets; and quick-dissolve, extruded, effervescent, powder products.

Current OSD manufacturing is regulated for quality by the U.S. Food and Drug Administration (FDA) and more strictly by international regulatory agencies. Quality and compliance, coupled with selling drugs at affordable prices, provide the background for the development and upgrade of OSD manufacturing facilities with new technology. The variety of products range from highly regulated, branded, and generic drugs to a variety of over-the-counter nutritional products, which have recently been challenged by regulatory concerns and newly enacted compliance mandates.

OSD products (also referred to as small molecules) will continue to be the major source of drug product delivery in the near future. The OSD products are a stable drug delivery form, the least expensive to produce in large quantities, and simpler to produce than sterile injectable products. The future extension of the product life span will revolve around development and approval of newer methods of extended release and formulations that prohibit tampering with the finished dosage form.

Currently, innovations related to tamper-resistant OSD products have proved to be effective in preventing the removal of active ingredients from the finished dosage forms that have contributed to illegal substance abuse in this country.

REGULATORY CHALLENGES

Current Good Manufacturing Practices (cGMPs) related to the elimination of cross-contamination, resulting from airborne exposure, material transfer, and mix-up, are paramount. The increased use of ingredients that are active, potent, cytotoxic, or sensitizing agents has increased the need for upgraded employee health and safety precautions that impact the design of individual processing spaces. This chapter explains the current and imminent changes in the regulatory requirements that are raising the bar of the overall drug manufacturing industry.

MANUFACTURING PROCESSES

DRUG DELIVERY TECHNOLOGIES

Drug delivery technologies are diverse for the various manufacturing operations that range from unitary, manual processes to automated, integrated processes. The technologies revolve around the processes needed to produce both the physical unit dose form and the method of active drug release. Sizes, shapes, and novel forms of delivery provide increased complexity of manufacturing facilities. Alternative methodology for immediate- and sustained-release characteristics for active ingredient absorption creates a range of manufacturing environments for finishing processes, driving OSD development and its subsequent manufacture.

The technologies required for dedicated large-volume operations differ from those used in small-volume, multi-product facilities. The differences in the scale of production are the driving force behind the strategic planning process for successful facility design. The collaboration between the research and development (R&D) scientists of a pharmaceutical organization and the realities of the operations and engineering project delivery requires early intervention to secure the technologies that meet the industry and market needs for quality, compliance, and the best-cost end result. The technology transfer process must consider new systems, processes, and formulations to meet the facility needs of the future.

New OSD technologies that have resulted from the proliferation of novel drug delivery systems and devices provide multiple challenges to the design of OSD facilities. The addition of newly developed technology into the design of a new or renovated facility, before the completion of the product's development or regulatory approval, creates a need for flexibility in the design, which, in turn, requires an early interface between the facility design team, R&D, and operations staff.

REGULATORY PRESSURES ON OSD MANUFACTURING

International regulatory bodies have established recommendations and requirements for OSD manufacturing, demanding compliance worldwide. Facility-related requirements, based on regulations of the FDA, Saudi Food and Drug Authority (SFDA), Ministry of Health, Labour, and Wealth (MHLW), European Medicines Agency (EMA), Medicines and Healthcare Products Regulatory Agency (MHRA), Therapeutic Goods Administration (TGA), Brazilian Health Surveillance Agency (ANVISA), and other international regulatory agencies, bring a global focus to the critical utility systems, layout, inclusion of airlocks, and single-direction flows throughout facilities. Concerns related to filtration, purified fluid and gas, air installations, cross-contamination, product mix-up, processing visibility, cleaning facilities, and personnel protection for high-potency and sensitizing products, along with gowning facilities, all present differing levels of concern or compliance to different agencies. Multinational product distribution has created the challenge of multiagency compliance at facilities located around the world. Good design practices enable facilities to meet the current design standards that are being harmonized for worldwide conformance.

ENVIRONMENTAL HEALTH AND SAFETY

Environmental health and safety (EHS) play a major role in the design of all facility projects. Involvement of EHS programs ranges from tackling actual risks in manufacturing to the waste stream emanating from liquid and airstreams. Requirements of EHS start from baseline requirements of the Occupational Health and Safety Administration (OSHA) and the Environmental Protection Agency (EPA) in the United States and end with the company standards that are developed. Standards include risk-based requirements for personnel safety from inhalation or skin contact with particulate material that may cause allergic reactions or ingestions that may cause illness. The EHS standards play a significant role in the design of personal safeguards and the segregation, cleaning, storage, and distribution of identified materials produced.

CONTAINMENT FOR HIGH-POTENCY COMPOUNDS

The pharmaceutical industry has established categorization systems to help manage exposure and contamination risks. A typical pharmaceutical company has either a four- or five-band system. For each band, guidance is provided on engineering control measures to be implemented to mitigate exposure risks. Some international regulatory agencies have expressed concern over certain therapeutic drug classes, for example, antibiotics, specifically penicillin; these agencies have therefore demanded a dedicated facility for the production of this antibiotic. Other drug classes, such as cytotoxic compounds, also require dedicated or segregated facilities, depending on the market distribution and regulatory authority. The discovery and registration of drugs that include potent compounds have been on the rise. As a result, many new facilities have implemented enhanced control measures for both a primary (where the product is exposed) and a secondary (where the product has been packaged in a final form but has not received secondary packaging for final shipment) containment. Most process handling for potent compounds is designed for closed operations to provide primary containment through the equipment, and secondary measures are taken in the design of heating, ventilation, and air conditioning (HVAC) systems and airlocks.

CONTINUOUS PROCESSING

Continuous processing is commonplace in most chemical industries; however, it has been slow to be adopted in the pharmaceutical industry. There has been a recent surge in interest as the benefits to scaling out versus scaling up are realized. A few challenges that have held the pharmaceutical industry back from adopting this technology include regulatory aspects of batch definition and process variable changes. The regulatory agencies and pharmaceutical companies are working together to provide new directions on these issues. It is anticipated that in the near future, the industry will register more and more products, implementing continuous processing technologies. This issue is discussed in detail in Chapter 10.

SPECIALTY PROCESSING SYSTEMS

Systems used in specific steps of OSD manufacturing are primarily selected during the development phase of drug R&D. The selection of specific processing technologies is a critical step in the development process. Each new equipment technology or vendor becomes a specific part of the validated drug manufacturing process during the development phase; it is scaled up to commercialized batch sizes during the submission process for a new drug application (NDA) for a branded drug and an abbreviated new drug application (ANDA) for a generic drug.

The vendor-specific technical requirements become a critical part of the design for OSD facilities, in terms of the size, weight, access, and mechanical, electrical, and critical utility loads. Connections to the coordination of the engineered processing systems are the major focus of the planning of the OSD facilities. These spaces must not only meet initial processing requirements but also may be the baseline for creating more flexible space that may be required if equipment changes or modifications are required for future OSD products.

Sustainability

Sustainability in the design of pharmaceutical facilities is reviewed on a project-by-project basis. Today's design goals for energy conservation have a direct impact on the cost of products due to the high cost of utilities to drive the critical engineered systems in these facilities. The inclusion or exclusion of these sustainable features is driven by the client's corporate philosophy and also by the restrictions of the return on investment (ROI) in terms of months or years achievable. Sustainability is discussed in detail in Chapter 16.

Smart Buildings

"Smart buildings" have become a critical aspect of some large pharmaceutical OSD manufacturing facilities, primarily for large-scale, dedicated product plants. The initial capital costs, which are large, and the subsequent challenges to validating these facilities have minimized their presence in the industry. The ongoing challenges of maintaining the buildings in a validated state, combined with the rapidly advancing changes in building management technology, have created an environment that may make it difficult to maintain these buildings both financially and operationally.

MEETING INDUSTRY AND MARKET NEEDS

The business climate in the pharmaceutical industry has changed as a result of mergers and acquisitions of large and small manufacturers and also the international nature of the pharmaceutical business. The international approval and distribution of products requires that manufacturers adjust their supply chain philosophies to meet a variety of needs. Different regulatory agencies require different manufacturing mandates as to where drugs are manufactured, as well as regulations of products that are imported. Transfer of product formulations between countries can be limiting factors in the exportation of drug manufacturing technologies. This international business transition has also created a lower cost of goods, as certain locations and labor for manufacturing are more profitable, which is reflected in the bottom line of the business. The shift in the locations of manufacturing has created a need to design facilities that are technically equivalent, yet meet local construction material and system availability for installation, maintainability, and overall quality standards. These new challenges require vigilance during the design effort to ensure the long-term capability of these installations.

Advances in Drug Delivery Technologies

Drug delivery technologies have changed over the past 30–40 years. While the basic technologies have not changed, the equipment advances have increased throughput and improved overall manufacturing speed, consistency, and quality.

To minimize cross-contamination, equipment has been developed to contain particulate material. Advances in equipment design to meet handling requirements have resulted in fully contained equipment with sealed product transfer, both loading and unloading of equipment, and wash-in-place (WIP) systems that provide product cleaning without the need for human intervention. With the increasing need for equipment to handle the highly potent, sensitizing, and cytotoxic products, these contained, self-cleaning additions to equipment have increased the need for space and segregation to accommodate the equipment sizes, needed clearances, and significant increases in capital spending requirements.

Primary equipment selections no longer focus on exposed product processing equipment, such as open dispensing, sieves, milling, open blenders, hand-scooped transfers, and drying ovens. Any point of open product to the airstream should be avoided to eliminate cross-contamination of materials and products.

IMPACT OF NEW DRUG DELIVERY SYSTEMS

Some of the new forms of drug delivery include products that dissolve transmucosally for a convenient and faster method of reaching the bloodstream. Other new forms include dissolvable strips with active medication, micronized powder inhalation devices, and extruded formulations that limit the adulteration or tampering with the final dosage form. These tamper-resistant drug delivery forms are used with highly addictive products, such as fentanyl (Actiq and Durogesic), and are becoming the preferred method of dosing-controlled substances.

The ability to re-create and reformulate existing drug molecules, especially those reaching their patent expiration, enables drug producers to file with the FDA for a NDA, thus extending the life of their proprietary product or converting a generic product into an ANDA for higher profitability.

REGULATORY ADVANCES OF INTERNATIONAL HARMONIZATION

Harmonization of international regulatory agencies has been a movement that has spread over the past 10 years, affecting both aseptic manufacturing and OSD manufacturing, which has achieved greater harmonization in international arenas than in the United States. International regulatory bodies have expectations for the harmonization of many products, including segregation of high-risk product processing, while the FDA has mainly addressed only penicillin and cephalosporin products.

Due to the international distribution requirements for most drug products, high-level international standards are the preferred method of achieving current and potential future compliance, anywhere in the world. Concurrence with the most stringent international area served would be the most prudent direction to take, whether it is the European Union (EU) for Europe or ANVISA for South America. These organizations generally are the most prominent and specific in defining design requirements.

BUSINESS SEGMENT SPECIALIZATION

Branded, Generic, and Contract Manufacturers

Distinctions among branded, generic, and contract OSD manufacturers historically were common in their manufacturing facility design. The cost of goods was a driving force among these business segments, primarily as a result of the total ROI each segment was able to generate. As the level of regulatory compliance has risen worldwide, the disparity in the facility attributes has narrowed significantly. Branded drug producers have streamlined their operations and facilities to lower the unit cost of the goods produced.

Branded Drugs

These drugs are still under a patent. These drugs have received NDA approval from a governing regulatory body and been approved after a three-phase clinical trial process by that regulatory body.

Generic Drugs

These drugs are similar to NDA drugs and have been approved through an ANDA application after the expiration of the drugs' patent. These drug "similars" are approved without clinical studies and contain within 10% the equivalent active content of the NDA version of the drug. Generic manufacturers are constantly raising their level of compliance and parity with branded manufacturers.

Their need to improve their image, relative to agency compliance and rapid response to aggressive ANDA product introductions, together with ANDA approval exclusivity, is mandated to garner market share for a limited window of commercial opportunity.

Contract Manufacturers

Contract manufacturers pose the greatest challenge. Facilities must remain in full regulatory compliance, while at the same time reaching levels of compliance to meet various customer audit mandates. Combining the regulatory and customer requirements with an industry that is driven by a competitive cost of goods requires manufacturing facilities to be the most cost-effective in the pharmaceutical industry. The expanding world of pharmaceutical outsourcing to contract manufacturers is creating a new class of facilities that must meet the regulatory requirements to satisfy customers and service providers alike (Table 9.1).

Sales Forecast Effect on Optimization of Processing Equipment

Sales forecasts are the baseline capacity requirement for most OSD facilities. Sales forecasts are based on data that are driven on anticipation of usage by government agencies, hospitals, physicians, and consumers, along with the realities of competition. Government agencies are by far the largest purchasers of drug products in the United States, in particular. The forecasts are initially based on timelines relating to regulatory approvals and projected launch dates. Many factors impact the accuracy of the sales forecasts; thus, great care must be exhibited in using these data at face value.

Operations and engineering professionals, who must quantify the relationship between the dosage unit requirements and the sizing of the manufacturing facilities, must understand the assumptions of the forecast baseline requirements. This understanding is vital in producing a consensus as to the quantification of the manufacturing equipment need and the overall optimization of the facility design. The company philosophy related to batch sizes, equipment sizing, capacity utilization, changeover, and WIP abilities plays a role in the development of a strategic plan for purchasing manufacturing equipment.

Optimization of manufacturing equipment, upon acceptance of a sales forecast by management, is a balance between operations, quality assurance, quality control release, and actual order receipt or inventory requirements. The sizing and optimization of equipment are calculated based on a downstream evaluation of increased run capacity to minimize bottlenecks and maximize the output of the entire process.

TABLE 9.1

Comparison of Branded, Generic, and Contract Manufacturers

	Branded	Generic	Contract
Single product	■		
Multiproduct		■	■
FDA compliance	■	■	■
International compliance	■		■
High-volume products	■		■
Unit processes		■	■
Automated processes	■		
Capital intensive	$$$	$$	$
Engineered solutions	■	■	
Procedural solutions		■	■
Large engineering and operations staff	■		

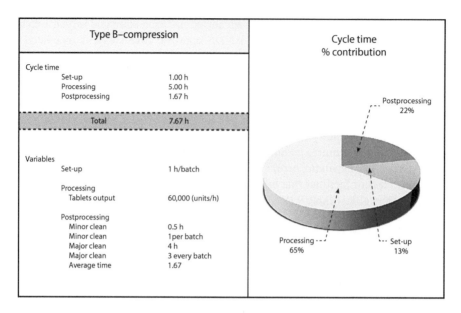

FIGURE 9.1   Static simulation graph for a typical tablet product.

A typical optimization model is illustrated by the static simulation graph for a typical tablet product (Figure 9.1).

Similar models are performed for individual processing steps, including multiple products, with simultaneous manufacturing operations. This is discussed in more detail in Chapter 10.

Management Preferences

Branded manufacturers develop products for both large-scale production and small, niche markets. Each of these widely divergent markets requires significantly different types of facilities to optimize manufacturing and maintain the lowest cost of goods produced. Large, branded manufacturers with large-volume products traditionally have made large capital investments in their facilities. Large investments are usually directed at creating automated, high-throughput facilities, increased yield rates, and a reduced labor cost per unit produced, thus minimizing the risks in achieving the major financial objectives for the drug.

Small-volume, niche market–focused branded drugs are traditionally manufactured in older, less automated facilities, with unit operations. The concerns for volume throughput and major financial objectives relegate this segment of their brands to their "dog and cat" operations (this refers to products that have a small demand and sales volume). The small-volume products are important segments of a company's market penetration strategy, especially if they are for unmet medical needs (i.e., an orphan drug).

Generic manufacturers focus on a product mix that is usually driven by a specific segment of drugs, for example, oncology, hormone replacement, cardiology, beta-blockers, gastroenterology, and dermatology. Their choice of drug type relates to the complexity of its manufacturing level to reduce potential competition or simplified compounds, requiring shorter ANDA approval schedules, or the specific branded competition resistance to potential patent challenge litigation.

The manufacturers of ANDA drugs traditionally use unitary processes because of the financial viability and life cycle of their products. Multiple product plants are commonplace and require a level of investment that keeps their profit margins at the very highest level possible. Modest capital investments in facilities and overall facility overheads are commonplace in this arena. Manufacturing equipment for generic manufacturers and the overall level of regulatory compliance have risen over the past decade to a level equivalent to that of branded manufacturers.

Contract manufacturers are a growing resource to both branded and generic manufacturers. Whether it is an outsource manufacturer for a single product, an overflow resource, or the expert in specific processing and drug delivery technologies, the primary focus is on speed to market and cost of goods. Quality assurance is considered a baseline expertise that is built into the manufacturing operations of the contract manufacturer.

Unitary capabilities (i.e., individualized processing capabilities) with a high degree of cross-contamination controls are a requirement that is paramount. The manufacture of multiple products in adjacent spaces creates the need for facilities with validatable HVAC and critical utility systems that ensure compliance with each of their customer's quality concerns. Quality and regulatory compliance are givens and are mandated in each of these distinctly different manufacturing segments.

Single-Product versus Multiproduct Environment

Single-product facility design provides a platform for the innovations that enable a branded producer to maximize throughput, without the restrictions created in a multi-product plant. Manufacturing equipment selections are driven on product transfer capabilities that maximize equipment use and reduce downtime. Special material handling issues, related to potent and cytotoxic compounds, are more readily achieved in single-product plants due to the clear definition of a single process. Manpower and personnel protection issues can be dealt with one well-thought-out method, thus minimizing risk.

The multi-product plant environment is one that must deal with competing needs on a regular basis. Cross-contamination, product mix-up, and cleaning issues are just some of the issues that must be addressed through engineering and procedural solutions. The life of a multi-product facility design is ever changing and requires an adaptable layout; a set of critical utility and HVAC systems; and purified water, gases, steam, and hot water that can meet changing capacities and distribution needs. Quality assurance concerns for this changing work environment are vital components of a design solution that maintains regulatory compliance.

PRODUCTION TECHNOLOGY: YESTERDAY, TODAY, AND TOMORROW

Drug manufacturing processes have made a gradual transition over the past century. While tablets or soft gelatin capsules have been the principal dosage forms used for many years, new OSD forms have evolved, including quick-dissolve tablets or wafers, sustained-release capsules, and film technologies for rapid drug solubility. The manufacturing technology that produces these drug forms is primarily divided into the following categories: (1) sampling, dispensing, or handling of active solid or liquid chemicals and excipients; (2) alteration of particle size, granulating, mixing, drying, and milling; (3) compression and encapsulation; (4) coating and printing; and (5) primary and secondary packaging.

MANUFACTURING FLOWS

Currently, OSD facilities are designed with distinctive flows to minimize cross-contamination and meet the intent of cGMPs for separation of products and activities. Flows related to personnel movement, gowning facilities, materials management, waste removal, and cleaning have become major components of pharmaceutical facility design. *The flows that are mandated for sterile manufacturing should not be equated to the design of OSD facilities.* The design of flows for OSD facilities should be weighed against specific project concerns related to cross-contamination and product mix-up, while maintaining the physical environment for each specific project. The relative throughput of the facility must be a governing factor in the design of all OSD facilities. The actual traffic of materials, personnel, and waste should dictate the degree of concern for the crossing of flows and the risk that is present during day-to-day operations (Figure 9.2).

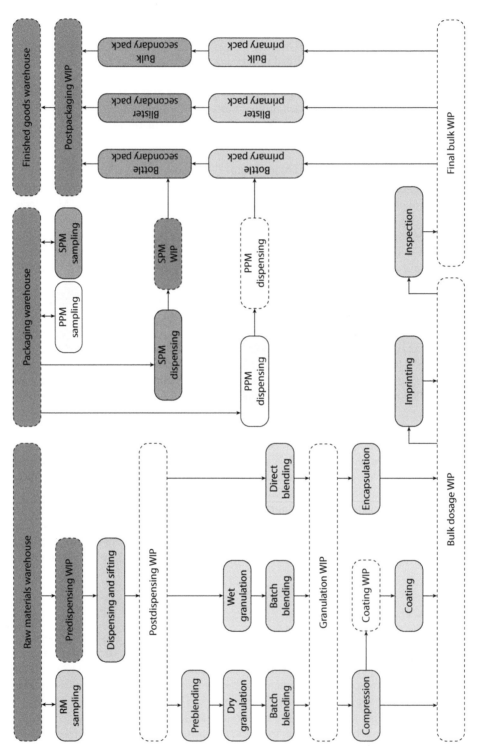

FIGURE 9.2   Typical OSD manufacturing block flow diagram (BFD); other BFDs are discussed in Chapters 4 and 10.

Employee Health and Safety Concerns

Requirements for personnel protection have evolved from those of governmental regulatory agencies and pharmaceutical companies. The design challenges presented in OSD projects for health and safety are significant and increasingly important. Because of the use of potent and cytotoxic materials, significant concerns about exposure have been raised. The level of experience and documented research on the short- and long-term health concerns that were present in the past and will be present in the future has affected all design solutions.

Engineered and procedural solutions are commonplace, coupled with specific employee health and safety policies. Determining the hazard levels present, through either physical testing or empirical modeling, has provided matrices for the levels of risk that must be addressed. Determination of the policies and procedures and the physical facility design is the most important aspect of OSD facility design. The issues relating to the employee health risks will grow with each year of experience in the manufacture of drug products.

Challenging Preconceptions

Preconceptions of the mandated requirements for OSD manufacturing facilities have exceeded the practical requirements for facility design. Concerns related to layout, critical system specifications, and scope of required validation all have exceeded true regulatory compliance. The thoughtful balance of interpretive procedural compliance versus "brick-and-mortar" solutions can provide sound methods of preserving precious capital resources. Thus, balance in challenging preconceptions is a major risk management issue that should be discussed, analyzed, and determined early in the design process. This is one of the costliest issues to be dealt with in determining the scope of an OSD project. Sample layouts of various processing operations can be seen in Figures 9.3 and 9.4.

IMPLICATIONS FOR PERFORMANCE AND COMPLIANCE

New Greenfield versus an Expanded or Renovated Facility

Most major OSD projects present the choice of building a new facility or renovating and expanding an existing one. The cost and schedule implications of this decision are irrevocable. Strategic decision making must bypass personal agendas. Decision making that revolves around reductions in capital investment can create long-term problems in creating a facility that can still meet long-term needs and flexibility for changing product pipelines.

Identification of realistic short-range, mid-range, and long-range business plans must be prepared, and they must receive the support of senior management. The plans will be based on current manufacturing issues, forecasts, and long-term visions based on the organization's strategic plan. The final decision will be based on the organization's capital spending resources or philosophy, or it may simply be a vision.

Designing a facility that meets the requirements for production capability, cost, schedule, and compliance is paramount. The design of facilities that provide the flexibility to adapt to the changing product types, product capacity needs, personnel protection needs, and regulations is a task that requires experience, vision, and an understanding of the direction of the industry—a difficult but achievable goal.

Production Requirements

Planning an OSD facility begins with the drug product or products forecasted for inclusion in the facility. Correlation of a production forecast with the reality of a production environment requires a strategic plan specific to the facility. Production requirements range from high-volume, large-batch products to small-volume, small-batch products. The facility design philosophy requires a direction

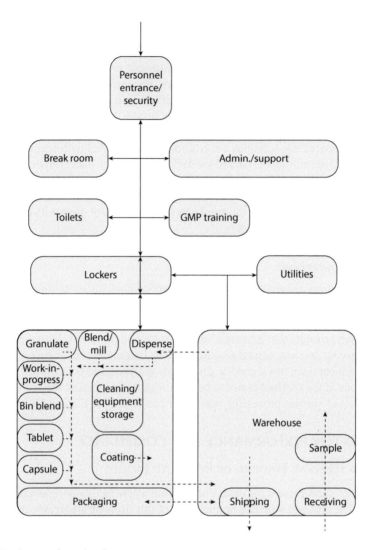

FIGURE 9.3   Basic manufacturing flows.

modeled on the volume and batch-size parameters. This production order of magnitude sets the platform for the manufacturing equipment quantification, facility staffing, materials management capabilities, and support requirements. The "domino effect" of the production requirements initiates a large group of design variables that determine a cause and effect that will create a unified approach to meeting the production requirements.

MANUFACTURING EQUIPMENT

Manufacturing equipment requirements are primarily driven by the R&D of a drug product. The process is primarily developed on equipment selected by the product development team. Engineering and operational staff are encouraged to participate in the equipment selection; this interaction, during a product's development, depends on the drug manufacturer's internal philosophy of collaboration. This area of internal politics can produce valuable insights into equipment selection, the ease of manufacturing, quality assurance issues, and the cost of goods produced. The quality organization should be involved at every step of this decision-making process. Because of inherent EHS issues, the use of open, exposed product equipment should be excluded from the development

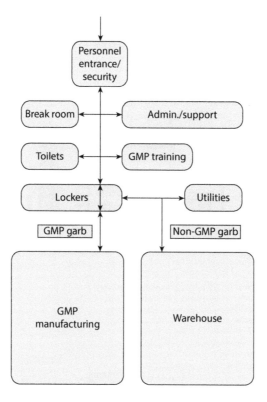

FIGURE 9.4 Basic personnel flows.

process of new or reformulated products. The personnel liability issues that can develop from exposure to chemicals are not acceptable risks.

Upon resolution of the process, it is incumbent to determine an equipment train that maximizes the output, through balancing the overall throughput of the multistep process. This balancing process is dependent on rate of production, the batching philosophy, the cleaning and changeover logistics, the timing, and the quality assurance and quality control constraints that are imposed at each step of the process.

The actual manufacturing equipment includes both dry and wet processes. Dry processes offer a containment challenge for dust migration, while wet processes require purified water or solvents to achieve their desired processing step. The discussion below covers the types of equipment that are typically used in OSD manufacturing.

Delivery and Measurement of Chemical Ingredients, Excipients, Liquids, and Fillers

The manufacturing equipment used for dispensing, weighing, or pharmacy areas includes material handling devices, which can be both horizontal and vertical for dispensing, and scales, which can be in-floor scales, pit- or surface-mounted scales for large quantities, pedestal models for mid-range quantities, and bench-top models for small quantities (Figure 9.5).

Released bulk raw materials are delivered to the predispensing WIP area as necessary. These released bulk raw materials are retrieved from the predispensing WIP area and transmitted into the selected dispensing room through the dedicated material airlock. Once transitioned, the bulk material is staged for dispensing.

Following the dispensing operation, any unused bulk material is returned to the predispensing area through the dedicated material airlock. Only one ingredient is handled in the dispensing room at any given time. Any waste generated is also removed through the material airlock.

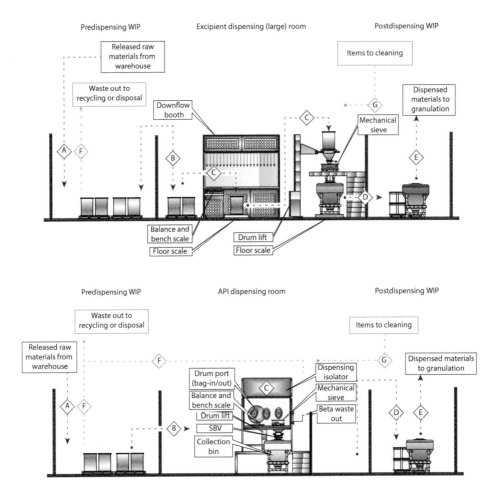

FIGURE 9.5 Manufacturing equipment for dispensing chemical ingredients and excipients and weighing these products. A: Released bulk raw materials are delivered to the predispensing WIP area as required. B: Released bulk raw materials are retrieved from the predispensing WIP area as required and transmitted into the selected dispensing room through its dedicated material airlock. Once transitioned, the bulk material is staged for dispensing. Following the dispensing operation, any unused bulk partial material is returned to the predispensing area through the dedicated material airlock. Only one ingredient is handled in the dispensing room at any given time. Any waste generated is also removed out through the material airlock. C: Raw material is dispensed and weighed as required by the batch record into intermediate drums. The drums are then lifted, inverted, and discharged through a sieve and collected into a bin. D: Once all of any given raw material has been dispensed and sifted, the bin is transitioned out of the dispensing room through the dedicated material airlock and staged with the other materials associated with the batch in the postdispensing WIP area. E: Once all batch materials are dispensed and kitted and required in manufacturing, they are retrieved from the postdispensing WIP area and delivered to the required processing room (i.e., blending or wet granulation). F: Waste is removed and properly recycled or disposed. G: Following processing, equipment and parts are wetted down and, as required, bagged and sent to the washroom for final cleaning.

Raw material is dispensed and weighed as required by the batch record into intermediate drums. The drums are then lifted, inverted, and discharged through a sieve and collected in a bin. Once all of any given raw material has been dispensed and sifted, the bin is transitioned out of the dispensing room through the dedicated material airlock and staged with the other materials associated with the batch in the postdispensing WIP area. Once all batch materials are dispensed and kitted, they are retrieved from the postdispensing WIP area and delivered to the required processing room (i.e., blending or wet granulation). Waste is removed and properly recycled or disposed. Following processing, equipment and parts are wetted down, bagged, and sent to the washroom for final cleaning.

Milling, Blending, Mixing, Granulating, Compacting, Drying, and Formulation

Production rooms can be separate or combined for individual pieces of equipment, depending on the batching philosophy, volumes of products produced, material transfer technology, and transport container type. Material handling for all steps may be performed using a mechanical device, gravity fed from an elevated platform or floor above, or a manual device. The means and methods depend on the quantity of material, its particle flow characteristic, the ergonomic and personnel issues, and the ability to meet a validated cleaning process. Lift trucks, pallet jacks, drum dumpers (portable or fixed), handling "super sacks," and drums (lined fiberboard, stainless, or a polymer), along with metal or polymer tote bins, are the primary mode of transport and container.

The following manufacturing steps are paired with the equipment most likely to be used for that step:

- Milling is performed in sifters, co-mills, separators, and comminuters.
- Blending is performed in a twin-shell V or cone, ribbon, or tote blender.
- Granulating is done in a low-shear or high-shear fluid bed or interplanetary kneader.
- Compacting is performed by roller compactors or tableting compaction.
- Drying occurs in a fluid bed, oven, microwave, or vacuum, among others.
- Gelatin preparation occurs in tanks or mixers.

Preblended materials are delivered from the bulk granulation WIP area and staged in the dry granulation room (Figure 9.6). Bins are fed to the roller compactor via the lift, and compacted and milled materials are collected in bins. Following processing, the filled bins are moved to bulk granulation WIP, awaiting the final blending operation.

Following processing and under closed-system conditions, equipment and parts are wetted down, bagged, and sent to the washroom for final cleaning, which may or may not be necessary. Waste is removed and properly recycled or disposed.

For direct-blend operations or dry granulation preblends, predispensed batch materials are delivered from the postdispensing WIP area and staged in the blending room. For the final blend of granulation batches, predispensed batch materials and in-process granulated materials are delivered from the bulk granulation WIP area and staged in the blending room (Figure 9.7). As required, materials are changed into the blend shell, using the lift of a vacuum, and transferred to the batch bin, using a portable platform (small additions only). A portable access platform is used to make vacuum connections. Materials are blended for the prescribed period of time.

Following blending, the blender is raised to allow the bins to be filled, and then bins are moved to bulk granulation WIP, awaiting dry granulation, compression, or encapsulation. Following processing and under closed-system conditions, equipment and parts are wetted down and, as required, bagged and sent to the washroom for final cleaning, which may or may not be necessary. Waste is removed and properly recycled or disposed.

Predispensed batch materials are delivered from the postdispensing WIP area and staged in the granulation room. The granulation is formulated within the granulation room and lifted to the granulator access level (Figure 9.8). Batch solids are charged in the high-shear granulator via the lift, and granulation solution is supplied as required; granulated materials are discharged through an in-line wet mill into the fluid bed for drying. Dried material is discharged out of the fluid bed through an in-line dry mill and collected into a bin. Transfers are all closed systems. In-process materials are moved to the bulk granulation WIP area, awaiting final blending. Following processing and under closed-system conditions, equipment and parts are wetted down and, as required, bagged and sent to the washroom for final cleaning. Waste is removed and properly recycled or disposed.

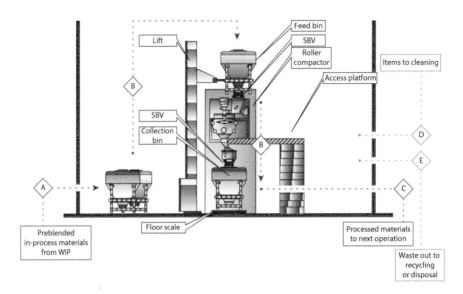

FIGURE 9.6 Dry granulation room. A: Preblended materials are delivered from the bulk granulation WIP area and staged in the dry granulation room. B: Bins are fed to the roller compactor via the lift, and compacted and milled materials are collected in bins. C: Following processing, the filled bins are moved to bulk granulation WIP, awaiting final blending operation. D: Following processing and under closed-system conditions, equipment and parts are wetted down and, as required, bagged and sent to the washroom for final cleaning. This may not be required. E: Waste is removed and properly recycled or disposed.

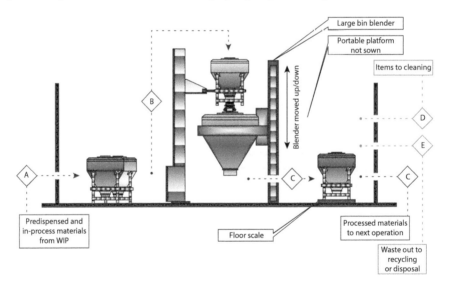

FIGURE 9.7 The blending room. A: For direct-blend operations or dry granulation preblends, predispensed batch materials are delivered from the postdispensing WIP area and staged in the blending room. For final blend of granulation batches, predispensed batch materials and in-process granulated materials are delivered from the bulk granulation WIP area and staged in the blending room. B: As required, materials are changed into the blend shell utilizing the lift of a vacuum, transferred, and added to the batch bin utilizing a portable platform (small additions only). A portable access platform will be used to make vacuum connections. Materials are blended for the prescribed period of time. C: Following blending, the blender is raised to allow filling of bins, and then bins are moved to bulk granulation WIP, awaiting dry granulation, compression, or encapsulation. D: Following processing and under closed-system conditions, equipment and parts are wetted down and, as required, bagged and sent to the washroom for final cleaning. This may not be required. E: Waste is removed and properly recycled or disposed.

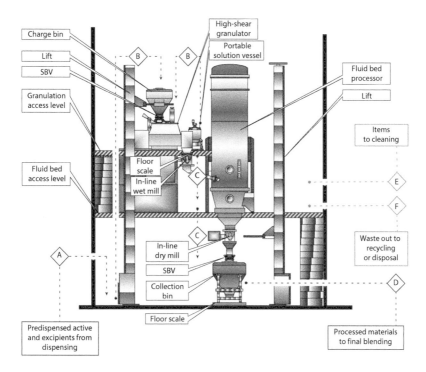

FIGURE 9.8 Wet granulation room. A: Predispensed batch materials are delivered from the postdispensing WIP area and staged in the granulation room. B: Granulation solution is formulated within the granulation room and lifted to the granulator access level. Batch solids are charged into the high-shear granulator via the lift, and granulation solution is supplied as required. C: Granulated materials are discharged through an in-line wet mill into the fluid bed for drying. Dried material is discharged out of the fluid bed through an in-line dry mill and collected in a bin. Transfers are all closed systems. D: In-process materials are moved to the bulk granulation WIP area, awaiting final blending. E: Following processing and under closed-system conditions, equipment and parts are wetted down and, as required, bagged and sent to the washroom for final cleaning. F: Waste is removed and properly recycled or disposed.

Compression, Encapsulation, and Specialty Drug Delivery Unit

Primarily equipment is housed in individual rooms to limit cross-contamination and product mix-up. During compression of single or layered tablets, the equipment has a de-duster, a weight check, or other quality or discharge devices. Encapsulation is performed with hard-capsule powder and liquid fill and is equipped with a discharge device. Gel tabs are dipped in a liquid gelatin coating to simulate capsules; soft gelatin capsules are filled with liquid.

Final blended bulk batch bins are delivered from the bulk granulation WIP areas and staged in the compression room. Empty capsule shells are delivered to the compression room. Bins (product and empty capsule) are fed to the filter via lifts, and filled capsules are ejected from the filter and vacuum transfer through a metal check to a weight check. Weight-verified capsules are collected into bins or buckets. Processing bins or buckets are moved to bulk dosage WIP, awaiting the inspection operation. Following processing and under closed-system conditions, equipment and parts are wetted down and, as required, bagged and sent to the washroom for final cleaning, which may or may not be necessary. Waste is removed and properly recycled or disposed (Figure 9.9).

Final blended bulk bins are delivered from the bulk granulation WIP area and staged in the compression room. Bins are fed to the press via the lift, and compressed tablets are ejected from the press through a de-duster or metal check and collected into tablet bins or buckets (Figure 9.10). Following processing, bins or buckets are moved to coating WIP or bulk dosage WIP, awaiting coating or the inspection operation.

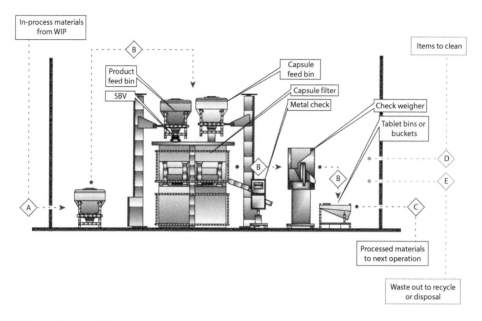

FIGURE 9.9 Capsule filling and weight check room. A: Final blended bulk batch bins are delivered from the bulk granulation WIP area and staged in the compression room. Empty capsule shells are delivered to the compression room. B: Bins (product and empty capsule) are fed to the filter via lifts and filled capsules are ejected from the filter and vacuum transfer through a metal check to a weight check. Weight-verified capsules are collected into bins or buckets. C: Following processing, bins or buckets are moved to bulk dosage WIP, awaiting inspection operation. D: Following processing and under closed-system conditions, equipment and parts are wetted down and, as required, bagged and sent to the washroom for final cleaning. This may not be required. E: Waste is removed and properly recycled or disposed.

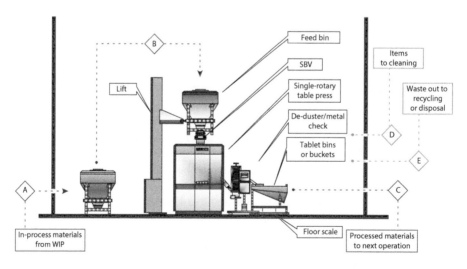

FIGURE 9.10 Compression room. A: Final blended bulk bins are delivered from the bulk granulation WIP area and staged in the compression room. B: Bins are fed to the press via the lift, and compressed tablets are ejected from the press through a de-duster and metal check, and collected into tablet bins or buckets. C: Following processing, bins or buckets are moved to coating WIP or bulk dosage WIP, awaiting coating or inspection operation. D: Following processing and under closed-system conditions, equipment and parts are wetted down and, as required, bagged and sent to the washroom for final cleaning. E: Waste is removed and properly recycled or disposed.

Following processing and under closed-system conditions, equipment and parts are wetted down and, as required, bagged and sent to the washroom for final cleaning. Waste is removed and properly recycled or disposed.

Coating, Printing, and Inspection

Primarily, equipment is housed in individual rooms to limit cross-contamination and product mix-up. The coating and printing equipment use dedicated air handling systems. Either conventional rotating coating pans, using aqueous or solvent-based coating solutions, or cylindrical, perforated, revolving coating pans are used.

Fluid-bed coating uses an internal coating column, with aqueous- or solvent-based coating solutions. Solvent-based systems have building code implications.

Printing equipment consists of ink-jet, laser, or other marking systems. Inspection can follow, using a wide range of techniques, from random visual inspection to automated vision systems.

Packaging

Manufacturing equipment ranges from hand packaging operations to fully integrated filling, bottling, and blister lines, with cartoners, case packers, and palletizers.

Bottling lines consist of the following: bottle unscramblers, blow and vacuum, accumulation tables, desiccant loader, slat filler or photo eye counter, cottoner, tamper-evident sealer, capper, retorque, labeler, leaflet inserter, cartoners, case packer, case sealer, bar code printer or labeler, palletizer, and stretch wrapper. Blister lines consist of a blister former, filler, foil sealer, card applicator, and cartoner. Processing equipment clearances for operational space related to height and room width and depth must be carefully planned to permit installation, operation, and maintenance.

Manufacturing Flows

Flows through OSD facilities are categorized as material flows, personnel flows, equipment flows, and waste flows. Material flows consist of incoming raw material, sampling, incoming packaging components, work in progress (operations and quality assurance), and finished goods (shipping and distribution). Personnel flows consist of changing or uniform facilities, manufacturing personnel (operations and quality assurance), material handling personnel, support personnel (maintenance), administrative personnel, and quality control personnel. Flow of equipment that needs to be cleaned consists of dirty equipment, equipment cleaning, inspection, assembly, cleaning validation, clean equipment, and parts storage. The flow of waste material (i.e., liquids, solids, and trash) consists of the following: waste neutralization, waste holding, waste removal, waste disposal, and recycling.

It should be noted that the once-through, noncrossing flow patterns are ideal within a given design. The reality of operational flows typically does not warrant the total once-through philosophy. Analyzing the actual material throughput, in terms of pallet counts, per shift or hour, for raw materials, work in progress, finished goods, and waste flows, rarely creates instances of extensive traffic within OSD manufacturing areas. Modeling of the concurrent material quantities flowing through an OSD facility will provide a more commonsense approach to the level of segregation of flows that is truly required.

Airlock, Garb Change, and Gowning Requirements

The functional need for airlocks to segregate areas of facilities translates into separate zoning for HVAC systems. Division between nonclassified areas, such as a warehouse, and classified manufacturing areas is mandatory to preserve the integrity of manufacturing operations. Airlocks for materials and personnel garb change are required universally, with the exception of nonpotent drug products. Potent drug manufacturing facilities require airlocks in all regulatory jurisdictions for material transfer and personnel garb change to eliminate the possibility of cross-contamination of particulate matter. The garb-change philosophy should include the capability to divorce the

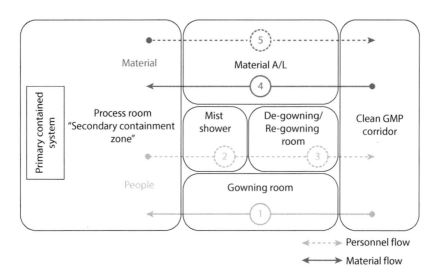

FIGURE 9.11 Conceptual personnel and material flow diagram.

ability of employees to enter manufacturing areas in any garb other than dedicated uniforming and dedicated safety shoes or disposable shoe covers. Uniforms, specifically footwear, are the single greatest liability in tracking particulate matter throughout a facility.

As cross-contamination risks have grown, secondary garb additions, such as disposable Tyvek suits, have become procedural additions to safeguard employees and diminish the risks of cross-contamination. Additionally, equipment has also been added, such as misting showers, to minimize the transport of potent materials from the secondary garb, before leaving the de-gown rooms and exiting the processing operation. Examples of airlock and gowning and de-gowning arrangements are shown in Figure 9.11.

Misting showers, shown in Figure 9.11, are primarily used to contain potent compound particulate matter. Gowning is further discussed in Chapter 4.

QUALITY ASSURANCE REQUIREMENTS

Quality assurance is an all-encompassing design consideration in an OSD manufacturing facility. The facility-related quality assurance or regulatory compliance design inclusions relate to many of the facility's physical attributes, such as flows and layout, specific employee change philosophy, sampling and testing locations, label storage and distribution, and office and workstation space. Requirements also revolve around critical utility design parameters for temperature, humidity, pressurization differentials, and other vital validation criteria.

Standard operating procedures (SOPs) and their link to the physical design are vital information that should be formulated at the inception of the project to gain the greatest advantage during the design process. Traditionally, many SOP considerations are not developed until the design is far along or the facility is actually under construction. A proactive approach can generate many collaborative ideas that can simplify the design and even eliminate the need for compromise and concessions late in the project delivery process.

PHYSICAL MANUFACTURING ENVIRONMENT

The physical manufacturing environment can vary greatly, depending on the nature of the business, the philosophy of the manufacturer, and the available capital resources. Compliance is not directly proportional to the magnitude of the investment or the sophistication of the facility. The balance of creating the ideal manufacturing environment is a point of discussion that should occur very early in the planning process. The short- and long-term goals for each facility require analysis of many influences, including whether there will be a new or an existing facility; the life span of the facility; whether there will be a single- or multiproduct output; the hazard level of products to be manufactured; the volume of products to be produced; the breadth of regulatory compliance; the attributes that affect the complexity of the design, such as flexibility in its long-term use; the risk tolerance to meet stated manufacturing criteria and regulatory compliance; and the staffing philosophy, including projections for supervision and level of daily operations.

SPECIAL PRODUCT CONSIDERATIONS

Special product considerations can range from protection of employees to the physical ability to manufacture in a given space. Potent compounds range from category 1 products to high-hazard category 5 products and cytotoxic compounds, the production of which requires an analytical approach to the facility design. Consideration of the hazard level is an important component of the risk assessment required by a manufacturer of OSD products. The legal liability for the manufacture of these drug products warrants consideration by senior management and legal opinions to ensure that the correct course of action is taken. For cytotoxic drug cross-contamination, the FDA and other regulatory agencies, such as the National Institute for Occupational Safety and Health (NIOSH), also merit an analytical approach to define the true hazard versus the implied hazard and to determine whether a separate facility is necessary.

Special product considerations should be determined by fact, not speculation. Gaining specific data relating to the specific product hazard level or difficulty to manufacture must be determined early in the design process. Testing the effect of the special product on the facility design is critical in developing a commonsense approach to meeting the stated level of the necessary manufacturing capabilities.

Personal protection equipment (PPE) affects the level of safety for personnel. Combining the specific equipment capabilities with the recommended exposure levels and with the limitations on personnel mobility and productivity requires careful analysis. Respirators, breathing air systems, and barrier-type garb are examples of individual PPE.

Engineered solutions for process containment focus on equipment design that provides containment during charging, processing, sampling, discharging, cleaning, and maintenance. Primary containment solutions for high-potency processes entail closed-system designs and isolation technologies. For less potent processes, primary containment control can be achieved through the use of airflow technologies, including local exhaust ventilation and downflow booths. Secondary containment measures are engineered through the facility design, including HVAC and architectural elements. Combining engineering control measures with precautionary PPE and procedures can result in a robust, safe, and cost-effective design.

PROVISIONS FOR CONTROLLED SUBSTANCES

Controlled substances are a significant portion of the product mix in many OSD facilities. The regulations are contained within the U.S. Department of Justice Drug Enforcement Administration (DEA) Title 21 of the U.S. Code (USC) Controlled Substance Act. Sites of manufacture and storage must be registered and approved by the DEA before initiating manufacturing and storage.

The definitions of the controlled substances are defined by the DEA in classes. The classes range from 1 to 5, depending on their requirements for storage, security, surveillance, and documentation at every level of operation throughout the manufacturing process (Table 9.2).

The security provisions for controlled substances are clearly defined in Part 1301 of the DEA regulations (§1301.72, "physical security controls for non-practitioners; narcotic treatment programs and compounders for narcotic treatment programs; storage areas"). The provisions for security controls are defined for the specific designs of caging, vaults, locked areas, and surveillance hardware that are appropriate for the classes of drug products present. International regulations, on a country-by-country basis, define similar regulations for the local area of manufacturing or storage.

TABLE 9.2

Definitions of Controlled Substances as Defined by the Drug Enforcement Administration

Schedule I	(1) The drug or other substance has a high potential for abuse. (2) The drug or other substance has no currently accepted medical use in treatment in the United States. (3) There is a lack of accepted safety for use of the drug or other substance under medical supervision.
Schedule II	(1) The drug or other substance has a high potential for abuse. (2) The drug or other substance has a currently accepted medical use in treatment in the United States or a currently accepted medical use with severe restrictions. (3) Abuse of the drug or other substances may lead to severe psychological or physical dependence.
Schedule III	(1) The drug or other substance has a potential for abuse less than the drugs or other substances in schedules I and II. (2) The drug or other substance has a currently accepted medical use in treatment in the United States. (3) Abuse of the drug or other substance may lead to moderate or low physical dependence or high psychological dependence.
Schedule IV	(1) The drug or other substance has a low potential for abuse relative to the drugs or other substances in schedule III. (2) The drug or other substance has a currently accepted medical use in treatment in the United States. (3) Abuse of the drug or other substance may lead to limited physical dependence or psychological dependence relative to the drugs or other substances in schedule III.
Schedule V	(1) The drug or other substance has a low potential for abuse relative to the drugs or other substances in schedule IV. (2) The drug or other substance has a currently accepted medical use in treatment in the United States. (3) Abuse of the drug or other substance may lead to limited physical dependence or psychological dependence relative to the drugs or other substances in schedule IV.

CLEAN DESIGN

Implications for Performance and Compliance

Assigning Proper Level of Design to the Solution

Architectural solutions to clean pharmaceutical design can be costly to design and install. This is an area of differing perspectives on the ideal solutions. The materials and finishes also can be expensive and play a vital role in how well an area can be cleaned. Solid dosage projects are facilities with varying degrees of dust accumulation as a result of the product processes and the dust collection systems employed.

The true risk associated with clean detailing is a balance between the actual clean detail and the SOPs for the actual room housekeeping. Flush details improve the ability to keep a vertical or horizontal surface clean. The SOPs for the scheduled cleaning procedure can be the true test of the extent of the flush or ledge-free detailing. Frequent quality cleaning procedures are a vital link in the quality assurance program for housekeeping, and thus a more important fact than the detail itself. Examples of clean detailing can be found in Chapter 4. The level of solution, in great part, is in proportion to the level of quality assurance protocols and procedures that are set forth by the facility operations. The costs of capital, cleaning labor, and cleaning requirement conformance are a delicate balance that requires economical analyses. Determining the proper level of physical solutions and ensuring that they are appropriate are extremely important risk assessments on every project. The level of engineered solutions is proportional to the capital resources available. The burden of right or wrong rests in the overall engineered solution, combined with SOPs, leading to the quality assurance and regulatory compliance of each product produced.

Value-Added Solutions

Examples of value-added solutions for OSD manufacturing facilities can include:

- Equipment selections that use the least amount of equipment to produce the largest volume of product
- Capacity modeling that provides data to maintain output levels going downstream in all steps of the process, to yield alternatives for bottlenecking and unitary operations and to provide a consistent throughput at all stages of operation

- Layouts that reduce the overall number of personnel required to operate a facility
- Material handling systems that maximize throughput, diminish operator ergonomic issues, and minimize opportunities for dust migration and cross-contamination
- Solutions that provide containment of product particulate matter within each processing room
- Installation of an adequate quantity of light fixtures and light levels in manufacturing rooms for supervision and regulatory observation of operations
- Design and installation of Part 11—compliant, validatable building automation systems (BASs) that control and monitor critical utilities

Balance of Engineered Solutions to SOP Solutions

Common evaluations that are performed during the design of OSD facilities are listed below:

- BASs versus manual documentation of critical utilities, using independent Magnehelic gauges. These gauges are visually read versus automated, integrated differential pressure sensors, integrated to BAS for control and monitoring.
- Flush double glazing in manufacturing rooms versus sloped sills that require scheduled SOP housekeeping to maintain dust-free surfaces.
- Wash-down of manufacturing rooms versus dry wipe or vacuum of particulate matter.
- Use of PPE by manufacturing personnel, with once-through HVAC systems compared to recirculating HVAC systems.
- Electronic, interlocked magnetic locks for airlocks versus red light–green light.

SOP-focused operation of interlocked airlock doors.

PROJECT MANAGEMENT ISSUES

Appropriate Level of Capital Investment

Early in the life of a project, a determination of the funding limitations, scheduled completion, and level of quality needs to be established by senior management. The level of funding can set many of the variables that must be selected to quantify an overall facility philosophy. The philosophy can be a determination between first cost and long-term cost of the capital investment. Typical decision points relative to this determination include the following: sizing of utility systems for future capacity; levels of redundancy of critical and noncritical engineered systems for chilled water, steam, compressed air, and electrical systems (including emergency power); overall sizing of the individual space components of the facility for future growth and flexibility; and quality of materials, finish selections, types of doors, extent of vision lights, and flush details. There are no correct or incorrect choices here. Determining the level of acceptable risk combined with the available capital is the baseline criterion upon which a facility's long-term standard for flexibility, space, finish, and capability is built.

Schedule Advancement Ahead of Scope Definition

Inevitably, pharmaceutical OSD manufacturing projects advance before goals related to products, their capacities, and the product processes and their required manufacturing equipment are solidified. Quantifying the specific quantities and sizes of processing equipment is vital to the planning process. Delays in determining these data can create additional costs and delays in meeting the project milestones.

Fast-track projects may be conceived before establishing the long-term employee health and safety capabilities necessary to mitigate risk for potent compound manufacturing. EHS procedures and powered air-purifying respirators (PAPRs) can be mated at various levels of complexity to match the eventual product mix versus product categorization that is be added to the facilities.

Project end dates are regularly set without regard to determination of the issues discussed above. The initiation of facility design in this case requires a thorough risk assessment to guide the inclusion or exclusion of flexibility, space, and engineered system concepts to contemplate the unknowns that will inevitably present.

Some key factors that should be reviewed during the initiation of projects where schedules are a driving force include the following: the business objectives and drivers for the project; the ability to leverage an existing building shell or build a new one; the impact to ongoing operations and schedule coordination with construction; the coordination of scheduled plant shutdowns; the anticipation of processes requiring air and wastewater abatement, combined with local, state, and federal regulatory approvals for construction and operations; and the compliance conformance to federal and international regulatory bodies for facility design and operation.

REASONABLE LEVEL OF QUALITY FOR THE DESIRED END PRODUCT

Quality is an attribute that can range from the life expectancy of facility-related equipment, such as air handling units, to the durability of wall, floor, and ceiling systems. Quality can be dictated by corporate standards, plant standards, or industry standards. Conformance to SOPs can help achieve levels of serviceability that can also be attained by procurement of more sophisticated designs. The overall quality must be determined on a system-by-system basis or on the attributes of a specific material of construction. Examples of typical quality ranges can include

- USP water piping, ranging from polypropylene to polished stainless tubing
- Flooring materials from painted epoxy to epoxy terrazzo with integral base
- Wall coatings from water-based epoxy coatings to heat-welded polyvinyl chloride (PVC) materials
- Active-pressure-control HVAC systems, with supply and return variable air volume boxes, and hard-balanced, to damper-controlled HVAC systems
- Integrated BASs for control and monitoring to unitary control systems on each air handling unit with a freestanding environmental monitoring system not connected to the system controls
- Variable-frequency electric drives to fixed-frequency drive motors

The benefit of each quality decision can be determined independently or in the context of an overall facility design philosophy.

FUTURE DEVELOPMENTS

REDUCING THE COST OF PRODUCTS PRODUCED

Reductions in the costs of goods produced often lie outside the design parameters of an OSD facility. The areas of cost savings that result from the design process include the energy efficiency of the utility-related engineered systems; the systems that require less frequent maintenance and less costly spare parts for repair; reductions in the physical layout to reduce travel distances for material, personnel, and waste, in both cGMP and non-cGMP areas of the facility; and standardization of equipment and procedures.

INTERNATIONAL COMPLIANCE

Individual pharmaceutical regulatory agencies are primarily concerned with regulating specific design parameters that focus on cross-contamination, product mix-up, and facility cleanliness.

The FDA guidelines, listed in the *Federal Register*, for facility design are very general, while international agencies may set specific thresholds for design. Care must be taken to ensure that each design for each facility meets the intent of the country or countries to which manufactured product is destined for distribution or sale.

Regulations for controlled substances, such as those of the DEA, set highly specific design standards. These standards deal with the handling, manufacture, and short- and long-term storage of controlled substances. The DEA standards are categorized by drug classes, from class 1 to 5. Storage may vary from locked rooms to cages or vaults. Most specifications are contained within the regulations in the *Federal Register*.

OUTSOURCING TO LOW-COST PROVIDERS

The manufacture of OSD products is frequently outsourced to contract manufacturers. The contract manufacturers can be either independent contractors or major branded manufacturers with excess production capacity. As the concern for the cost of goods increases, the pressure on all manufacturers is to seek their best option to improve their bottom line, without creating risk for their brand.

Facility design for contract providers is subject not only to the regulatory bodies but also to the quality audits of potential customers. In many cases, potential customer requirements exceed the requirements of the regulatory bodies. This increase in facility scrutiny creates a need for designs that at times exceed industry standards to meet the customers' quality and risk avoidance standards.

CHALLENGING THE MORES AND PRECONCEPTIONS

A fundamental strength of an experienced OSD facility designer is to challenge a manufacturer's operation. This challenge provides the dialogue necessary to test the validity of current manufacturing practices, facility flows, and SOPs. The ideal separation of cGMP and non-cGMP zones of activity requires detailed discussions related to material handling, from its receipt at the loading dock through all of the manufacturing steps to its departure as a finished drug product from the loading dock. Personnel flows, including gowning, transitioning between differing zones of cleanliness, and their interface with the actual manufacturing process, all require challenges to determine the most reasonable solution for the specific project. The challenge of mores and preconceptions can make the difference between facilities that can meet the expectations of the manufacturing environment of the future and facilities that cannot.

SPECIAL DISCUSSION

BENCHMARKS TO OTHER INDUSTRY

Solid dosage manufacturing can be compared to the food industry, in terms of the unitary processes, standard of care, and fact that the products are ingested. The primary differences are the lack of validated processes and the creation of a regulated environment that ensures the long-term quality of the products produced. The regulatory statutes mandated by each country are the crux of the framework for the faculty's design and operation. The regulatory scrutiny and enforcement placed on the pharmaceutical industry by individual countries provide a much higher level of compliance than virtually any industry that affects human welfare on a continuous basis. The nuclear industry is the only other highly regulated industry. The primary difference is protection of the public welfare through the physical environment versus the manufacture of a consumable product. The benchmark of the pharmaceutical industry is a quantifiable series of activities, under the scrutiny of the manufacturers and regulators alike. This standard is one that provides ongoing, consistent safeguards for the end user of drug products.

PROJECT TEAM SUGGESTIONS

Peer reviews should be conducted with operators, quality staff, and subject matter experts to ensure that all facets of operation have been addressed programmatically and operationally. Code reviews are related to local and national codes, in addition to mandatory regulatory agency requirements. Quality checklists should be developed to facilitate all facility design, quality assurance, and validation and EHS requirements.

Sessions covering lessons learned should be scheduled at the conclusion of all projects to ascertain the successes as well as problems encountered when completing projects. Specific references to agency checklists, violations, and recommended practice sources should always be assembled during the programmatic phase of each project. Third-party reviews are always beneficial in developing differing philosophies and ideas from other projects, clients, and industry experts. Sit-down reviews with an agency are prudent and should be scheduled as early as possible, once the scope has been defined.

COMPARISONS TO OTHER TECHNOLOGIES

The comparisons and contrasts to OSD manufacturing relate primarily to the differences in drug delivery technologies. Solid dosage drugs are delivered through absorption into the body's system of organs or absorptive surfaces, such as the tongue. Compliance concerns relate to cross-contamination. Manufacturing concerns revolve around particulate control, through containment and cleaning procedures. Solid dosage drugs are among the simplest to manufacture and deliver and provide consistent quality.

Sterile aseptic or sterile liquid drugs are delivered parenterally via direct injection through the skin, directly into the bloodstream, through transfer or direct contact with absorptive surfaces, such as the eye. These drugs can be delivered in either single or metered-dose delivery systems. Compliance concerns are highly stringent, in terms of personnel garb, air filtration, positive pressurization, microbial control, and air changes, tied to regulatory "grade" definitions. Manufacturing concerns include airlock separation of cascading grade areas, cleaning procedures, and stringent monitoring of all environmental and product specifications.

Transdermal and surface-applied drugs are delivered on adhesive patches or topically through the skin in either short- or long-term delivery methods. Compliance concerns relate to the technology that permits consistent delivery of the active drug product from the patch into the dermatologic membrane or the rate of absorption with topical application. Manufacturing concerns primarily relate to the uniform method of drug application. Manufacturing issues can relate to the high quantity of solvents required to compound the active drug products that may create safety issues for the facility or personnel involved with the manufacture.

FURTHER DISCUSSION

1. What are the similarities and differences between single-product and multiproduct facilities?
2. Describe what goes on in an excipient dispensing room. How does this differ from an API dispensing room?
3. Describe what goes on in a dry granulation room. How does this differ from a wet granulation room?
4. Describe what goes on in a blending room.
5. Describe what goes on in a capsule filling and weight check room.
6. How are gowning requirements determined?

ABOUT THE AUTHORS

Edward J. Tannebaum has more than 45 years of experience as an architect, construction manager, and corporate facilities lead, primarily focused on the pharmaceutical industry. As the head of facility design and construction for Johnson & Johnson, McNeil Consumer Healthcare Division, he was responsible for the planning and execution of facilities, both domestically and abroad. His comprehension of the OSD business from the owner's, designer's, and constructor's perspectives has provided him with a unique perspective into operational issues that are critical to address in these projects. His knowledge of domestic and international statutes and trends has become a larger and larger focus in recent years of consulting. As a senior principal of Integrated Project Services (IPS) for many years, he led design and build efforts and many conceptual design activities related to OSD and novel drug delivery facilities. For many years, he was a frequent speaker at International Society for Pharmaceutical Engineering educational programs related to design and project facilitation. His role as a principal of Strategic Planning Initiatives, LLC, provides him with a platform of expertise to continue assisting pharmaceutical management with strategic master planning to coincide with their business needs. Tannebaum was the author of the OSD chapter for the first edition of *Good Design Practices* and has provided input to bring the publication to its current level of information.

Samuel Halaby is a recognized subject matter expert in OSD processing and potent compound handling. He has more than 20 years of experience in the design and qualification of pharmaceutical and biotechnology facilities, ranging from clinical to full-scale production plants. Halaby's experience is international, and he has filled the role of project manager and process lead on major capital projects through to construction. Halaby is heavily involved in evaluating and establishing the design basis of many of the new state-of-the-art OSD manufacturing facilities located in the United States, Europe, India, China, and South America. In addition, Halaby has presented and lectured on various technology subjects, including continuous processing, containment of highly potent compounds, trends in regulatory requirements, and aseptic design strategies.

10 Continuous Oral Solid Dose Processing

Michael Rooney

CONTENTS

INTRODUCTION

Oral dose delivery of active pharmaceutical ingredients (APIs) is the oldest, simplest, and most common means for delivering a drug into the human body. An oral solid dose (OSD) product is defined as any solid pharmaceutical product ingested by mouth to be absorbed in the gastrointestinal (GI) tract. With the advent of modern clinical methods and achievements in scientific research and development (R&D), the delivery method of OSD products has become as critical as the API itself. How to deliver the APIs to specific target zones without losing their efficacy is at the heart of the OSD industry.

The first oral delivery systems were simple mixtures of ingredients that were compressed into a pill for ease of swallowing. This process, which involves mixing ingredients and then milling the mixture to reduce all particles to a consistent size, is called direct compression; the milling operation is continuous, whereby material is fed to a mill and processed particles are collected from the discharge of the equipment. While direct compression is the simplest and most cost-effective process, it has performance limitations. Dry granulation was developed to increase the amount of API per dose, known as drug loading, and to aid in manufacturing. Dry granulation increases the density of the mixture with a roller compactor, which, like a mill, is a continuous process.

Dry granulation was an improvement, but to meet product performance demands, wet granulation was developed. Wet granulation requires multiple steps. These three processes have been used for years to make most OSD products consumed worldwide (Figure 10.1).

Despite the various options available to a modern product formulator, OSD facilities predominantly use batch processing. Even though both direct compression and dry granulation are based on continuous processing, the facility layouts are based on batch manufacturing. Facility layouts and process flows are impacted by the individual process steps, quality testing, and indirect requirements, such as market demand. The critical product attributes associated with OSD products are particle size, concentration, and moisture content, all of which impact product efficacy, dissolution, GI track targeting, and onset of action. The OSD facilities also include many stopping points in the process where the quality of the product is evaluated. Downstream operations are dependent on the testing results of intermediate steps, and subsequent additions might require adjustments based on data from previous steps in the process.

Recently, continuous processing, using direct compression, dry granulation, and wet granulation, has been suggested for OSD manufacturing; thus, the individual processing steps would occur without incremental steps. Quality testing would still occur, but with data resulting in real-time control of the critical process attributes. This chapter explores continuous processing and its impact on quality, facilities, operations, equipment, and the future of the OSD business [1]. It addresses the developments in the industry that are responsible for the change. This chapter justifies the use of continuous granulation, identifies the risks, and provides the development necessary to support these changes. After reading this chapter, readers should have a good understanding of the benefits of continuous processing.

EXECUTIVE SUMMARY

Continuous processing, a cost-effective method for manufacturing certain pharmaceutical products, feeds raw materials into an integrated system and a finished dosage comes out, with no stops at the end of each step. Critical quality parameters are measured in-line, and process attributes are adjusted automatically by the control system to keep the process within specifications. Batch processing is typically scheduled to correspond to operating shifts, while continuous processing typically operates 24 h a day.

Continuous processing is not new. The food industry has been using vertical, gravity-fed processing trains for years. In a typical commercial food facility that handles dry powders for products, such as Jell-O (R) and cake mixes, the process starts many stories up in the facility and

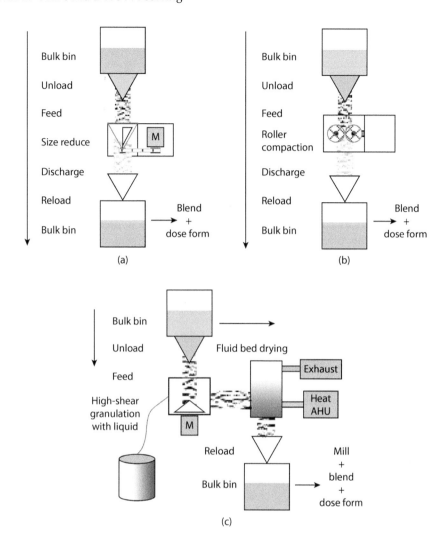

FIGURE 10.1 (a) Direct compression, (b) dry granulation, and (c) wet granulation.

ends on the ground floor in the high-speed packaging line. There are no queuing steps or holding for testing. The food industry perfected vertical continuous granulation years ago to reduce operating costs. The challenges and design considerations associated with any continuous process are the same.

- Critical quality attributes must be monitored in-line, and correction algorithms to adjust the process automatically must be developed and validated in real time.
- Product demand must be high to justify such costly technology. Not all pharmaceutical products have the market pull to justify the complexity and cost of a continuous granulation process.
- When a problem appears in the continuous process flow, it must be determined how much of the process has to be quarantined and how to get the process back into steady state.
- Development data must support an understanding of continuous processing in real time.
- Capital costs for continuous processing equipment are high.
- Vertical integration of any continuous solid processing is recommended, so the facility arrangement must be able to accommodate the height to maximize the benefits.

- Regulatory requirements defined by the Food and Drug Administration (FDA) are very strict regarding the approval of drugs and manufacturing facilities to ensure the safety of the patient. A thorough understanding of regulations, validation, and quality systems is necessary to develop any compliant manufacturing operation.

The pharmaceutical industry was reluctant to implement continuous processing because of the lack of adequate process automation tools. Process automation technology (PAT) is the ability to measure critical process attributes in-line and then control the parameters that affect these attributes in real time. The standards to meet FDA regulations for a pharmaceutical manufacturing operation are significantly higher than those of a food production line; for example, the FDA requires that the amount of an API per dose must be within 10%. The dissolution of the finished product in the GI tract has to be repeatable. These are specific requirements that guarantee that our drug industry is safe and provides a consistent product. In cake mix processing, for example, if there is 15% more of one ingredient than necessary, the result may not be satisfactory to the customer, but the consumer's health is not compromised. The pharmaceutical industry has traditionally manufactured with a batch format with quality checks and quarantine steps between each process step to ensure quality and minimize losses. Wet granulation further necessitated the practice of batch processing (Figure 10.2).

PAT is the most significant technological advancement in the evolution of continuous granulation. Continuous processing can reduce labor costs, necessary facility space, quality assurance (QA) testing, purified water use, waste, and yield loss, all while providing tremendous scaling capabilities. Continuous granulation requires a high initial capital cost for equipment, but less capital for facilities. Depreciation of equipment and facilities is typically 15 and 25 years, respectively, so the offset of capital between equipment and facility is not equal.

The amount of historical and developmental data required to use PAT for control of a commercial process cannot be underestimated. If a commercial process is monitored in real time, the controller needs a validated developmental database to evaluate the performance. Without a real-time baseline, the PAT monitoring system cannot effectively control the commercial process. This presents a significant challenge if the application for continuous granulation and in-line PAT is for an existing commercial batch process. New benchmark data are required to retrofit the process, which would require a significant investment.

Continuous granulation is best applied to pharmaceutical products that meet the following three criteria: (1) Product demand should be large enough to justify the extra capital expense. (2) Developmental data should be available due to scale-up and clinical development. (3) A facility must allow for vertical integration to maximize the integration of the continuous processing equipment.

Table 10.1 compares a 25 kg/h continuous granulation train with a traditional batch process. Assuming the continuous process operates 24 h a day, the basis of this analysis is 600 kg/batch.

These data show a significant reduction in operating costs for continuous processing, but the numbers are also based on a product demand of 1 billion tablets a year for each process train, which requires an appropriate business plan to support the investment.

Continuous granulation can have an impact on more than just manufacturing commercial products. Continuous granulation is based on a feed rate and time. When developing a new pharmaceutical product, one must scale the process up to prove the process is viable and repeatable and supply product to various clinical trials. As the product development progresses, the volume and equipment for a new product progress with it. In the case of a batch process, the product development sequence must find bigger and bigger batch equipment until the product is approved and then commercialized. During this development phase, the scientists conduct countless experiments to optimize product performance. With a continuous process, the design of experiments (DOE) is simpler and less costly in labor and API materials because the only parameter to change during development is time. The equipment is the same for development as it is for commercial use. This approach can reduce the need for new expensive APIs and labor to run many experiments on equivalent

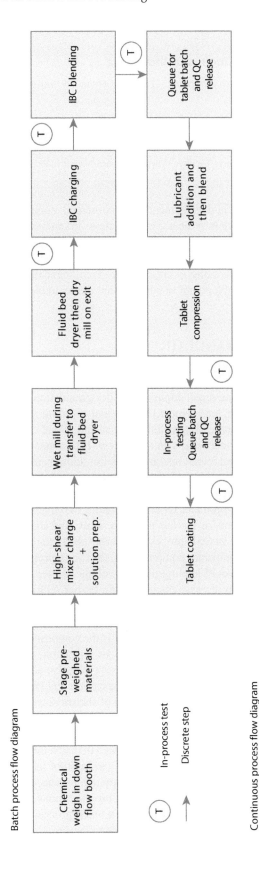

FIGURE 10.2 Process flow diagrams. IBC, intermediate bulk container; PAT, process automation technology; QC, quality control.

TABLE 10.1

Batch Processing versus Continuous Processing

	Batch Processing	Continuous Processing
Equipment cost	$8.5 million	$13.5 million
Facility area	8,320 ft^2	4,000 ft^2
Facility cost	$2.5 million	$1.2 million
Utility consumption	$47,753/year	$27,698/year
Staffing estimates	77 man-hours/1 million tablets	37 man-hours/1 million tablets

batch equipment trains. The money saved in development and commercial manufacturing of a product forms a very compelling reason to dive into the use of continuous granulation technology [2].

Continuous granulation is not the answer for all products, but given certain criteria, it can result in significant efficiencies and improve business performance. The assumption that all products can be processed in batch or continuous processing is not realistic. Significant testing is required to develop and validate products during development to confirm that the technology is capable, controllable, and repeatable.

OVERVIEW OF CONTINUOUS GRANULATION

Batch Processing

Most OSD products are manufactured using direct compression, dry granulation, or wet granulation. Most of the unit operations are the same; for example, milling and blending are used in all three operations. Each unit operation in batch processing includes unload and reload steps, which result in yield and time losses that are additive throughout the entire process. If the product is hazardous and requires containment, then each unload and reload operation requires additional containment equipment, which reduces yield and adds operating costs, which significantly increases capital costs.

The objective of OSD processing is to create a specific mix of APIs and excipients that can be compressed or encapsulated in a way that produces repeatable results. Mixing technology is a challenge when working with many ingredients of various particles, sizes, and shapes. Particle sizing with milling equipment is a common step in OSD processing that results in particles of similar size and shape for a consistent blend. Roller compactor equipment is used to compress a powder mixture, influencing its density and increasing the API loading per unit volume. A wet granulation process adds moisture to bind particles together to increase the density for higher API loading. These various steps are used uniquely or in combination to obtain a repeatable product.

Due to the yield losses associated with the many steps of a batch process, maintaining the correct formulation throughout the process requires testing at each step. If the composition of an in-process batch is not monitored, the consistency of the mixture may not be repeatable as required by FDA regulations. Since the formulation of most OSD products requires progressive additions of materials during the process, quality checks are required after each unit operation and before the addition of materials. For example, a formulation might require the addition of sucrose late in the process in an amount based on the percentage of the total weight, which is critical to the performance of the product. If the yield loss varies between 10% and 20%, then the additional weight is based on the actual yield of each batch; thus, the batch is weighed and the added amount adjusted to match the critical percentage.

To ensure the consistency and quality of a product, the yield and mixture integrity is checked at each step in a batch process. Each quality test point includes sampling, testing, and release by quality control (QC). Thus, in addition to the unloading and reloading operations for each step, there is sampling and testing, which requires time between steps of a batch process. The results of the testing might determine a pass–fail result or weight adjustments for downstream material additions.

Technologies and Improvements

In-process testing performed during a batch operation has traditionally been completed in a lab, either within the production area or in a separate lab building. A critical element of continuous processing is in-line and real-time data collection and analysis. The three most important process parameters are particle size, blend composition, and moisture content, with each parameter monitored, using size analyzers, near-infrared, and loss in drying, respectively. The instruments associated with measuring these parameters have significantly improved over the years to be capable of in-line testing in real time. These instruments are the basis of the OSD PAT program.

The next challenge is to impact the process with a conclusion from the data. Historically, operators made adjustments to the process based on test results. Over the past 10 years, there have been significant improvements in the analytical instrument and data collection industry that allow the equipment to adjust itself instead of requiring human intervention. Changes in the instruments have given them the ability to (1) measure the key process parameters in-line without disrupting the process, (2) evaluate the data against a standard that confirms that the present state is within a validated range, and (3) modify the inputs into the system before the actual values exceed alarm limits, known as correction algorithms.

The use of continuous processing was very limited until these three issues were resolved, which allowed the various process steps to be integrated into a continuous process equipment system. Equipment suppliers began to convert batch equipment to continuous equipment. The direct compression and dry granulation processing were already based on continuous processing: milling and roller compaction. Additionally, the dosage operations, such as tablet compression and encapsulation, were based on continuous processing.

The first step toward this development was the improvement in raw material feeders and in-line blending systems. Product raw material formulations do not come in equal parts; some of the excipients might have a 10:1 ratio between the largest and smallest raw material components. However, the feeding and mixing of each component must be consistent despite the various component ratios. Significant improvements have been made to allow accurate feeding of large variations in formulation. When engineers consider using continuous processing, they must know the formulation requirements and the limitations of each feed station so that the formulation matches the feeder capability and accuracy. The engineer must also consider potential conditioning steps that some material might require before the feeding process, such as sieving, screening, and de-lumping.

Improvements have also been made to the granulation and drying equipment systems used for wet granulation processing. New proprietary screw-type granulators can now complete the work of a high-shear granulator. These in-line continuous granulators can compress the powder, add moisture, and thoroughly mix multiple ingredients to specific process requirements, completing multiple steps of the process that previously required additional equipment. The discharge of this unit operation can now use PAT to check moisture and composition as the material leaves the twin-screw granulators. The signal is compared to the standard, and then the system makes adjustments to the feeders of raw material automatically (Figure 10.3).

The last step in the restructuring of a batch of a wet granulation process is the conversion of the typical batch drying fluid bed to a continuous product dryer. Suppliers have come up with two basic methods as of the writing of this chapter; cyclical segmented fixed volume and linear continuous flow fluid bed drying technique.

- The rotary segmentation design converts a traditional batch-type, fluid-bed bowl and expansion chamber volume into small pie-shaped segments. Repeated processing of small segments of a typical fluid bed simulates continuous manufacturing.
- The high-shear granulator feeder can feed all segments of the fluid bed, one segment at a time.
- A rotating diverter system is used to divert the flow of material from the high-shear mixer to the various segments.

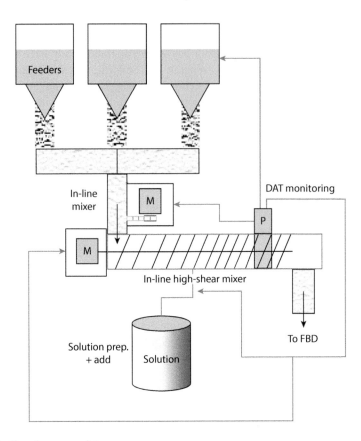

FIGURE 10.3 In-line shear granulator.

- The high-shear mixer and the fluid bed are stationary. The diverter between the two coordinates the flow to each segment.
- The discharge of all segments of the fluid bed is collected in the same position for transfer liner continuous fluid bed to the next processing step (Figure 10.4).
- The design is based on a linear fluid bed instead of a round bed. The narrow and long bed transports the material through the linear fluid bed with a stainless steel screw conveyor located in a linear fluid-bed dryer system.
- The high-shear granulator deposits the moist intermediate product into the linear fluid-bed dryer continuously.
- The screw feed transports the particles across the entire bed as the product is dried in transit (Figure 10.5).

These new processing concepts represent the critical changes and equipment developments necessary to allow the development of a continuous processing system capable of processing direct compression, dry granulation, and wet granulation, all on the same processing equipment platform.

CONTINUOUS GRANULATION

The ideal arrangement for a continuous OSD processing system is to supply all powdered raw materials to the top of the system and discharge the product at the lower production level. The raw materials can be charged directly into the feed systems or can be pneumatically transferred to surge

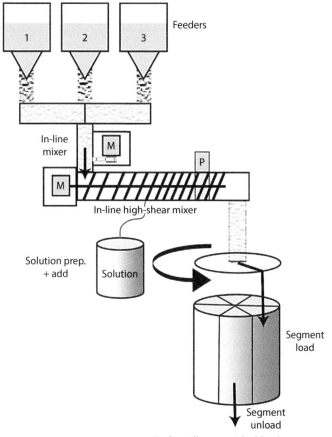

FIGURE 10.4 Segmented fluid-bed dryer concept.

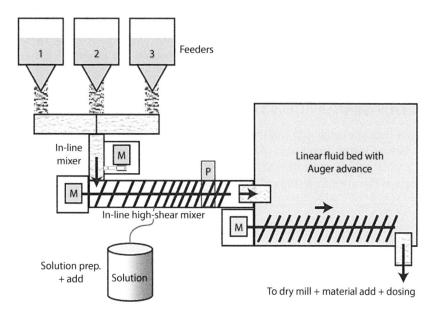

FIGURE 10.5 Linear fluid-bed dryer concept.

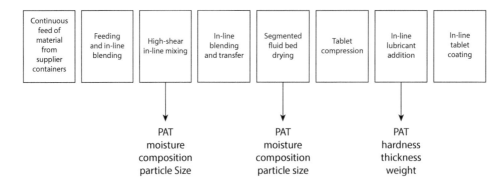

FIGURE 10.6 Continuous process flow diagram.

hoppers on top of the equipment train. The feed systems feed each of the materials into the collection hopper in their correct proportions. The control of this feed is based on PAT measurement and correction algorithms.

- If the product is based on direct compression, the raw material dispensing systems feed an in-line blender and mill configuration and then transfer directly to the tablet press.
- Dry granulation requires an in-line roller compactor, which then feeds an in-line mill, after which more material is added and blended on the way to the tablet press.
- Wet granulation requires an in-line high-shear mixer that compresses the mixed powder and adds water. The discharge of the mixer feeds segments of a fluid-bed dryer for product drying. After drying, the product is milled in-line, mixed with more raw materials, and then sent to the tablet press.
- After tablet compression, the tablets are de-dusted and then sent to an in-line continuous coater, after which the finished product exits the process train and is ready for packaging. The granulation can also be filled into gelatin capsules in an encapsulator instead of compressing into a tablet.

The PAT sensors are located strategically in the flow of material to measure moisture and blend uniformity, including API concentration. The PAT data are compared to historical data, and the upstream parameters are adjusted to keep the critical attributes within acceptable specifications (Figure 10.6).

CONTINUOUS GRANULATION VERSUS BATCH PROCESSING

A comparison between batch and continuous OSD processing must include the consideration of equipment, facility layout, operation, utility use, staffing, and capital costs. The advantages of a continuous process will become obvious as the various aspects of the design are examined. This section compares the manufacturing of 600 kg of a granule product by a batch and a continuous process.

Equipment Requirements

The assumptions associated with both batch and continuous processing include the following: Each day a batch of 600 kg is processed. The bulk density of the granulation product compressed or encapsulated is 0.6 kg/L. The final tablet dose is 150 mg, and the final number of tablets per batch is 4 million each calendar day. A wet granulation process is used as the basis for comparison.

The finished product will be coated tablets. There will be a 50% API–excipient blend plus 50% sucrose added before tableting. The rotational speed for tableting, using a double-sided press, is 60 rpm (750,000 tablets/h). None of the products are hazardous.

The batch process train runs two batches per day of 300 kg each.

- Raw materials are weighed per batch in a downflow booth and then staged in an assembly area until use.
- Raw material processing steps, such as sieving and de-lumping, occur next.
- Batch high-shear granulator (batch weight/bulk density/% full = working volume): 300 kg ÷ 0.5 kg/L ÷ 0.6% full = 1,000 L mixer.
- Fluid-bed dryer: 1,200 L bowl.
- In-line sizing mill.
- Intermediate bulk container (IBC): 2,000 L bin.
- Blender: IBC.
- Storage and QC testing.
- Material addition: 50% sucrose.
- Blender: IBCs.
- Storage and QC testing.
- Lubricant addition.
- Blender: IBCs.
- Tablet press with wash-in-place (WIP) system takes 6 h.
- Tablet transfer: IBC for tablet cores.
- Tablet coating with WIP system.
- Finished product transfer container.
- Support equipment.
- WIP system for high-shear granulation, fluid-bed processing equipment, and co-mill.
- IBC washer for granulation and tablet core bins.
- The total capital estimate for all equipment systems is $8.5 million, including 6% for engineering support, 5% for shipping, 25% for an installation allowance, and an 8% qualification cost.

The continuous process equipment train runs at 600 kg/day.

- Dumping stations for drums and super sacks direct raw materials to feeding stations. Depending on the API loading or potential hazard of the API, a small isolator is used to fill small quantities into disposable feed bags; multiple feed stations are used, as there is one per ingredient.
- Continuous high-shear granulator.
- Continuous fluid-bed dryer.
- In-line sizing mill.
- Additional feeders for second adds.
- In-line mixer.
- Tablet compression system.
- Continuous tablet coater.
- Finished product transfer container.
- Support equipment: WIP system for high-shear granulator, fluid-bed dryer, and sizing mill.
- The total capital estimate for all equipment systems is $13.5 million, including 6% for engineering support, 5% for shipping, 25% for an installation allowance, and an 8% qualification cost.

FACILITY REQUIREMENTS

The equipment requirement list illustrates the simplicity of a continuous process train. The reduction in process steps, equipment, and associated space results in a more efficient operation. In the case of batch operations, storage, testing, and release can be complicated by testing logistics and data analysis. Facility layouts typically include extra floor space to accommodate unexpected testing results during storage and testing. Typically, the bins on-test are stored in the same area as clean and ready bins with an additional 50% space for the unexpected. Thus, the required storage space is much greater with a batch process than with a continuous process. There are also safety considerations due to movement of IBCs and equipment that do not exist with a continuous process.

Both batch and continuous processing can be designed on one level if necessary, but integrating either process into a vertical orientation maximizes the advantages when handling powders. With batch processing that uses an upper floor for unloading and the lower floor for processing the intermediate material and reload, the processed material must travel from the lower floor to the upper floor after each step in the batch process. This takes both time and labor. Because of the nature of batch processing and in-process transfers in IBCs, empty IBC bins end up on the upper floor. It is advantageous to place the IBC washing system on the upper floor adjacent to the unload stations to minimize the travel of dirty bins.

By comparison, the continuous process uses vertical integration and gravity flow to contain the transfer of intermediate product within the process equipment. The infeed to the process is continuous, and all of the raw materials are charged from their commercial containers, such as 200 L drums or large super sacks. Once these containers are emptied, they are removed as waste. The continuous process has no intermediate product or stopping points, so there are no IBCs or holding containers. The output of the continuous process is coated tablets that are ready for packaging so the containers used for transport are also disposable. Gravity and vertical integration are ideal for both batch and continuous processing, but the inherent discontinuity of the batch process, the in-process storage requirements, and the reusable IBCs add space, labor, and complexity, which do not exist within the continuous process.

The impact of continuous processing on water use is quite substantial. Washing and cleaning each of the process units is essentially the same with batch and continuous processing. However, the containers entering and exiting the continuous process are single-use or disposable (SUD) systems and do not require cleaning. The batch process includes many IBCs, which must be cleaned using process water. The process water savings are significant with continuous processing when you consider the amount of water needed to wash and clean the IBCs in batch processing.

Batch Processing and Continuous Processing Facility Layouts

The layouts in Figures 10.7 through 10.10 are schematic for the purposes of providing a relative size and functional comparison between a two-story batch process and a two-story continuous process.

FACILITY LAYOUTS

OPERATING REQUIREMENTS

Continuous processing eliminates many of the steps and intermediate handling of product, which has a direct impact on staffing and labor costs. A smaller staff can manage many process steps simultaneously. Tables 10.2 and 10.3 give a rough estimate of labor required for the two process types. Each application has a unique perspective regarding staffing and operating cost. Processing, testing, and transfer times are all affected by the specific product being manufactured, the local labor structure, and the constraints of the facility layout.

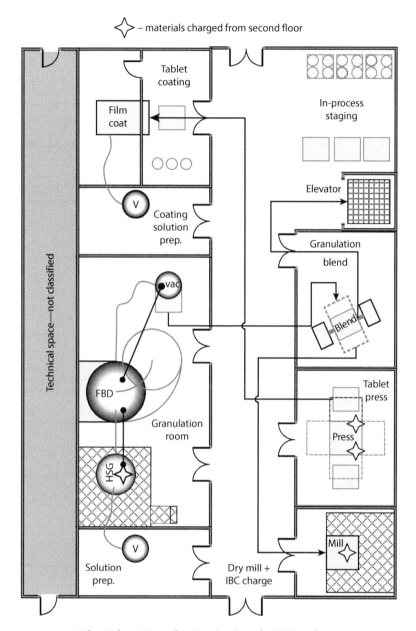

$\diamondsuit$ – materials charged from second floor

FIGURE 10.7 Wet granulation: batch processing first floor.

Equipment, facility, and operating differences are significant between batch processing and continuous processing. The capital requirement to commit to continuous processing is quite large due to the complexity of the equipment, PAT, and associated control systems. Batch processing does not require a lot of communication between steps, in-line analysis, or large control systems. Each unit operation essentially operates as an island of automation. Continuous granulation is essentially one machine that takes raw material in, monitors its performance, and self-adjusts to meet specifications (Table 10.4).

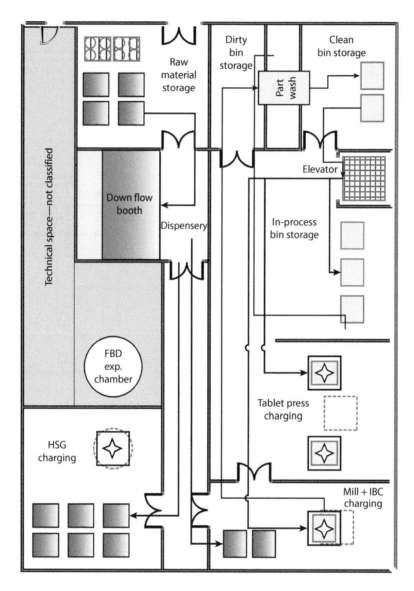

4000 sq. ft/ceiling height 10 ft/CNC classification

FIGURE 10.8 Wet granulation: batch processing second floor.

Constraints

Based on the comparisons above, why would one not use continuous granulation for all processing needs? The following constraints should be considered for the potential application of continuous processing of OSD products.

Product Volume

In this chapter, a continuous granulator size of 25 kg/h was used. This rate can produce 1 billion tablets a year, based on a tablet weight of 150 mg. The rate of 25 kg/h is just one example, as there are systems that can produce more per hour. The first question to ask when considering use of a continuous process is whether 1 billion or more tablets a year is necessary; thus, it is important to note

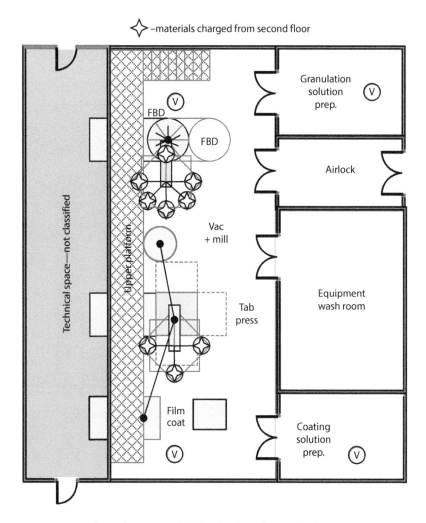

FIGURE 10.9 Wet granulation: continuous processing first floor.

the following: (1) One billion tablets can be distributed across multiple products. (2) The continuous granulator can allow all three process types to be used on one equipment platform. This lowers the volume requirement across multiple products and processes. (3) Repeat manufacturing of the same product, or campaigns, and an excessive number of products on one platform are not ideal due to downtime between each campaign. Processing multiple products on one system has limits.

Product Development Data

When PAT is applied to granulation, data is available in real time. Once the data is understood, an algorithm has to be built to adjust the critical parameters and ignore the noncritical anomalies. This accumulation and analysis of data and knowledge takes time. This is why applying PAT and continuous granulation while developing and scaling the product is the only practical way to implement the technology. If you applied continuous granulation and PAT to an existing commercial product, how would you establish robust algorithms?

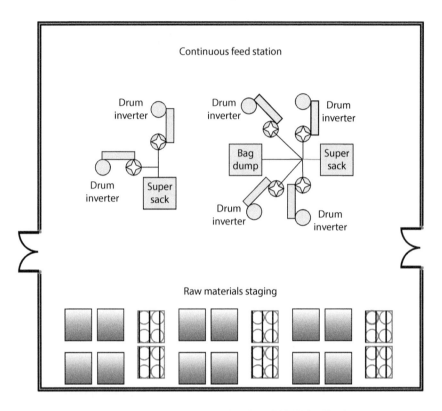

50 ft × 45 ft = 2250 sq. ft/ceiling height 12 ft/CNC classification

FIGURE 10.10   Wet granulation: continuous processing second floor.

TABLE 10.2

Labor Requirements for Batch and Continuous Processing

	Batch Processing	Continuous Processing
Total production area	8,050 ft^2	4,000 ft^2
Support QA testing area	100 ft^2	100 ft^2
Total HVAC air	24,220 cfm	13,513 cfm
Chiller size	75 tons	42 tons
Plant steam size	21 BTU	10 BTU
Annual energy cost	$47,753/year	$2,769/year
Total facility cost ($400/ft^2 without equipment)	$3.2 million	$1.6 million

Note: QA, quality assurance; HVAC, heating, ventilation, and air conditioning; cfm, cubic feet per minute; BTU, British thermal unit, measures heat energy.

Process Recovery

Continuous processing in steady state produces a good product, but problems can develop with the equipment, or there may be an equipment failure. Clearing a mishap on a continuous processor is like loading bad product into current Good Manufacturing Practice (cGMP) equipment. The intermediate material does not meet specifications because of the failure, but clearing the material might

TABLE 10.3
Labor Analysis for Batch and Continuous Processing

	Batch Processing	Continuous Processing
Staffing		
Dispensary	2 man × 2 shift	
Raw material feed		2 man × 3 shift
Granulation and fluid-bed drying	2 man × 3 shift	2 man × 3 shift
Milling, charging, and blending	2 man × 3 shift	
Tableting	2 man × 3 shift	
Tablet coating	2 man × 3 shift	
Material handling	2 man × 3 shift	2 man × 3 shift
Support		1 man × 3 shift
Supervision	1 man × 3 shift	
Total hours per 600 kg	296 h	192 h
Tablets/batch (150 mg/tab)	4 million	4 million
Hours/million tablets	74 h	48 h
Percentage reduction		35%

TABLE 10.4
Summary of the Various Design Aspects of Batch and Continuous Processing

	Batch Processing	Continuous Processing
Equipment requirements	$7.5 million	$11 million
Facility requirements	8,050 ft^2	4,000 sq^2
Facility cost	$3.2 million	$1.6 million
Operating requirements	74 man-hours/1 million tablets	48 man-hours/1 million tablets

require sending the bad material through the entire machine. Validating that all of the bad material is out of the machine is possible for most failure modes, but part of validating the system has to include running each failure scenario, establishing a validated clearing method, and then validating the results.

Definition of a Batch

One challenge associated with using continuous granulation is the definition of a batch. If the system can operate continuously, what constitutes a batch? The FDA recalls are usually based on batch numbers, so defining a batch is important. Batch definition includes tracking the excipient lots that feed the process. The system is fed continuously with containers that are from multiple lot origins or one lot from many batches. Raw material subbatch tracking is not unique to continuous processing; batch processing is required to do the same. The unique aspect of the continuous process is that the operator has to manage it as a continuous stream. A high degree of control is required to manage batch documentation. Strong standard operating procedures (SOPs) and a potentially more automated manufacturing execution system (MES) are required to support management of the constant flow of materials.

Financial Justification

Payback might be a struggle due to the capital requirements of continuous granulation. The business environment is very competitive in the pharmaceutical industry, and a strong payback might be hard to develop, considering all the factors that influence the business case, such as volume, depreciation, and so forth.

DESIGN DETAILS AND COMPLIANCE CONSIDERATIONS

EQUIPMENT AND UTILITY REQUIREMENTS

Integration of a complete continuous granulation process requires coordination among material-handling equipment companies, PAT system suppliers, granulation equipment companies, and dosage processing equipment companies. The present industry offerings for most continuous granulation systems include the granulation equipment and PAT as part of an integrated system. Some of the granulation equipment suppliers may not be able to offer a tablet press or a continuous coater, so they cannot supply a fully integrated system through continuous coating; however, as the demand for these systems grows, the supply of equipment promises to grow as well.

The integration of the PAT system is typically coordinated by the granulation equipment supplier. The PAT data are communicated from the PAT controller to the granulator controller, whereby actions are made to the process based on the PAT data. Integration between the two is critical. The idea of collecting data with PAT while in development and scale-up was discussed earlier; scale-up of the PAT monitoring is critical. The end user could commit to an instrument and supplier for its PAT during development before considering the selection of commercial processing equipment. To minimize technical transfer problems, it is recommended that a user select a PAT system that is common and proven with the process equipment suppliers.

While design and integration of the material handling systems are less complicated, the design of these stations is influenced by the formulation, supplier, and MES procedures. The formulation dictates separate and unique feed stations for each of the material additions. The material containers received must be standardized and cannot change without a full analysis of the impact to the material handling equipment. Some material might only be available in bags, requiring continuous feeding of the bagged material to the systems, typically by a manual operator. Super sacks (i.e., 300 kg or greater) can be used to reduce handling by connecting the super sack directly to the feeders. Some formulations might require very small quantities that have to be weighed in a transfer container to interface with the automatic material feed systems. To further complicate the material handling design, each formulation may have unique requirements, and if an equipment train is to manufacture many products, change between products has to be carefully considered (Figures 10.11 through 10.13).

Cleaning a continuous granulator is typically semiautomatic. The system supplier provides a WIP system for completing a product rinse or wash of the system. An initial wash removes most of the residual powder. After the initial WIP, the operators dismantle the system and complete the cleaning by hand. Use of detergents to clean the system is based on the product formulation. Chemicals are typically avoided, as all traces of the cleaning chemical must be removed, and for this reason, water is the ideal cleaning solution. The WIP system is typically located in a utility space adjacent to the equipment. Utility stations with water drops with heat-mixing devices are included in the design of the room to provide a water source for cleaning during manual cleaning by the operator. Drains are necessary to manage the wash water in the room.

ARCHITECTURAL CONSIDERATIONS

Gravity and vertical integration increase the efficiency of a continuous OSD system. However, in a horizontally oriented system, the equipment can be installed on one floor under a 15 ft ceiling. The product is transferred between each unit operation by pneumatic conveying. The equipment must include the pneumatic transfer systems and the separation filtration, along with the controls. This type of system has to be cleaned and maintained properly. Including a filtration system is challenging when switching between products. A single-level system might be the best solution if the system is being installed in existing cGMP space, but it is not the best arrangement.

Physical arrangements can range from a single-level facility to a completely vertical integration with the tablet coater on the ground floor, tablet presses on the second level, granulators and fluid bed on the third, and material handling on the fourth. This arrangement provides complete vertical

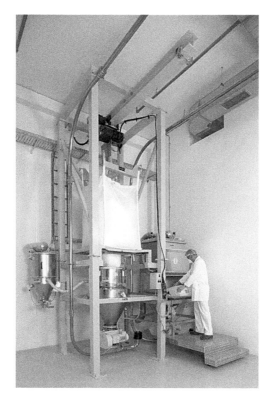

FIGURE 10.11 Super-sack unload station.

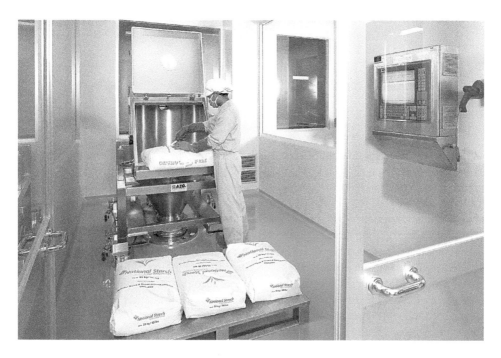

FIGURE 10.12 Drum inverter.

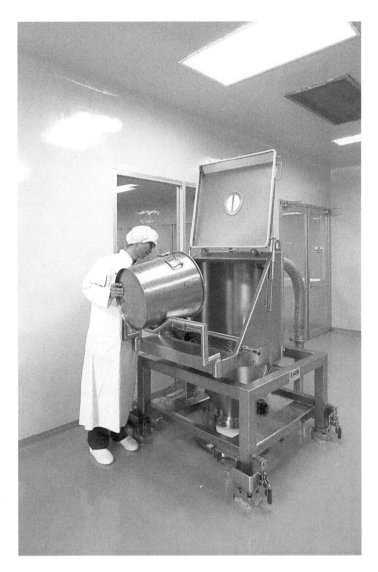

FIGURE 10.13 Bag station.

integration (much like a food facility), but the number of floors is impractical relative to the area per floor. The facility would be 20 ft × 20 ft × 4 stories 20 ft tall, or 80 ft tall. This might be reasonable if the plan is to install half a dozen continuous granulator systems, but not for just one.

A typical arrangement for a continuous processing suite is to use gravity for material changing, but then pneumatic transfer of product from each unit operation on the ground floor. The ground level will have a high ceiling (about 15 ft) to accommodate the pneumatic transfers on top of all the process equipment. The second level is reserved for material movement and feeding the processes below. Remember that the process accepts a constant flow of material in the SUD containers supplied by the material supplier. There is no weighing or reconfiguration of the material before entry into the process. Having a direct adjacency between the feed level and the warehouse is ideal for efficient material flow (Figure 10.14).

To leverage gravity, a fully integrated facility includes packaging on the lowest level, granulation on the second level, and material feed systems on the third level. The warehouse can be located adjacent to the three-level stack so that an automated storage and retrieval system can be leveraged

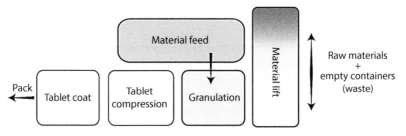

FIGURE 10.14   Vertical and horizontal continuous processing facilities.

for efficient material movements. An automatic crane system in the warehouse can move the materials up to the third level without interaction with personnel. The only intermediate storage step would be between the tablet coating process and the primary container fill operation (Figure 10.15).

HVAC Design Considerations

The space for OSD manufacturing is designed to meet an ISO 8 or grade D environment, but there is no clam of classified space as there is in a sterile manufacturing facility. The European Union, FDA, and World Health Organization currently do not state that OSD products have to be manufactured in classified space unless the safety of the product requires such an environment. The specific needs of a product might dictate a higher level of environmental integrity, but typically OSD manufacturing space is controlled nonclassified (CNC) space. Unlike a batch process, there are no loading and unloading operations within the process, and therefore, there is better containment of the product when manufacturing in a continuous process. The pneumatic transfer designs have to be considered when developing the air-balance design. Some pneumatic transfer systems extract air from the clean room and then expel the air outside of the room envelope demanded by cGMPs.

Pressurization of the cGMP rooms is not unique between batches and continuous processing. The cGMPs say that the pressurization of the rooms should not promote dust migration out of the rooms. There is not a lot of dust associated with the continuous process, but the pressurization of

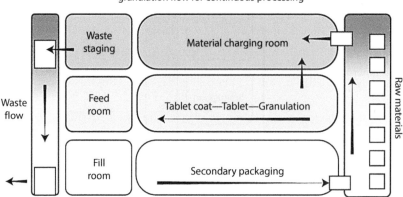

FIGURE 10.15   Fully integrated facility.

adjacent rooms around the main processing room should be positive to the main room. If airlocks are used to enter the main process room, the pressurization should be cascading.

UTILITY REQUIREMENTS

The utility requirements to support a continuous granulator depend on the process being considered. Direct compression and dry granulation processing require only electrical power and compressed air. For wet granulation, the utility requirements are more diverse. The wet granulation process includes a liquid compound addition that produces a granulation that gets removed from the product by heat in a fluid-bed dryer. The mixing process requires USP water for compounding. The drying process uses a dedicated air handler that heats air to dry the product to a specific moisture level. The air handler required to support drying needs plant steam and chilled water. The heat is required to elevate the temperature, and the chilled water is used to remove moisture and control the heat. A tablet coater has requirements similar to those of a wet granulation process; if tablet coating is included, then plant steam and chilled water are required.

Dust collection is required to control the migration of dust. The continuous process is essentially closed, yet dust collection is still necessary. In the case of pneumatic transfers, there is a separation filter in the system, but not all of the air removed from the product is dust-free. Under normal running conditions, a dust collector is required to manage the dust within the equipment and create an appropriate pressure differential to contain the unwanted dust.

PROJECT MANAGEMENT ISSUES

Incorporation of continuous OSD processing requires careful integration into the design of the building and transfers from development to commercial phases. The facility design should focus on the integration of the processing equipment and material handling equipment in a way that provides as much flexibility as possible. Technical transfer of the product from development to commercial, using PAT in a commercial setting, is actually more critical than the physical plant itself. If the development work does not provide comprehensive data of critical parameters, it is very challenging to validate the PAT system, even if the equipment and facility integration are well executed.

If a two-level equipment arrangement is selected, then both the material handling equipment and granulation equipment companies must provide significant detail early in the program to develop a strong facility design. Details regarding the PAT system are also critical, but the timing regarding the development of control algorithms to communicate between the PAT system and the equipment can be delayed until late in the program. The PAT instrument integration does not affect the facility design in a significant way during the early conceptual phase of the design.

Because of the nature of the equipment and integration challenges, the following project management issues should be considered at the beginning of the project:

- It is essential to establish a strong process design basis. Continuous OSD processing is not necessarily a flexible process. For example, if the number of ingredients is not defined well at the beginning of the project, then adding another product to the project that has $n + 1$ ingredients will likely not be easy. Some materials include in-line sieving or de-lumping before additions, and adding this to an established design would be difficult. Material weights, accuracy, and supplier configurations all affect the material handling systems.
- Containment requirements need to be well defined. The addition of a hazardous or low-dose API will also have an effect on the design. Depending on the hazard level, the system might require a support isolator or high-containment transfer bags. It is most efficient to establish the containment requirements in the beginning of the design because adding the requirement after the design is complete will have an impact on the cost and schedule of the project.
- Once the process is defined, a cGMP risk assessment should be conducted to identify the critical process parameters, to develop a plan to mitigate and monitor them, and then to validate each critical parameter. The most important aspect of this effort is to correlate the critical process data and the data generated in the development stages so that the appropriate PAT systems can be selected [3]. This approach is critical for the technical transfer of the project from the development or clinical stage to commercial approval.
- Continuity in data is important for a successful technology transfer. While it is possible to use one specific brand of instrument for process data collection during development or clinical work and then select another instrument brand for the commercial system, it may result in more validation work. Validated data from two independent instruments should be interpreted similarly, but changing PAT platforms between the data development and commercial integration should be done after considerable analysis. An equivalency test should be completed before commitment to the commercial system.
- As of the end of 2014, there are a number of continuous granulation suppliers on the market, and the numbers are likely to grow. The process equipment supplier selection should be completed before the beginning of conceptual design. This is not typically required for a batch-based process because the equipment systems used for batch processing are well established and have not changed significantly in more than 20 years. Continuous granulation equipment is new technology. As this technology grows in popularity, all systems might migrate to the same arrangement, and then it will be possible to wait to select the supply at the end of the basis of design (BOD) phase, also known as preliminary engineering. Until the equipment evolves to that point, selection of the continuous granulators should occur before the beginning of the conceptual design.
- Most equipment suppliers can supply the facility design team with three-dimensional models that represent their equipment. Because of the vertical integration challenges, it is advisable to require three-dimensional models of the selected systems at the beginning of the preliminary engineering phase, or BOD phase. Both the process equipment and material handling suppliers should provide models at the end of the conceptual design phase in preparation of design development during preliminary engineering.
- Due to the integration of multiple equipment systems, such as the PAT system and related control systems, material handling systems, and support equipment, establishing boundary limits and scope is important. Most suppliers of equipment install all interconnecting wires between their various pieces, but the boundaries of responsibility must be delineated.

A user requirement specification (URS) is developed as the basis for validation of the system and development of equipment specifications. The URS in this case describes the granulation equipment, dosing equipment, coating equipment, material handling equipment, PAT instrument, and most importantly, the control system that monitors and actively controls the process. The URS should be issued with development data included and an instrument reference for the PAT instrument used in the development and clinical manufacturing states. The risk assessment should be included to define the critical parameters associated with the system. Because the system is continuous, the URS will be quite complicated with many systems included within the document. The boundaries of the URS might not correspond with the supplier boundaries and need to be evaluated early in the program.

THINGS TO CONSIDER

SCALING OF CONTINUOUS PROCESSING

Continuous processing is based on a set process, producing material at a consistent rate. Capacity is only defined by the duration of a run. Assuming raw materials can supply the continuous process without any interruption, the capacity of the system is limited only by time. Traditionally, the industry has used incremental batch sizes to scale up and commercialize products. For example, a phase 2 clinical batch might be based on a 40 kg batch, but the commercial version might be based on a 400 kg batch. Significant investment will be required to prove that the process and product quality of the 40 kg batch is the same as that of the 400 kg batch.

As an alternative, a continuous process operates at the same rate, such as 25 kg/h. If 40 kg/h is required, then the equipment will operate for 1.6 h. Commercial quantities are obtained with the same process and same equipment, but a run time of 16 h. In this case, there is no scale-up, just an increase in production time, and the effort required to show equivalence is significantly reduced.

COST SAVINGS DURING THE DEVELOPMENT STAGE

During the scale-up phase and through manufacturing of clinical materials, the product developers constantly perform testing to further their knowledge of processing the product. For new chemical entities, the supply of the API is usually very small, extremely expensive, and hard to get. If a developer has batch-type equipment for developing experiments, the requirements for the API can rise quickly, and the cost and schedule can become prohibitive. The use of continuous granulation optimizes the use of the API and can reduce changes to the process to complete DOE testing to a fraction of the traditional methods.

The savings in this case can vary dramatically, depending on the cost of the API, but the justification of continuous granulation is much stronger if the development savings in time and API are combined with the manufacturing savings.

DEFINITION OF BATCH SIZE

Since the continuous process can operate for hours and days, there is no natural break to define a batch. Defining a batch is necessary to run a business and comply with regulatory requirements. Each unit of sale requires a lot and expiration date stamped on each sale package. They must be labeled on each unit of sale so that if there is a quality issue, the entire batch can be recalled. If a company makes one batch over a 1-month period, the recall of that batch would involve a tremendous amount of product and would not be good business or good for the patient. A recall of mega-batches could result in temporary product shortages.

Defining a batch based on the calendar is a reasonable method of batch identification. A method or SOPs must be developed to clear the equipment and then restart the equipment to define a batch separation. The ultimate decision about batches will be based on a business analysis, including risk to and impact on the patient.

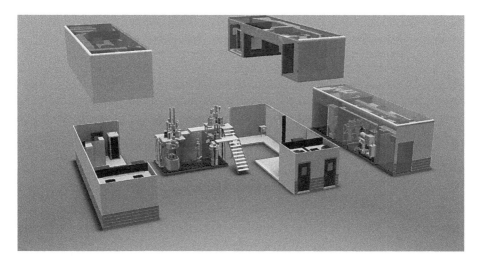

FIGURE 10.16 Pod-based mobile facility containing a continuous process. (Courtesy of G-Con Manufacturing, Inc., College Station, TX, and GEA, Columbia, MD.)

SPECIAL DISCUSSION: PORTABLE GRANULATION SUITE

Previously, the relative size of a continuous OSD process was demonstrated. The footprint of a 25 kg/h process system is quite small, that is, small enough to consider installation into portable cGMP facilities, referred to as pods [4]. These self-contained pods include all the necessary support systems, such as electric systems, fire protection, and HVAC systems. The pods are self-contained and only require connection to utility supply systems to operate within cGMP requirements. These pods can be removed and relocated to another site, reconnected, and started within a matter of weeks. Since the pods can be arranged to contain a fully functional continuous process, the combination of process and portable facility can result in a mobile OSD manufacturing facility (Figure 10.16).

FURTHER DISCUSSION

Readers should be able to answer the following questions based on the information provided in this chapter:

1. What are four considerations or concerns that would prevent manufacturers from applying continuous OSD processing? Consider market volumes, scale-up, and campaign length.
2. Why would manufacturers not integrate a continuous OSD process across many vertical floors?
3. How would an engineer design a system to recover from an equipment error or an "out-of-specification" associated with a continuous OSD process?
4. What products currently on the market would be good candidates for continuous OSD processing?
5. What products would be less than ideal candidates for continuous OSD processing?
6. Can capsules be used as the dosage form associated with continuous OSD? If yes, what limitations might there be?

ABOUT THE AUTHOR

Michael Rooney is the founder of MSR Consulting, LLC. He is presently a subject matter expert for OSD for Jacobs Engineering, Conshohocken, Pennsylvania. His 25-year career includes product development support, clinical equipment scale-up, design and implementation of commercial systems, and integration into cGMP facilities. He has designed commercial facilities in the United States, Europe, China, and South Korea. His specific experience includes nano-OSD products, potent products, wet granulation, dry granulation, dosing technology, and packaging line design. He has worked for both operating companies, such as Elan, Bayer, and McNeil Consumer Products, and architectural design firms that specialize in pharmaceutical manufacturing facility design. Most recently, Rooney was involved in the integration of continuous granulation into a pod facility. He has been the lead process engineer for OSD projects for AbbVie, Bayer, Eisai, Bristol-Myers Squibb, and Novartis.

FURTHER READING

American Society for Testing and Materials, ASTM E2968-14: Application of Continuous Processing in the Pharmaceutical Industry, American Society for Testing and Materials, West Conshohocken, PA.

REFERENCES

1. Rockoff JD, Drug Making Breaks Away from Its Old Ways, *The Wall Street Journal*, February 8, 2015.
2. Palmer E, Vertex, J&J, GSK, Novartis All Working on Continuous Manufacturing Facilities, *FiercePharma Manufacturing*, February 9, 2015.
3. U.S. Food and Drug Administration, Power Blends and Finished Dosage Units—Stratified In-Process Dosage Unit Sampling and Assessment, Guidance for Industry, U.S. Food and Drug Administration, Silver Spring, MD, October 2003.
4. Almhem P, Lemperle R, Sivertsson C, Using Modular Systems in Solid-Dosage Manufacturing, *Pharmaceutical Technology*, Solid Dosage and Excipients Issue, 2014.

George Wiker

CONTENTS

INTRODUCTION

The goal of this chapter is to provide a good design practice guideline for developing a sterile manufacturing facility. It focuses on the final formulation, filling, and finishing (initial packaging) of injectable products. Other products, such as inhalants, medical devices, and cell therapy, may be manufactured similarly to injectables, requiring a high level of integrity and protection. Thus, some of the principles and ideas presented here are applicable to those products. This chapter may help anyone who is developing a sterile manufacturing facility project to realize good design practices. It should be read in tandem with related agency guidelines and other guides, such as the International Society for Pharmaceutical Engineering (ISPE) Baseline Guide series.

Injectable products typically function by targeting specific regions or indications within the body. Such drugs, like vaccines and genetic therapies, are introduced directly into the bloodstream to be most effective and do not pass through the body's natural defense mechanisms when ingested. The impact of a defective sterile manufacturing facility on injectable drug products can be catastrophic, so maintaining a very high level of control of product integrity and mitigation of risk is essential to human safety.

The term *sterile manufacturing facility* is used throughout this chapter as a description of a range of facilities that produce injectable products for humans. Chapters 10 and 18 have information regarding upstream (drug substance) processing and downstream (secondary) packaging of typical sterile manufacturing operations.

EXECUTIVE SUMMARY

By introducing a drug directly into the bloodstream, it reacts faster and with more intensity than other dosage forms. Therefore, the dosage must be free of any by-products or microorganisms that may adversely affect the body [1]. Also, many injectable products have limited stability, making the shelf life and storage conditions critical elements to the product's effectiveness. Manufacturing and storage of these products are subject to regulatory compliance, and thus a high degree of effort is centered on current Good Manufacturing Practices (cGMPs).

The differences between sterile and aseptic processing are discussed, which is critical to understanding how these processing methods affect the design, operation, and testing of injectable products. The reader should be attentive to these processing methods.

Injectable dosage forms, or parenterals, comprise the largest portion of these manufactured products, and typically fall into one of two categories: large-volume parenterals and small-volume parenterals, which are composed of cytotoxic and noncytotoxic drug substance matrices. Other forms of injectable products include inhalants, cell therapy products, diagnostics, and compounded products. The facilities in which these products are processed are discussed in this chapter. The processing technologies have been influenced by developments in the processing of biologics and dairy products, where product sterility is essential. The design, construction, validation, and operation of these facilities have greatly contributed to the success of pharmaceutical sterile manufacturing facilities today.

In Western medicine, the use of injectable products first began in 1796 with Edward Jenner's vaccination for smallpox (Figure 11.1) [2]. The use of injectable products expanded to include delivery of anesthetics, transfusions, and a variety of delicate drug matrices. The processing of these products expanded over the decades, and in 1987, the U.S. Food and Drug Administration (FDA) issued the "Sterile Drug Products Produced by Aseptic Processing" guideline. This guideline was issued under Title 21 of the U.S. Code of Federal Regulations (CFR), Part 10.90, and while it did not set legal requirements for aseptic processing, "it states the principles and practices of general applicability … acceptable to the Food and Drug Administration" [3]. With new and more delicate drug matrix developments comes a surge in the use of injectables as a method of effective drug delivery into the human body. Today, injectable products represent a significant portion of the total prescription drug delivery methods and are regulated by agencies all over the world. "Injectable dose formulation is the fastest growing segment, with a projected growth rate of 12.2% in 2012" [4]. "The global injectable drug delivery market [has] reached a value of around $22.5 billion by the end of 2012 and is forecast to grow to $43.3 billion by 2017. This estimates a compound annual growth rate of 14% between 2012 and 2017" [4].

"The increased focus on cytotoxics (toxic to cells to develop a therapy), lyophilized (freeze-dried) prefilled syringes, and reformulation of existing products is expected to drive the remarkable success of injectables. Lyophilization and manufacturing of sterile products, such as cytotoxics, are likely areas of growth potential, given the demand for oncology and high-potency drugs. Key growth drivers include increased pharmaceutical and biotechnological focus on complex disease areas, trends in disease control, growth in emerging markets, the pharmaceutical patent cliff (i.e., several blockbuster

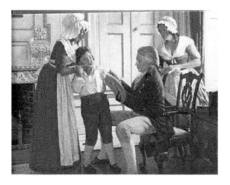

FIGURE 11.1   A child receiving a smallpox vaccination. (Available at http://www.blatner.com/adam/consctransf/historyofmedicine/3-immunology/3-lecture.html.)

drugs losing patent protection), and reformulation of existing products. The major growth is expected to be cytotoxics as both cancer research and the development of new cancer therapies are driving growth in this area" [5].

"The number of injectable drugs to be introduced in [the] long-term is expected to be significant [and] to outweigh the threat from advanced alternative drug delivery technologies. Additionally, increase[d] innovation in alternative technologies has [heightened] the focus of injectable market participants on issues, such [as] injector design, convenience, and painless modes of injectables" [6].

INJECTABLE PRODUCTS

Injectable products come in a variety of primary package forms, including ampules, vials, syringes, bottles, and bags (Figure 11.2). Injectable products, as defined by the characteristics of the drug matrices, are often rendered sterile via a number of qualified methods: suitable membrane filtration (i.e., 0.2 μm pore size or smaller to remove all microorganisms), ionizing radiation, dry or moist heat, and chemical sterilization.

Not every injectable product, due to the nature of the drug matrices, can be rendered sterile through the methods listed above, in which case the product must be processed aseptically. This often applies to vaccines, cell therapy processes, or drug matrices that are damaged or impacted by the above-mentioned sterilization methods.

UNDERSTANDING THE PRINCIPLES OF STERILE AND ASEPTIC

When discussing the processing of injectable products, it is very important to understand the definitions and differences of the terms being used; for example, the terms *sterile* and *aseptic* are often misused. *Aseptic* is an adjective that describes a condition where a substance or item is free of pathogenic microorganisms, as proven by appropriate sterility testing, showing a log reduction (see testing guidelines as defined by the agency with jurisdiction). *Sterile* is an adjective that describes a condition where a substance or item is free of all microorganisms, as proven by appropriate sterility testing (see testing requirements as defined by the agency with jurisdiction).

STERILE MANUFACTURING FACILITIES

In the spectrum of pharmaceutical manufacturing facilities, injectable product manufacturing facilities represent the most sophisticated and challenging to design, build, qualify, and operate,

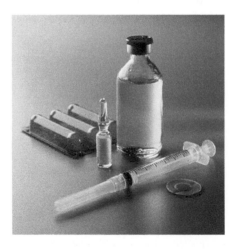

FIGURE 11.2 Packaging for injectable products.

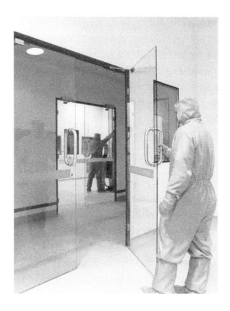

FIGURE 11.3 Controlled room environments.

particularly when products manufactured in these facilities are rendered sterile and ready to inject directly into a human when complete. For this reason, very careful consideration is necessary when developing such a facility. Key measures that make sterile manufacturing facilities unique include highly controlled room environments (equal to Grade A or C Class A/ISO 5), unidirectional flow of materials and personnel, highly sophisticated and controlled sterile or aseptic filling systems, clean-in-place (CIP) and steam-in-place (SIP) systems, complex equipment and components, and intensive utilities and heating, ventilation, and air conditioning (HVAC) systems (Figure 11.3).

Generally, there are two types of processing operations within a sterile manufacturing facility: primary bulk processing of the drug substance, and the formulation, filling, and finishing of the drug product into its final dosage form. Testing of diagnostic kits, medical device assembling, cell therapy processes, and in-process product testing are examples of other types of operations carried out in a highly controlled sterile or aseptic manner.

Major sterile manufacturing operations include component preparation in ultrasonic sinks, autoclaves, and other wash and preparation equipment; compounding and formulation by mixing and blending several product components in either fixed or portable tanks or mixing systems; filling, which ranges from hand-fills under a hood to a fully automated high-speed container filling system; freeze drying (lyophilization) or removing water from a drug product or dose for greater stability and longer shelf life; inspection, ranging from a manual inspection by operators to a fully integrated multifunctional inspection system; and process utilities by direct-impact systems, which support manufacturing, including water-for-injection (WFI) and clean steam generators, as well as the supply of sterile air or gases and other product contact utility supply systems.

PROCESS TECHNOLOGIES

At the core of the sterile manufacturing operation, process technology drives the ability to safely, efficiently, and repeatedly produce sterile products. Early sterile manufacturing facilities centered on aseptic processing (often open processing) in a clean room environment with personnel in the critical work area. This approach created the risk of particulate and bioburden contamination. Thus, as sterile manufacturing technologies and practices developed, the drive to close the process and separate the critical manufacturing environment from personnel became a key driver in the development of the core process technology. Today, the most commonly prescribed approach is to close the manufacturing process and locate it behind a fully contained International Organization for Standardization (ISO) 5 isolator system in an ISO 7 or ISO 8 background clean room environment. In contrast, when the ISO 5 zone is open to the surrounding environment, the background environment is commonly designed to meet ISO 5 or ISO 6, thus increasing the complexity and management of materials and personnel.

DRUG PRODUCT PROCESSING

The principles and approaches to cleaning and sterilization are the centerpiece of technological development, evolving from manual operations recorded on paper (by hand) to fully automated cleaning and sterilization systems with compliant electronic recording devices. The primary drug substance is made from either a biological or chemical process, producing a bulk active pharmaceutical ingredient (API). These processes are discussed in detail in Chapter 10.

Table 11.1 outlines the major steps for the secondary processing of the drug product and shows typical room cleanliness classifications for European Commission (EC) guidelines.

Primary Drug Product Processing

Drug product compounding, also known as formulation, is the basic preparation of a drug product for final filling. It includes the final preparation of a product through the dilution, concentration, or other preparation of a mixture of approved pharmaceutical ingredients into a bulk quantity. This process

TABLE 11.1
Room Function and Classifications

Function	Compounding Operations	Filling Operations	Typical Room Cleanliness Classification
Gowning	✓	✓	Varies to support functional room
Staging and storage	✓	✓	Varies, best to locate outside core area, Grade D at most
Raw materials staging	✓	✓	CNC or Grade D
Materials dispensing/weighing	✓		Grade C or D, depending on the nature of the process
Component preparation		✓	Grade D
Equipment preparation	✓	✓	Grade D
Product preparation and transfer	✓	✓	Grade C or D
Filling		✓	Grade A local, Grade A or B background
Sampling and testing	✓	✓	(Part of other functions)
Lyophilization		✓	Grade A local, Grade A or B background
Capping		✓	Grade B Local, Grade B or C Background
Terminal sterilization		✓	Grade B, C, or D, depending on the locale
Inspection	✓	✓	Grade D
Packaging		✓	CNC
Cleaning and sanitization	✓	✓	(Performed in functional rooms)

Note: CNC, controlled not classified.

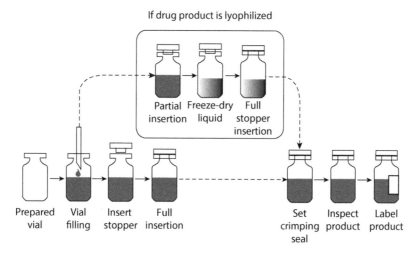

If drug product is lyophilized

Partial insertion / Freeze-dry liquid / Full stopper insertion

Prepared vial / Vial filling / Insert stopper / Full insertion / Set crimping seal / Inspect product / Label product

FIGURE 11.4 Vial filling operation.

can range from a simple, one-step dilution to a multistep process of homogenization. The batch is sampled, and when the process is complete, it is then quarantined, tested, and released for final filling and finishing.

Drug product filling in a sterile facility consists of the transfer of a bulk formulation (prepared in the same facility or elsewhere) into a dosage form for patient administration. Dosage form containers typically consist of bags, vials, and syringes, and the final product may be either in liquid form or lyophilized (freeze-dried) if required [4,5]. Figure 11.4 is a simplified diagram showing a vial filling operation.

Processing Scales

When developing a facility program, the intended scale of manufacturing drives many decisions that impact design and operation. The scale of manufacturing determines the methods and approaches. In a developmental-scale facility, design solutions may call for manual operations and administrative procedural solutions rather than fixed, automatic, or complex engineering solutions. In a commercial-scale facility, the design leans toward automatic operations and engineered systems, including redundancy and robustness. There are four main scales of processing of products that are described below.

1. *Developmental scale.* This is a processing scale where the drug or drug matrix is developed from the bench scale to a measured quantity. Considerations of eventual scale-up to larger volumes are essential. Many processes are carried out manually, so having a firm grasp on standard operating procedures (SOPs) is prudent. Careful consideration of drug toxicity is also critical here, since the process may need to be highly contained to protect operators. In this case, creating a contained process that is also scalable is essential.
2. *Clinical scale.* A clinical scale concerns the manufacture of product for integrity and patient testing. Processing is still manual and controlled through procedures. Engineering systems and controls, however, are employed, especially for critical steps and data collection. Some automatic features may also be included as the process develops through clinical trials, along with tighter controls in practice. The scalability of the process is further developed, so that when the product reaches agency approval, the process capacity is scalable to meet market launch demand. As the product progresses through clinical trials, the process typically moves toward a more uniform, consistent, and repeatable operation.

3. *Launch scale.* Once a regulatory body has approved a product for commercial use, larger quantities are needed to satisfy product launch into the marketplace. Launch-scale quantities are often made from the clinical-scale facility. Typically, as a product moves through phase 3 clinical trials, sourcing decisions are made to either build a dedicated facility or contract with another company for large-scale manufacturing capacity. Some companies have operations set up specifically for new products being introduced into the marketplace, while a full commercial-scale facility is prepared for operation.

4. *Commercial scale.* Commercial scale is a full-scale process operation designed to meet marketplace demands for one or more products. The process operations are well defined and developed, with automatic or engineered methods of processing employed. The facilities are large and expensive, providing high reliability with risk managed through complex engineered solutions and administrative procedures.

Process Equipment

Sterile manufacturing operations are rigorously scrutinized for integrity and consistency to maintain patient safety. Accordingly, process equipment supporting or controlling sterile operations is designed to meet strict regulatory guidelines and design requirements. Major design considerations in process equipment include operability and ergonomics; cleanability of the system; ability to sterilize the system; drainability; smooth, hard, and crevice-free finishes of all product contact surfaces; fully controllable, consistent, and repeatable functions (manual or automatic); closed versus open process systems; and the ability to control the manufacturing environment to a prescribed level.

Materials of construction for sterile manufacturing equipment typically comprise 316L-grade stainless steel, designed for cleanability, strength, durability, and especially sterilizability. Stainless steel contact surfaces often meet very high standards, consistent with interior surface finishes as defined in Part SF, "Stainless Steel and Higher Alloy Interior Surface Finishes" [6].

Process Design of *Open versus Closed* Systems

Issues related to *closed* versus *open* systems significantly affect the development, size, cost, and operation of a sterile manufacturing project and, as such, become a top priority in the design of a process. In comparison, while closed process systems require greater design and operational integrity to function consistently in a controlled manner, *open* systems often require more real estate in a facility and add complexity of access or egress into a critical environment, so a comparative understanding of each approach is very important in the development and operation of a facility.

An *open* process system is a system that is exposed to the background environment in a processing facility. Such examples include final filling into dosage forms, loose connections in a process system, testing of samples, and open transfer of product within a clean room or biosafety cabinet (BSC). An *open* system used to process an injectable product that cannot be maintained in a closed state is typically located within a Grade A or ISO 5 environment. This approach requires rooms and functions to support this critical operation. For example, a closed process system, occupying 500 ft^2, may grow to as much as 2,000 ft^2 to accommodate support and background features for an open system.

A *closed* system is commonly defined as a process that has no normal potential exposure to the surrounding environment. This system may comprise multiple- or single-unit operations. A closed system can be opened initially for cleaning or product or parts changeover, but it is then intrinsically closed and SIP before use in a process operation. When a system can be operated and maintained in a closed state, it has been proposed that the background environment may be significantly downgraded. In most cases, though, the background is maintained to a determined level regardless of a closed process state due to conservative design practices (i.e., engineering solutions over procedural solutions) and conservative risk management considerations.

The design should reflect the number and frequency of connections made to the process system, as well as the method of connection, before declaring a system closed or open. The design should consider that the system may be required to be closed to contain a process because of operator exposure limits to certain drugs and drug matrices. When a level of segregation is required, barrier or isolation systems should be considered along with personnel protection (see Chapter 14).

Processing in Barrier and Isolation Systems

Barrier and isolation systems represent the most common approach in the design and operation of sterile facilities. A restricted access barrier (RAB) isolation system is a barrier system consisting of a set of glass doors set into a stainless steel frame that surrounds the critical filling environment. Due to the nature of this system, interventions during processing, as well as the loading and unloading of material, must be clearly understood, since these aspects often require the background environment to be highly controlled to mitigate risk caused by the opening of the RABs into the room (Figure 11.5).

An isolation system consists of a stainless steel and glass enclosure system, with glove ports, creating a totally sealed system for the critical environment. These technologies are very different, so a comprehensive understanding of the impact of either technology selection is a key part to following good design practices (Figure 11.6).

Benefits to these technologies include protection of product, containment of potent and cytotoxic compounds, protection of personnel, and the potential ability to reduce the environmental classification level of the background environment.

While an isolation system may cost more than a RAB system, the positive effects of both reduced background environmental requirements and operational benefits often exceed the additional initial cost as measured by life cycle costs. Some process systems and unit operations may require a variety of interventions during an operational run; thus, understanding the benefits, limits, and risks of barrier and isolation systems is important during early conceptual design and development. Integration of a barrier or isolation system with process equipment often requires the process equipment to be fabricated and then sent to a vendor specialist to locate the process component in the barrier or isolation system. Consideration of schedule and cost should be made when considering process equipment vendor options. Further dialogue on barrier, containment, and isolation systems can be found in Chapter 14.

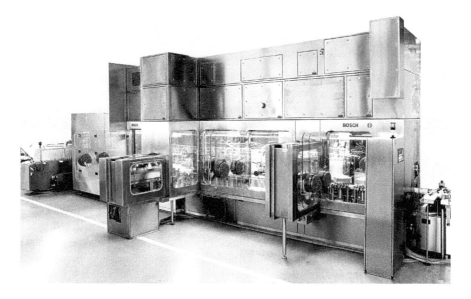

FIGURE 11.5 An isolation system. (Courtesy of Bosch Technologies, Palo Alto, CA.)

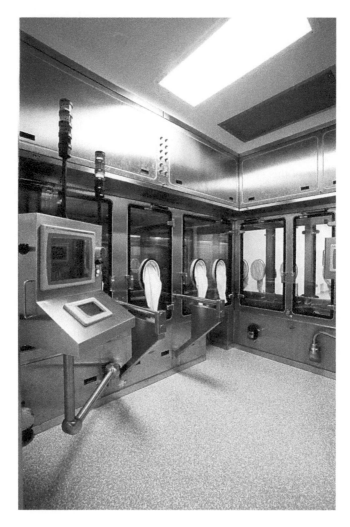

FIGURE 11.6   Barrier and isolation systems. (Courtesy of Cook Pharmica, Bloomington, IN.)

CLEANING, SANITIZATION, AND STERILIZATION

Any equipment, materials, and systems that offer product contact surfaces in a sterile manufacturing facility must be free of all viable microbial organisms on or in inanimate surfaces [7]. To achieve this, any contact surfaces must be thoroughly cleaned and sterilized. Consistent and thorough preparation of product contact surfaces represents a great challenge, so intensive design efforts are required to achieve a fully qualified operation. To mitigate risk or achieve an economic advantage, a company may opt to purchase rather than produce certain sterilized raw materials and disposable products.

Cleaning Process Equipment

While nonproduct contact equipment, such as tables, racks, carts, and so forth, is cleaned at intervals, product contact equipment, such as tanks, pumps, and piping, must be cleaned routinely (between different product runs or batches). Product contact equipment also consists of fixed and portable equipment. Fixed equipment is disassembled with some components removed from the room for cleaning-out-of-place (COP) in a purpose-built room. This also includes the removal of portable equipment for cleaning, typically in the same location. Remaining components are CIP by flushing the system with a series of solutions and rinses while the system is closed. Control of cleaning fluids is managed by both the process equipment and CIP system (typically a skid) control units. The COP typically consists of further disassembly of equipment, where it is cleaned along with an ultrasonic-type or detergent-flushing cleaning cycle (semiautomatic or automatic). A final rinse and drying step completes the cleaning process. Cleaned equipment is then reassembled (if required) and may be placed into a container or bag for protection and sterilization. As the equipment moves through the cleaning process, the surrounding environment increases in cleanliness to correspond with the state of the equipment being cleaned. This typically means that the rooms will be designed to meet a Grade D or C environment, with local Grade B or A areas as required.

Sanitization

Sanitization, in comparison to sterilization, is the "process of substantially reducing or destroying a number of microbial organisms to a relatively safe level." Sanitization "generally requires a 99.9% or greater reduction of a test organism." The "test organism should be agreed upon with the inspecting agency" before completion of the design and validation of the process [8]. In general, most agencies, designers, quality assurance (QA) personnel, and operators prefer that a product is rendered as being sterile as close to the end of a process cycle (i.e., bioburden is controlled throughout the process) as possible. Ideally, this is realized through terminal sterilization, in which filled containers of product pass through a prescribed process, consisting of heat sterilizing the product at a fixed range of parameters (Figure 11.7).

Equipment Sterilization

In the development of a sterile facility and operation, understanding the meaning of a term and the effect of declaring it in a cGMP environment is extremely important since once that term is declared, it must be maintained. This is similar to the previously discussed difference between the terms *aseptic* and *sterile*. One such declaration is the need to declare a system either sterilizable or sanitizable.

Once a process room and equipment have been cleaned, product contact components and other critical items are sterilized. To claim that a system or unit operation is sterilized or sterilizable, one must prove that the system can consistently and repeatedly "destroy all forms of viable microbial organisms on or in inanimate surfaces." Sterilization is usually required for the following reasons: to prevent contamination, to protect product, to protect the patient, and to ensure that only a certain product is present [8]. Critical design factors for sterilization are the

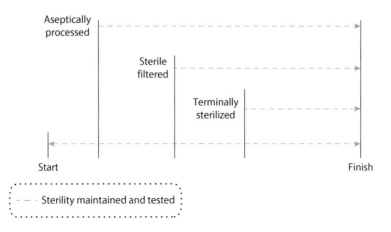

FIGURE 11.7   Aseptic process cycle.

material compatibility with the sterilization method, the design elements of time, the environmental conditions, the temperature, and the chemical contact [9].

Equipment SIP is typically achieved through the introduction of pure steam in a closed system for a prescribed interval of time and temperature. Equipment and components that cannot be sterilized in this manner must be removed from the system and installed in an ISO 5 environment before a process operation. These typically consist of silicon or plastic materials used for disposable tubing, containers, or other components; they can be chemically sterilized, irradiated, or purchased already sterilized.

Once a level of sterility has been achieved in an injectable operation, that level must be maintained from that point forward to maintain that product's declared integrity. Thus, having a clear understanding of why, when, and how a product in a process is to be sterilized is very important.

Monitoring Sterility

Once a product is rendered sterilized, that level of purity must be maintained and tested to ensure product integrity, so a clear understanding should be had early in the development of a project as to the method of monitoring batch integrity.

The QA team will verify that a process room has been cleaned through testing before commencement of a process operation, through the sampling of surface areas in a room, as well as the measurement of microbial organisms and particles. This is typically performed in accordance with the environmental tables of classifications (i.e., tables D and E). In a sterile manufacturing facility, process utilities, such as water, steam, air, and other gases, are rendered as pure or sterile so that the product integrity is not compromised during processing.

Primary and Secondary Containment

Every process operation in place today essentially has a primary and a secondary level of containment. The most common type of primary containment is a process equipment or system (ideally closed), and the process room and surrounding environment are the secondary level of containment. Examples are given in Table 11.2.

When targeting an efficient cost structure for a project, a review of the background environment (the secondary containment) should be done first, since often this costs more than the process equipment (the primary system), while offering no more manufacturing capacity. For example, in a typical sterile manufacturing facility, the process equipment consumes 10%–35% of the total cost of the project, compared to 30%–60% for the background environment and other costs. Thus, any reduction in the background environment is significant to the overall cost of the project, while not affecting process capacity. Space planning and management continue to be critical aspects of understanding the best approach to designing an efficient sterile manufacturing facility.

Often, the secondary containment element (i.e., the room or local protection) is required to perform at a certain level, since the primary containment system may require an opening or break in the

TABLE 11.2
Primary and Secondary Containment

Primary Containment and the Associated Classification	Secondary Containment Surrounding the Primary Mechanism
Open process system	Process room, Grade A
Open process system in a Grade A hood	Process room, Grade B or C
Closed process system in a process room	Process room, Grade B or C
Process system in a Grade A isolator	Process room, Grade C
Process system in a Grade A RAB	Process system, Grade A or B

system during a process run, or the product may have a containment or exposure limit requirement. In this case, the secondary containment element becomes an important line of protection to maintain product integrity, protect operators, and contain a product within a certain boundary.

DESIGN CONSIDERATIONS FOR OPERATION INTERVENTIONS

A manufacturing process typically has materials introduced to and taken from the process area during an operation. These activities include (1) initial material additions, (2) material additions made during a process operation, (3) sampling of in-process product, (4) transfer of product from one system to another, and (5) integrity testing of a process system. While these activities may seem at times insignificant in the overall manufacturing effort of a sterile product, any intervention like those listed above can destroy the integrity of the process environment and a product batch if not well understood, designed, and operated properly.

Sampling of product and utilities also represents a significant portion of a daily manufacturing operation. Routine sampling requires careful design consideration to afford the operators reasonable access, while preserving the integrity of the process. A review of sampling requirements and locations should be conducted before the commencement of construction.

Process and Plant Utilities

Process utilities are those systems that directly support manufacturing and also come in contact with product. According to the ISPE Baseline Guide *Commissioning and Qualification*, these systems are considered direct-impact systems, and therefore need to be validated in cGMP operations [10]. These systems must provide a utility supply that does not contaminate or damage the integrity of a sterile product in manufacturing.

Process utility systems are generally expensive; therefore, careful design is required to balance demand of capacity as well as cost to the project. On small projects, such as developmental and clinical manufacturing, alternative considerations to developing a process utility within a project include the purchase of prepared products, as well as the more extensive use of disposable processing products.

Examples of process utilities include the United States Pharmacopoeia (USP) WFI, clean steam, process gases, and process vacuum and extract systems (in product contact conditions). Applicable regulatory guidelines and engineering texts should be considered when designing these systems. Also, sampling of utilities and maintenance must be considered before the completion of the design.

Utility systems supporting process and facility demands that do not come in direct contact with product are considered indirect-impact systems. These systems typically include plant utilities, process water, steam and hot water, chilled water, potable water, compressed air, lubricants, and water pretreatment.

IMPLICATIONS FOR COMPLIANCE

APPLICATIONS FOR cGMP

A foremost consideration in the design and operation of a sterile manufacturing facility is the identification of which regulatory bodies have jurisdiction. This is decided by determining where the final product will be distributed on a global basis. Since most products are distributed to the United States and Europe, the FDA and the EC are widely recognized as leading agencies with jurisdiction over the review, qualification, and inspection of sterile manufacturing facilities. The facility professional must master the vast array of guidelines and standards to ascertain which rules and principles are applicable to a given project.

PATIENT SAFETY

Sterile products are manufactured worldwide, and for this reason, agencies governing the development and manufacture of these products have been established for major regions. These regions have adopted guidelines for the development and operation of sterile manufacturing facilities. Table 11.3 provides an overview of regions, along with the governing agency.

Balance of Engineering with Procedural Solutions

Throughout the development of a sterile facility project, many issues surface, and solutions to these problems generally fall into two categories: engineering and procedural. Engineering solutions mitigate processing risk through the inclusion of physical elements or engineering controls. Procedural solutions manage risk through the development of SOPs, which require an operator or process to work in a certain manner. The facility professional must strike a balance between engineering and procedural solutions, since engineering solutions can drive up the cost of a project significantly, and procedural solutions may be more scrutinized in certain situations (Figure 11.8).

TABLE 11.3
Regulatory Agencies by Region

Region	Agency
United States	Food and Drug Administration (FDA)
Europe	European Commission (EC)
Europe	European Medicines Agency (EMA)
International	Pharmaceutical Inspection Convention and Pharmaceutical Inspection Co-operation Scheme (PIC/S)
International (Ireland)	Medicines and Healthcare Products Regulatory Agency (MHRA)
International	World Health Organization (WHO)
International	International Organization for Standardization (ISO)
Japan	Ministry of Health, Labor and Welfare (MHLW)
China	China Food and Drug Administration (CFDA)
Argentina	Argentina Administración Nacional de Medicamentos, Alimentos y Tecnología Médica
Australia	Therapeutic Goods Administration (TGA)
Brazil	National Health Surveillance Agency of Brazil (ANVISA)
India	Ministry of Health and Family Welfare

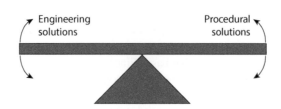

FIGURE 11.8 Engineering versus procedural solutions.

Risk Created and Mitigated by Personnel

Often, the single largest source of particulate and bioburden contamination comes from personnel working in clean room environments. Good design practice should be routinely implemented to remove personnel from a critical process environment whenever possible. This may add some initial capital costs or complexity to a facility program; yet the risk mitigated will often reduce operating costs, which should offset any impact of employing this approach.

Risk Created and Mitigated by Equipment

The equipment used in a sterile manufacturing facility is the cornerstone to safely, effectively, and routinely producing injectable products. When developing an equipment design and operational approach, it is very important to understand the characteristics of the drug matrix being processed, and then set that drug matrix process into an equipment configuration that best fits without creating risk. This understanding starts in process development, so streamlining the process at this stage provides benefit as the process is scaled up and commercialized.

Designing a sterile manufacturing facility requires careful consideration of basic engineering principles and details, particularly in rooms containing critical process operations. It also requires not only particular focus and attention to each design discipline, but also considerations in construction, qualifications, and operation of the facility. Critical cGMP design elements include room finishes, such as hard finishes that are easily cleanable with minimal or no crevices; material and personnel flows, such as unidirectional flow of air in critical environments; equipment placement and ergonomics to maintain product and process integrity and safety; HVAC, controls, zoning, and pressurization to protect product, control contamination, and employee comfort; protection of product exposed to the room environment; and risk assessment, management, and mitigation to control risk by procedural or engineering solutions to make the sterile product safe for the marketplace.

DEVELOPING PROJECT DRIVERS AND OBJECTIVES

This section discusses common concepts, principles, and design considerations for the following major design disciplines: programming, process, process architecture, architecture, mechanical, electrical, plumbing, instrumentation, and controls.

This list also indicates the general order of involvement for each discipline. Good design practices require each discipline to address specific concepts and principles, and in an iterative manner, each discipline should review and understand that each person has a direct effect on the ability to construct, qualify, and operate a sterile manufacturing facility successfully.

Project Concepts, Principles, and Considerations

The participating facility professional requires clear direction (and agreement) regarding the basic concepts, principles, and considerations that directly affect the outcome of a project. From the start of a project, a team must work through a series of discussions and, as a team, identify the drivers of a project by answering a series of questions that begin broadly and then focus particularly on vernacular drivers that relate specifically to a project. When a project begins, usually a new team is assembled to deliver the project. They must meet and discuss the drivers, goals, and objectives of the project. This is typically achieved during intensive kickoff sessions, where everyone in the group participates by identifying the basic components in the project, as well as understanding and agreeing to general ideas, terms, and expectations. This approach should flush out basic decisions and factors in the project, including the purpose of the project, concerns about the project (risk analysis), basic goals and objectives, functionality, compliance requirements, cost, schedule, quality, and safety.

Project Philosophies

At the beginning of a project, the team must develop basic project philosophies, which are brief statements about each major project factor. These philosophies become part of the basis of design (BOD), which serves as the record and source of team and project scope information. Developing a project philosophy provides a platform for future project decisions over the life span of a sterile operation, assists operators with complying with inspections, and allows operators to modify and maintain the facility. Some examples of philosophies for a sterile manufacturing facility are discussed below:

1. *Processing.* It is important to determine process operating conditions and approaches, such as whether the process is open or closed, primary and secondary containment, multiproduct or single product, integrated or stand-alone processing operation controls, and campaign or concurrent batch processing.
2. *Functional zoning.* The general cGMP zones and critical functions in a project must be determined. This affects the scope of the project, the general composition of the layout, and basic environmental design principles.
3. *Product flow and management.* The basic logic for the general flow of critical and noncritical materials throughout the facility must be developed, as well as how the overall project flows integrate into the surrounding environment.
4. *Personnel flow and gowning.* How people enter and exit operating areas must be defined, as well as how they move from street clothes to critical sterile operations. The logic developed here should be consistent with similar operations within the company's domain.
5. *Cleaning.* A simple logic as to how product and nonproduct contact surfaces will be cleaned must be developed. This philosophy also includes ideas, such as CIP and COP, the use of prepared or disposable items, and the general flow during cleaning conditions.
6. *Sterilization.* The boundaries of sterilization must be defined, as well as the general criteria for sterilization, in a simple and basic manner. A well-developed sterilization plan is essential to good facility operating practice.
7. *Waste management.* How the waste will be managed in a sterile facility operation must be delineated.
8. *Constructability.* The execution approach for how the project will be built must be defined, not only the cost, schedule, and quality but also the basic ideas of modularization, facility life span, and how any adjacent operating areas will be managed during project delivery. Construction should be considered early in the design phase to ensure it does not become an issue of cost and scheduling further into the project.
9. *Commissioning and validation.* A realistic validation master and execution plan must be developed, clearly describing direct and indirect systems and boundaries, as well as an agreement on basic performance requirements, acceptance criteria, definitions, and terms.

Process Design and Architecture

With the philosophies, drivers, and project goals identified, the design may begin. The design effort commences with the development of core process functions and, in an iterative manner, progresses from process systems to primary environments and secondary support mechanisms and finally to the external project components.

The overall program begins with the definition and configuration of the process. In this regard, one key aspect in configuring a sterile manufacturing facility is to determine the process containment technology for the project. In this regard, there are three options: isolation containment, RABs, or open processing in a process room. Since all three of these options require an ISO 5 or Grade A environment, it is important to minimize the size of this critical environment and remove personnel from this environment whenever possible. The author recommends that isolators be used whenever possible to remove personnel from the critical process environment and reduce the overall footprint of a sterile manufacturing facility. With the process technology identified and the process operations developed, the integration of the process into a facility environment may commence.

Proper Material and Personnel Flows

In sterile manufacturing facilities, the flows of materials and personnel are very influential on product integrity, and regulatory agencies and quality personnel often scrutinize these flows. This is particularly true in rooms involving product contact and critical operations. In these cases, unidirectional flow of personnel and materials is very important to minimize the risk of product contamination. This principle is applied from room to room, as well as within the room whenever possible.

Proper material and personnel flows are essential in pharmaceutical operations. Good flows efficiently manage and control the movement of people and materials through processing operations, minimizing the risk of contamination whenever possible. Flow patterns to be addressed typically include employees entering and exiting an operation, clean equipment entering an operation and dirty equipment exiting for cleaning, raw materials and components supply, prepared equipment for processing, materials in process, finished goods, and waste materials (Figure 11.9, unidirectional airflow).

Room Layout and Facility Configuration

Since operator and maintenance personnel in a critical operation represent one of the more significant sources of contamination, careful consideration must be made to minimize risk through good ergonomic design and operation of a sterile process. When developing a program for a sterile facility project, careful consideration is required for the placement of equipment and people within segregated process operating rooms. In a critical operation, the location of the supply and return air grilles must be integrated with equipment locations and operations, since it is essential that the clean airstream flows in a unidirectional pattern across the critical operation with minimum interference from people or other obstructions.

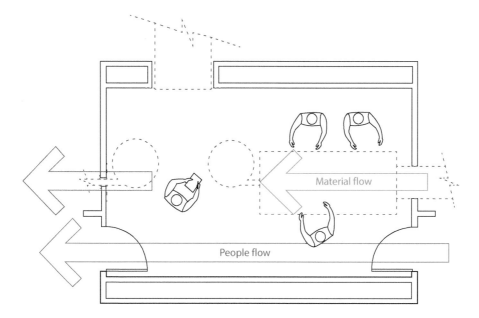

FIGURE 11.9   Unidirectional airflow.

Room Volumes and Geometry

The footprint of a room affects the capacity of an HVAC system. Additionally, even though the height of a room does not affect the number of air changes per hour in a room, it does affect the capacity of the heating and cooling system required to maintain a set temperature. Thus, a facility professional should drive a coordinated effort to minimize the height of a ceiling in a processing room.

When designing a room for a critical operation where unidirectional airflow is included, the design and layout of the room should carefully balance process equipment and ergonomics, as well as the ability for the critical environment to meet airflow design. For example, a room that is 16 ft wide by 22 ft long will perform better than a room that is 22 ft by 22 ft. Also, the simpler the room footprint (i.e., a rectangle) and the fewer openings there are into the room, the easier it is to design the HVAC system. The variation of the geometry for air filters should be considered, so that only one or two sizes of replacement high-efficiency particulate air (HEPA) filters will be required.

Architectural Design

The design of surfaces in clean rooms requires careful attention to detail, construction methodology, and characteristics of smooth and hard surfaces, as well as the ability to withstand frequent cleaning with chemicals. "Sterile Drug Products Produced by Aseptic Processing—Current Good Manufacturing Practice" states that "clean rooms are normally designed as functional units with specific purposes. A well-designed clean room is constructed with materials that allow for ease of cleaning and sanitizing. Examples of adequate design features include seamless and rounded floor to wall junctions as well as readily accessible corners. Floors, walls, and ceilings are constructed of smooth, hard surfaces that can be easily cleaned" (§211.42) [11].

In general, epoxy-coated materials and stainless steel dominate the finish types in sterile manufacturing facilities. Common materials of construction exposed in clean rooms typically include epoxy paint on gypsum board and steel studs for walls and ceilings; epoxy terrazzo or resinous flooring on concrete; an epoxy-coated suspension grid system, with smooth ceiling tiles sealed to the grid; epoxy-coated steel for doors and frames, with stainless steel hardware; stainless steel for doors, frames, panels, and escutcheon plates; glass and plastic for vision panels and barriers; and modular panel systems. While most of these items are readily available, the challenge is to integrate them in such a manner as to minimize joint failures and other crevices. Such conditions are prone to cause microbial and other contamination problems.

The designer must also understand that as construction progresses to completion, the construction tolerances become much tighter. From a construction standpoint, the ability for an architectural system to accept and absorb these tolerances, while minimizing and eliminating joints and seams, is essential to a successful completion of a clean room fit-out.

The failure of surface finishes typically stems from a lack of integration of process equipment into architecture; varying tolerances of systems (±1/8 in. epoxy on ±1/2 in. concrete); improper installation or application of materials; impact of architectural finishes on other systems (an ability to balance room air pressure due to air bleeding through tile and grid ceilings); different material types expanding and contracting at different rates, causing cracks and crevasses; incomplete consultations about materials and surface connections; degradation of surfaces due to chemicals in cleaning; and a lack of understanding of basic design ideas. There are many ways to complete architectural details in clean rooms, but only through good communication (i.e., good documentation and communication between the designer and builder) can the systems be completed successfully.

Room Finishes

The level of clean room finishes varies for room functions and particular conditions. In general, one could consider the room grades in Table 11.4 as a starting point when developing a sterile manufacturing facility.

TABLE 11.4

Airborne Particulate Classifications (EU cGMP Annex 1)

	Maximum Permitted Number of Particles/m³			
	At Rest		In Operation	
Grade	≥0.5 µm	≥5 µm	≥0.5 µm	≥5 µm
A	3,520	20	3,520	20
B	3,520	29	352,000	2,900
C	352,000	2,900	3,520,000	29,000
D	3,520,000	29,000	Not defined	Not defined

Note: EU, European Union.

Modular Wall Systems

Modular facility systems should be considered in place of stick-frame construction materials and methodologies, especially when quality control and speed are essential. Modular wall systems have developed significantly to provide factory-built panels and systems of high quality and performance.

Room Design Considerations

Sterile manufacturing facilities consist of an intensive design array of utilities, environmental controls, and access requirements. At the conceptual design stage, careful consideration is given for access to mechanical systems serving clean rooms. Whenever a cGMP spatial envelope is broken to provide access to utilities, the room must be reestablished per approved SOPs before beginning a following operation. Thus, good access design, while maintaining the cGMP envelope and ongoing operations, can be achieved through the inclusion of such items as technical spaces, walkable ceilings, and controlled, unclassified, peripheral spaces to afford necessary access to mechanical systems.

MECHANICAL DESIGN

Design of Utility Systems

One of the significant development challenges of a sterile manufacturing facility is the design of utility systems. The facility professional should drive the design to be as simplistic as possible, by using readily validatable technologies, as well as proven off-the-shelf skidded systems provided by qualified vendors. A system can fail qualification because the design is not coordinated with expectations. Early design activities should establish clear objectives and criteria for systems, with proper documents of these basic decisions collected into user requirement specifications (URSs). This approach increases the probability of success through clearer communications.

HVAC Systems

Control of Room Environments and Pressurization

The establishment and control of room classifications, pressurizations, and monitoring are based on the process risks and requirements within a room. Tables 11.4 and 11.5 set the basis for establishing control in a process room.

Classification of air cleanliness for clean rooms and associated controlled environments are defined by ISO 14644.1 in Table 11.6.

To provide clarity for those not fully familiar with the ISO and European classifications, Table 11.7 shows the nearest equivalents related to the old withdrawn U.S. Federal 209E classification system. It should be noted that U.S. customary classifications only address in-operation conditions. As such, near equivalency is only for in-operation conditions.

TABLE 11.5

Recommended Limits for Microbial Contamination (EU cGMP Annex 1)

	Recommended Limits for Microbial Contamination			
Grade	Air Sample, cfu/m³	Settle Plates (Diameter 90 mm), cfu/4 hours	Contact Plates (Diameter 55 mm), cfu/plate	Glove Print, 5 (Fingers, cfu/glove)
A	<1	<1	<1	<1
B	10	5	5	5
C	100	50	25	—
D	200	100	50	—

Note: cfu, colony-forming units.

TABLE 11.6

ISO Airborne Particulate Cleanliness Classes

Classification Designation	0.5 μm (Particles/ m³ of Air)	5.0 μm (Particles/ m³ of Air)
ISO Class 5	3,520	29
ISO Class 7	352,000	2,930
ISO Class 8	3,520,000	29,300

TABLE 11.7

Clean Room Classification Equivalencies

ISO 14644.1 Classifications		EU and U.S. Nearest Equivalent Classifications	
At Rest	In Operation	EU Grade	U.S. Customary (Old FS 209E)
ISO 5	ISO 5	Grade A	100
ISO 5	ISO 7	Grade B	10,000
ISO 7	ISO 8	Grade C	100,000
ISO 8	Not defined	Grade D	N/A[a]

[a] Recognized by industry and baseline guides, such as the International Society for Pharmaceutical Engineering Baseline Guides, as pharmaceutical or controlled unclassified; however, not defined by classification systems.

In addition to agency-identified classification, this facility uses an enhanced classification program to address specific needs. This program includes an additional designation of local protection and controlled nonclassified (CNC). Local protection is a localized zone providing enhanced protection for nonaseptic operations to reduce the risk of exposure. The local zone has different qualifications and design criteria from its background environment but is not defined by the FDA or the EU grading system (e.g., final rinse and wrapping of component and parts before autoclaving). The design criteria for local protection are defined as follows: total particulate is ISO Class 5 at rest, micro is Grade C, and unidirectional airflow is from the ceiling to 30 in. above the finished floor.

"Design of a given area should be based on satisfying microbiological and particle standards defined by the equipment, components, and products exposed, as well as the particular operation conducted in the area" [12]. When the product is exposed or opened to the surrounding environment, the room must be designed to meet substantial mechanical performance minimums, to satisfy regulatory agency guidelines, such as Class 100, Grade A, or ISO 5.

Achieving a compliant sterile manufacturing operation requires the use of increasing levels of environmental cleanliness or zones. Using a design of increasing levels of zones facilitates the ability for product and people to enter and exit the facility.

Figure 11.10 illustrates a generic clean room zoning cascade, along with typical air pressurization differentials from critical to noncritical zones. In noncritical peripheral areas, a design can be downgraded to a CNC state, where the room is designed to meet Grade D performance parameters but may not be validated. A CNC room classification should be used whenever practical in a sterile manufacturing facility.

Pressurization

Room pressurization and pressure differentials are usually a highly scrutinized element in design. This is the case since there are times when BOD philosophies may contradict each other or, when followed rigidly, may put the design into an impractical design or operational state. Room pressurization in a sterile manufacturing facility is controlled typically by the difference between the pressure in a particular process room and a fixed atmospheric point outside the core processing area. Through this approach, the HVAC system is more likely to remain stabilized in normal operating conditions since all monitoring points are tied back to a single reference datum. Room pressurization values are generally determined through the analysis of clean room zones and process functions within a conceptual floor plan for a manufacturing environment. Typically, air cascades from the cleanest and controlled operating environment to an uncontrolled area. Exceptions to this approach stem mainly from the requirement to contain a process environment due to potency, containment of an open process (e.g., dispensing of powders), or other operator exposure limitations. In such a case, an additional airlocking level or zone is included to achieve the design objectives.

The challenge in designing a pressurization scheme is to balance practical design with published regulatory guidelines. For example, if a designer were to rigidly follow superseded guidance, such as the FDA's 1987 issue of the "Guideline on Sterile Drug Products Produced by Aseptic Processing," then design professionals would develop a minimal and relative pressure differential (between two different area classifications) of 0.05 in. of water [13]. Compounding this instance is that the QA group may also refer to the same text body and require that the differential should never go below that value. This approach compounds itself in Figure 11.11.

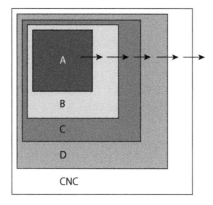

FIGURE 11.10 Generic clean room zoning cascade.

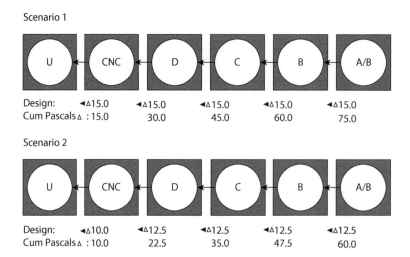

Scenario 1

| U | CNC | D | C | B | A/B |

Design: ◄▲15.0   ◄▲15.0   ◄▲15.0   ◄▲15.0   ◄▲15.0
Cum Pascals▲ : 15.0   30.0   45.0   60.0   75.0

Scenario 2

| U | CNC | D | C | B | A/B |

Design: ◄▲10.0   ◄▲12.5   ◄▲12.5   ◄▲12.5   ◄▲12.5
Cum Pascals▲ : 10.0   22.5   35.0   47.5   60.0

FIGURE 11.11 Pressurization schemes.

Thus, with a typical cascade effect from a Grade A room to an uncontrolled space, the resultant pressure value for the Grade A room may be 0.31 in. of water to meet a minimal operating differential of pressure between areas of 0.05 in. of water. This can become an unmanageable operating condition within a sterile manufacturing facility.

Our recommendation here is to first balance realistic design with good procedures and operations, to achieve a good pressure regime at a reasonable value. Future trends in guidance documents and agency reviews are based on process risk, rather than prescribed numerical values. Good design practices here would be based on the establishment of clear design values and ranges of control, and then one can logically broaden the ranges of control in qualification and operation (e.g., two times those of the design) to avoid alert and alarm conditions, while maintaining a safe processing environment for the injectable products.

Air Filtration and Airflow Movement

To achieve the various grades of spaces, it is necessary to filter the incoming air supply to remove airborne particulate and microbial forms (Figure 11.12). Most regulatory texts offer guidelines for airflow and filtration that represent a good starting point for design. In Grade A spaces, for example, airflow should be HEPA filtered, unidirectional, and moving at a higher velocity at the working elevation, especially when sterile product is exposed to the room environment.

Supply Air

Most of the supply air in a sterile facility operation is HEPA filtered. Only in nonclassified and uncontrolled areas should less clean supply air rather than HEPA air be considered, provided there is no significant adverse risk put on the systems or operations. Ultra-low penetration air (ULPA) filters are also used in this application. An ULPA filter is capable of removing at least 99.999% of dust, pollen, mold, bacteria, and any airborne particles with a size of 0.1 μm or larger from the air (Figure 11.12).

Airflow Control over a Supply Grille

Part of the qualification of a critical environment includes the measurement of airflow over an entire area of supply. With a plenum supply design, airflow may vary over the total surface, which at times can cause problems due to perceived (and at times real) inconsistencies. To achieve an acceptable design, the facility professional must decide on the design and operational tolerances for the

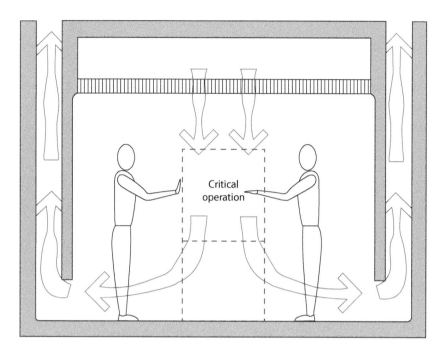

FIGURE 11.12 Air filtration and air movement.

rate of supply. Additionally, a design may include an airflow control device, such as an adjustable baffle plate, to create a more uniform and consistent rate of airflow over an entire surface.

Recirculating versus Once-Through Air

Typically, in a sterile facility project, the room environment air conditioning is recirculated, mainly to reduce utility demand and operating cost. Only in exceptional circumstances, such as open potent or biological processing operations open to the room environment, should a once-through air system be considered for part (or all) of the HVAC design.

Velocity of Air at the Working Elevation

For a Grade A critical process, the desired unidirectional airflow at the location where product is exposed to the environment is driven by the process functions within the critical process zone. As general guidance, airflow design typically starts in the range of 90 ft/min (0.45 m/s) and is adjusted as needed to achieve a Grade A condition based on the process. To achieve that level of airflow at a working level, a higher velocity of air is often required at the face of the supply air discharge point, reaching as high as 120 or more feet per minute (0.60 m/s). These levels should be considered a starting point in design development, and the actual level should be raised or lowered to satisfy the particular design condition for a project (Figure 11.13).

Prefabricated HVAC Modules

Prefabricated airflow modules offer a good solution to achieving local A or B conditions at a good value. These units can be designed to fit a certain operating condition or purchased as a standard size and set up. The boundary between this local Grade A environment and the surrounding area is typically achieved with prefabricated transparent partition barriers commonly referred to as RAB (Figure 11.14).

These units typically use a large plenum box where fan and filter units are located. Return air is typically brought from within the room where the unit is located and filtered through the unit to

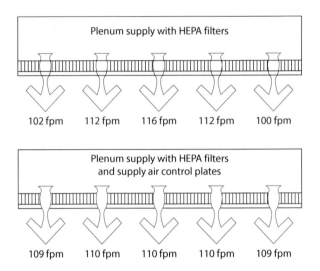

FIGURE 11.13 Plenum supply with HEPA filters.

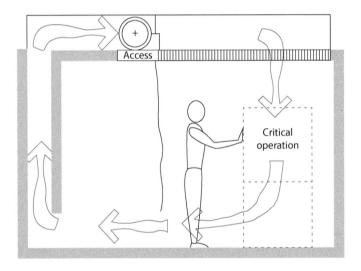

FIGURE 11.14 Prefab airflow modules.

supply clean, laminar flow air necessary to achieve a Grade A operating condition. Access for maintenance to the unit is necessary, as well as the need to provide space for filter-monitoring devices and an electrical service disconnect.

Return Air

Low-wall returns are used in Grade A spaces to achieve unidirectional airflow and are typically used for Grade B spaces as well to maintain proper airflow turbidity. Grade C and D spaces typically use ceiling returns, but may also use low-wall returns when required for a particular operation or circumstance.

Since Grade A spaces with unidirectional airflow often move a tremendous amount of air, the amount of low-wall return area required to meet the desired air-change rate is significant, often occupying two entire sides of a process room.

Electrical Design

The electrical service in a sterile manufacturing facility is not usually readily visible in an operation, but critical process and building functions rely on consistent power to keep process equipment programmable logic controllers (PLCs) and building management systems (BMSs) working properly. Any glitch in the quality of the power supply can significantly affect an operation.

When power must always be available for certain electronic recording devices or control equipment, the facility professional may decide to use an uninterruptable power supply (UPS) with emergency power backup. These two utilities in combination can keep critical operations functional until the operators can properly and safely shut them down. These systems are expensive, so a clear understanding of which items need these services and the associated cost should be reviewed and agreed on early in the design process.

Lighting for operators in process rooms is typically designed for 70–100/candle watts at a working elevation. Consider this measurement as a starting point, and then adjust the level to suit real operating conditions and applicable codes.

Lighting systems in critical process rooms, classified as Grade A, are typically integrated into the HVAC supply system, since that system occupies most of the ceiling surface. These lights are gasketed and sealed, and typically are either fluorescent or light-emitting diode (LED). Lighting in Grade B and less controlled areas typically consists of fluorescent tubes in a sealed prefabricated housing that is then inserted into either a ceiling tile, grid system, or gypsum board ceiling. These light fixtures must be cleanable and designed with minimal crevasses, as well as resistant to the cleaning agents used in process rooms. Good design coordination is required to achieve proper lighting levels, as well as locations for other services in the ceilings of process rooms.

Electrical devices in process rooms typically consist of power connections to equipment, as well as any electrical control and supply boxes located in walls. As with all other materials and surfaces, these items need to comply with basic design guidelines for cGMP process rooms. Items that require electrical service include door interlocks, automatic doors, safety devices, telephone and intercom, and clocks. These systems must comply with applicable regulatory guidelines and codes. While purchasing these devices for clean rooms has been difficult in the past, vendors have now developed complete product lines designed exclusively for clean room applications.

International power requirements can be an issue when process equipment is purchased from different countries. A careful understanding of electrical engineer terms (e.g., Conformité Européenne [CE] and United Laboratories [UL]) and local and state code requirements is essential to successful design of a system. An electrical engineer should review the type of power required for each process system (e.g., volts or hertz), the process equipment specifications, and the design criteria before final development and procurement.

Power for manufacturing equipment typically is supplied locally to the equipment, from either a disconnect switch or a control panel. Connections to freestanding components in rooms are often made from overhead, with a flexible line connecting directly into the equipment. The cleanability and safety of flexible connections must be considered before completion of design and engineering.

Instrumentation and Controls

In the design and construction of sterile manufacturing facilities, instrumentation component and control (I&C) systems have developed significantly. Developments in I&C systems include (1) the establishment of Good Automated Manufacturing Practices (GAMPs), (2) a better understanding of direct (cGMP) and indirect (non-cGMP) instruments and controls, (3) the availability of electronic batch records and recording devices, and (4) better software and hardware designs, affording greater control capability and quality.

In a facility, instrumentation components monitor systems in operation to verify that the system is performing as planned. Instruments typically monitor particles, microbial levels, pressure, temperature, humidity, flow, volumetric levels, mechanical settings, and status conditions. These monitoring points are essential to monitor and trend the performance and quality of product, process utilities, process manufacturing, and room environments.

Control Systems

Control systems collect information gathered from instruments and then monitor, record, and control the systems to meet prescribed performance settings and requirements. Within a sterile manufacturing facility, typically there are control systems set up for direct-impact operations, such as control of process equipment and cGMP room environments, as well as indirect-impact operations, such as plant steam, potable water, and chilled water. The level of complexity for control systems can vary greatly, but typically a company will opt to separate cGMP controls from non-cGMP controls. This approach enables a programmer to manipulate non-cGMP system programs more freely than a change-control-managed cGMP system modification. An additional consideration here is to create a mirror image of the controls software for each system. This allows programmers to tweak the software more easily in the non-cGMP system, and then they can very quickly make the proven modifications in a cGMP system under change control.

Data Recording

Data recording in cGMP operations is a topic of much discussion. When a company decides to include electronic data recording for batch records and trending, much work must be done to prove the integrity of the data collected and stored. Books such as the ISPE Baseline Guide *Good Automated Manufacturing Practices* [14] provide excellent information and guidance for the development of such systems. When the islands of automation approach is used, data are typically printed out at the completion of each process unit operation and collated into the process batch record. All data are subsequently erased from the controller the next time it is used.

Plumbing

Plumbing systems in sterile manufacturing facilities typically consist of domestic cold and hot water and waste drainage. While these systems are widely used in noncontrolled environments, such as utility rooms, washrooms, and cleaning stations, they are not typically used or exposed in a controlled environment due to the risk of contamination. Often, when a drain is required in a cGMP operation, it is limited to Grade C or D spaces and is designed to be a contained connection with the proper air break to comply with codes. Alternatively, drains can also be located in adjacent technical spaces to manage risk.

Many drainage system designs are specialized in sterile manufacturing facilities, since the liquid introduced may be very hot, slightly corrosive from cleaning materials, or mineral deficient. Such considerations as specialized pipe materials or quench (or flash) tanks can be used to render the waste safe for disposal into the common waste system.

Any water for use in general cleanup in noncritical areas is typically treated, while water used in critical operation rooms is sterilized.

PROJECT MANAGEMENT ISSUES

BALANCING QUALITY, COST, AND SCHEDULE WITH NET PRESENT VALUE

When developing any facility, understanding the aspects of cost, schedule, and net present value (NPV) is very important. This is particularly important when developing a sterile manufacturing facility, since the cost per square foot and the process equipment cost can be very high. When (typically) a company waits as long as possible to develop such a facility, schedule planning and management are just as critical to realize a successful project and drive a beneficial NPV assessment.

The project team should use the NPV assessment as a primary driver to understand how to best develop such a facility; this assessment may, in fact, indicate that an additional capital investment will yield a very positive return.

Quality

Pharmaceutical clients demand a high-quality sterile manufacturing facility, at an efficient cost and fast-track schedule. For a facility professional, balancing these three points can be difficult. It is therefore essential that the project management team connect the design and execution team with the particular cost, schedule, and quality drivers in a project (Figure 11.15).

Cost

Sterile manufacturing facilities are high-cost facilities. The direct facility cost (i.e., all the physical elements) alone can be an average of US$500–$1,000 per square foot ($5,382–$10,764 per square meter), and the process equipment can cost millions more. Add to these costs the allowances for indirect service costs and contingencies, and the total facility cost is significant.

The profiles of the projects above are diverse, so before a comparison can be made between any facility projects, a clear understanding of the factors that drive the cost must be understood. In a review of a sterile manufacturing facility cost, there is a need to consider the following: (1) facility, process, and indirect services costs; (2) greenfield, retrofit, or renovation projects; (3) the project execution approach (i.e., integrated or phased execution); (4) the scale of the project (i.e., there are some economies with large-scale projects); (5) the location of the project (i.e., the availability of skilled labor and the cost of materials and labor); (6) the targeted speed of the project completion; (7) the extent of modularization; (8) the sophistication of the facility and process design; and (9) product containment requirements (e.g., potent or cytotoxic). Only when a project is broken down into its components can a team understand the significant design factors that drive the ultimate cost of a project.

Schedule

Sterile manufacturing facilities are complicated projects, and therefore sterile projects typically take a significant amount of time to design, build, and qualify. For a greenfield project, the duration for a new sterile manufacturing facility may take as long as 48 months to realize full operational readiness (ready to manufacture). Since many clients seek to complete a project as fast as possible, the facility professional must develop an execution approach that balances schedule targets with cost and quality.

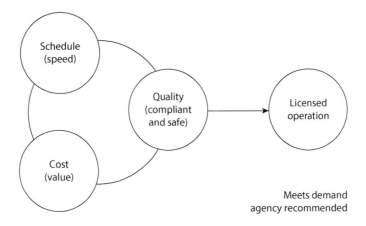

FIGURE 11.15 Schedule, quality, and cost of a licensed operation.

Schedule is particularly driven by the project execution approach. When a fast-track project schedule is essential, then the client may choose an integrated engineering, procurement, construction management, commissioning, and validation execution. This is commonly referred to as an integrated project delivery (IPD).

Schedule is also greatly affected by the delivery of long-lead equipment. Typically, the long-lead equipment is the core of the sterile manufacturing operations, which can also be the most difficult to install. A filling system alone can take 12–24 months to design, fabricate, test, and deliver to a project site for installation. In this case, select equipment packages may be ordered very early in the project schedule, and the surrounding components are then designed to fit the purchased equipment configurations.

As with cost, it is essential to connect the entire team to the importance of schedule so the team may account for schedule drivers in the design of a sterile manufacturing facility. When accelerating a project schedule, one should consider using some level of modularization to deliver a project faster than a conventional stick-frame approach. This notion assumes, though, that the project may be broken into parallel tracks in which process, utility, and facility components are designed by vendors into skids, fabricated in a controlled facility environment, and tested prior to delivery to the project site. In fact, some of the testing done in the factory may help accelerate the qualification process at the site. Meanwhile, the main facility components can be constructed at the site. When completed, the modularized systems are then delivered and installed in the facility.

Lastly, when a project schedule is accelerated significantly, completing all the preferred paperwork, such as URSs, may be difficult. An execution approach should be developed, using interim (draft) documents, which capture the essence of a system, with additional and more particular information to follow.

Good Design Practice Guidance

It is important to organize a core team comprising personnel representing all phases of the project to develop a program and execution approach. This team should describe the essential goals of a project.

Understanding the importance and limits of compliance and establishing a group within the facility to monitor and ensure compliance in a cGMP project are crucial steps. Also, the design team must be connected to the importance of compliance to ensure the successful qualification and operation of a facility. Lastly, a sensible approach to compliance must be developed, first by understanding what compliance is and second by determining what level of compliance is necessary for a given project.

Often, the validation group may use design ranges to qualify a facility, when a broader operating range is certainly acceptable. It is important to take time early in the design to develop a matrix, comparing design ranges to acceptable operating and qualification ranges for regulated systems. To create a better product and an operating facility, the design team should be connected to the aspects of product quality and facility operability.

Many times the designers and engineers are not "connected" to the project. They need to be connected not only in terms of understanding the drivers, goals, and particular conditions within a project, but also in terms of understanding the effect of a design decision on a project. The management team should maintain a consistent connection of project drivers to the design team.

When sterile filling equipment takes a year to be delivered to a project site, the project should be designed so that this equipment can be successfully installed and connected at the site, by working with the management team to understand the project execution sequence. These critical milestones must be identified early, integrated into the schedule, and expeditiously managed. In many respects, good quality management in the development of a sterile facility operation drives the successful completion of a project.

With every additional surface introduced into a critical process room, the need to clean frequently and maintain it increases. Every exposed surface must be accessible for routine cleaning, so every effort should be made to minimize the amount of surfaces through the relocation of nonessential components to an area outside the room, as well as the concealment of components in cabinets and panels. Cleaning equipment and the formulating and dispensing of cleaning solutions consume a significant amount of space in a sterile facility. Careful consideration should be made to include space allocations in the program for these operations. In large-scale operations, a cleaning system or area may be designated specifically for the preparation and storage or staging of cleaning components.

Agencies understand that the basic context of a project affects the solutions generated for a project. It is therefore essential to document that something was done so a representative may better defend a position taken in the project. Sometimes space limitations may require an airlock regime or process flow to be nonstandard, relying more on SOPs for control of product integrity.

PROCESSING RISKS AND ISSUES

Contamination Sources

People represent the single most significant source of contamination in a sterile manufacturing operation. This is the case due to particle shedding, microcontamination, and airflow disturbance due to fast movements by operators. Thus, proper gowning, the minimal presence of operators in critical rooms, and proper training for the movement of operators are necessary.

Unvalidatable Systems

Process systems are often unvalidatable because the major phases in a project are not properly coordinated; for example, a design may be developed without an understanding of how it will be managed, cleaned, and inspected, thus creating significant challenges to the construction, qualification, and operation teams. If documentation is not properly maintained over the course of a project's development, significant voids will be left in the document trail of a project. A construction team may not install the equipment as designed, thus creating significant challenges for the commissioning and validation team. A validation team may attempt to force a system to perform within unreasonable ranges, as well as qualify parameters that do not need to be validated, because the team was not properly engaged and managed.

FUTURE DEVELOPMENTS

Trends in sterile manufacturing facilities include more potent drug matrices, cell therapy technologies, combination sterile product and medical device products, new filling techniques, new sterile container types, the ability to purchase prepared sterile containers and ready-to-use components, improved environmental system controls, virtual modeling of the project, modularization and standardization, harmonization of regulatory bodies, and a risk-based approach and risk management.

NEW AND MORE POTENT DRUGS

As biotechnology and more sophisticated pharmaceutical APIs are developed to target specific regions in the body, the need to deliver the drug directly into the body is imperative to its efficacy. Many of these new products, though, are either very delicate or potent and, as such, have required engineers to be far more cognizant of their design for sterile filling of these products. Isolation technologies, highly controlled filling systems, more robust room environments and controls, and better-trained operators are but a few of the implications of such new drug developments.

CELL THERAPY TECHNOLOGIES

On the forefront of oncological therapeutic developments is the commercialization of cell therapies. Cell therapies, or immunotherapy, typically consist of the aseptic processing or manipulation of autologous or allogeneic (i.e., tissue, blood, or cells) material, which is then administered intravenously or subcutaneously into the patient. These processes are still in development, and at this time, the processes are typically manually based and, at times, open, requiring the work to be completed in an ISO 5 (or Grade A) local environment, that is, a BSC, with an ISO 6 (or Grade B) background environment.

NEW FILLING TECHNIQUES AND STERILE CONTAINERS

Filling techniques and container types have dominated new trends in sterile manufacturing facilities. At this time, new and more accurate filling methods, such as pressure-sensitive filling, have enabled pharmaceutical companies to safely fill vials and containers with new and more delicate drug matrices. New filling systems, based on compact, monoblock robotic arm filling systems, are becoming more readily available. These systems, typically set into an isolator, can be combined with ready-to-use filling container components to enable companies to provide very cost-effective sterile filling services and capabilities. These systems will change the landscape of sterile filling, providing more compact and efficient filling capacity globally. New fill techniques, such as the aseptic filling of closed primary containers (e.g., vials and bags), will help to reduce the background environment and other typical constraints, while maintaining product integrity and personnel safety.

In addition to the above-mentioned developments, advances in plastics and other material technologies have allowed companies to sterile-fill complex bags and containers, as well as actually form and fill a container in one step (referred to as blow–fill–seal).

IMPROVED ENVIRONMENTAL SYSTEM CONTROLS

Minimizing contamination of product exposed to the environment has always been an issue. With the advent of more reliable and sophisticated control capabilities, the designer is able to create a system and facility that will work reliably and effectively. Since the actual operating environment is also difficult to predict before it is built, new software developments have enabled designers to create virtual simulations of an actual room condition, through computational fluid dynamics (CFD). The CFD technology allows engineers to review how airflow, temperature, and humidity within an environment are projected to behave. This allows designers to make adjustments to the design before it is built, thus improving the chances for a successful operation. This, in combination with more robust and reliable environmental control systems, has helped to produce more reliable and consistent sterile operations.

MODULARIZATION

Applying various levels of modularization in the development of sterile manufacturing facilities has become an increasing trend. Vendors and designers have responded to this trend by developing process unit operations within a skid, as well as offering a modular wall and ceiling panel system and fully functional facility or process operating modules. Examples of modularization include modular wall and ceiling panel enclosure systems, facility modules integrated with process systems, facility pods integrated with process systems, and complete modular solutions with integrated process systems.

From skidded systems to fully developed process environments, pharmaceutical companies are looking to modularization as a means of improving quality, performance, cost, and schedules for the development of projects, as well as significantly improving the NPV assessment. As new sterile manufacturing facilities are constructed globally, applying modular concepts will improve the success potential of projects. Where experienced and skilled labor is at a shortage or where material availability is an issue, modular facility systems provide an excellent solution to a real problem.

Skidded systems promise to grow in size, and pharmaceutical companies will continue to look at this idea as a means of leveraging skilled labor working in a more controlled environment to produce a better system. Also, these skids will be better qualified and tested before installation in the field, thus improving overall completion time of a project.

STANDARDIZATION AND HARMONIZATION

As pharmaceutical companies have grown and expanded operations, some companies have developed different practices and techniques for manufacturing sterile products. This is an issue with regulatory agencies, especially as products are further distributed to many global regions. The need to harmonize operations from location to location will become even more important, since regulatory agencies will look for more consistent operations and practices in sterile manufacturing operations.

In the past, pharmaceutical companies have developed sterile manufacturing facilities to meet only local regulatory compliance guidelines. As product demand broadens across multiple regions, the demand for a sterile manufacturing facility to comply with a variety of different agencies is increasing. Over the past few years, a concerted effort has been made by regional agencies, particularly in the United States and the EU, to work toward a more unified set of guidelines for sterile manufacturing facilities. The trend for harmonization of regulatory agencies is already in process. This trend should continue into the future to make new drug products available globally.

RISK-BASED APPROACH AND RISK MANAGEMENT

To assist in the approval process of new drugs and new facility operations, regulatory agencies (e.g., the FDA) will employ a new risk-based approach to cGMPs. Pharmaceutical companies will have greater abilities to modify a process or enhance a process at their own risk. Proof of equivalency, safety, and compliance is still necessary, but with this growing trend, companies will be better able to capitalize on new trends in processing and operating technologies. The EC will be updating and issuing the EudraLex, "The Rules Governing Medicinal Products in the European Union," Volume 4, "EU Guidelines to Good Manufacturing Practice: Medicinal Products for Human and Veterinary Use, Annex 1: Manufacture of Sterile Medicinal Products". Reportedly, these updates include a more risk-based approach to the design and operation of sterile manufacturing facilities, particularly as they relate to the basis for air changes within a clean room.

SUMMARY

The reality of our profession today is that most people learn how to manage and design a sterile manufacturing facility project through on-the-job training. Thus, this chapter is a starting point for learning the basic practices, guidelines, and drivers behind the development of sterile manufacturing facilities, as well as identifying some of the key issues that are important to the overall success of the project.

FURTHER DISCUSSION

1. How do sterile products function?
2. Why is it so important to design, build, and operate sterile manufacturing facilities safely?
3. What are three or more injectable product forms?
4. What are the two main types of processing operations within a sterile manufacturing facility?
5. What is the primary difference between aseptic and sterile?

ABOUT THE AUTHOR

George Wiker is the executive director at AES Clean Technology, Inc. Wiker has more than 24 years of experience in the programming, design, construction, and operation of manufacturing operations worldwide. His particular focus has been in the programming of cGMP-regulated facilities for the manufacture of biological and chemical drug substances, as well as OSD and injectable drug products. Wiker promotes the application of standardized and modular solutions to develop clean manufacturing facilities rapidly and predictably. Wiker is a member of ISPE, Parenteral Drug Association (PDA), and Bio-Process Systems Alliance (BPSA) and is a contributing author of published articles and publications. He has also been a speaker at ISPE, PDA, and FDA educational seminars.

REFERENCES

1. U.S. Food and Drug Administration, Guidance for Industry, Sterile Drug Products Produced by Aseptic Processing—Current Good Manufacturing Practice, Draft Guidance, U.S. Food and Drug Administration, Silver Spring, MD, August 2003.
2. International Society for Pharmaceutical Engineering, *Baseline® Pharmaceutical Engineering Guides for New and Renovated Facilities*, Vol. 3: *Sterile Manufacturing Facilities*, 1st ed., International Society for Pharmaceutical Engineering, Tampa, FL, 2009.
3. World Health Organization, Good Manufacturing Practices for Sterile Pharmaceutical Products, Annex 6, WHO Technical Report Series No. 902, World Health Organization, Geneva, 2002.
4. Health & Medicine, Business, Jennifer Carson, 2013. http://www.slideshare.net/FrostandSullivan/global-pharmaceutical-contract-manufacturing-market-injectable-dose-formulations-will-likely-spur-the-growth-of-cm-os.
5. http://www.pharmaceutical-journal.com/research-and-development-in-novel-injectable-formulations-and-devices/11107939.article.
6. http://www.companiesandmarkets.com/Market/All-Sectors/All?Keywords=injectable+drug&SearchType=Phrase&AZKTCode=AZ1005&AZKCode=AZ21502.
7. American Society of Mechanical Engineers, ASME BPE-2014: Bioprocessing Equipment, An International Standard (Revision of ASME Bpe-1997), American Society of Mechanical Engineers, New York, 2014.
8. Warf TR, ASME Bioprocess Technology Seminars, Facility Design, San Diego, CA, October 28–November 1, 2002.
9. Warf TR, Engineering for Sterilization, ASME Bioprocess Technology Seminars, Facility Design, San Diego, CA, October 28–November 1, 2002.
10. International Society for Pharmaceutical Engineering, *Baseline® Pharmaceutical Engineering Guides for New and Renovated Facilities*, Vol. 5: *Commissioning and Qualification*, 1st ed., International Society for Pharmaceutical Engineering, Tampa, FL, 2001.
11. U.S. Food and Drug Administration, Guidance for Industry, Sterile Drug Products Produced by Aseptic Processing—Current Good Manufacturing Practice, Draft Guidance, U.S. Food and Drug Administration, Silver Spring, MD, August 2003, Section IV, Part E, Design, Paragraph 7.
12. U.S. Food and Drug Administration, Guidance for Industry, Sterile Drug Products Produced by Aseptic Processing—Current Good Manufacturing Practice, Draft Guidance, U.S. Food and Drug Administration, Silver Spring, MD, August 2003, Section IV, Paragraph 1.
13. U.S. Food and Drug Administration, Guideline on Sterile Drug Products Produced by Aseptic Processing, U.S. Food and Drug Administration, Silver Spring, MD, 1987.
14. International Society for Pharmaceutical Engineering, *Good Automated Manufacturing Practices*, International Society for Pharmaceutical Engineering, Tampa, FL, 2003.

12 Biotechnology Facilities

David M. Marks, PE

CONTENTS

INTRODUCTION

Biotechnology is an applied science that is generally regarded as new and rapidly evolving advanced technology. Contrary to popular perception, biomanufacturing is as old as the production of fermented drink, but it has in recent decades undergone a renaissance of new applications, resulting from the development of recombinant DNA technology (Figure 12.1). Biotechnology facilities today produce a diverse array of products, from yogurt to biofuels. The focus of this chapter, however, is on the particular application of biotechnology facilities to produce products for the prevention and treatment of disease. These biopharmaceutical products are extending and improving lives and are transforming the practice of medicine at a meteoric rate.

The therapeutic products produced by biopharmaceutical facilities fall into the category of regulated substances known as biologics. The U.S. Food and Drug Administration (FDA) considers a wide range of products to be biologics, including "vaccines, blood, blood components, allergenics, somatic cells, gene therapy, tissues, and recombinant therapeutic proteins. Biologics can be composed of sugars, proteins, or nucleic acids or complex combinations of these substances or may be living entities, such as cells and tissues" [1]. Biologics may be isolated from many natural sources, including humans or animals. The focus of this chapter, however, is on biotechnology facility design for manufacturing biological products derived from microorganisms through fermentation or cell culture. An introduction to the basic principles and key concepts associated with current Good Manufacturing Practice (cGMP) biomanufacturing is covered first. Since the design of biotechnology facilities is fundamentally process driven, an overview of bioproduction systems and bioprocess manufacturing operations is provided. Additional background on bioprocess unit operations is provided in the appendix. This establishes a foundation for a discussion of the biotechnology facility programming, including area requirements, layout, and the flow of people and materials through the facility. The specific regulatory requirements that affect the design of biotechnology facilities, including cGMP and containment issues (e.g., cytotoxic and highly potent compounds and biohazardous materials), are covered. This chapter also discusses the unique challenges to the design and delivery of biotech facilities from a project management perspective. A discussion of the emerging industry trends concludes the chapter.

This chapter provides the reader with a foundational understanding of the history, technology, engineering principles, and good design practices employed to design modern biopharmaceutical plants. The strategic approach to biomanufacturing is rapidly evolving because of new technologies, such as disposable or single-use systems (SUS), continuous bioprocessing, and modular construction, all of which are discussed. The globalization of regulatory requirements and biopharmaceutical engineering

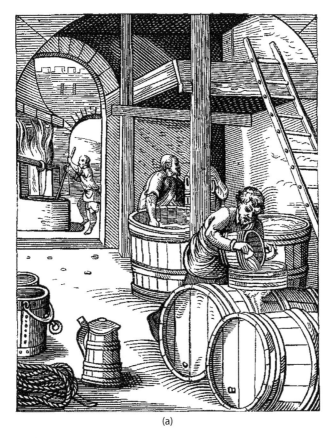

(a)

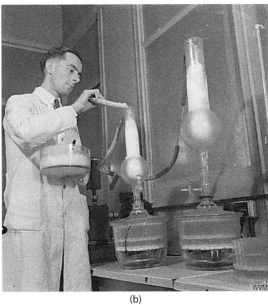

(b)

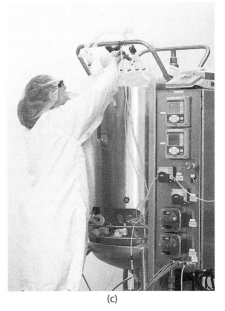

(c)

FIGURE 12.1 (a) "The Brewer," designed and engraved in the sixteenth century (courtesy of J. Amman). (b) A technician preparing penicillin in 1943 (courtesy of Ministry of Information, Photo Division. Photographer: Stone Richard). (c) Laboratory-scale cGMP bioreactor in 2015 (Xcellerex photo courtesy of GE Healthcare Bio-Sciences Corp., Pittsburgh, PA.).

standards is covered as well. The strategies being used to deliver future biomanufacturing capacity faster, better, and cheaper are presented. The next generation of biopharmaceutical manufacturing facilities will need to be more flexible and cost-effective; the objective of this chapter is to provide the reader with the concepts and tools needed to meet this challenge.

EXECUTIVE SUMMARY

Overview

Biotechnology facilities are fundamentally different from other pharmaceutical manufacturing facilities because they are required to harness the inherent complexities and variability of living things. Biologics are large and complex molecules that are difficult, if not impossible, to characterize completely [2]. In contrast to traditional pharmaceutical facilities that manufacture small-molecule drugs via chemical synthesis, biotechnology facilities produce large-molecule biologics (i.e., proteins with a molecular weight greater than 5,000 Da). For comparison, a typical monoclonal antibody (mAb) weighs 150,000 Da and contains 20,000 atoms. Most biological drugs have the ability to generate a significant immune response in the human body. Relatively small changes to the manufacturing process can have a significant effect on the efficacy or immunogenicity of the drug. In most cases, biologics are also unstable over time and require special handling and storage to protect the product from degradation. In comparison with small-molecule drugs, some manufacturing processes are more susceptible to microbial contamination. Bioburden control is required from the initial manufacturing steps through the final fill. Aseptic processing (i.e., process operations that are devoid of measurable bioburden) is required for many of these steps.

Biological therapies are the fastest-growing segment of the pharmaceutical industry. In most cases, biologics are also more profitable than small-molecule drugs due to the high cost and complexity of producing generic equivalents. Without biotechnology facilities, most of the lifesaving new drugs and revolutionary therapies introduced in the last several decades could not be manufactured.

Historical Context

Early applications of biotechnology to medicine relied on the extraction and purification of existing plant and animal sources for active ingredients. The use of microorganisms to produce drugs for medical applications in humans can be traced back to the early 1940s, when penicillin was first introduced to treat infection. Alexander Fleming's 1928 discovery of the antibiotic properties of the mold penicillium was largely a laboratory curiosity until Pfizer (New York) opened the world's first large-scale penicillin manufacturing facility in 1944. This facility employed deep-tank fermentation, an aseptic process for growing large quantities of microorganisms that require oxygen for survival [3]. A similar process is used to produce most commercial biopharmaceutical products today.

The scientific breakthroughs widely regarded as precursors for the modern biopharmaceutical industry are the 1953 discovery of the structure of DNA by James Watson and Francis Crick and the development of technology to transfer genetic material into bacteria by Stanley Cohen and Herbert Boyer in 1973. These discoveries led to the development of the field of recombinant DNA technology (i.e., genetic engineering), which ultimately enabled the expression of a variety of protein therapeutics through common microbial production platforms, such as *Escherichia coli* (Figure 12.2) fermentation. In 1978, a team of researchers from a start-up biotech company (Genentech, South San Francisco, California) and City of Hope National Medical Center, Los Angeles, developed the first viable biotechnology manufacturing process to synthesize a human protein (insulin). The resulting commercial product, Humulin, rapidly replaced animal insulin for the treatment of diabetes. In the decade that followed, several other biosynthetic manufacturing processes were developed, using recombinant DNA to introduce breakthrough therapeutics, including alpha-interferon in 1980, human growth hormone (hGH) in 1981, hepatitis B vaccine (Recombivax HB) in 1986, and tissue plasminogen activator (tPA) in 1987.

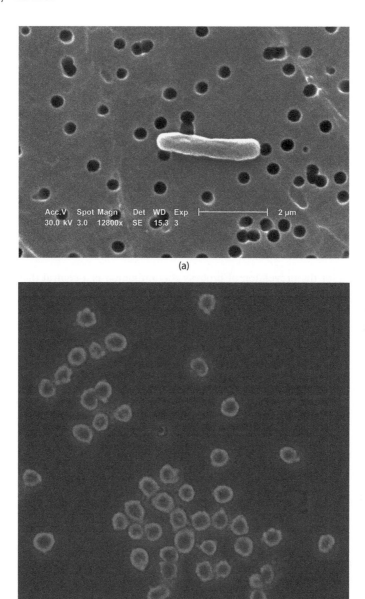

(a)

(b)

FIGURE 12.2 (a) Scanning electron micrograph of a rod-shaped *E. coli* bacterium; magnification, 12,800× (courtesy of CDC/Evangeline Sowers, Janice Carr). (b) A phase-contrast image of a monoclonal antibody, producing hybridoma cells grown in tissue culture. These cells are producing large amounts of monoclonal antibody, which can be readily purified from the culture media. Image taken on a Zeiss inverted microscope with 40× phase-contrast optics (photo by Gerry Shaw in the EnCor Biotechnology Lab via Wikimedia Common).

The first commercial bioprocessing used robust and fast-growing microbial production systems. However, microbial fermentation methods are not ideal for the production of some large, complex molecules. This situation led to the development of genetically engineered animal cells for the large-scale production of a new class of medicines, that is, biologics. In 1955, the first vaccine derived from mammalian cell culture was developed for polio prevention. Another significant development came with the 1975 discovery by Georges J.F. Köhler and César Milstein of hybridoma cell culture technology (see Figure 12.2) to produce monoclonal antibodies (mAbs). Cell culture is more susceptible to contamination than microbial fermentation due to a relatively long culture time in growth-promoting medium. Therefore, several advances in aseptic process technology were required before it could be implemented in large-scale cGMP manufacturing. Initially, the cell lines used were all anchorage dependent (i.e., required a substrate to attach to); thus, production was scale-limited to roller bottles or required the use of microcarrier beads in a stirred-tank bioreactor. To overcome these limitations, the ability to grow cells in suspension on a large scale was needed. By the late 1980s, suspension cell culture and aseptic process technology had developed to the extent that large-scale cell culture was a viable alternative to microbial fermentation and, in the subsequent decade, supplanted it as the predominant production system for large-scale manufacturing of new biological products.

KEY CONCEPTS AND PRINCIPLES

The design criteria for the prevention of process contamination is a central theme in this chapter. Biopharmaceutical manufacturing requires attention to the level of bioburden control that is appropriate for each step in the process. This is determined through a system of quality risk management (QRM), which ensures that the safety, identity, potency, purity, and quality of the drug substance are not compromised. The system of QRM is a regulatory requirement that involves systematic risk assessment, risk control, and risk review for every aspect of the manufacturing process, from supply train to delivery of the finished product. As it relates to the design of facilities and equipment, QRM requires particular attention to the flow of materials and personnel, and segregation of manufacturing operations, to prevent mix-ups and minimize contamination. Clean rooms, isolators, and closed process systems are employed to provide an appropriate level of protection from environmental contamination.

Contamination from bioburden is a chief concern throughout the manufacturing process. However, product contamination can also come from airborne particulates, raw materials, utility systems, product contact materials, and other products manufactured in the same facility. Therefore, the prevention of product contamination is the predominant principle driving every aspect in the design of biotech facilities. Table 12.1 presents an overview of the types of contaminants that must be considered when designing the biopharmaceutical manufacturing plant.

Contamination control is fundamentally different from *containment* control (as may be required for a biohazard or potent compound). Conceptually, it is the difference between

---

TABLE 12.1

Contaminants That Must Be Considered in Biotechnology Facility Design

Source of Contamination	Potential Risk	Facility Design Impact
Materials	Viruses, bacteria, and cross-contamination	Flow of materials, controlled raw material sampling and storage areas, quality control labs, and storage of samples, product, and waste
Manpower	Bacteria/particulate contamination and cross-contamination	Flow of personnel, gowning, and locker facilities
Equipment and environment	Bacteria and cross-contamination	Flow of product and waste, single use, closed systems, cleaning validation, utility design, air handling and room classifications, segregation of activities, and cleanable surfaces

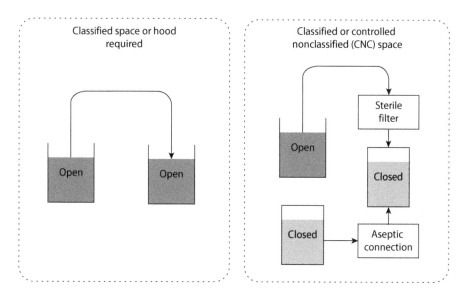

FIGURE 12.3   Open and closed processing.

protecting the product from the environment and protecting the environment from the product. Both principles require a barrier of some kind, which can lead one to confuse the requirements. Other design features, such as room pressurization gradients, may require a formal risk assessment and nuanced design discussions to identify the best method to protect both the product and personnel adequately.

One determining factor in the assessment of risk in biomanufacturing is the nature of process isolation from the environment. An open process has no physical barrier between the product and the local environment and relies heavily on clean room conditions to mitigate the risk of contamination. Critical open process operations are often performed in biosafety cabinets (BSCs) or restricted access barrier systems (RABs). Open processing is inherently less reliable than processing in a closed system, which relies on equipment to isolate the product from the environment (Figure 12.3). A *closed system* is defined as a "process system that is designed and operated such that the product is never exposed to the surrounding environment" [4]. When biomanufacturing is executed entirely in closed systems with material transfers performed in a completely closed fashion, a less stringent area classification may be employed.

Many bioprocess systems are routinely opened to prepare the equipment for processing, and then rendered closed through a validated cleaning and sanitization or sterilization step before process use. Such process systems are frequently referred to as functionally closed [5]. In some briefly exposed operations, such as buffer and media preparation, material is initially processed in an open bioburden-controlled environment and then rendered closed for subsequent process operations (Figure 12.4).

DEFINITIONS

An understanding of the contamination control terminology used to describe bioprocessing operations is critical to identify the design requirements for a biotechnology facility. Conversely, an incomplete understanding of these terms can result in facility features that are either inadequate or unnecessary. Even within the biotech industry, the terminology can be confusing. For example, some operations are described as *sterile* or *sterilized*; these terms do not, in this context, refer to the complete absence of life. In practice, the process of rendering something sterile, or *sterilization*,

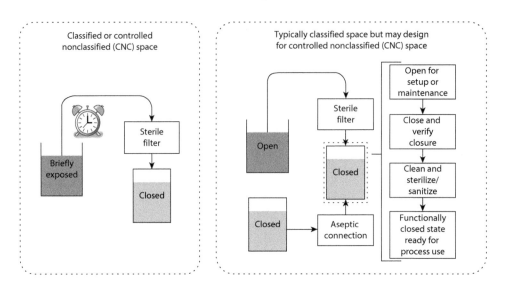

FIGURE 12.4 Briefly exposed and functionally closed processing.

refers to a condition where the probability of remaining bioburden (i.e., number of viable contaminating microorganisms present) is statistically insignificant. Most bioprocessing unit operations are bioburden controlled but not truly sterile. Often, the sterilization of equipment is used to assist in bioburden control.

The most accurate term for describing bioburden-free operations in biotechnology facilities is *aseptic*. Aseptic operations are considered devoid of detectable bioburden. Processing in bioreactors is occasionally described as aseptic but is more accurately described as *axenic*. The term *axenic* refers to a culture that contains a single strain of living organism (as intended in a bioreactor) but is entirely free of all other contaminating organisms.

The manufacture of drug substances from living organisms is often referred to as *bioprocessing*. Bioprocessing requires clean manufacturing under conditions of low bioburden. The term *hygienic*, as used in the biopharmaceutical industry, refers specifically to the maintenance of cleanliness so that the product does not adversely affect human health.

BIOTECHNOLOGY FACILITY DESIGN

A proper approach for biotechnology facility design starts with a thorough understanding of the manufacturing process (i.e., the process flow, the timing of operations, and the equipment and utilities that are required). From this foundation, designers can proceed with architectural programming, including adjacencies and transitioning to cGMP areas, to lay out the facility.

PRODUCTION SYSTEMS

The user requirements for biotechnology facilities are heavily influenced by the type of product (e.g., protein therapeutics, mAbs, vaccines, gene therapy, or stem cells), the propagation system (i.e., host microorganism used to produce product), and the final dosage form. Most biopharmaceutical products are delivered as a parenteral (i.e., injectable) dosage form, whereby the drug is injected directly into the bloodstream; thus, the level of contamination prevention and bioburden control required is much more stringent than that required for oral or topical dosage forms. Bioburden is a particular issue with injectable drugs for the following three key reasons:

- *Endotoxins* created by Gram-negative microbial contaminates can elicit an immune response with unwanted side effects (e.g., inflammation, fever, internal bleeding, and septic shock).
- *Exotoxins* from environmental bacteria, which are not routinely monitored, can cause cell culture death and are highly toxic to humans in small quantities.
- Bacterial action on the product may cause unwanted variants by clipping protein chains or changing the glycosylation pattern (neither of which may be readily detectable by analytical testing).

Product contamination can come from airborne particulates, raw materials, utility systems, product contact materials, and other products manufactured in the same facility. Therefore, the prevention of product contamination is the predominant principle driving every aspect in the design process of biotech facilities.

Biopharmaceutical products are diverse and are produced by a variety of methods. Therapeutic proteins and mAbs are typically produced by microbial or cell culture propagation systems. The first commercial biopharmaceutical products used microbial fermentation (e.g., bacteria, yeast, and fungi) for protein production. These simple and fast-growing production systems produce a high yield, but usually have the disadvantage of intracellular product expression. Since in this case the product is produced inside the cells, the cells must be lysed (i.e., ruptured) as part of the manufacturing process to release the protein being produced. Unfortunately, this process also releases cell debris from the host cell, which requires relatively extensive purification to reduce impurities to safe levels in the bulk product. A cell culture production system, on the other hand, has the advantage of extracellular expression. During cell culture, product expression is by secretion of protein through the cell wall. Instead of lysing the cells to harvest product, the product is drawn from the media surrounding the cells. This significantly simplifies the process purification requirements. In addition, cell culture is capable of producing the biologically active pharmaceutical ingredient (API) in a form that is more usable by the human body, which also simplifies downstream processing and improves product potency. Cell culture production systems are usually based on mammalian cell lines, such as Chinese hamster ovary (CHO) and hybridoma cells, although some cultures use insect or plant cells. Both microbial and cell culture protein production systems are in common use today, although microbial propagation systems are best employed for production of simple proteins that do not require significant posttranslational modifications to activate the product. This discussion is relevant to the topic of biotechnology facility design because the choice of propagation system has a significant impact on the manufacturing process, which, in turn, affects the equipment requirements, process utilities, area classification, flows, and space planning for the facility.

Vaccine manufacturing, originally produced from live animals or fertilized eggs (Figure 12.5), involves the production of an antigen that triggers an immune response in the patient. Today these products are also manufactured using microbial and cell culture production platforms. The method of production has a huge impact on facility design, particularly if the manufacturing process uses live viruses, which must be processed in a segregated area.

BIOPROCESS MANUFACTURING OPERATIONS

In comparison with other chemical process industries, unit operations for biologics manufacturing are typically executed on a relatively small scale. Following the commercialization of blockbuster drugs in the first couple of decades after the introduction of recombinant DNA technology, biopharmaceutical manufacturers became increasingly reliant on product portfolios that include drugs for

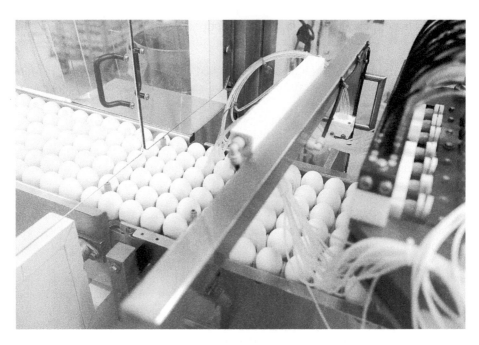

FIGURE 12.5 Flu vaccine production: eggs being inoculated with the seed virus (Val de Reuil, France, March 2009). (Courtesy of Vincent Moncorgé; copyright Sanofi Pasteur, Lyon, France.)

small patient populations (requiring small volumes of product per batch). In addition, optimized biomanufacturing has yielded improvements in the process titer over the past decade, further reducing the manufacturing scale required for many high-value biologics.

Batch processing has historically dominated biotechnology manufacturing because of available technologies, risk aversion, and perceived regulatory difficulties associated with continuous manufacturing. The industry typically relied on existing batch technology to provide a safe and reliable process. However, emerging technology has opened up many options to make continuous processing more feasible in drug manufacturing. Bioprocess development for future facilities is expected to make greater use of continuous processing to enable more efficient manufacturing on a small scale.

As bioprocessing is a wet operation requiring frequent cleaning, cGMP bioprocess equipment is typically designed and constructed in a manner that facilitates external cleaning and sanitization. Likewise, the manufacturing areas that are designed to accommodate surface cleaning and the occasional spill typically have a floor drain, berm, or other architectural feature designed to collect fluids. Most bioprocess unit operations are aqueous processes, although small quantities of solvents may be used for downstream processing (e.g., organic solvents in operating buffers for some chromatography steps), which may require explosion-proof areas designed to handle flammables and combustibles safely.

Biotechnology manufacturing operations are typically categorized as *upstream* or *downstream* processes (Figure 12.6). Upstream bioprocessing refers to all of the manufacturing processes required to produce the biological APIs, including inoculum preparation, bioconversion (via fermentation or cell culture), and harvest steps (via centrifugation or filtration). Downstream bioprocessing refers to all of the processing required for the API to meet purity and quality requirements, including product recovery, purification, and polishing steps (via chromatography and filtration). After downstream processing, the purified drug substance is formulated (sometimes also conjugated) and filled into a bulk container for storage in a stable form. Upstream, downstream, and bulk filling processes are all supported by ancillary manufacturing activities, including weigh and dispense, media preparation,

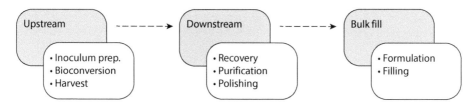

FIGURE 12.6 Typical biotechnology manufacturing operations.

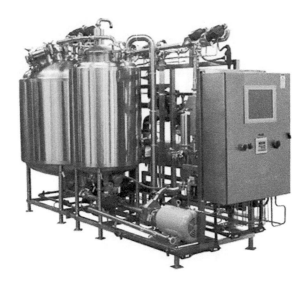

FIGURE 12.7 Typical central CIP system. (Courtesy of Sani-Matic, Inc., Madison, WI.)

buffer preparation, sterilization, and part washing operations. Refer to the Appendix for a more detailed discussion of bioprocess unit operations and their relevance to good design practice for biotechnology facilities.

Equipment Cleaning and Bioburden Control

Traditional biomanufacturing in stainless steel equipment requires facility infrastructure for cleaning and sterilization. Centralized clean-in-place (CIP) systems (Figure 12.7) are designed to prepare and distribute cleaning solutions throughout the plant to facilitate cleaning of equipment *in situ*. These systems are typically designed to recirculate cleaning solutions through the product contact areas of the process equipment, although single-pass systems may be required for cleaning areas with potential biohazard exposure. The design of distribution loops for CIP is critical because it requires piping that is correctly sloped and free of dead legs (i.e., pockets with stagnant areas). The CIP rinsing operations are typically the largest user of compendial water in a facility, so system drainability and minimizing holdup are important for economical and sustainable water use. This places some constraints on facility design, whereby it is often desirable to locate CIP systems in mechanical space near the equipment to be cleaned. In multilevel facilities, it may be advantageous to locate CIP areas in the space above or below the process to facilitate the drainability of distribution piping. For some small bioprocess systems, cleaning may be accomplished with temporary connections to portable CIP systems (Figure 12.8) or through disassembly and cleaning-out-of-place (COP) (Figure 12.9).

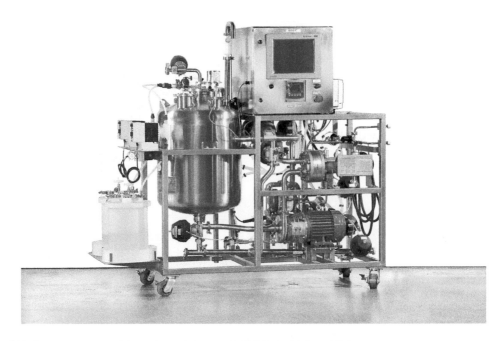

FIGURE 12.8 Portable CIP station. (Courtesy of ABEC, Bethlehem, PA.)

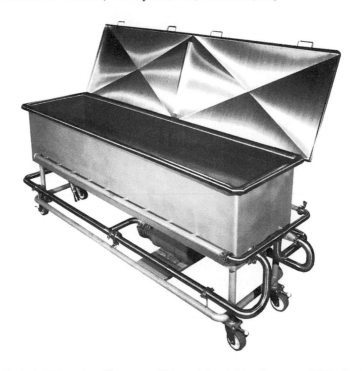

FIGURE 12.9 Typical COP station. (Courtesy of Electrol Specialties Company (ESC), South Beloit, IL.)

The number of CIP systems required for biomanufacturing is determined by production timing and process segregation requirements. As CIP systems can be a source of cross-contamination, separate systems are typically used for buffer or media preparation and upstream and downstream operations. Further process segregation may be required as determined by QRM assessment.

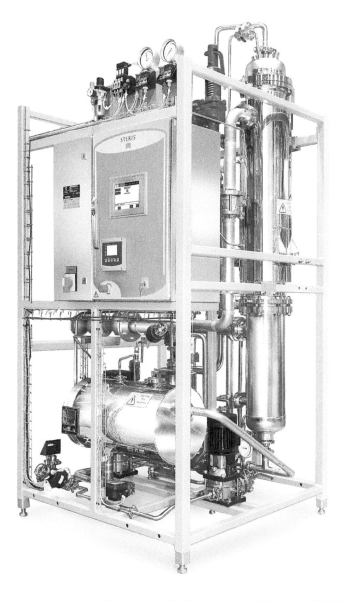

FIGURE 12.10 Pure steam generator without steam distribution piping. (Courtesy of STERIS FINN-AQUA, Tuusula, Finland.)

For equipment sterilization or sanitization, centralized clean steam systems (Figure 12.10) are typically connected directly to process equipment for automated steam-in-place (SIP) operations. In addition, SIP and CIP stations may be required to make temporary connections to mobile tanks or process systems for equipment sanitization, sterilization, or cleaning.

SINGLE-USE TECHNOLOGY

Single-use technology may be used for biomanufacturing in which materials in contact with the process are discarded after processing. This technology uses gamma-irradiated bags, connectors (Figure 12.11), and tubing (Figure 12.12) to enable aseptic closed processing without CIP or SIP requirements (Figure 12.13). The capital equipment investment for SUS is less than that for comparable stainless steel systems, but operating costs for consumable supplies and waste disposal are higher.

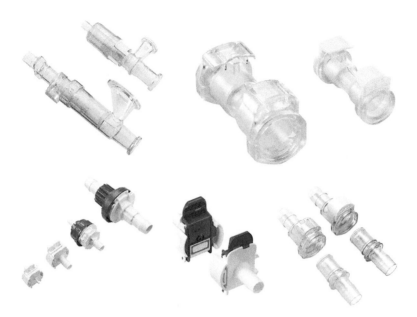

FIGURE 12.11   Typical single-use connectors: upper left, MPX quick connect; upper right, connected MPX connectors; lower left, aseptic connector family; lower middle, unconnected genderless aseptic connector pair; lower right, steam-through connectors. (Courtesy of Colder Products Company, St. Paul, MN.)

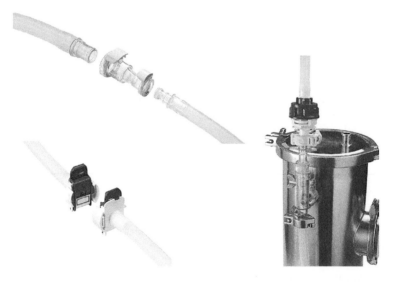

FIGURE 12.12   Tubing and attachments are critical aspects of single-use technologies: upper left, MPX and MPC quick connectors with tubing; upper right, aseptic quick and steam-through connectors connected to a tank assembly; and lower left, unconnected genderless septic connector pair with tubing. (Courtesy of Colder Products Company, St. Paul, MN.)

If single-use technology is deployed extensively in a facility, a significant reduction or elimination of CIP or SIP infrastructure requirements may be possible. Relative to traditional facilities that use stainless steel tanks and process piping, SUS technology also provides the advantages of faster turnaround times for process systems (increasing throughput), a reduction in compendial water and waste neutralization requirements, and greater process flexibility for multiproduct manufacturing. In addition, single-use technology may be used to simplify and facilitate closure of a process, thereby

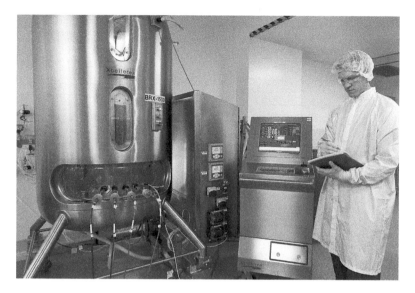

FIGURE 12.13   Aseptic closed processing with single-use or disposable technology. (Courtesy of FUJIFILM Diosynth Biotechnologies, Morrisville, NC.)

reducing facility segregation requirements and enabling manufacturing in controlled nonclassified (CNC) space or areas of lower classification. Reported benefits of this approach include a reduction in manufacturing area requirements by 15%–30%, a reduction in clean utility requirements by 80%–90%, and reductions in steam and chilled water requirements by up to 60% [6].

Single-use solutions are commercially available for almost every step in biomanufacturing (excluding only unit operations that require pressure or temperature extremes or handling of organic solvents). Manufacturing with SUS requires a commitment to robust supply train management to ensure the consistent quality of consumables (Figure 12.14). The handling for installation and removal of bioprocess bags is also critical to maintaining the integrity of SUS. Facilities that make extensive use of SUS will require additional space for controlled-environment storage and staging of consumables, as well as collection and disposal of disposables after use. Areas that use SUS in contact with biohazardous materials may require a decontamination autoclave to process disposable waste before it can be removed from classified space.

The application of SUS is limited by process scale. Manually installing and removing large bags, particularly when wet, is generally very difficult above a 2,000 L scale. Likewise, it is difficult to safely move materials in bags greater than 500 L due to limitations associated with the weight of materials being manually manipulated. Larger mobile containers are available, but they may require the use of motorized pallet jacks for safe handling. There are also limitations to the size of commercially available process transfer tubing that can facilitate aseptic connections.

Process suites designed for flexible use of mobile SUS may provide ceiling-mounted utility panels to facilitate easy connections to electrical power and process utilities at multiple stations within the processing area. The facility layout should take into account the most likely combinations of equipment arrangements and ensure that there is adequate space for the staging of material transfer bags. Equipment arrangements and adjacencies should also minimize the length of transfer tubing required between unit operations.

Product Transfer

The method of material transfer in a bioprocess facility has a large impact on its design. In production-scale facilities with hard-piped product transfer, a large network of highly automated

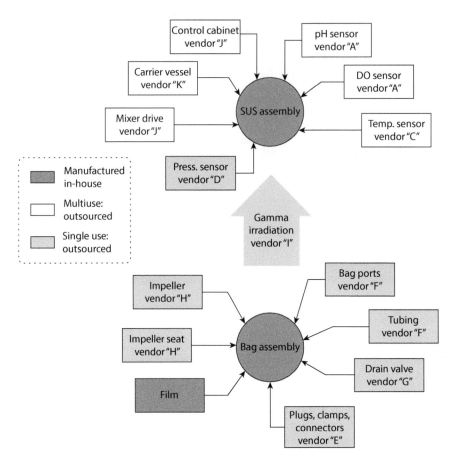

FIGURE 12.14 Typical SUS supply chain based on a single-use bioreactor example. Note that the out-sourced components usually are from multiple vendors and manufacturers.

process piping, requiring SIP and CIP, is needed. This may require a complex system of transfer panels and automated valve clusters for routing and isolation of process fluids. The impact on facility architecture and mechanical space requirements can be significant. Therefore, front-end process design is a critical component of space programming.

Facilities that rely heavily on single-use technology may eliminate much of the process piping infrastructure in a facility, but instead bring a relatively larger impact on loading docks, storage, and material transfer areas of the facility. Aseptic connections with single-use tubing are typically accomplished via a sterile tube welder or aseptic disposable connector. Material transfer between processing areas is usually executed by manual manipulation of mobile bag containers through airlocks and hallways, so the traffic in these areas may require additional consideration.

Where large volumes of process fluids are transferred between unit operations via disposable tubing, consideration should be given to the routing and support of flexible tube lines. The flexible tubing interconnecting SUS can create contamination and personnel safety issues if allowed to rest unsupported along the floor. The provision of cleanable racks or hangers to support flexible tubing is a good design practice. These may be mounted to the walls or ceiling to facilitate tubing support overhead. If disposable tubing is used to pass fluids between classified areas (e.g., bioreactor media charging), a sealed "mouse hole" or clean room pass-through system will be needed to feed the tube through the wall of an adjacent classified area.

PROCESS AUTOMATION

At the unit operation level, most process automation applications for batch processes are not complex. Automated system reliability and the integrity of data captured for the batch record are of paramount importance for cGMP manufacturing. This requires an automation development process that is highly structured, well documented, and validatable. Beyond the rock-solid robustness that is required for all cGMP pharmaceutical manufacturing operations, process analytical technology (PAT) is recommended by regulatory authorities to provide "a system for designing, analyzing, and controlling manufacturing through timely measurements (i.e., during processing) of critical quality and performance attributes of raw and in-process materials and processes, with the goal of ensuring final product quality" [7].

Bioreactor control systems present one of the more difficult bioprocess automation challenges because batch automation is required to accommodate a large load variance throughout the culture life cycle, from lag phase through exponential growth. Control parameters may be adjusted, according to bioreactor growth phase, by using time profiles or adaptive control to adjust for the anticipated growth curve and inherent variability of living organisms.

The next level up from basic process automation of unit operations is supervisory control and data acquisition (SCADA). The SCADA system provides a method to access equipment status, ongoing operations, and process variables for the entire manufacturing process. Human–machine interface (HMI) stations may be provided within clean manufacturing space to allow operators SCADA access to view and control local operations, as well as critical utilities and processes in other manufacturing areas. Since access to clean room areas is restricted and requires special gowning, control rooms are typically provided for personnel to view the process, respond to alarms, and access the SCADA data historian.

In traditional biomanufacturing facilities, the most challenging automation requirements usually come from the need for precision control of the sequential steps required for CIP and SIP of process systems. These automated operations require the concurrent, coordinated control of multiple unit operations and must mediate the usage of shared CIP systems and transfer lines. CIP and SIP automation can provide a safe and highly reliable cleaning and bioburden reduction capability with very little manual intervention.

Single-use systems require far less plant automation because the cleaning and sterilization of product contact services are essentially outsourced to the SUS vendor. However, the performance and reliability of these systems are far more dependent on manual manipulations (see Figures 12.11 and 12.12). In such facilities, the manipulation of SUS is a key component of the operator training program. Further risk reduction can be provided through automated materials tracking and tracing, including the many disposable components that are required for the SUS manufacturing process. Manufacturing execution systems (MESs) are the next level above SCADA and typically provide this function.

Process automation is a key enabler of continuous bioprocessing in regulated biotechnology facilities. Continuous processing in a cGMP manufacturing environment requires continuous monitoring and PAT, which enable parametric release. Parametric release (real-time release) is a quality assurance release program where demonstrated control of the process enables a firm to use defined critical process controls, in lieu of final quality control testing, to fulfill the intent of regulatory release requirements, such as 21 CFR §211.165 and §211.167. Essentially, PAT provides continuous assurance that a process is working correctly and that the product is of the right quality throughout the process.

PROCESS UTILITIES

The process utilities used in a biotechnology facility include general plant utilities, such as plant steam, chilled water, and compressed air, as well as clean utilities, such as compendial water, clean steam, and clean gas systems. The QRM method requires a criticality assessment of process utilities as part of facility design to identify the impact of utility systems on product quality. The reliability of process utility systems in cGMP biotechnology facilities can be every bit as critical as that of the process equipment for unit operations. Fermentation and cell culture operations can require sustained utility services for days, weeks, or months at a time. Therefore, system reliability, equipment redundancy, and ease of maintenance are key considerations during system design to mitigate the risk of failure and its impact on the product being produced. Biotechnology facilities are typically designed with backup electrical and mechanical systems for this reason (e.g., uninterruptible power supply [UPS] power, backup generators, redundant pumps, redundant boilers, and air compressors).

As cGMP biotechnology facilities typically produce parenteral products, the clean utility systems that have a direct path to product contact surfaces or that have the potential to come into direct contact with the product must be designed to operate free of contaminates that could be carried into the product stream. These systems are typically designed for sampling at use points to verify the consistent quality of clean utilities supporting the process. Unless the process is small enough to be supported by outsourced compendial water supplies, a utility system is typically required to generate, store, and distribute water for injection (WFI) for process formulation and for equipment and parts' final rinse during cleaning.

Biomanufacturing Area Requirements

Biotechnology facilities have distinctive areas for manufacturing and manufacturing support that can be characterized in terms of function, adjacencies, and typical user requirements (Figure 12.15). Depending on the spatial segregation and environmental requirements of the process, each of these areas may represent a separate room or, under certain conditions, several operational areas within a room. Typical operational areas for biomanufacturing are described in Table 12.2.

In addition to the core manufacturing areas typical to biotechnology facilities, several manufacturing support areas are necessary for cGMP operations. These are summarized in Table 12.3.

Facility Space Programming

Programming is a systematic process for decision making about organization and project values, goals, and requirements [8]. This is the process whereby required facility spaces are identified, and the size and relationships between these spaces are established.

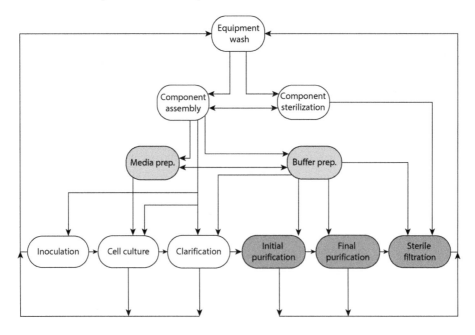

FIGURE 12.15 Overview of typical area adjacencies for biotechnology manufacturing.

TABLE 12.2
Biomanufacturing Area Requirements

Operational Area	Description	Adjacencies and User Requirements
Media preparation	Area where media (cell food) for the growth of cells is mixed and formulated.	Adjacencies: upstream processing. May require dust collection for open operations.
Buffer preparation	Area where buffer solutions are mixed, formulated, and staged for the purification process.	Adjacencies: downstream processing. May require dust collection for open operations.
Inoculum preparation	Provides benchtop equipment, BSC, freezer, and incubators to grow cells from a small frozen vial to a volume sufficient to inoculate a bioreactor.	Adjacencies: upstream processing. Typically classified space with ISO 5 BSC and ISO 7 background for axenic open process operations.
Upstream processing (cell culture and fermentation)	Area where cell material is grown to a targeted volume and concentration (titer). This area contains a seed train of progressively large-sized bioreactors plus full-scale production bioreactors.	Adjacencies: media preparation, inoculum preparation, cell separation. Typically ISO 8 or CNC space with process utilities supporting bioreactors.
Cell separation	Area where cellular material is separated from product. Frequently combined in same room as upstream processing. This area contains harvest equipment and clarified product-hold vessel.	Adjacencies: upstream processing, downstream processing. Segregated space with sound attenuation may be required for homogenization or centrifugation.
Downstream processing	Area where harvested material from cell separation is processed; involves multiple process steps for clarification, recovery, purification, and polishing operations (e.g., filtration, chromatography).	Adjacencies: cell separation, final purification, buffer preparation. Typically flexible classified space. May require segregated area for virus removal/inactivation before final purification.
Final purification	Area where final material is purified and transferred into bulk containers. Last step in drug substance manufacturing.	Adjacencies: downstream processing. May require classified space with ISO 5 BSC and ISO 7 background for aseptic open process operations.

TABLE 12.3

Manufacturing Support Area Requirements

Operational Area	Description	Adjacencies and User Requirements
Locker rooms	Area where personnel change from street clothes into low-lint scrubs to mitigate clean room contamination from operations staff.	Adjacencies: access and return corridors; close to manufacturing areas but not inside classified space. Typically, men's and women's locker rooms are provided with toilet and shower facilities.
Cleaning supply	A janitor's closet where cleaning and disinfectant supplies are kept.	Adjacencies: near area exit. Typically provided with potable water supply.
Returned equipment	Area where equipment used in manufacturing is returned for cleaning and sanitization.	Adjacencies: equipment preparation (and part washer), close to manufacturing areas.
Equipment preparation	Area where parts are unloaded from a part washer and typically assembled or placed in a clean bag in preparation for autoclaving.	Adjacencies: returned equipment, equipment staging. A local protection area is usually provided to keep parts free of particulates.
Equipment staging	Temporary storage area for equipment that has been autoclaved and staged until ready for reuse in manufacturing.	Adjacencies: equipment preparation. A local protection area is usually provided to prevent particulate contamination of parts as they cool down after autoclaving.
Column packing	Area where chromatography columns are prepared by transferring resin into a vertical pressure container (column).	Adjacencies: downstream processing. Typically classified space. May not be required if prepacked columns are used.
Cold room	Area for storage of processing intermediates. Occasionally purification steps may need to be executed in a cold environment.	Adjacencies: close to manufacturing. Typical environment validated for 2°C–8°C.
Freezer room	Area for dedicated product freezers.	Adjacencies: close to manufacturing.

(Continued)

TABLE 12.3 (Continued)
Manufacturing Support Area Requirements

Operational Area	Description	Adjacencies and User Requirements
Cell banking	Areas for master cell bank and working cell banks.	Adjacencies: none. Typically alarmed storage freezers, backup power supply.
Warehouse	Area for storage of raw material, intermediates, final products, and consumables.	Adjacencies: loading dock. Unclassified space with temperature, humidity, and access controls. Contains raw material receiving and sampling areas and segregated quarantined and released materials.
Weigh/dispense	Area for dispensing measured raw materials for manufacturing; often assembled in single-use kits for protection from contamination.	Adjacencies: warehouse. May require local protection area and dust collection for open operations.
QC laboratory	Area for processing samples for chemical/physical assays and microbiological assays (including EM and validation samples).	Adjacencies: none. Requires sample receiving and cold storage space. Typically contains segregated chemistry lab (with fume hoods) and microbiological lab (with BSC and incubators), both supported by autoclave, glass washer, purified water, and laboratory gases.
Document control	An administrative area for storage, review, and approval of new and executed QA documents.	Adjacencies: none. A secure and fireproof space for storage of master documents is required.
Maintenance and metrology	Areas for storage of spare parts, tools, and instruments, as well as bench calibration and repair activities.	Adjacencies: none.
Analytical support	Area for in-process testing by production staff.	Adjacencies: close to manufacturing.
Personnel support	Area for operations staff to gather for breaks, meetings, and computer access.	Adjacencies: none. Nonclassified space outside the gowned area.

Note: EM, environmental monitoring; QC, quality control; QA, quality assurance.

In cGMP biotechnology facilities, the manufacturing and regulatory requirements should always drive the space program. The starting point is the process. The manufacturing process must first be developed and documented at production scale with a process flow diagram (PFD) and mass balance. At this stage, an approach to risk-based process segregation needs to be developed to determine the philosophy of spatial separation required between manufacturing operations. This approach should consider both the risk of product contamination and safety risks from hazardous materials.

Process Segregation

Process segregation within biopharmaceutical facilities may include

- Segregation from environment
- Segregation from personnel
- Segregation by product
- Segregation by batch
- Segregation of concurrent operations
- Segregation of operations containing viable microorganisms
- Segregation between unit operations before and after virus removal or inactivation steps

The facility's process segregation approach determines where operational areas can be combined, and how people, materials, and equipment should flow through the facility (Figures 12.16 and 12.17). It also determines the personnel gowning requirements and procedures for concurrent and sequential operations.

The rationale and methods of process segregation are summarized in Table 12.4.

Area Adjacencies

Physical segregation in biotechnology facilities is typically developed using bubble diagrams to identify the discrete spaces required and their relationship to each other. These developmental

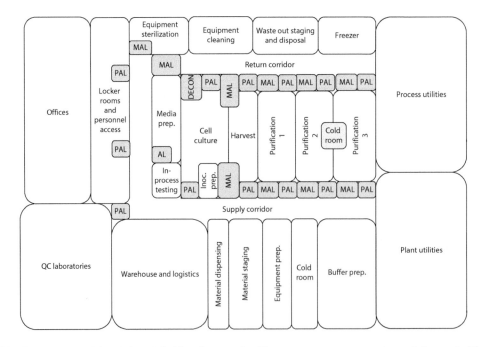

FIGURE 12.16 Traditional biotech facility diagram that illustrates process segregation, relying on facility or area environmental clean room classifications to protect the product.

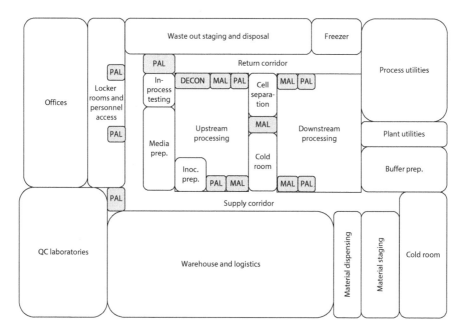

FIGURE 12.17 Ballroom biotech facility diagram that illustrates process segregation, relying on equipment or closed process systems to protect the product (note the consolidation of operational areas relative to the traditional layout relying on facility segregation).

diagrams are used to represent the program areas, their adjacencies, and clean room classification as determined by the risk-based process segregation philosophy of the facility. This is a critical stage in the design development of the facility because it has a direct impact on process contamination control and regulatory compliance. Once the area adjacencies are established, these diagrams can be used to illustrate room pressurization (relative to adjacent rooms) and the flow of personnel, equipment, materials, and waste through the facility (transition diagrams).

cGMP Area Transitioning

Spatial segregation within the facility is maintained by controlling the flow of people, material, and equipment through the facility. An assessment of contamination risk should drive the selection of clean space classification for each cGMP operational area. Particular attention should be given to the means of transitioning between areas of different classification. Airlocks (small intermediate rooms with interlocked doors) are used to maintain area classification by allowing people, material, and equipment to transition to a different classified space without disrupting the room pressurization. As gowning locker rooms, access and egress hallways, personnel airlocks, equipment airlocks, and material pass-through chambers are all required for cGMP area transitioning, these areas are a critical component of the programmed space for a biopharmaceutical facility and should be detailed on transition diagrams.

Area Sizing

In biotechnology facilities, the sizing of manufacturing space is driven by the sizing and selection of process equipment, in conjunction with an analysis of the staging space required to support materials for unit operations and process hold points. The PFD and mass balance are used to size and select the process equipment that will be installed in each room, taking into account requirements for throughput, number of batches, shift schedules, and so on. A major equipment list and utility matrix are developed to identify the requirements for facility integration with bioprocessing operations. These requirements are frequently documented on a *room card*, which illustrates the equipment footprint, area layout, and utility requirements for each space.

TABLE 12.4
Process Segregation Rationale and Methods

Type of Segregation	Rationale	Method
Segregation from the environment	Environmental particulates and bioburden can contaminate the manufacturing process.	Closed processing and/or clean rooms with HEPA filters and EM for nonviable particulates and microorganisms.
Segregation from personnel	People are the most common source of process contamination. May be required for handling low OEL materials, such as biohazards, cytotoxins, and potent compounds.	Closed process equipment, isolators, clean room gowning, and BSCs are used to isolate operating personnel from the process.
Segregation between products	Required to prevent mix-ups and cross-contamination between different products or their product intermediates; product segregation is particularly important for QRM when processing live virus vaccines and other processes involving infectious microorganisms.	Temporal (time-based) segregation, with decontamination and cleaning of process suites and equipment between production campaigns. Physical (spatial) segregation through clean space with segregated HEPA filtration and segregated flow of materials, people, and equipment.
Segregation by batch	Segregation is required to prevent carryover from one product to the next product or between subsequent batches of the same product.	Procedural, including cleaning and sanitization of the process suite between batches, including product contact process systems and centralized CIP systems. CIP and SIP of process contact surfaces on equipment, or use of SUS.
Segregation between concurrent operations	Required to prevent crossover from one operation to another operation in the same manufacturing process.	Isolated process systems, using piping panels or double-block and bleed piping arrangements (e.g., CIP distribution). Physical (spatial) segregation through clean space with segregated HEPA filtration and segregated flow of materials, people, and equipment.
Segregation of unit operations containing viable microorganisms	Required to isolate cell-containing from cell-free unit operations; the product must be separated from the live microbiological culture that produced it.	Closed processing or clean room segregation; upstream and downstream unit operations are traditionally located in segregated processing areas and serviced by separate HVAC and CIP systems.
Segregation between unit operations before and after virus removal/inactivation steps	Required to protect bulk product from viral contamination after virus inactivation/removal steps.	Closed processing or clean room segregation; previrus and postvirus reduced unit operations are typically located in segregated processing areas and serviced by separate HVAC and CIP systems.

Note: HEPA, high-efficiency particulate air; OEL, occupational exposure limit; HVAC, heating, ventilation, and air conditioning.

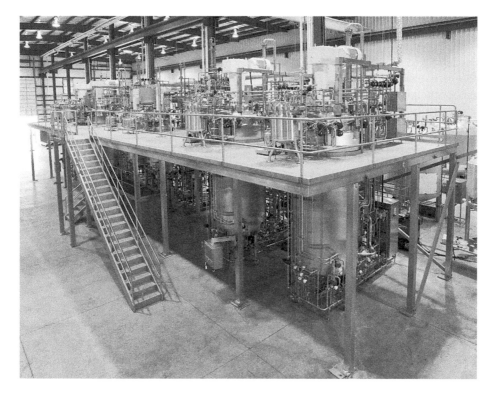

FIGURE 12.18   A 20,000 L insulin fermentation train under construction with mezzanine access. (Courtesy of ABEC, Bethlehem, PA.)

When developing the equipment layout, particular attention should be given to the arrangement and adjacencies of process systems to facilitate an orderly flow of materials, as well as access requirements for operations and maintenance. Some large-scale bioprocessing equipment requires platform or mezzanine access (Figure 12.18) and may be positioned so that part of the equipment may be located adjacent to unclassified gray space to minimize the equipment footprint in the clean room.

Mobile tanks and disposable bag totes are frequently used to transfer material into a manufacturing suite, so adequate consideration should be given to the area staging of material and waste required for bioprocessing. This may require the development of a dynamic process model to simulate the flow and accumulation of mobile containers and other manufacturing material. Material staging requirements can be particularly challenging in perfusion culture, tangential flow filtration (TFF), and chromatography unit operations. Adequate consideration should be given to the segregated staging of clean and dirty equipment in part washing and autoclave areas.

Building Systems

Many biomanufacturing processes require continuous operation for several days or weeks at a time. This requires a building infrastructure that is designed to support these operations without interruption. The building should be designed for generator and UPS backup of power to critical process systems; process utilities; clean room heating, ventilating, and air conditioning (HVAC) systems; and cold room, refrigerator, and freezer equipment containing valuable process materials. Critical building systems are commonly alarmed to provide critical notification and interlocks in the event of power or mechanical failure. These are typically connected to a computer-based control system or building automation system (BAS) to control and monitor the building's mechanical and electrical equipment, such as ventilation, lighting, power systems, fire systems, and security systems.

SUSTAINABILITY

Clean room operations are energy-intensive, so a focus on the facility programming and mechanical systems associated with classified space is a good place to start a sustainability initiative. Anything that can be done to reduce the size or classification level of manufacturing space reduces energy consumption and operating costs. As personnel are typically the primary generators of particulates in clean space, classified space can also be programmed for reduced air exchange rates during unoccupied periods.

Compendial water generation, such as WFI, is another energy-intensive operation. As the biggest consumer of compendial water in biopharmaceutical facilities is typically equipment cleaning, the development of optimized CIP cycles can substantially reduce water consumption and energy costs.

The SUS technology employed in modern biomanufacturing is a source of biowaste in the form of disposables that may require special handling and decontamination. In some cases, it may be possible to recycle this material or use it as fuel for cogeneration power. However, the sustainability of single-use technology should be evaluated on balance with full consideration of the potential benefits in terms of reduced classified space requirements and clean utility utilization.

IMPLICATIONS FOR PERFORMANCE AND COMPLIANCE

REGULATORY COMPLIANCE OVERVIEW

Regulatory authorities generally recognize that the manufacturing processes for biological products warrant "special treatment because of their distinct characteristics, such as their complex structures and susceptibility to variation during manufacturing" [9]. Thus, biotechnology facilities manufacturing drug substances are subject to some regulatory requirements that specifically address the challenges associated with biomanufacturing.

The regulation of biologically derived products was initiated in the United States by the 1902 Biologics Control Act, which required the licensure of facilities manufacturing these products. This law gave the FDA regulatory authority to ensure the safety and efficacy of biologics, that is, "medical products, such as vaccines, blood and blood derivatives, allergenic patch tests and extracts, HIV and hepatitis tests, gene therapy products, cells and tissues for transplantation, and new treatments for cancers, arthritis, and other serious diseases" [10].

The European Union (EU) also has special requirements for biotechnology products, which require a thorough description of the manufacturing process, including manufacturing facilities and equipment (see Annex I, Section 3.2.1.2 of [10]). The European Medicines Agency (EMA) specifically addresses biological products in Annex 2 to the EU GMP guidelines.

Increasingly, the cGMP requirements of the United States, EU, and other worldwide regulatory agencies are moving toward a more harmonized approach to international compliance. Notable initiatives toward global cGMP harmonization have been led by

- The International Conference on Harmonisation (ICH) of Technical Requirements for Registration of Pharmaceuticals for Human Use
- The Pharmaceutical Inspection Convention and Pharmaceutical Inspection Co-operation Scheme (jointly referred to as PIC/S)

CONTAMINATION PREVENTION

The design of biotechnology facilities, utilities, and equipment must take into account the risk of product contamination. This is of paramount importance, particularly in licensed multiproduct biopharmaceutical facilities, because of regulatory requirements for the safety and purity of the product. Product quality may be ensured by identifying the potential sources of product contamination and designing facility, equipment, and procedural controls to mitigate the risk at the source. Typical contamination sources and risk mitigation mechanisms in cGMP facilities are listed in Table 12.5.

TABLE 12.5

Typical Contamination Sources and Risk Mitigation Methods

Contamination Source	Risk Controlled By
Raw materials and process intermediates	Supplier certification, quality sampling and inspection, and controlled cGMP storage
Airborne viable and nonviable particulates	Closed process systems and HEPA-filtered clean rooms and isolators with environmental monitoring for particulates and viable microorganisms
Process utilities and waste systems	Clean utilities designed for low bioburden, quality sampling and inspection, and backflow prevention
Equipment, piping, and instrumentation	Materials of construction for process contact are designed and qualified for resistance to corrosion and particle shedding
single-use materials in product contact	Disposable materials sourced from a qualified supply chain with quality control of bioburden, particulates, leachables, and extractables (typically manufactured in a clean environment and UV irradiated); also must be free from animal-derived components
Crossover from concurrent operations	Facility and equipment segregated by design from concurrent operations
Carryover from prior operations	Qualified and validated cleaning and bioburden reduction processes (e.g., CIP and SIP); changeover procedures
Manufacturing and maintenance personnel	Closed process systems and personnel gowning and procedural controls
Rodents, insects, and other pests	Provisions for pest control, including detection and elimination of animal contamination sources

In general, contamination prevention requires a method to maintain segregation between the process and potential contamination sources. The most reliable means of segregation is through closed processing, whereby equipment is used to create and maintain a sealed process environment completely separate from potential contaminates in the room environment, including operators and airborne particulates.

CLOSURE ANALYSIS

As discussed in earlier sections of this chapter, closed processing provides greater flexibility when programming area classifications within a biopharmaceutical facility by placing the primary barrier for contamination prevention at the equipment level. However, successful implementation of a contamination-controlled biomanufacturing process requires a systematic means of evaluating closure requirements at each step of the process.

Closure analysis is a risk-based approach to evaluating the adequacy of process closure throughout the entire drug substance manufacturing process [11]. This takes into account the level of bioburden control required at each step, the presence of mitigating downstream operations (e.g., purification and sterile filtration), and the environmental controls in the manufacturing area. The scope of closure analysis should include all bioprocess unit operations, buffer and media preparation, clean utilities, intermediate process pooling, and transfers between unit operations. For each unit operation, the closure boundary must be established and each step of the operation evaluated. Closure analysis is intended to ensure that appropriate procedures, process systems, and environmental controls are provided to prevent contamination that may adulterate the product.

It is important to recognize that the mechanisms for process closure must be validated and maintained to support cGMP operations. This becomes an integral part of the manufacturer's quality management system. Functionally closed process systems require media challenge testing as part of their performance qualification and frequently incorporate integrity testing as part of normal operations to verify that process closure is established before exposure to the product. In addition, standard operating procedures should be in place to handle a breach of process closure, including procedures for decontamination and equipment return to its operational state.

PROCESS CONTAINMENT

Process contamination prevention should not be confused with process containment, although closure analysis may be required to address both issues. Some biopharmaceutical products are cytotoxic or highly potent compounds that present a significant safety risk to personnel. In addition, biotechnology facilities may be required to process live microorganisms that have the potential to infect humans and cause illness. Manufacturing safety considerations may require additional equipment and facility design features beyond what would otherwise be required to protect the product.

Infectious agents are categorized in risk groups by regulatory agencies, according to their potential hazard to personnel and the environment. The Centers for Disease Control and Prevention (CDC) and the National Institutes of Health (NIH) have established four biosafety containment levels for infectious agents [12].

The facility and equipment design requirements for biosafety containment in large-scale manufacturing operations are stipulated in Appendix K of the NIH guidelines [13]. This section provides a comparison between good large-scale practice (GLSP), recommended for well-characterized agents not consistently known to cause disease, and biosafety-level large-scale (BL-LS) practice, recommended for large-scale research or production of viable organisms containing recombinant or synthetic nucleic acid molecules.

The World Health Organization and other international agencies have risk group classifications that are similar but not necessarily equivalent to those of the United States for a particular pathogen. The American Biological Safety Association (ABSA) maintains a database of infectious agent classifications to identify an appropriate biohazard classification for laboratory and manufacturing space [14]. A summary of biosafety levels in the NIH guidelines is provided in Table 12.6.

TABLE 12.6
Summary of Biosafety Levels

NIH/CDC BSL Laboratory	Corresponding BL-LS Practice	Description
BSL 1	BL1-LS	Well-characterized agents not known to consistently cause disease in immunocompetent adult humans and presenting minimal potential hazard to laboratory personnel and the environment
BSL 2	BL2-LS	Agents that pose moderate hazards to personnel and the environment
BSL 3	BL3-LS	Indigenous or exotic agents that may cause serious or potentially lethal disease through the inhalation route of exposure
BSL 4	No provisions are made for large-scale research or production of viable organisms that require BL4 containment at the laboratory scale	Dangerous and exotic agents that pose a high individual risk of aerosol-transmitted laboratory infections and life-threatening disease that is frequently fatal, for which there are no vaccines or treatments, or a related agent with unknown risk of transmission

Note: BSL, biosafety level.

Large-scale BL2-LS and BL3-LS operations require processing in closed systems designed with containment provisions appropriate to the biosafety level. The facility typically provides a secondary level of containment in this case. It must be designed to contain spills and provide treatment of exhaust gases and liquid biowaste to prevent the release of viable organisms. In addition, BL3-LS operations require a clean room operating at negative pressure relative to the environment to contain any breach of the primary containment.

Risk Management

Risk management, if properly incorporated into the facility design process, can not only facilitate the difficult task of ensuring product quality but also present opportunities for improvement of the reliability and cost-effectiveness of a facility (Figure 12.19).

Following the landmark 2004 publication "Pharmaceutical cGMPs for the 21st Century—A Risk-Based Approach" [15], the FDA shifted its emphasis from inspection-based quality assurance to risk management systems as the foundation for evaluating and maintaining product quality. This was consistent with the parallel publication of ICH Q9, "Quality Risk Management," finalized in 2005 [16]. These documents articulate a risk-based philosophy of quality assurance that extends beyond the day-to-day quality management systems required for biopharmaceutical manufacturing compliance.

QRM provides a framework from which design criteria can deviate from the accepted norm represented by legacy facilities, thereby establishing a rationale grounded in good science to establish facility and equipment requirements that are directly linked to product quality. At the same time, the risk-based approach rightly impacts everything from facility programming (e.g., segregation and facility flows) to process systems design (e.g., process closure, cleaning, bioburden control, and single-use technology) to equipment verification for process validation (see ASTM E2500 [17]).

PROJECT MANAGEMENT ISSUES

As is evident in the prior discussion, good design practice for biopharmaceutical facilities requires a thorough front-end planning and risk assessment process, involving multidisciplinary owner personnel (e.g., engineering, operations, quality, and regulatory compliance). The design process is typically implemented in multiple phases, as is appropriate to the size and complexity of the effort, to develop user requirements, design criteria, cost estimates, and project plans. The biotechnology facility design is often executed in three phases: conceptual design, preliminary engineering, and detailed design.

Process item	Impact	Severity 1 = low 5 = high	Frequency* 1 = low 5 = high	Detectable 5 = low 1 = high	Risk priority 1 to 125	Mitigation
Loss of power to bioreactor	Loss of batch	3	1	1	3	No high risk; may choose to install on UPS connected to EPS, based on business driver
Single-use bag integrity breach	Personnel exposed to biohazard	5	1	3	15	Ensure secondary container protects bag; ensure operators use proper PPE; pre-use integrity test

*   Probability of occurrence.

FIGURE 12.19   Example of a qualitative process risk assessment.

The conceptual design phase is essentially a feasibility study to determine if the project is viable and to provide sufficient information to secure project approval and funding. In small and well-defined projects, this phase may be combined with preliminary engineering. The objective of the conceptual design phase is to define user requirements for the facility (e.g., products, processes, operations, throughput, manufacturing scale, and regulatory constraints) and to identify the best options to achieve the owner's goals for the project. The deliverable for this phase is typically a conceptual design report, providing high-level information that includes a general process description, process flow or block flow diagrams, space program requirements, general layout options, a preliminary major equipment list, preliminary utility descriptions, and schedule and construction cost estimates. A well-executed conceptual design clearly identifies the benefits and cost implications of the options presented.

After the desired facility concept is developed and a project is authorized and budgeted, the design process advances to the preliminary engineering phase. Preliminary engineering, sometimes referred to as basic engineering or schematic design, typically advances the engineering design of the facility to 30% completion. The objective of this phase is to establish a technical basis of design (BOD) for the selected design concept. The deliverables from this phase form the foundation for the detailed design. At this stage, the BOD is typically subject to a 30% design review, which may include further evaluation via process hazard analysis (PHA) or design qualification (DQ) to verify cGMP compliance. During this phase, it may also be necessary to expedite the development of specifications and bid packages for long-lead process equipment, such as production bioreactors. Upon completion of preliminary engineering, the BOD is locked in, and any subsequent changes to the scope or design basis will likely have a significant impact on the cost and schedule for the project.

The detailed design phase develops the BOD into a completed facility design package. The objective of this phase is to generate construction documents fit for permitting and building. Design reviews during detailed design are usually conducted at 60% and 90% completion.

The design process does not end with delivery of construction documents. Engineering support is typically required for procurement, construction, commissioning, and qualification activities. As the process systems for biotechnology facilities require specialized design and fabrication methods, shop drawing reviews and inspections should be conducted by qualified bioprocess design professionals where appropriate. Engineers should be available to answer requests for information (RFIs) quickly during construction and to support the development of a clean-build strategy to transition the facility from a dirty construction environment to a progressively cleaner state through commissioning and qualification. After construction is complete, as-built design drawings should be archived to support systems qualification and future maintenance of the facility.

The design phases described above are common but by no means universal. The design process should be defined as part of the overall project plan, which is subject to the unique requirements of the project and the conventions and preferences of project stakeholders. Throughout the entire design life cycle, it is imperative that the design effort is subject to good engineering practice (GEP) [18] to ensure that the deliverables support the requirements for qualification and validation.

As biotechnology facilities are frequently highly automated, a life cycle approach is also good design practice for the development of automation systems. Project management for automation development is particularly challenging because progress and project status are not easily visualized. In addition, process automation must be well documented and traceable to user requirements for validated manufacturing systems. The Good Automated Manufacturing Practice (GAMP) technical subcommittee of the International Society for Pharmaceutical Engineering (ISPE) has developed a set of guidelines [19] for defining user requirement specifications (URSs), functional requirement specifications (FRSs), and detailed design specifications (DDSs) for automated systems used for pharmaceutical manufacturing. These standards provide the project manager with a means to benchmark progress and ensure that automated systems can be qualified for a validated manufacturing process.

FUTURE DEVELOPMENTS

As discussed in the introduction to this chapter, the practice of harnessing biotechnology to produce useful products is not new, but the technologies that enable the manipulation of organisms at the genetic level, and provide groundbreaking medical therapies, are developing now at an accelerated pace. In this sense, the biopharmaceutical industry is young and constantly evolving to leverage the latest therapeutic approaches and drug delivery methods. Following the early success of large-market breakthrough drugs in the 1980s and 1990s (the low-hanging fruit), manufacturers increasingly have focused on orphan drugs and personalized medicine and therapies for niche markets. The effort has produced revolutionary new drugs for devastating diseases and intractable genetic disorders. These benefits come at a substantial cost. Future cost–benefit factors are anticipated to have a substantial impact on the design of biopharmaceutical manufacturing facilities.

BUSINESS DRIVERS

Although the pace of drug discovery and innovative new technologies continues to drive growth, the biopharmaceutical industry is maturing in response to business drivers to reduce cost (Figure 12.20). With the creation of a regulatory pathway for generic biologics (i.e., biosimilars, biogenerics, or follow-on biologics) and many of the blockbuster drugs that ushered in the biotech boom going off-patent, the need for efficient, flexible, and cost-effective biomanufacturing facilities has never been greater. Increasingly, the social pressure to control health care costs and the expansion of biologics into less lucrative emerging markets will add to the demand for economical alternatives to traditional manufacturing methods. In addition, the trend toward personalized medicine and the higher percentage of orphan drugs under development for niche markets run counter to the former paradigm that achieved economy through mass production. The resulting cost pressure is unprecedented in the biopharmaceutical industry. Manufacturers who want to be successful in this new economy must embrace lean manufacturing methods while refusing to compromise on product quality.

The need for lean operations drives greater scrutiny on capital spending, leading to a trend toward more risk-based design decisions in place of the old "that's the way we've always done it" rationale. However, the design decisions that optimize plant throughput and reduce ongoing manufacturing costs, thereby increasing the long-term return on investment, yield the most significant cost reduction.

Facility use has a huge impact on the cost of goods sold. This is a big issue with much of the legacy biomanufacturing infrastructure going into the twenty-first century because it was designed

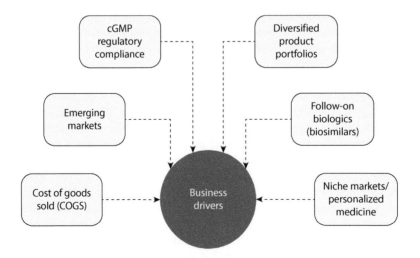

FIGURE 12.20   Business drivers influencing future facility design.

for single-product, large-volume manufacturing. These facilities are ill-suited to handle the diverse product portfolios of the modern biologics manufacturer. Batch sizes are getting smaller. This is due in part to an increase in selective therapies for niche markets and in part a result of the industry's success in optimizing biomanufacturing to produce higher yields. Consequently, many legacy facilities are poorly used and are not designed to transition from one product to the next quickly and efficiently. Poor facility use can also lead to quality issues because of the lack of consistency in manufacturing operations. All of these factors are driving a trend toward greater flexibility in new biofacilities to allow them to handle a more diverse mix of products with relatively small batch sizes. This capability, used in conjunction with traditional facilities that are efficient at large-scale production, provides a more cost-effective model for future operations that will be required to support both small- and large-volume biomanufacturing.

MANUFACTURING TECHNOLOGY

The biopharm industry today is focused on understanding the manufacturing process and critical quality attributes associated with product quality. The regulatory drive to develop more science-based manufacturing methods is well aligned with the need for greater process knowledge so that manufacturers can more effectively manage risk and better target investments to areas that really influence product quality. Ongoing improvements in analytical methods, adventitious agent detection, and product characterization provide tools for quantifying risk and verifying product quality. The commercially available technology for process instrumentation and control, PAT, and MES are also improving and enhance the ability of future facilities to demonstrate that they are in a state of control.

All of these enablers provide a framework from which product risk can be more easily assessed at each stage of the manufacturing process (Figure 12.21). This facilitates the selection of design features in future multiproduct facilities that are more efficient and reliable. It also provides an opportunity to challenge expensive industry design conventions that may have evolved because early manufacturers did not have a good understanding of their process design space. One of the trends facilitated by better process understanding is the migration to more closed processing and less reliance on classified space to protect products from contamination.

The technology that enables the biopharmaceutical industry to meet future challenges is evolving at a rapid pace. For example, the rapid development and commercialization of single-use technology for biomanufacturing has been a significant transformative factor, enabling future facility flexibility and improved utilization. The hard costs of going the single-use route are often a trade-off: lower

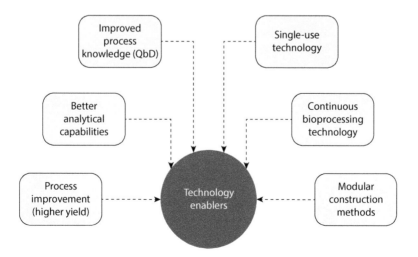

FIGURE 12.21 Technology enablers for future facility design.

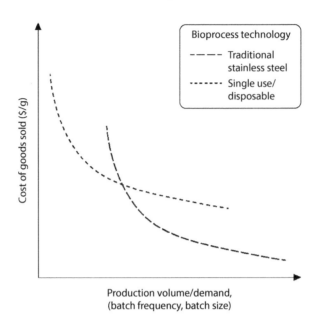

FIGURE 12.22   Relationship between bioprocess technology, production demand, and cost of goods sold.

capital costs but higher costs of consumables (Figure 12.22). However, the ability to modify SUS and adapt to a diverse product portfolio is unparalleled. In addition, the elimination of CIP and SIP operations can provide an opportunity for quicker changeover between batches, thereby increasing the overall facility throughput. There are scale limitations to single-use technology, and it is not a solution for every scenario. In many applications, a hybrid stainless steel and SUS approach is appropriate. Also, the traditional stainless steel and single-use process systems are not necessarily interchangeable for each unit operation. If the goal is to go 100% SUS and eliminate CIP and SIP infrastructure, then the manufacturer needs to be committed to that strategy throughout process development.

Another trend for future facilities is the use of continuous biomanufacturing to overcome the inherent scale limitations of SUS. Achieving a robust continuous manufacturing process is difficult, but the upshot is the ability to handle the same production throughput at a scale that is an order of magnitude smaller than what would be required for batch or fed-batch operations. Therefore, it is likely that there will be future expansion of the use of SUS, beyond pilot plant and buffer and media prep applications, into full-scale production.

Nevertheless, many production facilities will continue to use traditional stainless steel equipment for large-volume production requirements. These will be highly automated multiproduct facilities with design features intended to maximize flexibility and utilization.

MODULAR CONSTRUCTION

Modular construction methods can be used strategically to enhance the speed of facility delivery and overall flexibility of operations. Modularity, ranging from integrated super-skids to clean rooms to entire buildings, brings the advantage of precommissioned functional units that can be quickly assembled on-site. This is particularly useful in areas where local skilled trades at the construction site are scarce or where an aggressive delivery schedule is required.

Preengineered modules can further enhance the speed of delivery. The trade-off for this is that design options are limited to the selection offered by the solution provider. The growing selection of modular solutions will provide options for most manufacturing scenarios, but some elements of the design are fixed nonetheless, and the specific configuration of modules may need to be locked in earlier in the overall project schedule. Of course, modules can be customized, but the price for this is acceptance of delivery schedules that incorporate a more traditional engineering design process.

The portability of some modular units may allow them to be treated as an equipment asset. Many modular solutions are designed for ease of reconfiguration, expansion, or relocation in response to dynamic business needs. The ultimate example of this is the use of clean room pods, which are prefabricated manufacturing units that can be easily "docked" to the larger facility infrastructure and are designed for quick adjustment to meet dynamic manufacturing needs. Pod-type solutions are likely to expand in the future, particularly for small-volume segregated processing (e.g., viral processing, biohazards, and potent compounds) (Figure 12.23).

FACILITY DELIVERY

The development of new technology enablers to address regulatory and business drivers will require the implementation of new strategic and tactical approaches to biotechnology facility design and delivery (Figure 12.24). Strategically, the development of manufacturing capacity should be accompanied by a philosophical commitment to the technologies that will be employed and the tactical approach that will be used to deploy them. Decisions regarding manufacturers' approaches to risk management, process segregation, and manufacturing technologies employed should be an integral part of project planning and should be the guiding principles in every stage of the design development process.

In one survey of biopharmaceutical professionals, risk management was identified as the biggest challenge associated with implementing next-generation biomanufacturing (defined as biofacilities that use the technology enablers previously discussed) [20]. Future facilities will need to leverage new tools that are evolving in the industry while controlling the risks associated with using technology solutions that are still rapidly evolving. In the same survey, 49% of respondents indicated that the "need for flexibility" is the strongest driver for building next-generation biopharmaceutical facilities. Only 9% identified "lower capital cost" as the strongest driver. To achieve success in the dynamic economy of future biomanufacturing, project planning should focus on long-term return on investment and the development of manufacturing capacity that complements and efficiently leverages legacy facility infrastructure.

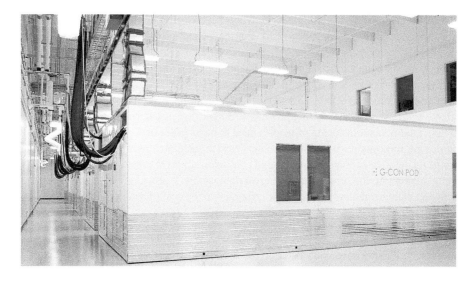

FIGURE 12.23 Prefabricated, autonomous clean room pod bioprocess. (Courtesy of G-CON Manufacturing, Inc., College Station, TX.)

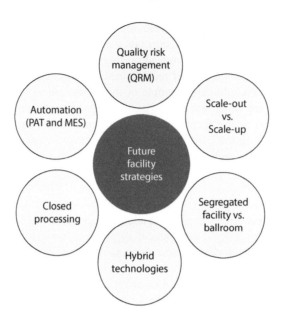

FIGURE 12.24   Strategies for design of future biopharm facilities.

SPECIAL DISCUSSION

One indicator of a maturing industry is the development of global guidelines and standards for manufacturing. The biopharmaceutical industry is maturing. Globalization is leading to a harmonization of regulatory expectations and the standardization of some design requirements for biotechnology facilities and equipment. The commercial environment increasingly resembles that of other mature regulated process industries, such as food and fine chemicals. In this economy, modern-quality manufacturing methods (e.g., quality by design, PAT, and lean six sigma) and global standardization are important factors in maintaining product quality, driving down production costs, and managing regulatory expectations.

The science-based methods and principles embodied in today's pharmaceutical quality systems were established and proven in other industries where high-quality products are now commodities [21]. While the manufacturing process for most biopharmaceutical products currently requires a degree of sophistication and proprietary know-how that is not characteristic of a commodity, the trend is clearly in that direction. As manufacturers adjust to dwindling drug pipelines, fewer blockbusters, and loss of product patent protection, the adoption of strategies that have been successful in other industries is imperative. In recognition of this business reality, regulatory agencies have encouraged a focus on efficient, effective, and lean manufacturing processes. Rather than attempting to control quality by testing the back end, quality manufacturing principles need to be incorporated in the front end, including planning and design. Biotechnology facilities are expected to facilitate the establishment and maintenance of a manufacturing state of control. A culture of continuous improvement is encouraged. This emphasis on building quality into the process achieves two noble goals: it provides both a method for protecting the patient population and a mechanism for driving down the cost of drug products.

INDUSTRY GUIDELINES

Many industry guidelines have contributed to the harmonization of biopharmaceutical manufacturing practices, although a few nicely summarize the requirements for biotechnology facilities. While guidelines do not have the regulatory teeth of a standard or code, they are useful tools for building industry consensus and provide a harmonized approach for dealing with ambiguous regulatory statutes.

A good primer for understanding the impact of modern quality initiatives on cGMP facility design can be found in the ISPE guide *Science and Risk-Based Approach for the Delivery of Facilities, Systems, and Equipment* [22]. This document nicely summarizes the project life cycle for delivery of a biopharmaceutical facility, including planning, design, construction, verification, acceptance, and release. It also provides an overview of GEPs, design review, and change management processes, which are crucial elements of the design process for such facilities. The guide presents a structured approach to the delivery of regulated facilities that aligns well with the latest industry and regulatory initiatives.

Perhaps the most useful design reference for both new and veteran professionals is the ISPE Baseline Guide *Biopharmaceutical Manufacturing Facilities* [4]. This guideline directly addresses the key programming issues associated with biopharmaceutical facility design. It provides an in-depth discussion of the unique requirements for biopharmaceutical operations, risk management, process closure, cGMP facility layout, and architectural and mechanical design considerations.

ENGINEERING STANDARDS

The most notable engineering standard applicable to biotechnology facilities of all stripes is the Bioprocessing Equipment (BPE) Standard from the American Society of Mechanical Engineers (ASME) [23]. This is an international consensus standard for the design of process systems in biotechnology facilities, including materials, fabrication methods, components, and equipment. The ASME has established an expanding certification program to identify vendor compliance with BPE. The BPE identifies key requirements for the design and construction of new fluid processing equipment used in the manufacture of biopharmaceuticals, where a defined level of purity and bioburden control is required. It is an excellent reference document for the design of process systems and components that are subject to cleaning and sanitization or sterilization, including CIP, SIP, and single-use technologies.

APPENDIX: BIOPRESS UNIT OPERATIONS

UPSTREAM BIOPROCESSING

Upstream bioprocessing starts with inoculum preparation, where cells are taken from a working cell bank and thawed (Figure 12.25). These cells are resuspended and cultivated to grow sufficient volume to inoculate a small bioreactor. Cells are cultivated in a series of progressively larger bioreactors, commonly referred to as a *seed train*, until there is sufficient volume to transfer to a production bioreactor at manufacturing scale. The term *bioreactor* is sometimes

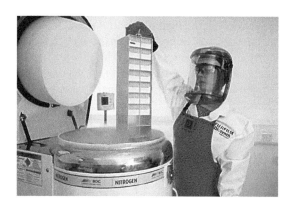

FIGURE 12.25 Cell bank being lifted out of a liquid nitrogen freezer. (Courtesy of FUJIFILM Diosynth Biotechnologies, Morrisville, NC.)

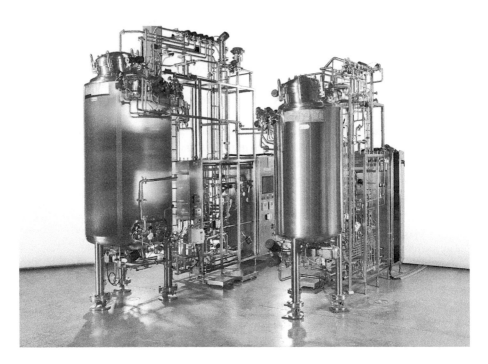

FIGURE 12.26   A 1500 L and a 500 L bioreactor system. (Courtesy of ABEC, Bethlehem, PA.)

used synonymously with the term *fermentor*, although by convention, bioreactors are typically associated with cell culture and fermentors typically refer to microbial fermentation. The most common bioreactor design used for large-scale manufacturing is a stirred tank due to its simplicity and ease of scale-up (Figure 12.26). A typical culture growth profile includes a lag phase, where cells are acclimating to a new environment after inoculation; a log phase during which cells are growing exponentially; a stationary phase where maximum cell density is maintained; and a death phase after nutrients have been depleted.

Fermentation

Microbial fermentation is used to cultivate prokaryotic cells, such as bacteria, yeast, and fungi. Prokaryotic cells require relatively simple media formulations to grow. Fermentors are typically designed for measurement and closed-loop control of temperature, pressure, aeration rate, agitation rate, pH, and dissolved oxygen within the culture. Control of pH typically requires additional acid and base tanks to be located nearby for aseptic additions to the fermentor. A reservoir for an anti-foaming agent may also be required to control the foam level in the fermentor. Most fermentors are operated in a fed-batch mode in which a medium or nutrient feed is established to supplement the media in later stages of fermentation, requiring additional containers for local storage and aseptic transfer of media and nutrients.

As prokaryotic cells grow relatively fast, the utility demands for aeration, agitator power input, and process cooling can be substantial and peak when the maximum cell density is reached near the end of fermentation. Fermentation media are typically heat sterilized *in situ* within the bioreactor prior to inoculation and axenic fermentation. This batch sterilization has a direct impact on the heating and cooling utilities within the fermentation area, as well as the peak heat load that the HVAC system is required to handle. Stirred-tank production fermentors typically have an aspect ratio of approximately 3:1, so it is common for production bioreactors to be located in high-bay areas with fixed platforms to provide access to the top of the vessel. The agitator assemblies on production fermentors can be quite large and heavy, and they require regular maintenance to maintain mechanical seals. Therefore, the fermentation production area should be equipped with a means to lift the agitator assembly and should provide sufficient clearance to remove it from the tank if necessary.

Cell Culture

Cell culture bioreactors are designed to grow eukaryotic cells that contain a nucleus, mitochondria, and other membrane-bound organelles. In contrast with microbial fermentation runs, which are timed in hours and typically complete within 2 days, cell culture operations can last for days or weeks, depending on the mode of operation and the growth rate of the microorganism. Bioreactors share many of the same control parameters as fermentors, but the utility requirements are an order of magnitude less due to the slower growth rate of the culture. In addition, cell culture media are much more complex and cannot be steam sterilized *in situ* because they are heat labile. Therefore, stainless steel bioreactors are typically sterilized empty, and sterile filtration is used for aseptic addition of media. In addition to clean air, cell cultures typically require additional specialty gases (e.g., O_2, N_2, and CO_2) for control of dissolved oxygen, dissolved carbon dioxide, and pH within the bioreactor.

Single-use (disposable) bioreactors are commonly used for cell culture clinical manufacturing and increasingly for cGMP production up to a 2,000 L scale. As single-use bioreactors use disposable gamma-irradiated bags for axenic culture, there is no need for a SIP or CIP system to sterilize and clean the bioreactor.

Perfusion Culture

As cell culture does not require destruction of the host cells in order to extract the product, it can be executed as a continuous manufacturing process. Continuous (perfusion) culture requires maintenance of an axenic environment in the bioreactor over a long period. Following expansion to a predetermined cell density, a cell culture may be maintained for weeks or months if fresh media are continuously perfused into the system and spent (depleted) media are removed along with the secreted product in the harvest stream. This enables the production of a large volume of product over time by a relatively small bioreactor. In order to operate continuous cultures economically, a perfusion system is required to separate the viable cells in the bioreactor from the harvest stream. The cell separation device may operate on the principle of cellular size exclusion (e.g., membrane filtration) or density (e.g., settlers and centrifugation), but in either case, it probably requires a long-term aseptic connection and additional space adjacent to the bioreactor. As perfusion processes require a continuous stream of fresh media and accumulate a large volume of product over time, the location and sizing of adjacent media preparation and harvest space are critical. Perfusion technology is frequently used to manufacture therapeutic proteins that are sensitive to heat degradation, so an adjacent cold room for product pooling may be required.

Harvest

Harvest is the process by which product is recovered from the bioreactor, clarified, and concentrated before transfer to downstream unit operations. Products that are produced by microbial fermentation require an initial cell disruption step to lyse the cells and release the product so that it can be harvested. Cell lysis can be accomplished chemically (e.g., detergent) or physically through mechanical disruption, requiring the fermentation broth to pass through a homogenizer or microfluidizer. This process releases a large amount of DNA and cell debris (relative to cell culture) that needs to be removed as part of the harvest process. In this scenario, depth filtration, flocculation and precipitation, or centrifugation may be used to remove large insoluble particles before secondary clarification [24].

Cell culture operations produce a harvest stream with a lower particle load in comparison to fermentation, but the challenge here is to remove the cell mass *without* breaking the cells and minimizing released cell debris. Primary recovery is typically via depth filtration, tangential flow microfiltration, and disk-stack centrifugation, followed by a secondary clarification step to remove colloids, lipids, DNA, residual cells, and other particles that were not removed by primary recovery. In most scenarios, the product is recovered in the filtrate or centrate (supernatant) stream; however, in some cases, the product may be in the retentate or heavy process stream (e.g., production of viruses or virus-like particles). Following recovery and secondary clarification of the harvest stream, a terminal clarification and polishing step is typically executed via membrane filtration.

Harvest operations are frequently executed in the same room as cell culture or fermentation, with the possible exception of centrifugation, which may be located in a separate processing area to contain any aerosols produced by the operation and attenuate noise from the machinery. The facility programming for harvest and recovery areas requires sufficient space for these unit operations. TFF, in particular, may require substantial floor space, depending on the amount of membrane surface area required, as well as when buffer storage for diafiltration is required. This area usually contains a harvest tank for product pooling before transitioning to downstream purification.

DOWNSTREAM BIOPROCESSING

Downstream unit operations receive the clarified cell-free harvest from cell culture or fermentation and execute further purification of the drug substance. In some cases, downstream operations also modify or combine desired proteins. The objective of downstream processing is to reduce contaminates and manufacturing by-products in the harvest to acceptable levels, including removal of endotoxins, DNA, host cell proteins, aggregates, and viral particles. Downstream processing may also include conjugation, concentration, and formulation steps to create a stable product for bulk filling. Most downstream operations are bioburden controlled (i.e., maintained at low bioburden within controlled limits) before terminal sterilization of the bulk drug substance at the end of the purification process. However, in the case of products containing live cells, live or attenuated viruses, or virus-like particles, manufacturing must be executed aseptically throughout the entire purification process because bioburden and endotoxins cannot be removed by a final filtration step.

As the bulk drug substance may be processed in a more concentrated form, downstream bioprocessing equipment is typically smaller relative to upstream process systems and may use a mobile skid to allow for equipment removal and replacement to accommodate diverse manufacturing processes. Therefore, the facility should be designed to accommodate equipment storage and transfer through equipment airlocks into and out of the downstream process suite. The primary process utilities typically used in downstream processing areas are compendial water, instrument air, clean air, nitrogen, clean steam, and chilled water or glycol. Some biopharmaceutical products degrade at room temperature and may require cold space, typically at 2°C–8°C, for pooling and purification operations.

Chromatography

Liquid chromatography is the primary method used to purify biopharmaceuticals and can achieve very selective and efficient separation of the target product protein from other proteins and non-protein species. Most downstream biomanufacturing processes include two to four chromatography steps.

There are two basic systems used in commercial manufacturing: size exclusion chromatography (SEC) and adsorption chromatography. SEC, sometimes called gel filtration, is used to isolate proteins based on their physical size relative to the pore sizes in the resin matrix. Adsorption chromatography achieves separation based on the protein's hydrophobicity, charge, or other chemical interaction with the resin. This category includes ion exchange (IEX) chromatography, hydrophobic interaction chromatography (HIC), reverse-phase chromatography (RPC), and affinity chromatography. Affinity chromatography, using protein A, is by far the most selective of the chromatographic methods and is the industry's workhorse for mAb purification [25].

In addition to traditional bind and elute systems, the use of flow-through chromatography to bind impurities is also very common. In flow-through systems, the resin is not eluted but cleaned free of the impurities. Membrane chromatography is increasingly used for both viral clearance and disposable capture chromatography and provides solutions that address some of the mass transfer limitations inherent in conventional resin-based chromatography. Most chromatography operations in the biopharmaceutical industry are batch processes. However, simulated moving-bed chromatography (SMCC), also called periodic countercurrent (PCC) chromatography, is gaining acceptance and offers a continuous processing alternative.

Chromatography unit operations are typically scaled up by maintaining the bed height and increasing the diameter of the column. Therefore, large-scale processing typically does not require high-ceiling clearance but can take up considerable floor space. In addition, the floor space required for product pooling and buffers typically exceeds that of the equipment itself. A segregated classified space is often provided for column packing as part of the facility.

Filtration

Filtration is used in downstream processing to reduce bioburden, clarify precipitates, concentrate proteins, exchange buffers (via diafiltration), remove viruses, and terminally sterilize the bulk drug substance. Filtration unit operations work on the size exclusion principle, whereby the product protein either passes through the filter membrane into the permeate stream or is retained by the membrane in the retentate. Microfiltration, which employs membrane pore sizes ranging from 0.5 to 10 µm, will remove larger particles and allow the protein to pass through into the permeate. Downstream microfiltration is commonly used for bioburden reduction and precipitate clarification. Ultrafiltration, with membrane pores from 1 to 20 nm, is effective for product concentration and buffer exchange because most biopharmaceutical products are retained by the membrane in the retentate. These operations typically use Tangential Flow Filtration (TFF), in which the retentate stream (passing cross-flow) sweeps the ultrafiltration membrane to prevent filter fouling and increase throughput.

The cell culture manufacturing process can produce endogenous retroviruses and may be infected with other viral adventitious agents during processing. This requires virus removal and inactivation steps as part of downstream purification to ensure product safety. Virus retention filters with ultrafiltration or microfiltration membranes may be used as part of the manufacturer's viral clearance program. Viral filtration typically precedes a final ultrafiltration concentration and diafiltration step, followed by terminal sterilization by a 0.2 µm sterile filter. Downstream operations following viral clearance are frequently processed in a segregated area to prevent cross-contamination.

CONJUGATION

Conjugation is required for manufacturing for many vaccines, PEGylated proteins, and antibody drug conjugates (ADCs). Conjugation processes are essentially chemical reactions whereby two different molecules are covalently linked to each other. Temperature control, mixing, and component additions are particularly critical in this unit operation. The conjugation process may require the addition of organic solvents, reagents, or other chemical constituents that are toxic or sensitizing to personnel, requiring additional segregation to limit exposure. In the case of ADCs, the product may be cytotoxic or a highly potent compound requiring closed processing and additional design measures to prevent operator exposure.

BULK FORMULATION AND FILLING

Bulk formulation and filling is the process whereby the drug substance is prepared for storage in a stable form prior to fill or finish processing to deliver the drug in the form received by the patient.

During bulk formulation, additional components (e.g., buffering salts, amino acids, sugars, and surfactants) are blended with the drug substance to adjust physical properties and enhance the stability of the product. Following bulk formulation, the drug substance typically undergoes terminal sterilization before filling into an appropriate storage container. The formulated drug substance may be stored in a cold room at 2°C to 8°C, or in a –20°C to –30°C freezer for long-term storage. The reliability of this storage environment is critical due to the high product value at this stage, so cold environments are typically equipped with backup power and are tied into the BAS to trigger an alarm in the event of failure.

PROCESS SUPPORT

Process support operations include weigh and dispense, glass and part washing, sterilization (autoclave), sterile assembly preparations, and buffer and media preparation. In addition, biotechnology facilities require space for warehousing, maintenance, spare parts, cleaning systems, and utility production.

Weigh and Dispense

Weigh and dispense and buffer and media preparation areas should be designed to handle powder components in a closed or contained manner to prevent cross-contamination from airborne particulates. A central weigh and dispense area near the warehouse is commonly provided to support open processing with dust collection in weigh booths, followed by kitting so that materials can be transported to manufacturing areas in the plant in a closed container.

Media Preparation

Media preparation systems provide nutrients to support growth and product expression in fermentation and cell culture operations. These systems are designed to blend media components in solution and adjust physical parameters, such as temperature and pH. If media constituents are heat labile, as is typically the case for cell culture operations, the media are passed through a sterile filtration system to facilitate aseptic transfer to the bioreactor seed train. As media components are growth promoting, any open processing associated with this unit operation should be executed in a segregated area to prevent contamination of other elements of the manufacturing process by adventitious agents. This may be a *briefly exposed* operation, meaning that the media preparation process may include some open operations in a CNC or bioburden-controlled area, but the formulated media are held for a limited, validated time before the process is *functionally closed* through terminal sterilization. Media preparation areas are typically located adjacent to cell culture or fermentation.

Buffer Preparation

Buffer preparation is the process whereby reagents are prepared and staged for use in the manufacturing process. This is primarily a blending operation requiring mix and hold tanks. If organic solvents are required for the manufacturing process, this area may require an explosion-proof design.

Sterilization and Part Washing

Sterilization and washing areas are typically required to clean and reduce or eliminate bioburden on small parts or containers used in the manufacturing process. Production-scale cGMP part washers and sterilizers are typically integrated with the building architecture to allow maintenance access to the mechanical components without entering clean space that requires gowning. This equipment is often specified as a "pass-through" design to segregate items in a separate room after sterilization or cleaning. Localized ventilation is typically provided above the exit door to draw vapor from the chamber and maintain a clean environment for cooling exposed items after cleaning or sterilization.

FURTHER DISCUSSION

Questions for further discussion include the following:

1. How is the manufacturing process for biologics different from that for other pharmaceutical API products, and what are the unique challenges associated with biotechnology facility design?
2. What are the most common contamination sources in biotechnology facilities, and how are they mitigated through facility design?
3. What is process closure, and how does it affect the layout of biotechnology facilities?
4. How are process risks managed through space programming in biotechnology facility design?
5. What are the business drivers affecting the future direction of biotechnology facility design, and how will new technologies enable manufacturers to address future challenges?

ABOUT THE AUTHOR

David M. Marks, PE is principal and founder of DME, an engineering and consulting firm serving the regulated life sciences industry (www.DMEforLife.com). He has 30 years of experience with process systems and facilities in the biotechnology and pharmaceutical industries. His professional experience is concentrated in the design of bioprocess systems and FDA-licensed commercial manufacturing facilities. Marks is an active member of the ASME BPE standard committee and serves as chair of the process systems design subcommittee. He is a frequent author, speaker, and consultant on bioprocess technology, facility design, and cGMP regulatory compliance topics.

ACKNOWLEDGMENTS

I wish to thank Carol Nolan and Timothy J. Hancock, Ph.D. for their assistance on reviewing this chapter.

REFERENCES

1. U.S. Food and Drug Administration, Resources for You (Biologics), U.S. Food and Drug Administration, Silver Spring, MD, http://www.fda.gov/BiologicsBloodVaccines/ResourcesforYou/.
2. Generics and Biosimilars Initiative, Small Molecule versus Biological Drugs, June 2012, http://www.gabionline.net/Biosimilars/Research/Small-molecule-versus-biological-drugs.
3. American Chemical Society, Development of Deep-Tank Fermentation, American Chemical Society, Office of Communications, National Historic Chemical Landmarks Program, 2008.
4. International Society for Pharmaceutical Engineering, *Baseline® Pharmaceutical Engineering Guides for New and Renovated Facilities*, Vol. 6: *Biopharmaceutical Manufacturing Facilities*, 2nd ed., International Society for Pharmaceutical Engineering, Tampa, FL, 2013.
5. Chalk S, Taber R, Probst S, Gil P, Palberg T, Kennedy M, Rogalewicz J, Johnson J, Green K, Challenging the Cleanroom Paradigm for Biopharmaceutical Manufacturing of Bulk Drug Substances, *BioPharm International*, August 2011.
6. Nelson KL, Approaches for Flexible Manufacturing Facilities in Vaccine Production, *BioPharm International*, November 2011 (Single-Use Technology and Facilities Supplement).
7. U.S. Food and Drug Administration, Guidance for Industry: PAT—A Framework for Innovative Pharmaceutical Development, Manufacturing, and Quality Assurance, U.S. Food and Drug Administration, Silver Spring, MD, September 2004.
8. American Institute of Architects, *Architect's Handbook of Professional Practice*, 13th ed., John Wiley & Sons, New York, 2000.
9. Wang W, Singh M (eds.), *Biological Drug Products: Development and Strategies*, 1st ed., John Wiley & Sons, New York, 2014.

10. U.S. Food and Drug Administration, Science and the Regulation of Biological Products, U.S. Food and Drug Administration, Silver Spring, MD, April 2009, http://www.fda.gov/AboutFDA/WhatWeDo/History/ProductRegulation/100YearsofBiologicsRegulation/ucm070022.htm.

11. International Society for Pharmaceutical Engineering, Closure Analysis Strategy, in *Baseline®* *Pharmaceutical Engineering Guides for New and Renovated Facilities*, Vol. 5: *Biopharmaceuticals*, International Society for Pharmaceutical Engineering, Tampa, FL, 2013, Section 4.4.1.

12. Centers for Disease Control and Prevention, *Biosafety in Microbiological and Biomedical Laboratories*, 5th ed., HHS Publication No. (CDC) 21-1112, Government Printing Office, Washington, DC, 2009. (Section III describes the principles of biosafety and Section IV establishes biosafety-level criteria.)

13. National Institutes of Health, Guidelines for Research Involving Recombinant or Synthetic Nucleic Acid Molecules, NIH Guidelines, National Institutes of Health, Bethesda, MD, November 2013, http://osp.od.nih.gov/office-biotechnology-activities/biosafety/nih-guidelines.

14. ABSA International, ABSA Risk Group Classification for Infectious Agents, ABSA International, Mundelein, IL, http://www.absa.org/riskgroups/.

15. U.S. Food and Drug Administration, Pharmaceutical cGMPs for the 21st Century—A Risk-Based Approach, U.S. Food and Drug Administration, Silver Spring, MD, September 2004.

16. International Conference on Harmonisation, ICH Q9: Quality Risk Management, Technical Requirements for Registration of Pharmaceuticals for Human Use, International Conference on Harmonisation, Geneva.

17. ASTM International, *ASTM E2500: Standard Guide for Specification, Design, and Verification of Pharmaceutical and Biopharmaceutical Manufacturing Systems and Equipment,* ASTM International, West Conshohocken, PA, 2007.

18. International Society for Pharmaceutical Engineering, *Good Engineering Practice*, ISPE Good Practice Guide, International Society for Pharmaceutical Engineering, Tampa, FL, 2008.

19. International Society for Pharmaceutical Engineering, *GAMP 5: A Risk-Based Approach to Compliant GxP Computerized Systems*, International Society for Pharmaceutical Engineering, Tampa, FL, 2008.

20. International Society for Pharmaceutical Engineering, Biopharmaceutical Industry Polling of Over 70 Professionals at a DME Presentation on Next Generation Facilities for Biomanufacturing, ISPE Annual Meeting, 2014, Las Vegas, NV.

21. International Conference on Harmonisation, ICH Q10: Pharmaceutical Quality System, Technical Requirements for Registration of Pharmaceuticals for Human Use, International Conference on Harmonisation, Geneva.

22. International Society for Pharmaceutical Engineering, *ISPE Guide: Science and Risk-Based Approach for the Delivery of Facilities, Systems, and Equipment,* International Society for Pharmaceutical Engineering, Tampa, FL, 2011.

23. American Society of Mechanical Engineers, *ASME Bioprocessing Equipment (BPE) Standard,* American Society of Mechanical Engineers, New York, 2014.

24. Shukla AA, Kandula JR, Harvest and Recovery of Monoclonal Antibodies from Large-Scale Mammalian Cell Culture, *BioPharm International*, 21(5), 2008.

25. Liu HF, Ma J, Winter C, Bayer R, Recovery and Purification Process Development for Monoclonal Antibody Production, *MAbs*, 2(5), 480–499, 2010.

13 Codes and Standards

Eric Bohn

CONTENTS

INTRODUCTION

This chapter provides an overview of the building and zoning codes plus associated standards and regulations that impact the design and construction of pharmaceutical manufacturing facilities. Local municipal and state governments are the primary authorities promulgating these codes. In addition, there are agencies at the federal level developing regulations and standards that impact facility design and construction. Examples of these include the Americans with Disabilities Act (ADA), the Occupational Safety and Health Administration (OSHA), and many specialty concerns, such as the Nuclear Regulatory Commission (NRC) for control and use of radioactive materials and the Drug Enforcement Administration (DEA) for controlled substances.

Codes represent the minimum requirements required by local, state, and federal governments to legally construct a facility. A design for a new facility, as well as renovation of an existing facility, must be based on the codes that apply for that particular set of circumstances. As will be demonstrated, compliance with codes represents an extraordinary amount of information that must be incorporated into a design. Fortunately, on any given project, the responsibility for code compliance is divided between the numerous specialty designers engaged, such as the architect and the civil, mechanical, electrical, pumping, fire protection, and environmental engineers.

Besides building and zoning codes, there are numerous additional guidelines and standards that impact the design and construction of buildings. These generally fall into two groups. First, there are technical standards that are specifically referenced by the building codes and thereby supplement and extend the technical precision of the code. These include standards by organizations such as the American Society of Heating, Refrigerating, and Air-Conditioning Engineers (ASHRAE), American National Standards Institute (ANSI), American Society for Testing and Materials (ASTM),

FM Global (FM), and National Fire Protection Association (NFPA). The second class of standards are specific federal ordinances that apply to special and specific aspects of a building, especially manufacturing facilities. These include regulations from the ADA and the following government agencies: OSHA, Environmental Protection Agency (EPA), DEA, and NRC.

EXECUTIVE SUMMARY

KEY CONCEPTS

Codes represent the legal minimum for the design and construction of any facility. Codes cannot be avoided. They must be embraced, understood, and integrated into every facility design. There is a legal obligation to follow the code minimums; however, exceeding the codes is sometimes appropriate and may be in the owner's best interest.

The sheer number of codes that relate to facility design is daunting. In order to proceed in an effective manner, it is necessary to be familiar with all the codes and know when and where each is applicable. In this way, one can narrow the pursuit and make compliance a manageable endeavor.

There are many codes and even more standards. Continual updates and new editions of the codes are common. It is crucial to follow the codes that are adopted and enforced in the jurisdiction where a building is being built. Be careful—this is not necessarily the most recent code. Sometimes it is assumed that the new codes are better and therefore more appropriate. However, it is only the legally adopted code that has legal standing and is the legal basis for enforcement. Not following the adopted code can easily result in noncompliance even if it is more recent.

The written presentation of codes is not linear in manner. This is particularly true when you consider the many different codes that must be researched and addressed. However, it is also true within the individual codes themselves. A thorough code review is an interactive process, requiring one to work back and forth between the various parts of the code and testing the various options available before settling on an approach appropriate for the circumstances at hand and beneficial to the owner.

The language of codes tries to be precise. However, when applied to real-world situations, the code does not always provide a clear answer. At such times it is necessary to seek an interpretation of the code. The local code official is typically charged with the legal authority to make final interpretations of the code. However, the design professional makes code interpretations as a matter of course while developing a design and has a legal responsibility to provide a design that is code compliant.

HISTORICAL BACKGROUND

In the United States, all levels of government have a constitutional mandate to protect the health, safety, and welfare of the public. All codes are an outgrowth of this mandate. During the early years of the twentieth century, the public's health, safety, and welfare was increasingly interpreted as including minimum requirements for the construction of buildings and structures. This interpretation has largely been the result of large disastrous events. One of the earliest events was the Chicago Fire of 1871. After this disaster, where it has been estimated that 300 people died and 100,000 were left homeless, the city required all construction to be masonry. In the latter part of the twentieth century, regulations to protect the public health, safety, and welfare relative to construction spread until they have become an almost universal requirement in communities all across the nation. Interestingly, many of the events that encouraged code development were fires where large numbers of individuals were killed. The public outrage that followed such events led to an understanding that government has a role to play in guaranteeing minimal, consistent levels of safety in building construction. A current example of this historical process is the tragedy of September 11, 2001. The World Trade Center terrorist attack has been aggressively researched by the National Institute of Standards and

Technology (NIST) in its World Trade Center Disaster Study. As a result, new code requirements have been adopted, particularly in regard to high-rise buildings. In an August 2011 report by *Scientific America*, structural engineer Shyam Sunder, lead investigator for the NIST report, was quoted as saying that there have been "23 changes to the 2009 editions of the International Codes and another 17 changes to the 2012 editions" as a result of the NIST recommendations.

The first building codes were simple and direct, such as the Chicago Building Code of 1875 that was in response to the fire of 1871 mentioned above; the code mandated the use of masonry construction in an attempt to prevent more devastating fires. An example of the intent of a modern building code is the following excerpt from the International Building Code:

> The purpose of this Code is to establish the minimum requirements to safeguard the public health, safety and general welfare through structural strength, means of egress facilities, stability, sanitation, adequate light and ventilation, energy conservation, and safety to life and property from fire and other hazards attributed to the built environment and to provide safety to fire fighters and emergency responders during emergency operations. (International Building Code, 2015 Edition, Section 101, subparagraph 101.3 Intent)

In 1916, New York City adopted the first zoning ordinance. This was a revolutionary set of land use laws that were a response to the intense development occurring in lower Manhattan after the turn of the century. The zoning code initially established height and setback controls to ensure that neighboring properties had access to light and air. Also, the code separated what were considered to be functionally incompatible uses; thus, factories were excluded from residential neighborhoods.

While building codes ensure public health, safety, and welfare within individual properties, which is to say the buildings themselves, the intent of zoning codes is to ensure the health, safety, and welfare of entire communities. The concern here is how multiple properties interact with each other and what impact they have on the overall community. Zoning concerns include

- Encouraging appropriate land uses for the community
- Safety from fire, flood, panic, and other natural or man-made disasters
- Establishing appropriate population densities, thus preventing overcrowding of land
- Providing all properties with access to adequate light, air, and open space
- Convenience and coordination of transportation routes
- Encouraging efficient expenditure of public funds by coordination of infrastructure and public development
- The conservation of property values

ZONING CODES

Local codes addressing building construction are split between the issues of overall land use and that of the building itself. These are, respectively, zoning codes and building codes. Zoning codes regulate general land use and development issues for individual properties. They provide specific restrictions on the use of individual properties from the perspective of the "greater good" of the community. Zoning and land development is a transparent, public process. Depending on the specifics of a project, public hearings are often necessary. When changes or variances are being sought for a specific property, the public hearing process is usually measured in months. Large projects covering many acres can take a year or more before approval is granted, and very large projects, involving perhaps hundreds of acres, may take several years. In many jurisdictions, especially for commercial and industrial development, it is prudent to have legal representation. Occasionally, in order to establish the limits of the individual property owner's rights versus the governing authority, cases are adjudicated in the courts.

The fundamental component of land use regulations is the zoning district. Every acre of land within a community is categorized as to uses that are acceptable. In general, these districts are categorized as residential, commercial, retail, and industrial. Often these categories are further subdivided into levels or densities of use, such as industrial and light industrial. Also, special mixed-use districts can be created that combine several of the traditional uses. The zoning code details the uses that are allowed for each particular district and establishes specific design standards and regulations. Besides the main or primary uses that are allowed, each district usually includes certain other special uses. These are typically called conditional uses and are considered compatible with the main use or are allowed under certain specific circumstances.

The regulations pertaining to each zoning district are described within the text of that municipality's zoning code. Historically, there have been no nationally recognized model zoning codes that are ready-made for adoption by local communities. However, today the International Code Council publishes such a model code. Most existing zoning codes, however, have been developed by the individual jurisdiction and are specific to that locale. Local zoning codes have typically evolved over time and been modified many times in response to the changing needs, concerns, and circumstances of the community. Because of the preponderance of these existing codes, the International Zoning Code is not widely used. As a consequence, codes from different municipalities vary greatly, and it is necessary to consult the specific code of the jurisdiction where a project is located.

BUILDING CODES

Since the early part of the twentieth century, three regional organizations developed model codes that have dominated the building industry throughout the United States. These were the Building Officials and Code Administrators International (BOCA), International Conference of Building Officials (ICBO), and Southern Building Code Congress (SBCCI). While regional code development has been effective and responsive to the needs of the country, in time it became apparent that a single set of codes, applied across the country, would be beneficial. It was believed that uniform codes would allow consistent and efficient code enforcement, encourage greater commerce across state lines, and result in consistent and higher construction quality. In 1994, the three model code organizations came together and created the International Code Council (ICC) and developed the International Building Codes (IBCs). Since their issuance in 2000, these codes have become the standard throughout the country.

A second model building code also exists. The NFPA 5000: Building Construction and Safety Code™ has been developed by the National Fire Protection Association. However, it is not widely used. In this chapter, we focus on the IBCs, believing that these codes represent a more general set of standards at this time. The IBC is not just a single building code, but a complete set of coordinated codes designed to accommodate the complete code needs of every municipality and jurisdiction across the country. These model codes are listed in Table 13.1.

There also exist several other specialty model codes. These are often adopted in conjunction with the previously mentioned codes. Prime examples of these are the National Electrical Code, which is a popular electric code developed by the NFPA, and the National Standard Plumbing Code, developed by the National Association of Plumbing–Heating–Cooling Contractors. Both these model codes can be used, and frequently are, in place of the corresponding ICC codes listed above. Very often, the total package of model codes adopted by a jurisdiction is a mix from these and other organizations. As an example, see Table 13.2, which lists codes adopted statewide by New Jersey as of 2015. Note in the table that there are model codes from different years or "code cycles," as well as from different organizations. Also, there are two specialty codes written by the jurisdiction itself.

Model codes are designed to be adopted as is. However, in all cases, every jurisdiction adopts those codes they deem appropriate. Very often there are administrative modifications and additions. In some cases, for example, New York State, the jurisdiction modifies many details of the technical content and effectively publishes its own code, even though the majority of the model code remains. Therefore, it is important to verify the codes that are enforced for each given location. Also, the model codes change over time. The ICC is on a 3-year cycle with yearly supplements. Therefore, it is

TABLE 13.1

2015 International Building Codes

International Building Code®

International Residential Code for One- and Two-Family Dwellings®

International Mechanical Code®

International Plumbing Code®

International Fire Code®

International Fuel Gas Code®

International Energy Conservation Code®

International Existing Building Code®

International Wildland Urban Interface Code®

ICC® Performance Code for Buildings and Facilities

International Property Maintenance Code®

International Zoning Code®

International Private Sewage Disposal Code®

International Swimming Pool and Spa Code®

International Green Construction Code™

TABLE 13.2

Model Codes Adopted in New Jersey (2015)

Code	Originating Agency
International Building Code—NJ, 2009	International Code Council
National Electric Code, 2011	National Fire Protection Association
National Standard Plumbing Code, 2009	National Association of Plumbing–Heating–Cooling Contractors
ASHRAE 90.1–2007 (Commercial Energy Code)	American Society of Heating, Refrigerating, and Air-Conditioning Engineers
International Mechanical Code, 2009	International Code Council
International Fuel Gas Code, 2009	International Code Council
Rehabilitation Subcode 5:23–6	New Jersey Department of Community Affairs
Barrier-Free Subcode 5:23–7	New Jersey Department of Community Affairs
ANSI A117.1–2003	American National Standards Institute

important to determine if a jurisdiction has recently changed or is planning to change their adopted codes to a more recent edition.

Beyond the specifics of the building code itself are the requirements set forth in the other complementary codes. Most of these are specific to the various construction trades and cover code minimum technical requirements for the engineered building systems, including plumbing, mechanical, electrical, fuel gas, and private sewage disposal. In addition, the fire, energy conservation, property maintenance, and residential codes cover areas of construction of special concern that are not adequately covered in the other codes. Depending on the scope of the project, some or most of these codes may apply. Fortunately, on any given project, the responsibility for code compliance is divided among all the specialty designers engaged.

OTHER STANDARDS

In addition to the building codes listed above, there are numerous additional standards and regulations that must also be addressed. The IBC itself devotes nearly 20 pages to standards from 56 different organizations that are specifically referenced in the text of the code. Many of these standards are specific to the use and design of particular materials and systems, such as those from the American Concrete Institute (ACI) and the NFPA.

NFPA standards warrant a special note. The NFPA standards referenced in the code include many that are typical for all types of construction, such as NFPA 13: "Installation of Sprinkler Systems." However, due to the common use of solvents and powders in pharmaceutical manufacturing facilities, the following are of particular importance:

- NFPA 30: "Flammable and Combustible Liquids Code"
- NFPA 69: "Explosion Prevention Systems"
- NFPA 654: "Prevention of Fire and Dust Explosions from the Manufacturing, Processing, and Handling of Combustible Particulate Solids"

Additional codes and standards that deserving note are as follows:

1. *Elevator code.* ASME A17.1, "Safety Code for Elevators and Escalators," is a standard referenced in the building code. However, because historically the elevator was recognized as posing a potential life and safety danger long before the advent of most building codes, many states mandate compliance with their own code. Often this is ASME A17.1, but frequently the states add special, detailed requirements.
2. *FM Global.* FM Global has developed many construction-related standards. A few of them are referenced in the building code. However, if a company is insured by FM Global, then compliance with these standards must be explored. In any case, it is always important to check with an owner's insurance carrier to see whether they have special requirements that will impact the facility design and construction.
3. *Occupational Safety and Health Agency.* A portion of 29 CFR 1910 addresses design of buildings and structures. Usually, the building codes cover the same ground and are more stringent. However, in practice there are times when the building code does not cover a particular situation. It is not unusual to find such conditions when developing the layout of mechanical rooms and equipment platforms. At those times when the building code is not applicable, it is necessary to look to OSHA as a minimum standard.
4. *Drug Enforcement Administration.* When narcotics or other controlled substances are present in a pharmaceutical facility, the DEA provides guidance. These provisions usually focus on security of the controlled substances and include the need and special criteria for the design of secure storage vaults.
5. *Americans with Disabilities Act.* This is a unique regulation that impacts the design and construction of pharmaceutical manufacturing facilities. Unlike any other standard, this is a federal civil rights law. The intention is to guarantee accessibility to the public realm for all people with disabilities. As such, it extends well beyond building design and construction, addressing issues such as hiring and firing, as well as the working conditions of disabled employees and potential employees.

   The ADA addresses the design and construction of public and commercial buildings through a set of design guidelines. The ADA design guidelines are based on a previous edition of the ANSI handicapped standards. Although these design guidelines are not dissimilar from other existing handicapped design standards that are familiar to construction and design professionals, the ADA must be addressed independently. The ADA design guidelines carry the weight of a federal civil rights law but are not enforced at the local level. As a civil rights law, these design standards are enforced only in the courts, that is, only when an accusation of discrimination occurs. It should be reiterated that this law goes well beyond the design guidelines for a facility and may impact a company's hiring and other operational considerations.

6. *Environmental Protection Agency and State Department of Environmental Protection permits.* When working with new or continued development of a site, there can be environmental restrictions and guidelines that must be followed. These issues can affect how a building is situated on the property. Examples include the presence of adjacent wetlands and, in some locations, endangered species. In addition, the various discharge potentials for a site, such as sanitary waste and storm drainage, may be an issue that needs careful consideration. The air discharge for a facility, if it contains potentially dangerous substances, may also be a regulated issue. In more urban areas, these issues are sometimes addressed locally, but often the permits are required at the state or even federal level.

CODE INTERPRETATION

Reading and understanding the various codes is an involved and intricate process. While much of the codes are reasonably clear, inevitably there are areas and situations that require interpretation. Because the origin of codes arises from the government's duty to provide for the public's health, safety and welfare, interpretations must be objective and not just made in the building owner's favor. Enforcement and interpretation of codes for the public good are provided through the building plan review and building permit process. It is a long-established principle that the local code authority responsible for enforcement is the final authority and arbiter of any code. This is clearly stated in the International Building Code. However, it is not appropriate or practical to look to the local code official for continuous code input during the lengthy process that is design. Likewise, it is the design professional that holds the legal responsibility to provide a code-compliant design. By necessity, the design professional provides code interpretations whenever he or she develops a design and can be called upon to consider various options and implications regarding the codes. When an unusual or particularly difficult situation arises that is outside the design professional's experience or expertise, it is possible to hire a consultant who specializes in code interpretation. Finally, the model code organizations provide code interpretation services for individuals and firms who are members. In fact, design professionals often take advantage of such interpretive services as a normal part of their design work.

To summarize, there are four primary sources for code interpretations:

- The design professional
- Specialty code consultants
- The model code organizations
- The local code official

ROLE OF THE DESIGN PROFESSIONAL

Licensed by the individual states, design professionals have a legal responsibility to provide designs that meet the codes that are enforced within their state. On a daily basis, the design professional deals with the codes and their design implementations. Their experience with the codes and the code officials, and the resulting impact on design, can be extensive. As a result, they are usually the best first source for interpretations, especially when dealing within their areas of expertise.

ROLE OF THE SPECIALTY CODE CONSULTANT

Due to the complexity and potentially intimidating quality of codes, a code consultant industry has developed. For these professionals, working with the code is a daily endeavor. Due to the intensity and singular nature of their practice, they are capable of acquiring an extraordinary depth of knowledge about the details of the codes.

ROLE OF THE MODEL CODE ORGANIZATIONS

As noted before, the ICC and the NFPA are the primary organizations responsible for the two competing groups of building codes. Both organizations have procedures designed to help the design professional and building owners interpret their codes. These include informal interpretations via the telephone, as well as formal, written interpretations.

ROLE OF THE CODE OFFICIAL

The code official is the public entity entrusted with enforcement of the code and has the legal authority to make code interpretations. Section 104.1 of the IBC states:

> The building official shall have the authority to render interpretations of this code and to adopt policies and procedures in order to clarify the application of its provisions. Such interpretations, policies and procedures shall be in compliance with the intent and purpose of this code. Such policies and procedures shall not have the effect of waiving requirements specifically provided for in this code.

The normal procedure is for the final construction documents to be submitted to the code official for review and approval, which is a prerequisite for issuing a building permit. Only when there is nonconformance does the code official make a statement about the code. Typically, the code official requests that changes be made to bring the design into conformance with specific code citations. While this is the formal procedure, it is often advisable and appropriate to request an informal meeting or even a number of meetings with the code official. These meetings should be used to review code issues early in the development of the design and perhaps again during the construction documents.

As with any opportunity for interpretation, agreement among all parties is not assured. Sometimes the design professional and the code official will not agree on a particular interpretation. When this occurs, the owner can choose to accept the code official's interpretation or to work with the design professional to change the code official's opinion. Sometimes this is as simple as asking the code official to use the text of the code to demonstrate the basis and logic of his or her interpretation. At other times, such situations amount to a negotiation. In those situations, it is always advantageous for the owner to state how the code official's interpretation may cause hardship or injury to the owner. Also, it is necessary for the design professional to use the text of the code to demonstrate the logic of his or her counterinterpretation. Providing the code official with an interpretation from the appropriate model code organization can also be a powerful argument. Although the code official, as the local authority with jurisdiction over interpretations, has no obligation to accept the interpretation of the model code organization, it is hard to refute the opinion of the organization that actually developed the code. And finally, some jurisdictions allow for the appeal of rulings by the building official. At such times a third-party panel is empowered to resolve the conflict.

A different case is when a clear conflict arises between the owner's needs and the requirements of the code. In cases where this conflict is clear, the only means of resolution is to apply for a variance. It is advisable to meet with the code official prior to a variance application and use this opportunity to understand, from the code official's view, what the issues are and the potential for awarding the requested variance. In such a case, the building owner may be required to provide certain additional measures beyond the letter of the code in order to mitigate what would otherwise be a non-code-compliant condition.

PROJECT MANAGEMENT ISSUES

The code issues that affect the management of a construction project are primarily time and schedule. Understanding what reviews, public meetings, and variances are required and then allotting enough time for these requirements is key. Establishing an effective sequencing of activities that moves the project forward, but does not expose the owner to project redesign, and therefore unnecessary financial expense, is also important.

The land development process is complex. It includes formal and informal submissions and reviews (often from several public agencies), as well as public meetings. For small projects, it is common for the land development process to take a minimum of 3 months. While a simple project can be submitted and approved in as little as a month, 2 or more months is a more reasonable estimate, especially when considering the time for initial contact and discussions with the jurisdiction. Affecting this too is that the schedule for public meetings is usually on a monthly cycle. As a consequence, when a submission date is missed by 1 day, the schedule is set back an entire month.

Large or complex projects almost always take more time. Large complex projects on a new site can easily take a year or more. And there are cases where the owner has opted to take the community to court instead of accepting the jurisdiction's decision. Due to the public nature of the review process, when the project is controversial within the community, the public meetings can become difficult, emotionally charged, and highly political. Identifying such potential very early in the project and perhaps avoiding sites and communities with this potential should be a consideration undertaken by the management team. On top of all this, there is the variance process. The same considerations for public meetings occur with a request for variance and additional time should be allocated. Therefore, except for the simplest of projects, it is best to allow a minimum of 3 months for land development review.

The plan review and building permit process is not a public review process. Because this process is essentially administrative in nature, the duration for submission, review, and issuing of building permits is usually measured in weeks. However, in jurisdictions that are experiencing rapid development, the building official's backlog of work can greatly slow the process. Understanding such local dynamics can be crucial for developing an accurate schedule. Of course, as with land development, variances will take longer. In many jurisdictions, the body responsible for granting variances meets monthly, and the potential to slip a month, if a submission date is missed, exists here also.

Another project management concern is developing a strategic concept for the facility in respect to the codes. This is necessary in order to align the desired result with the requirements of the building code. Such early conceptual work can facilitate optimization of the building size, allow for effective future expansion, and increase the flexibility in the use of the facility, especially regarding the use of hazardous materials such as solvents.

TRENDS AND FUTURE DEVELOPMENTS

Today, codes are a fact of the construction industry. During the twentieth century, codes became a prominent factor and represented the minimum standard for health and safety in building design and construction. Codes will continue to be influenced by major building disasters that result in lost lives. In addition, the drive for sustainability and business innovation is stimulating the development of new building materials. Science-based research into every aspect of facility design has become commonplace, and our knowledge of the optimum use of materials and building systems is increasing. As the original code issues of egress and fire-resistant construction become highly refined and deeply entrenched in the construction industry, the other less obvious areas of the code come to the fore. Some past examples include the relatively new and changing developments in accessibility standards and the accommodation of hazardous materials.

A clear future trend, then, is the refinement of the codes resulting in more precise definition of their requirements. Greater and clearer definition of the codes results in fewer questions; however, it usually simultaneously expands their restrictions. As we demonstrated in the introduction to the chapter, this is a historical trend that shows no sign of changing.

An interesting example is found in hurricane safety. The decade 1996–2005 was an intensely destructive period for hurricanes. With damage totaling $198 billion, it was one of the most destructive decades of the last century. There are numerous institutions, including the University of Florida and the Institute for Business & Home Safety, that are researching how to create more durable communities with the intent of providing an objective, sound foundation for enhancements to the building codes.

Since the adoption of the ADA in the early 1990s, accessible design has been vigorously embraced. However, due to the nature of the act as a civil rights law versus a technical design standard, when and to what extent the ADA design guidelines is applied is not completely clear. Over the last years, there have been a number of lawsuits that have begun to define these limits. These sometimes unsettling developments will continue until the law is more clearly defined or the courts provide that definition. There is also debate about the adequacy of some of the detailed requirements commonly found in the current accessibility standards, and more research will, undoubtedly, lead to more effective and appropriate design standards.

Over the last years, there have been many changes to the hazardous material portions of the codes. With the introduction of the IBC, a major step has been taken in clearly defining these requirements, especially regarding the need for explosion control. However, this clarity has also resulted in more restrictions. Due to the highly variable chemistry of hazardous materials in a room environment, facility design for hazardous materials is a particularly difficult endeavor. The physical characteristics of the particular material, the details of the handling and processing of that material, and the particulars and environmental conditions of the room itself all contribute to the potential hazard and mitigation of hazard. These highly variable circumstances seem to leave a lot of room for more code precision. Therefore, it seems likely that further changes are possible here, too.

There has been much discussion through the years about the prescriptive nature of the building codes—how this stifles creativity and denies alternatives to both designers and owners. In Europe, performance-based codes are common and represent an alternative to our approach in this country. The ICC and NFPA are both researching and experimenting with performance-based codes. Their current building codes actually allow for performance-based design, but only at the discretion of the local enforcement agency and with appropriate substantiation of the validity of the design. Supporting this trend is a growing number of specialty buildings that necessitate such an approach. In response, an experienced and knowledgeable group of consultancies is emerging. To what extent performance-based design will replace the prescriptive approach of the dominant codes remains to be seen, but the discussion is far from over.

Sustainable design is another trend. In the construction industry, the development and codification of "green" design has become part of the mainstream. Public and private organizations have embraced green design, including various branches of the U.S. government that have responsibility for a large quantity of construction. On this front, energy savings have seen the biggest advancements. The International Energy Code and ANSI/ASHRAE/IES 90.1–2013, "Energy Standard for Buildings Except Low-Rise Residential Buildings," have become the standard for building energy savings throughout the United States. While sustainable design is here to stay, it remains to be seen what other sustainable features, if any, will be taken up as code requirements by the individual jurisdictions.

SPECIAL DISCUSSION: HAZARDOUS MATERIALS

Hazardous materials are common in the pharmaceutical industry, in both manufacturing and research. With the intent to mitigate the potential for dangerous conditions, the ICC codes address facility requirements for the storage and use of hazardous materials.

When dealing with hazardous materials, the precise materials or chemicals must first be identified. In identifying chemicals, it is necessary to categorize them per the definitions provided in Section 307 of the IBC. The Department of Transportation hazard classifications that are easily found on material safety data sheets (MSDSs) do not usually have a direct correspondence to the categories used in the code. Instead, the physical properties of the material must be reviewed and compared to the code definitions in order to determine their proper definition. For instance, isopropyl alcohol is a liquid with a closed-cup flash point below 23°C and a boiling point above 38°C. These criteria define a Class IB flammable liquid. Table 13.3 gives a list of the categories of hazardous materials defined in the IBC.

TABLE 13.3
Hazard Classifications

Material	Class
Combustible dust	NA
Combustible fiber	Loose baled
Combustible liquid	II
	IIIA
	IIIB
Consumer fireworks	1.4G
Cryogenic inert	NA
Cryogenic oxidizing	NA
Explosives	Division 1.1
	Division 1.2
	Division 1.3
	Division 1.4
	Division 1.4G
	Division 1.5
	Division 1.6
Flammable gas	Gaseous
	Liquefied
Flammable liquid	IA
	IB and IC
Flammable liquids in combination (IA, IB, IC)	NA
Flammable solid	NA
Inert gas	Gaseous
	Liquefied
Organic peroxide	UD
	I
	II
	III
	IV
	V
Oxidizer	4
	3k
	2
	1
Oxidizing gas	Gaseous
	Liquefied
Pyrophoric	NA
Unstable (reactive)	4
	3
	2
	1
Water reactive	3
	2
	1

Next, the maximum quantity of each material that will be in use and storage must be determined. Current and accurate information of this sort should already be available within the company since OSHA, as part of its employee safety mandate, requires that a detailed hazardous material inventory be maintained. However, this information must still be properly categorized in terms of the code and the type of use: storage or open or closed use.

Table 307.1 of the IBC establishes a threshold below which materials are allowed in the building without changing the primary use group, that is, the amount of material that can be maintained in an F-factory or S-storage use group. This threshold corresponds to what the code terms a control area. A control area is a portion of a building that is enclosed in fire-rated construction. A building can contain more than one control area. Table 414.2.2 of the IBC defines the maximum number of control areas allowed per floor within a building. When floors occur above or below grade, Table 414.2.2 reduces the quantity of material allowed. Maximizing the use of control areas is sometimes all that is necessary to accommodate the anticipated amount of hazardous material for a facility.

Regardless of the quantity of hazardous material, the codes establish certain basic requirements that must be followed. Chapter 4 of the IBC covers general requirements for the use of the various types of material. In addition, the International Fire Code (IFC) devotes entire chapters to the various types of material covered in the code and establishes more detailed requirements. Therefore, it is important to review both the IBC and the IFC when coming to terms with hazardous materials.

When the quantity of hazardous material exceeds those listed in IBC's Table 307.1, the use group must be changed to the appropriate high hazard use group. Because of the common use of solvents, the most dominant high hazard use groups found in the pharmaceutical industry are H-2 and H-3. H-2 applies to flammable liquids that are in normally open containers (dispensing is a good example) or are pressurized at more than 15 lb/in.^{2}. H-3 corresponds to use and storage in normally closed containers or systems pressurized at 15 lb/in.^{2} or less. Storage is typically H-3.

Under all high hazard use groups, the allowable building areas are greatly limited per Table 506.2 of the IBC. This, in turn, limits the final size of the building even when it is a mixed-use structure. The alternative approach is to make the facility an unlimited area building or, alternately, to make the building highly fire resistant. In the end, it is clearly the intent of the code to restrict high hazard uses to a manageable size. In fact, as an example, an H-1 use is not allowed to be mixed with any other use group. An H-1 use is dedicated to detonation hazards and must be in a completely separate building. However, H-1 is a nontypical use for the pharmaceutical industry.

Another important consideration is whether a material is in storage, being dispensed, or used in processes that are open or closed. The code has specific requirements for each of these applications, and again, the code must be consulted for the particulars. When it comes to the dispensing and use of flammable materials, the need for special electrical classifications must also be considered. Chapter 5 of the National Standard Electric Code refers to hazardous location Classes I, II, and III. Here the parameters of each class are clearly defined and relate directly to the conditions of the materials being used.

A critical issue that must be reviewed when the quantities of hazardous material exceed those listed in Table 307.1 of the IBC is that of explosion hazards. When an explosion hazard exists, explosion control must be provided. Under the code, explosion control systems are defined as barricade construction, deflagration venting, or explosion prevention systems. NFPA 68, "Venting of Deflagrations," and NFPA 69, "Explosion Prevention Systems," provide the full requirements for explosion control. IBC Table 414.5.1, "Explosion Control Requirements," indicates where these controls are required. The IBC, IFC, and appropriate referenced standards, such as NFPA 68 and 69, must be consulted when dealing with explosion hazards.

The need for explosion control is not just triggered by the quantity of hazardous material. A process itself can be an explosion hazard even when the quantities of hazardous materials are below the threshold values of IBC Table 307.1. Therefore, if those responsible for a process know or believe that an explosion hazard exists, regardless of the quantities, then code-compliant explosion control

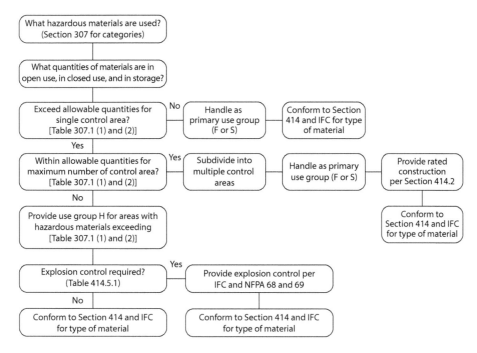

FIGURE 13.1 International Building Code hazardous materials decision tree.

must be provided. Of course, this determination is outside the expertise for most construction design professionals. Usually individuals trained in chemistry and industrial hygiene are required to analyze such situations.

As demonstrated in the example above, the IBC and IFC reference several NFPA standards in regard to hazardous materials. All such standards need to be reviewed when they are referenced. As another example, NFPA 30, "Flammable and Combustible Liquids Code," regulates the distance from a building that bulk tank storage of hazardous material must be located.

Figure 13.1 presents a decision tree that outlines a logical sequence that can be helpful when reviewing the code requirements for hazardous materials.

FURTHER DISCUSSION

The following questions are intended to prompt further discussion regarding building codes:

1. Does it matter which codes are used on a project?
2. Should building and zoning codes ever be exceeded?
3. How do building codes develop?
4. Would the public be safer without building and zoning codes?

ABOUT THE AUTHOR

Eric Bohn is a licensed architect with more than 35 years of experience designing and building facilities for corporate and institutional clients. For the last 20 years, he has focused on the pharmaceutical and biotechnology industry, bringing his broad range of construction experience to these technologically intensive facilities. His designs include renovations and additions to existing facilities across the nation, as well as internationally. His master planning efforts have helped numerous clients understand the potential of their legacy facilities, as well as bring them back into compliance with current Good Manufacturing Practices. In 2011, his architectural design work was recognized when the Merck Global Clinical Supply Facility won the ISPE Facility of the Year Award for Integration. Eric is a long-standing member of ISPE and has lectured on design issues for his local chapter, as well as at the annual meeting. In addition, he is the author of numerous articles for industry publications, including *Pharmaceutical Engineering* and *Pharmaceutical Technology*. Mr. Bohn is a partner with JacobsWyper Architects, an architectural firm located in Philadelphia, Pennsylvania, that specializes in the design of facilities for pharmaceutical research and manufacturing.

FURTHER READING

International Code Council, *2015 International Building Code*, International Code Council, Falls Church, VA, 2014.
International Code Council, *2015 International Fire Code*, International Code Council, Falls Church, VA, 2014.
International Code Council, *2015 International Mechanical Code*, International Code Council, Falls Church, VA, 2014.
International Code Council, *2015 International Plumbing Code*, International Code Council, Falls Church, VA, 2014.
National Fire Protection Association, *NFPA 30: Flammable and Combustible Liquids Code*, National Fire Protection Association, Quincy, MA, 2015.
National Fire Protection Association, *NFPA 68: Venting of Deflagrations*, National Fire Protection Association, Quincy, MA, 2013.
National Fire Protection Association, *NFPA 69: Explosion Prevention Systems*, National Fire Protection Association, Quincy, MA, 2014.
National Fire Protection Association, *NFPA 70: National Electric Code*, 1999 ed., National Fire Protection Association, Quincy, MA, 2014.
New Jersey Department of Community Affairs, New Jersey Administrative Code Title 5:23, Uniform Construction Code, New Jersey Department of Community Affairs, Trenton, NJ.
Occupational Safety and Health Administration, 29 CFR, Part 1910, Occupational Safety and Health Standards, Occupational Safety and Health Administration, Washington, DC.
Ching FDK, *Building Codes Illustrated: A Guide to Understanding the 2012 Building Code*, John Wiley & Sons, New York, 2012.
Kardon R, *Code Check Complete: An Illustrated Guide to Building, Plumbing, Mechanical, and Electrical Codes*, Taunton Press, Newtown, CT, 2012.
Shyam-Sunder, Sivaraj (December 1, 2005) "Federal Building and Fire Safety Investigation of the World Trade Center Disaster: Final Report of the National Construction Safety Team on the Collapses of the World Trade Center Towers" (NIST NCSTAR 1)
Choi, Charles Q. (August 11, 2011) "Twin Towers Forensic Investigation Helps Revise Building Codes, Despite Critics" Retrieved from http://www.scientificamerican.com/article/twin-towers-forensic-investigation-revise-building-codes/

14 Containment Technology

Hank Rahe and Brian G. Ward

CONTENTS

INTRODUCTION

Containment technology reaches across the entire health care spectrum, ranging from discovery to patient delivery. New drugs and delivery systems for drugs require the two critical elements that containment (or isolation) technology provides, namely, protection of the product and protection of personnel who produce the drugs. Since drugs are becoming more potent, exposure to small amounts can result in deleterious effects. Innovative delivery technologies create an even greater challenge, with final dosage forms that focus on specific targets in the body, creating a higher risk of exposure for health care personnel involved in the delivery of these drug forms to the intended patient.

The ability to measure small quantities of the active pharmaceutical ingredient (API) has resulted in a closer examination of the potential for cross-contamination. Drugs that can cause an adverse reaction or, even more critical, a nonreversible effect at low doses are becoming more common. The potency of these new drugs has added new dimensions for cleaning validation. Detection in the picogram (one trillionth of a gram) range of the drugs has also created new concerns with sample collection, measurement, and evaluation.

Additional factors that have created a need for isolation technology are waste minimization, which has become a priority, increased cost of raw materials, and the need for more extensive processing, all of which add significantly to the cost of the final product. The combination of the need for product protection and personnel protection, cross-contamination risk, waste reduction, and cost of the drug results in the need for isolation systems. The capability of the isolation system must meet the need for containment of airborne active drug substances to less than 1 ng/m^3.

Terms such *high containment* have little value when determining an effective approach to product or personnel protection. Defining the risk potential by using risk assessment tools leads to better solutions. This chapter addresses the technological solutions for minimizing drug exposure from material release. It also explores the means of evaluating the capabilities of isolation technology solutions, measurement techniques to determine how much drug is present, and the risks created by cross-contamination of the drug.

DEFINING DRUGS IN TERMS OF CONTAMINATION RISK

"The dose makes the poison" was first expressed by Paracelsus (Philippus Aureolus Theophrastus Bombastus von Hohenheim, 1493–1541), who intended the comment to communicate a basic principle of toxicology, which is that a substance can produce harmful effects associated with its toxic properties only if it reaches a susceptible biological system within the body in a high enough concentration. The basic principle of pharmaceuticals is to create a positive, not negative, effect on the patient. To accomplish the positive effect, the correct dosage for the intended patient is carefully designed and tested by the pharmaceutical manufacturing company. Extensive testing is conducted also to determine what quantity of the drug will create a negative effect. The negative effect can come in several different ways: a person can consume a higher than intended dose, or personnel working with and around the drug can be exposed to a level that will create a negative effect. The entire life cycle of the drug, from discovery to administration to the patient, is associated with exposure risks.

Understanding of the difference between the dose that makes the poison and that which benefits patients is far from simple. At the early stages of drug development, researchers are looking for a compound that creates a focused positive effect on a given category of disease. This process results in searches of thousands of compounds, looking for one that has the desired effect on the target disease. Along with the positive effect also comes a negative effect based on the quantity of the compound to which one is exposed. Once a compound is selected for further evaluation, testing begins and follows an extensive routine to determine both effectiveness and side effects. Initial containment assessments include only information available from limited toxicology tests and compounds that are chemically similar to determine the hazard potential of a compound.

Initial dose–response studies help to determine the point at which a positive effect is observed. As the dose is increased, there is an increase in the incidence and severity of adverse effects. Containment protection of personnel working with the compound at this stage is most important because the exposure risk is not well understood. In these early stages of drug development, a risk factor that fits the class of compound should be assigned based on worst-case assumptions, and the proper engineering controls that limit exposures should be implemented.

COMMUNICATION OF RISK

Communication of risk, using banding, was created in the 1990s in an attempt to place compounds in groups or bands that could then be associated with specific engineering technologies. A typical band defines a range of occupational exposure limits (OELs) that the given engineering control is capable of achieving. Individual companies created definitions of bands, ranging from three to six categories of exposure limits. Depending on category or band assigned to a specific drug, there was a significant economic impact on facilities that handled the drug.

The early primary containment focus was on powders, as it was believed that airborne particulates represented the greatest risk of exposure to workers. Studies were conducted to determine why different compounds produced greater exposure risks when processed in identical equipment. The results of the studies concluded that particle characteristics play a critical role with airborne emissions in terms of particle size, shape, and density that directly impact the ability of the particle to become and stay airborne [1]. The "dustiness index" describes the results of testing dust, using a Heubach dust meter. The Heubach method most appropriately simulates the particle behavior characteristic of those generated during drug manufacturing processes.

Liquids were considered a lower risk of airborne exposure until studies showed that when a liquid was placed under pressure, such as during the filling operation, liquid that detached from the filling needles could produce airborne aerosols. This risk also exists in the compounding transfer from drug vials to the final delivery package. Concerns about the risk of compounds transforming into vapors have been raised with the antineoplastic drug class by the National Institute for Occupational Safety and Health (NIOSH). Vapors can only be created during a phase change from solids and liquids to a gas as a result of pressure and temperature changes. Therefore, it is very unlikely that this phase change is significant at room temperature during normal manipulations that occur in transferring the drug from a vial to the final patient delivery package. An article written by a NIOSH team member stated that vapors could be produced during manipulation of some antineoplastic drugs, but this process required elevated temperatures [2].

Containment equipment manufacturers, engineering firms, and engineering societies wanted a definitive means of describing achievement levels of the engineering control and uniform test methods to validate the level of control capability of a specific engineering control configuration. In 2001, a book entitled *Containment in the Pharmaceutical Industry* was published, outlining containment control strategies based on hazard bands that addressed the potential solids, liquids, and vapors have to create hazardous emissions [3].

Risk Assessment by NIOSH and the European Medicines Agency

In August 2009, NIOSH published "Qualitative Risk Characterization and Management of Occupational Hazards: Control Banding (CB): A Literature Review and Critical Analysis" [4]. The scope of the publication includes CB strategies, presented within the context of qualitative occupational risk management concepts. The risk management strategy associated with CB is characterized by selection and implementation of appropriate control solutions.

In November 2014, the European Medicines Agency (EMA) finalized a guideline on setting exposure limits for use in risk identification in the manufacture of different medicinal products in shared facilities [5]. The guideline addresses management of cross-contamination based on risk assessment to ensure the safety of workers exposed to residual substances.

Measurement Techniques

Empirical methods are used to check the integrity of an enclosure before putting it in service. Acceptance by the quality organization is the main criterion for method selection. Test procedures include pressurized leak testing; ammonia leak testing, using ammonia-sensitive strips; aerosol fog leakage, using a particle counter; and pressurized sound sensing. Methods not involving chemicals contacting enclosure inner walls are more suitable for small enclosures with simple designs.

Quantitative methods have been established for measuring potential personnel exposures and engineering performance. The International Society for Pharmaceutical Engineering (ISPE) Good Practice Guide entitled *Assessing the Particulate Containment Performance of Pharmaceutical Equipment* [6] details the measurement of worker exposure within the test environment. A statistically robust engineering approach is described in *Containment in the Pharmaceutical Industry* [3]. The procedure can be used to create reference performance data against which further testing throughout the life of a containment device can be established (e.g., after a maintenance event).

TABLE 14.1
Hierarchy of Containment Technologies

Technology	Contamination Control Capabilities[a]
Isolators	Less than 0.1 ng/m³[b] (both personnel exposure and engineering capability data)
Glove bags	Less than 0.1 ng/m³[c] (both personnel exposure and engineering capability data)
Open-front, unidirectional airflow devices (includes downflow booths and biological safety cabinets)	Approximately 10 ng/m³
Local/point exhaust	30–100 µg/m³

[a] Capabilities are expressed in levels in the breathing zone of a person over an 8 or 12 h exposure time frame.
[b] The use of PPE as the primary engineering control is unacceptable to either the Occupational Safety and Health Administration (OSHA) or the Canadian Centre for Occupational Health and Safety (CCOHS).
[c] Below the quantification limit of the methodology.

COMPARISON OF EXPOSURE RISK TO ISOLATION TECHNOLOGY SOLUTIONS

Exposure risks are based on a number of factors, including engineering controls, personal protective equipment (PPE), quantity of compound present, and sampling and measurement sensitivity. The basic premise of the engineering control strategy should be to contain the compound as close to the source as possible. If the process equipment is able to provide adequate containment, the challenge becomes transfers and sampling of the compound during processing and equipment servicing. These are the points where additional isolation technology is required.

Engineering controls used for containment of the exposure risk can be categorized based on the effectiveness of the control device. Banding of compounds into groups with a given level of exposure allows engineering controls to be matched up with the bands. An example of this approach is expressed in a hierarchy of the containment capabilities of given engineering control technologies (Table 14.1). It should be noted that the level of protection afforded by the engineering technology is only a guide and needs to be verified by validation of the engineering control.

TECHNOLOGY DESCRIPTIONS

Within a given containment technology, there are a number of key elements that impact performance. This section explores not only the different technologies but also the configuration of the technology that impacts the containment ability of the engineering control device.

ISOLATORS

All isolators are constructed with four basic components: the physical structure, the internal environment, interaction components, and monitoring systems. The choices selected for alternative components in each of these categories determine the overall capability of the isolator. A mock-up of the isolator is an effective means of determining functionality of the isolator and should consist of easily modified materials, such as polystyrene panels defining the boundaries of the isolator and clear polycarbonate for the window. The mock-up is likely a throwaway item, not creating a look-alike piece to the isolator, but focused on testing functionality. The bottom should be capable of supporting the intended objects that will be placed into the isolator for manipulation. The mock-up offers several other uses, including ergonomic evaluations and as a training tool.

Physical Structure

The physical structure is made up of a variety of materials broken into two basic classes: hard shell or soft shell. The selection depends on the following three issues: durability, cleanability of internal surfaces, and line-of-sight visibility of the inside of the isolator. Typical hard-shell materials are various grades of stainless steel, plastic, and polycarbonates. Durability requirements, such as the environment in which the isolator is placed, equipment to be used in the isolator, internal environment in terms of heat and chemical compatibility, and cleaning requirements, impact the type of material used to construct the physical structure of the isolator.

Internal Environment

The internal environment requirements are a function of the processes to be performed inside the isolator. Requirements include air quality in terms of particulates; incorporation of special gases, such as nitrogen or argon, for product protection; the risk of flammability or explosion; and humidity control required by the process. Passing the air entering the isolator through high-efficiency particulate air (HEPA) or ultra-low penetration air (ULPA) filters removes particulates, controlling particulate air quality requirements. Air handling systems recirculate the air through either redundant filters or a once-through system. The recirculation system is typically used if special gases are required inside the isolator or if the location of the isolator makes exhausting to the outside difficult. The once-through systems are typically used for removing heat from the isolator or reducing cycle times if a Vapor Hydrogen Peroxide (VHP) biodecontamination system is used to decontaminate aseptic operations.

Transfer Technologies

Transfer technologies are the means of introducing materials into or taking materials out of isolators and range from opening a door to access the interior of the isolator to double-door transfer systems. A single-door access offers no level of separation between the outside environment and the interior of the isolator; however, if the process does not result in any hazardous gases or particulates, it would be acceptable when all materials are placed in the isolator and the door is closed. The double-door transfer system creates a transition space, or airlock, that contains an environment that differs from the outside environment. Typical applications for this are an aseptic transfer, an inert environment, or manipulation of hazardous compounds (e.g., weighing, mixing, or product additions). ISO 14644-7, "Cleanrooms and Associated Controlled Environments (Part 7): Separative Devices (Clean Air Hoods, Gloveboxes, Isolators and Mini-Environments)," contains descriptions of a number of transfer devices [7] (Figure 14.1).

Interaction Components

Interaction technologies are the means by which personnel exterior to the isolator perform operations inside the boundary of the isolator. Table 14.2 describes types of interaction technologies and their applications to different types of isolator structures.

Robotics

The use of robotics has made advances in a number of applications. Robotics offers a consistent means of performing a repetitive task that can reduce ergonomic stress as well as personnel error. Applications include sampling and personnel assist with heavy or hard-to-reach areas in isolators (Figure 14.2).

Flexible Membranes

Flexible membranes allow enough pliability to extend manipulation through the membrane wall. This technology has very limited applications.

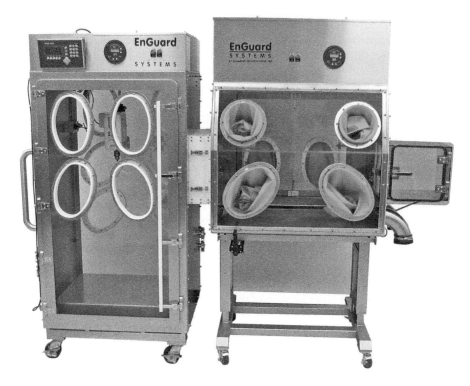

FIGURE 14.1   Containment weigh and mix isolator.

TABLE 14.2
Interaction Technology Applications

Interaction Technology	Hard Shell	Soft Shell	Glove Bag
Robotics	Yes	No	No
Flexible membranes	Yes	Yes	Yes
Half suits	Yes	Yes	Yes
Glove ports	Yes	Yes	Yes

Half Suits

The conventional half suit has both advantages and disadvantages. The advantages are an increased range of motion and allowance for increased lifting capabilities by personnel. The disadvantages are that textured flexible surfaces are difficult to clean, and personnel may experience problems adjusting to the confined space of the half suit. To reduce the cleaning issues, disposable half suits have been developed, but use of half suits increases disposable waste quantities.

Glove Ports

The glove port is the most common interaction technique. The ports can be different sizes as well as shapes. The size of the opening in the viewing panel of the isolator should consider two factors: the negative impact of the port on the ability to see inside the isolator and the positive impact of large ports in terms of reach and mobility (Figure 14.3).

Glove-port placement and shapes are the keys to a functional isolator. It is critical when designing locations and shapes to understand what is to occur in the isolator and how it is to occur. It is helpful to lay out the items to be used routinely on the floor of the mock-up without the viewing

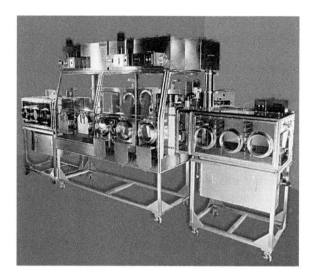

FIGURE 14.2 Automated aseptic vial filler.

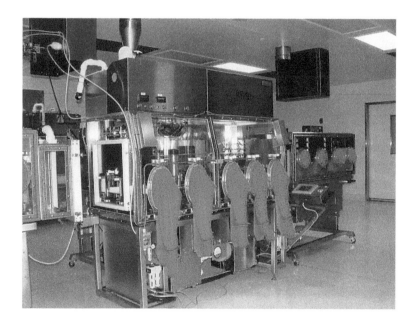

FIGURE 14.3 Aseptic filler isolator with docking. (Courtesy of Schaefer Technologies, Indianapolis, IN.)

window where the glove ports are to be and then to perform the intended steps, being careful not to breach the boundary that would be created by the viewing window. If this step is performed several times, it can help to establish a specific sequence of activities. Once the activities and sequences are understood, then the final locations for the glove ports in the viewing panel can be determined.

The required reach range determines both the shape and size of the ports. If the required reach does not necessitate a large range of motion inside the isolator to perform operations, a round port would be a good choice. The most common size of a round port is 8 in., but they are available in diameters of 6, 8, 10, and 12 in. If the operation requires either greater ranges of motion or nonroutine activities, the oval glove port offers a better choice. Ovals also can be mounted vertically, at an angle, or horizontally.

The glove-port design should allow as much surface as possible for operators to rest their forearms. This helps with arm fatigue and minimizes pressure points on the forearm. The ergonomic section provides additional details on the balance of providing temporary relief for the arms and shoulders versus leaning heavily on the supports, thereby creating a pressure point.

Glove-port height has been a subject of much debate, with a typical distance from the standing surface of 48–52 in. To establish the most ergonomically favorable height for a given operation, a survey of the personnel population working in the isolator should be taken. Height ranges across the personnel population help to determine optimum placement of glove ports, with the centerline of the port always the correct distance from the floor.

If possible, it is most desirable to equip the isolator with height adjustment to compensate for individual personnel. Adjustment is typically achieved by mounting the isolator on a hydraulic stand. Depending on weight and size, the hydraulic can be manually or electrically operated.

Sleeves and Gloves

Sleeves and gloves are the means by which glove ports are closed, allowing personnel to interact with the interior of the isolator. The factors to consider in selection of the sleeves and gloves are the chemical resistance to the materials being processed, the cleaning materials used in the cleaning process, the thickness of both the gloves and sleeves, and the durability of the materials. Chemical compatibility is critical in terms of both contamination of the materials being processed, which could be affected by leached materials from the sleeves and gloves, and permeability of the sleeve and glove material, which may breach containment of the isolator. ASTM D6978-05 (2013) is a means to determine the permeability of a given glove and sleeve material of a given thickness [8]. There are also a number of compatibility charts available from glove and sleeve manufacturers, and the many commercially available CDs based on the NIOSH database.

Gloves and sleeves are available in two configurations: one-piece or two-piece. The one-piece system has the advantage of a uniform surface, but has a number of disadvantages. The one-piece gloves and sleeves are manufactured using a dipping process; the thickness is determined by the number of times the mold that determines the shape and hand size of the glove portion is dipped. The thickness of the glove affects the flexibility and tactility of the glove, which has a major impact on the ability to manipulate objects in the isolator. The two-piece sleeves and gloves are also manufactured using the dipping process. The two-piece system has several advantages: different thickness of the gloves versus the sleeves, glove fit for different personnel, and cost. The thickness of the sleeves is typically greater than that of the gloves in the two-piece system, allowing increased flexibility and tactility when performing fine motor skill manipulations. Glove fit is another advantage of the two-piece system since gloves can be selected based on the hand size of the individual performing the manipulation, to reduce stress on the hands and allow for an easier grip of materials inside the isolator. Cost is another factor since gloves receive more stress and potential for wear, and the ability to replace them is much less expensive than replacing the one-piece configuration. There are several commercially available tools and techniques for a safe change of the gloves and sleeves of both types without breaching containment (Figure 14.4).

Monitoring Systems

Monitoring strategies for isolators cover a broad range based on the purpose of the isolator. Monitoring for containment of a specific compound online involves a sampling and analytical strategy selected for specific compound identification. Monitoring internal conditions inside the isolator is an easier task. Monitoring for temperature, humidity, gases, oxygen content, and particulates can be accomplished by selecting proper instruments and internal probes to collect the samples for analysis. Strategies for online monitoring for viable organisms attached to particles have shown promise for aseptic isolators. External monitors can be used to alert personnel of gas leaks that can lead to an unsafe condition.

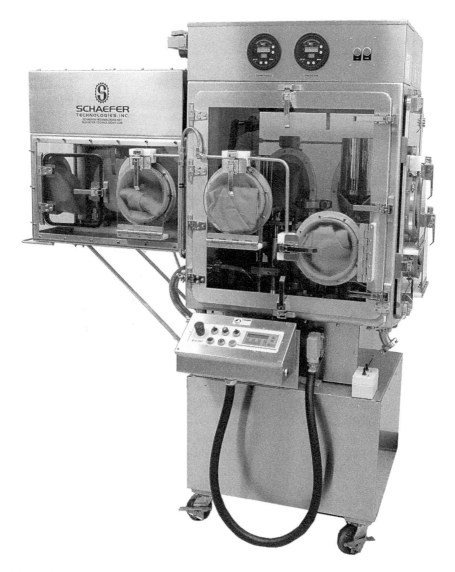

FIGURE 14.4 Wash-in-place isolator.

Examples are oxygen monitoring of an inert gas atmosphere inside an isolator, and hydrogen peroxide monitoring when a VHP system is being used for decontamination in aseptic operations.

ISOLATOR ERGONOMICS

Ergonomics play an important role in the correct design and use of isolators. Sound ergonomic principles based on human factor engineering have the potential to decrease injuries that can occur because of improper use of an isolator. There are a number of guides on the proper design and use of isolators, including human factor recommendations published by several universities, plus society publications such as "Guideline for Glovebox Ergonomics" from the American Glovebox Society (AGS) [9].

Training in the proper use of an isolator is critical. Several factors in the proper use of isolator systems, such as the ability to sit and stand when working in the isolator for long periods of time, proper working height through adjustment of the isolator or platforms, correct reach techniques, the need for reach-assist tools, and provision of proper exercise information that will reduce stress on the body, need to be addressed.

Glove Bags

Pliable plastic films can be configured into a broad range of sizes and shapes. This allows for solving containment challenges for many applications not addressed by other containment techniques. Sizes range from small, portable, utility glove bags for protecting processing tickets to room-sized enclosures, multichamber processing suites, and multilevel enclosures for maintenance access to complex processing equipment.

Several films are available. Linear low-density polyethylene (LLDPE) glove bags are available at low cost for laboratory applications. Both the LLDPE and polyurethane, with and without antistatic additives, are most commonly used in laboratories, pilot plants, and industrial settings. The LLDPE and polyurethane formulations have new drug application listings and meet regulatory criteria. With the exception of virgin polyurethane, all film formulations incorporate catalysts or plasticizers. All additives display low levels of volatility, which can become an issue when potential product contact is involved.

Tensile strength and chemical resistance of a film are key criteria in film selection. Film properties are available from the vendor. Regulatory agencies require supporting data developed by the user or independent testing laboratories for product contact films, including electrical conductance, incendivity, solvent compatibility, and short- and long-term material contact stability testing.

Flexible enclosures require structural support. Inflatable bladders integrated into the design allow for the ultimate in mobility and versatility. Internal and external frame supports are required for large enclosures. Grommets sealed into the external surfaces provide the most flexible means of support, using adjustable tie methods. Velcro strips integrated along the edges are convenient for rigid frame mounting and allow use of positive and negative internal pressures. The absence of gasket seals, such as windows and attachments, minimizes leakage potential and provides unobstructed lighting and visibility.

Flexible containment usage is a fairly new technology, which is undergoing rapid evolution. Regulations for use are constantly changing. Manufacture of flexible enclosures is best left to commercial manufacturers versed in the unique properties relating to the selected film and its sealing requirements.

Open-Front Unidirectional Airflow Devices

Open-front containment devices can include downflow booths, biologic safety cabinets (BSCs), and fume hoods, and all are dependent on both the external environment and personnel following proper procedures. With all of these factors in place, using this type of containment technology has a capability approaching an average of 10 ng/m^3 in the person's breathing zone over an 8 h exposure period. Technique dependency of open-front downflow and horizontal airflow–dependent booths and fume hoods was highlighted by data-supported examples contained in *Good Design Practices for GMP Pharmaceutical Facilities* [10].

Class II BSCs have been tested by the National Sanitation Foundation (NSF) [11]. Testing was performed under static conditions, and the data clearly showed that technique plays a major role in the containment capabilities of an open-front containment device. Studies have shown that a person passing within 3 ft of the open front of a Class II BSC can cause discharge of inside air into the room. Qualification methods developed by the American Society of Heating, Refrigerating, and Air-Conditioning Engineers (ASHRAE) use a vapor emission within the enclosure and a static dummy in place of personnel [12]. Testing has shown that the vapor-release method is not representative of particulate behavior, given that particulate characteristics have a profound effect on airflow capture and transport. Long-duration use results in visible deposition patterns on surfaces in front of a worker. A worker's hand and midriff are in the path of the particle flow, resulting in the worker contributing to room contamination by particle shedding when moving away from the enclosure. Major disruption to streamline airflow and particle dispersion occurs due to internal surface deformation and cutouts provided for utilities (e.g., electrical, computer, vacuum, and air or gas ports). Efficient use of airflow containment is degraded by both the size of material containers and the equipment placed inside the enclosure.

Local or Point Exhaust

A local or point exhaust system consists of a capture device or enclosure supported by ductwork and filtration. The design of the capture device is the most important element in the effectiveness of this type of system. Air velocity at the opening of the capture device is decreased with increased distance from the source of contamination. The environment in which a local or point exhaust is used can have a considerable effect on the efficiency of the engineering control. Local or point exhausts have been employed inside downflow booths to improve localized efficiency within the booth.

The relationship to the sources of contamination is important. Modeling of the impact of the local or point exhaust system helps to determine location. There are several ways that modeling can occur, with the basic means being use of smoke to provide a visual perception of the pattern created by the exhaust. It is important to remember that smoke does not represent the actual compound being exhausted because particle weight and shape impact behavior in the exhaust stream. Computer modeling, using tools such as computational fluid dynamics, is useful in the design of a local or point exhaust system because it allows shapes to be placed into the airflow. When the air hits a shape, it interrupts the dynamic flow and redirects the direction of the air. An example is a manual scooping operation where the scoop interacts with the airflow patterns. A well-designed local or point exhaust system can achieve containment levels in the range of 30 $\mu g/m^3$ in the breathing zone of a person based on an 8 h exposure time.

Typical slot-type design efficiency is a function of slot opening and distance from the point source of the contamination. The entry of air into the exhaust slot likely will produce turbulent zones, which can allow the contaminant to escape the capture device. Factors to consider when designing a slot-type exhaust are the shape and size of the slot, volume of air exhausted, control of velocities, distance of the slot above the supply, and receiving containers.

Cross-Contamination

Managing the risk of cross-contamination of other drugs begins with a risk assessment of a combination of factors, such as the type of contaminate, medical and safety risk, and the profile of the facility in terms of engineering controls at all steps of the operation to produce the drug that could be contaminated.

In November 2014, the EMA finalized a guideline on setting health-based exposure limits for use in risk identification in the manufacture of different medicinal products in shared facilities [13]. The guideline addresses the management of cross-contamination based on risk assessment to ensure the safety of personnel exposed to residual substances.

The greatest level of risk from cross-contamination is considered to be APIs with genotoxic potential. In the EMA guideline "Genotoxic Impurities in the Form of Threshold of Toxicological Concerns," it is suggested that the genotoxic threshold is 1.5 μg/person/day [14]. The International Conference for Harmonisation (ICH) finalized Q9, "Quality Risk Management" [15], and this document set the stage for risk assessments and the risk-based approach. The ICH document is a harmonized approach to risk management in the pharmaceutical industry and has been adopted by the Food and Drug Administration (FDA) [16], EMA [17], and the Japanese Ministry of Health, Labour and Welfare (MHLW). The ISPE published the *Risk-Based Manufacture of Pharmaceutical*

Products [18] in 2010, which was reviewed by the FDA. The consensus of these regulatory agencies is that the risk-based approach through risk assessments is acceptable and encouraged as an overall strategy to prevent cross-contamination.

SUMMARY

Paracelsus, who said "the dose makes the poison," communicated a basic principle of toxicology; that is, a substance can produce the harmful effect associated with its toxic properties only if it reaches a susceptible biological system within the body in a high enough concentration. The basic principle of pharmaceuticals is to create a positive, not a negative, effect on the patient.

Containment as close as possible to the source will help to protect personnel and patients from the potential negative effects of a drug. Selecting and applying the correct technologies are the responsibility of the pharmaceutical industry. To achieve these goals means selecting a strategy that manages both the risk of personnel exposures and cross-contamination by, and of, other drugs. This begins with a risk assessment of a combination of factors, such as the type of contaminate, medical and safety risk, and the profile of the facility in terms of engineering controls used in all steps of the operation. The risk-based approach through risk assessments, as an overall strategy to prevent cross-contamination and protect personnel, is an effective tool in understanding and applying containment solutions.

FURTHER DISCUSSION

1. Containment protection of personnel working within the compound at the early stages of development is most important because the exposure risk is not yet well understood. Explain how risk factors are assigned to various substances.
2. Describe the pros and cons, and differing uses, of the different forms of interaction technologies (robotics, flexible membranes, half suits, and glove ports).

ABOUT THE AUTHORS

Hank Rahe is currently director of Technology Containment Technologies Group, Inc. He has more than 30 years of experience in the pharmaceutical industry: 4 years in academia and 10 years in contamination control in pharmacy applications. He has an excellent working knowledge of pharmaceutical Good Manufacturing Practices. During the last 7 years of almost 30 years with Eli Lilly, Rahe headed up the technology group for advanced sterile processing and containment of hazardous drugs. Rahe is a recognized expert in the area of containment of potent compounds and advanced aseptic processing. He has extensive experience in facilities design, including barrier and isolation technology and clean rooms. He has worked for extended periods in Puerto Rico, England, France, Germany, and Italy. Rahe was educated at Purdue University, Lafayette, Indiana, receiving both BS and MS degrees.

Since 1963, Brian Ward has had a career involved with containment in multiple applications, beginning in graduate school (e.g., airflow, rigid, and flexible containment approaches). His most recent experiences relate to all aspects of pharmaceutical research, animal husbandry, development, production, and downstream user needs. His first foray into pharmaceutical applications (1993) was consulting on the design of a four-rig, four-floor bulk facility for manufacturing two cancer drug moieties, which today operates in a shirtsleeve environment. The most recent project was enclosing a 10-ton scale for in-line dispensing, blending, and bagging of animal antibiotics in Brazil, reducing the operation from full personal protection to shirtsleeve status. Ward was previously involved in asbestos and human carcinogen issues across a wide range of concerns, from creation through remediation and legally defensible procedures. His early experiences include handling highly hazardous moisture and air-sensitive materials in low-humidity and inert atmospheres (e.g., radioactive materials, rocket fuels, and an open 1,700°C reactor source). For more than 20 years, Ward has been a proponent of containment for simultaneously minimizing cleaning and validation requirements, worker exposures, environmental releases, and materials migration (i.e., cross-contamination control). His personal goal has been and continues to be to share his learning experiences.

REFERENCES

1. Pujara CP, Determination of Factors That Affect the Generation of Airborne Particles from bulk Pharmaceutical Powder, Purdue University, Lafayette, Indiana, 1997, http://docs.lib.purdue.edu/do/search/?q=author_lname%3A%22Pujara%22%20author_fname%3A%22Chetan%20Pratap%22&start=0&context=119483.
2. Connor TH, Shults M, Fraser MP, Determination of the Vaporization of Solutions of Mutagenic Antineoplastic Agents at 23°C and 36°C, Using a Desiccator Technique, *Mutation Research*, 470, 85–92, 2000.
3. Wood JP, Ed., *Containment in the Pharmaceutical Industry*, Marcel Dekker, New York, 2001.
4. National Institute for Occupational Safety and Health, Qualitative Risk Characterization and Management of Occupational Hazards: Control Banding (CB): A Literature Review and Critical Analysis, National Institute for Occupational Safety and Health, Washington, DC, August 2009, stacks.cdc.gov/view/cdc/5369.
5. European Medicines Agency, Setting Health-Based Exposure Limits for Use in Risk Identification in the Manufacture of Different Medicinal Products in Shared Facilities, European Medicines Agency, London, November 20, 2014.
6. International Society for Pharmaceutical Engineering, *Assessing the Particulate Containment Performance of Pharmaceutical Equipment*, 2nd ed., ISPE Good Practice Guide, International Society for Pharmaceutical Engineering, Tampa, FL, 2012.
7. International Organization for Standardization, ISO 14644-7: Cleanrooms and Associated Controlled Environments (Part 7): Separative Devices (Clean Air Hoods, Gloveboxes, Isolators and Mini-Environments), International Organization for Standardization, Geneva, 2004.
8. American Society for Testing and Materials, ASTM D6978-05: Standard Practice for Assessment of Resistance of Medical Gloves to Permeation by Chemotherapy Drugs, American Society for Testing and Materials, West Conshohocken, PA, 2013, www.astm.org/standards/D6978.htm.
9. American Glovebox Society, AGS-G013: Guideline for Glovebox Ergonomics, American Glovebox Society, Santa Rosa, CA, 2011.
10. Signore A, Jacobs T, *Good Design Practices for GMP Pharmaceutical Facilities*, Taylor & Francis Group, Oxford, 2005, p. 397.
11. National Sanitation Foundation, NSF 49: Biosafety Cabinetry: Design, Construction, Performance, and Field Certification, Ann Arbor, MI, 2014.
12. American Society of Heating, Refrigerating, and Air-Conditioning Engineers, https://www.ashrae.org/.
13. European Medicines Agency, www.ema.europa.eu.
14. European Medicines Agency, Genotoxic Impurities in the Form of Threshold of Toxicological Concerns, EMA Guideline, European Medicines Agency, London, November 20, 2014.
15. International Conference of Harmonisation, ICH Q9: Quality Risk Management, International Conference of Harmonisation, Geneva.
16. U.S. Food and Drug Administration, Guidance for Industry Q9: Quality Risk Management, U.S. Food and Drug Administration, Silver Spring, MD, http://www.fda.gov/downloads/drugs/guidancecomplianceregulatoryinformation/guidances/ucm073511.pdf.
17. European Medicines Agency, ICH Guideline Q9 on Quality Risk Management, European Medicines Agency, London, http://www.ema.europa.eu/docs/en_GB/document_library/Scientific_guideline/2009/09/WC500002873.pdf.
18. International Society for Pharmaceutical Engineering, *Baseline® Pharmaceutical Engineering Guides for New and Renovated Facilities*, Vol. 7: *Risk-Based Manufacture of Pharmaceutical Products (Risk-MaPP)*, International Society for Pharmaceutical Engineering, Tampa, FL, 2010.

15 Occupational Health and Safety

George Petroka CIH, CSP

CONTENTS

INTRODUCTION

Occupational health and safety pertains to all personnel who perform work at pharmaceutical facilities: it covers both company and contract employees working during routine, nonroutine, and construction activities. It addresses the chemical, physical, and biological hazards that may be handled and processed at the facility. It does not address the safety of the products, which are addressed through current Good Manufacturing Practices (cGMPs).

To effectively manage the occupational health and safety components of a pharmaceutical manufacturing facility, all potential risks must be assessed and controlled. Risk assessments follow a standard process and are performed by teams and competent staff having knowledge, experience, and understanding of their work activities and the hazards associated with those activities. Risk assessments provide a process that identifies and prioritizes the hazards, evaluates the effectiveness of existing controls, and identifies additional control measures as necessary. During the assessment, hazards are identified and their severity categorized, the adequacy of current and planned controls is analyzed, the probability of occurrence is assessed, and methods to eliminate or control the hazard are identified.

Risk assessments are important, as they form an integral part of a good occupational health and safety management program. Risk assessments systematically evaluate risks to employees and facility, create awareness of hazards and risks, identify who may be at risk (i.e., employees, cleaners, visitors, contractors, and the public), and determine if existing control measures are adequate or if an action plan to address identified gaps in control measures is needed. They also minimize risk of injuries or illnesses when done at the design or planning stage, prioritize hazards and control measures, and prioritize resources for continuous improvement.

The operation of a pharmaceutical manufacturing facility can present significant hazards and the associated risks. Internationally, occupational safety and health regulations, codes, and best industry practices have been developed to address many of the potential hazards. Many of the regulations require an assessment of risk in order to implement the appropriate controls. The facility occupational health and safety program must therefore include an effective risk assessment process that incorporates the applicable regulations, codes, and best industry practices. In addition, these risk management concepts and compliance requirements must be addressed during the design of the facility and through ongoing management of change.

OCCUPATIONAL HEALTH AND SAFETY MANAGEMENT

Health and safety management has the goal of providing guidance and direction in all phases of the safety program, including occupational safety and health, environmental control, fire safety, safety-oriented training programs, and building and equipment design criteria affecting safety codes and standards. Pharmaceutical companies must consider the health and safety of their employees to be of primary importance in the design, installation, and maintenance of all equipment, processes, and facilities, as well as during the performance of all operations.

From an occupational health and safety standpoint, the pharmaceutical company should comply with all country-specific, state, province, and local health and safety regulations in the design and operation of the facility. In addition, various organizations, including the International Society for Pharmaceutical Engineering (ISPE), publish consensus health and safety standards and guidelines having applicability to the pharmaceutical industry. Finally, the pharmaceutical company in many instances will adopt, as applicable, occupational health and safety regulations and guidelines as minimum requirements supplemented with pharmaceutical best industry practices. The most common example is the application of performance-based exposure control limits (PBECLs) for active pharmaceutical ingredients (APIs).

ACCIDENT PREVENTION SIGNS AND TAGS

Accident prevention signs and tags provide a method of warning of the presence of a hazardous material, hazardous condition, defective equipment, and so forth. Accident prevention signs are utilized in pharmaceutical facilities for normal operation, new construction activities, renovations, and emergency conditions. Minimum requirements for the wording, colors, and design for accident prevention signs and tags are specified by country-specific regulations and codes and include the following:

- ANSI Z53.1, "Safety Color Code for Marking Physical Hazards," and the identification of certain equipment, specifies standard colors and signs to be used in a safety and health program.
- U.S. Occupational Health and Safety Administration (OSHA) 29 CFR 1910.145 outlines specifications for accident prevention signs and tags.
- In Europe, the "Health and Safety (Safety Signs and Signals) Regulations 1995" implemented a European Council directive on minimum requirements for the provision of safety signs at work.

ACCIDENT PREVENTION SIGNS

Accident prevention signs provide a *permanent* method of warning of the presence of a hazardous material, hazardous condition, defective equipment, and so forth. The determination and use of accident prevention signs for a pharmaceutical facility should be identified during the design phase of a new facility or renovation. Accident prevention signs should be inspected and maintained as part of the facility's preventative maintenance (PM) program to ensure the accident prevention signs are accurate for the hazard and work area and are legible and in good condition (Figure 15.1).

In general, accident prevention signs can be classified according to use as listed below:

- *Caution signs:* Caution signs are used only to warn against potential hazards or caution against unsafe practices. Typically, the standard color of the background is yellow, and the panel is black with yellow letters.
- *Danger signs:* Danger signs are used only where an immediate hazard exists. Typically, danger signs consist of the colors red, black, and white.

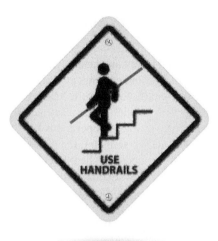

FIGURE 15.1   Accident prevention sign.

- *Directional signs, other than automotive traffic signs:* These signs are typically white with a black panel and white directional symbol.
- *General safety signs:* General safety signs are used where there is a need for general instructions and suggestions relative to safety measures. Typically, the standard color of the background is white, and the panel is green with white letters.
- *Slow-moving vehicle sign:* This sign typically consists of a fluorescent yellow-orange triangle with a dark red reflective border. The yellow-orange fluorescent triangle is a highly visible color for daylight exposure. The reflective border defines the shape of the fluorescent color in daylight and creates a hollow red triangle in the path of motor vehicle headlights at night. The emblem is intended as a unique identification for vehicles that, by design, move slowly (25 mph [40 kph] or less) on the public roads.
- *Specific hazard signs:* These signs utilize specific warning symbols (chemical, biological, and physical hazards; noise; laser; ultraviolet radiation; microwave radiation; etc.) to signify the actual or potential presence of a biohazard and to identify equipment, containers, rooms, materials, or combinations thereof that contain or are contaminated with viable hazardous agents.
- *Warning signs:* Warning signs are used to indicate a potentially hazardous situation that, if not avoided, could result in death or serious injury. Typically, they have the signal word *WARNING* in black letters within a safety orange truncated diamond on a black rectangular background.

Accident Prevention Tags

Accident prevention tags provide a *temporary* method of warning of the presence of a hazardous material, hazardous condition, defective equipment, and so forth. Accident prevention tags should not be used as a substitute for accident prevention signs. The designs of accident prevention tags should be the same as those of accident prevention signs. The messages on these tags will be removed or covered when the hazard no longer exists. Accident prevention tags should contain a signal word or emblem (such as *Danger*, *Caution*, or *Biohazard*) and a major message. The signal word should be readable from a distance of at least 5 ft and be understandable to all employees. The major message will indicate the particular hazard involved or instructions to the exposed person. Accident prevention tags will be located and secured as close as possible to the hazard (Figure 15.2).

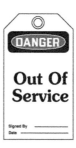

FIGURE 15.2 Accident prevention tag. (From Seton. Available at http://www.seton.net.au/lockout-tagout/lockout-tags/accident-prevention-tags/accident-prevention-tags-out-of-service-m3368.html)

COMBUSTIBLE DUST

When a combustible dust is processed or handled, a potential for deflagration exists. The degree of deflagration hazard varies depending on the type of combustible dust and the processing methods used. For a dust explosion to occur, the following criteria must be met:

1. The dust must be combustible.
2. The oxygen content of the atmosphere in which the dust is dispersed must be sufficient to sustain combustion.
3. The dust concentration must be capable of supporting combustion.
4. The particle size distribution must be capable of supporting combustion.
5. There must be an ignition source for sufficient energy to initiate the explosion.

A dust cloud explosion can be prevented if any of the above five conditions is not met (Figure 15.3).

In order to assess the risk potential for the likelihood of a dust explosion occurring, one needs to characterize the fire and explosion properties of the dust, determine the likelihood that a dust cloud with the properties and conditions to propagate a flame may form, determine whether adequate sources of ignition exist, identify the types and tasks of operations involved, and review the frequency and duration of the tasks.

Pharmaceutical facilities that handle raw materials, intermediates, and APIs in powder form need to assess the combustible dust risks associated with handling these materials. This should include the assessments and tests discussed in the following sections.

REVIEW AVAILABLE DATA FOR THE SOLIDS AND POWDERS HANDLED AND PROCESSED

A list of the raw materials, intermediates, and final products handled and processed at the facility should be assembled with the available dust combustibility and explosibility data on the solids and powders.

PERFORM DUST FLAMMABILITY AND EXPLOSIBILITY TESTING

Initial screening tests should include the following:

- *Explosibility screening test—A/B classification:* The explosibility screening test determines whether a powder or dust will explode when exposed to an ignition source when in the form of a dust cloud. The test results in a material are classified as either Type A (explosible) or Type B (nonexplosible). Thus, the test is also known as the A/B classification test. If the material is determined to be explosible, it will be further subjected to the minimum ignition energy and minimum explosible concentration tests described below.

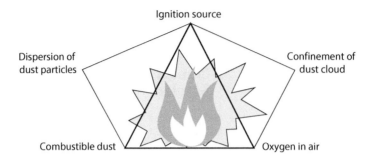

FIGURE 15.3 Fire and explosion pentagon. (From Airsystemsales, Inc. Available at http://www.airsystemsales. com/combustibledust/)

- *Minimum ignition energy (MIE) test—dust cloud:* The MIE test determines the lowest spark energy capable of igniting a sample when dispersed in the form of a dust cloud. This test is used primarily to assess the potential vulnerability of powders and dusts to electrostatic discharges, but is also relevant to frictional sparks.

Based on the data from these tests, additional testing may include:

- *Minimum explosible concentration (MEC) test:* The MEC test determines the smallest concentration of material in air that can give rise to flame propagation upon ignition when in the form of a dust cloud. This test involves dispersing powder or dust samples in a vessel and attempting to ignite the resulting dust cloud with an energetic ignition source. Trials are repeated for decreasing sample sizes until the MEC is determined.
- *K_{St} (DP_{max}) Test:* These tests are measures of explosion severity that are used in relief vent sizing and the design of explosion suppression and containment systems.

COMBUSTIBLE DUST EVALUATION AND RISK ASSESSMENT

A comprehensive combustible dust evaluation and risk assessment should be performed by first reviewing relevant solids and powder data (including material specifications); process equipment specifications; process, material flow, and equipment arrangement drawings; and safety procedures pertaining to handling combustible powders and dusts.

Following this review, a detailed site inspection of the facility, equipment, and operations should be performed. As part of the site assessment, key elements relating to powder handling, ignition sources, and electrical hazards and static electricity relating to the safe handling of combustible powders and dust explosion control and minimization will be evaluated utilizing best process engineering and chemical industry practices. These include

- Powder dust explosivity characteristics, including MIE, MIT, and K_{St} values
- Process batch size
- Charging and discharging of the equipment
- Grounding, bonding, and static dissipation of equipment and personnel
- Facility design issues, including conductive flooring and grounding bars
- Heating, ventilation, and air conditioning (HVAC) system, dust control and collection, and support utilities
- Personal protective equipment (PPE)
- Operability impacts to the process
- Equipment cleaning and maintenance activities
- Employee work practices

CONFINED SPACES

Confined spaces are defined as locations that meet the following criteria: they are large enough and so configured that they can be bodily entered, there is a limited means of access and egress, and they are not intended for continuous occupancy. Common examples of confined spaces in a pharmaceutical manufacturing facility include storage tanks, process vessels, tumble blenders, covered mixers, air handlers, and ductwork. Other less obvious confined spaces include manholes, vaults, pits, underground storage tanks, and trenches.

The hazards associated with confined spaces are potentially severe. Confined spaces may contain unknown or very high concentrations of airborne contaminants, including gases, vapors, and dusts at levels that are immediately dangerous to life or health; oxygen-deficient or oxygen-enriched atmospheres; potentially flammable or explosive atmospheres; contents such as liquids or powdered materials that could engulf a person; and a variety of other hazards, such as electrical, mechanical, thermal, or fall hazards. They may also have inwardly converging sides or a configuration such that a person could become trapped.

Pharmaceutical facilities that include confined spaces as part of the production or utilities should develop and implement the means, procedures, and practices necessary to ensure safe operations when employees must bodily enter confined spaces to perform cleaning, maintenance, and servicing activities.

The risks associated with potential confined space conditions should be assessed during the initial design phase for a new pharmaceutical facility or pharmaceutical process.

Because of the potential hazards associated with confined spaces, it is desirable to design the facility and select equipment such that the need to enter a confined space is eliminated. The need to enter a confined space can be eliminated for process vessels and tanks by designing and installing clean-in-place (CIP) capabilities to limit the need for entry to perform cleaning, and by identifying equipment with externally mounted features, such as magnetic stirrers, that do not require entry for servicing and maintenance activities. For manholes, pits, and so forth, the need can be eliminated by installing sensors and equipment that can be monitored and controlled remotely from outside of the confined space. For air handlers and ducts, select equipment that will facilitate maintenance and filter changes to be performed externally, and provide clean-out openings for ducts (Figure 15.4).

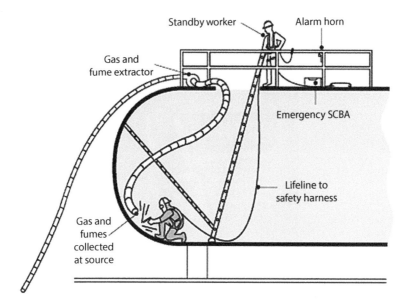

FIGURE 15.4 Confined space. (From Canadian Centre for Occupational Health and Safety. Available at http://www.ccohs.ca/oshanswers/hsprograms/confinedspace_program.html)

CONTROL OF HAZARDOUS ENERGY (LOCKOUT OR TAGOUT)

Pharmaceutical personnel servicing or maintaining machines or equipment may be seriously injured or killed if hazardous energy is not properly controlled. Injuries resulting from the failure to control hazardous energy during maintenance activities can be serious or fatal and may include electrocution, burns, crushing, cutting, lacerating, amputating, and fracturing body parts (Figure 15.5).

These hazardous energy sources include

- Electrical energy, including stored electric charges
- Hydraulic pressure
- Pneumatic pressure
- Pressurized gases and steam in process lines and piping systems
- Chemical energy
- Potential energy from suspended parts or springs under pressure
- Kinetic energy from moving parts
- Thermal energy

The risks associated with these hazardous energy sources must be assessed and controlled. In order to do so, it is imperative that all facility, maintenance, and production personnel have the ability to completely isolate equipment from all hazardous energy sources and achieve a zero energy state before commencing any servicing, maintenance, or cleaning activities. By rendering the equipment completely inoperative, affected personnel will be protected from injuries that could result from the unexpected reenergization or start-up of the equipment. To achieve a zero energy state, it is necessary to interrupt the transmission of all hazardous energy and physically prevent the restoration of that energy until the required work has been completed. Energy isolation devices, such as circuit breakers, electrical disconnects, and isolation valves, are the primary means for interrupting the transmission of hazardous energy. Locks should then be applied to the energy isolation devices to provide a physical barrier against the accidental restoration of energy (this is commonly referred to as lockout).

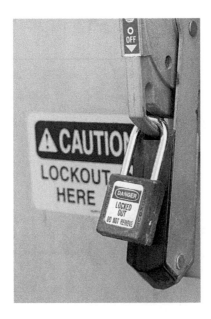

FIGURE 15.5   Danger: Use lockout before working on equipment. (From Ottawa Kent. Available at http://ottawakent.com/tag/lockouttagout/)

Hazardous energy control capabilities are an important factor in the design, selection, and operation of a pharmaceutical facility and its associated manufacturing equipment and utilities. In addition, prior to the designing of electrical and piping systems, the designers must anticipate the uses of the equipment and the maintenance, cleaning, and servicing needs to ensure that effective hazardous energy control can be designed into the system. Each process or piece of equipment must be equipped with energy isolation devices that are capable of being locked out. Energy isolation capabilities should be provided as close as possible to the individual process or piece of equipment on which work will be performed. In pharmaceutical facilities where APIs are being handled and equipment surfaces may be contaminated, it is desirable to provide localized lockout capabilities in each process room to eliminate the need for personnel to have to leave the room to implement the hazardous energy control procedures prior to servicing, maintenance, or cleaning.

All energy isolation devices must be readily accessible (e.g., located at ground level near equipment controls) with adequate clearance to accept the application of lockout devices. The design of the facility electrical and piping systems should be such that the application of any one energy isolation device will result in the minimal interruption of service to other equipment or processes. It is particularly important to provide an adequate number of isolation valves in pressurized liquid, gas, and chemical lines to help eliminate the need for hot tapping during maintenance activities. It is also important to plan for the ongoing maintenance of equipment and systems, including the changing of in-line filters and the removal and maintenance of in-line pumps. In these cases, the types of appropriate isolation devices, such as isolation valves or flanges, must be installed to limit the potential hazards associated with line breaking. Electrical equipment that is equipped with capacitors or otherwise has the ability to store or build up an electrical charge must have the capability to be easily grounded and the charge dissipated. Equipment with suspended parts, moving mechanical parts, and springs must have the capability to be physically restrained.

There are many possibilities when it comes to hazardous energy control capabilities, and "one size" certainly does not fit all. In all cases, engineers and designers should work closely with the building owners and end users to ensure that hazardous energy control capabilities are incorporated into the facility design in order to ensure safe and efficient operations during maintenance, cleaning, and servicing activities.

ELECTRICAL SAFETY

Electrical systems should be looked at from two perspectives during the design, construction, and operation of pharmaceutical manufacturing facilities: personnel safety and operational safety. Building and electrical codes essentially mandate safe installation criteria and practice; however, it is crucial that the proper operational intent be fully evaluated prior to detailed electrical system design. Designers, engineers, and environmental health and safety (EHS) personnel should try to anticipate future operations and electrical needs to reduce the need for costly infrastructure upgrades. The rapidly changing pharmaceutical manufacturing environment could lead to early obsolesce of an electrical system, particularly in multipurpose manufacturing suites and buildings. For example, consider a suite that is constructed for the manufacture of aqueous-based products. Typically, ordinary rated electrical equipment would be installed. However, if a flammable solvent is needed for equipment cleaning and decontamination purposes, there may be the need for the installation of hazardous-rated electrical devices in certain areas of the suite. Identifying this during the design is critical.

In the United States, all electrical installations must conform to the National Electrical Code (NEC). This standard specifies all installation requirements for equipment and wiring of all voltages. Other countries have similar regulatory requirements and electrical standards. Design and installation should only be done by qualified electrical engineers and licensed electricians. A valuable international reference is the International Electrotechnical Commission (IEC). The IEC provides

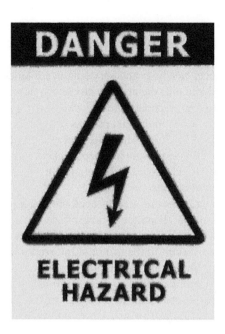

FIGURE 15.6 Danger: Electrical hazard. (From Ibex Tech Corp. Available at http://ibextechcorp.com/how-to-prevent-electrical-hazards/)

information on identifying and comparing electrical standards and equipment from varying countries (Figure 15.6).

Items that should be considered during the design of electrical systems and the installation of electrical apparatus are discussed in the next sections.

AREA CLASSIFICATION

Electrical equipment should be selected based on the hazards of the occupancy. Regulatory standards dictate the requirements for electrical equipment and wiring for all voltages where fire or explosion hazards exist due to the use or storage of flammable and combustible liquids, gases, dusts, or fibers.

The key is to ensure that electrical systems and apparatus are not potential ignition sources for hazardous materials. Process areas with hazardous-rated electrical equipment should be easily identified with warning signs to ensure that the basis of safety is not compromised.

STATIC ELECTRICITY

Static electricity can occur in all pharmaceutical manufacturing environments. Its presence not only creates safety risks, but also can affect product quality and process yield. Static electricity cannot be prevented; therefore, it must be controlled to reduce the risk of fire, explosion, personnel shock, and the effects on material handling. Static is generated any time dissimilar materials move together and are then separated. Typically, with more rapid movement of materials there exists greater potential for higher static charges. Static charges powerful enough to ignite flammable liquids, gases, and combustible solids can commonly occur in pharmaceutical operations such as liquid and powder transfer, on conveyor equipment, within ventilation systems, and by operators wearing synthetic garments and nonconductive footwear.

NFPA 77, "Recommended Practice on Static Electricity," is an excellent reference on the fundamentals of static generation and control methodologies. FM Global's Data Sheet 5-8, "Static

Electricity," also provides sound recommendations and practical guidance for static control. The more common control techniques are

- Electrically bonding and grounding (earthing) all equipment, walking and working surfaces, hoods, ductwork, and conductive objects to the same electrical potential with a resistance to ground not greater than $10^6 \, \Omega$
- Maintaining relativity humidity between 60% and 70%
- Installing conductive flooring, wearing conductive footwear, and using clothing that does not create static
- Installing static eliminators and dissipating devices
- Avoiding the use of insulating materials such as plastic ducts and piping, plastic drums, and plastic drum liners unless they are specifically designed for static control

The generation of static can also affect the quality of products and manufacturing process effectiveness. Static accumulations can prevent effective transfer of very fine powders, causing the material to cling to containers, weigh scales, and operator's hands and clothing. This can create risks of fire, explosion, and operator exposure, as well as loss of product into a process waste stream. With high-potency materials and high unit costs for active ingredients, these wastes can be very costly to the operation.

PROTECTING EMPLOYEES

Electrical installations that are completed in accordance with a recognized standard typically result in the proper level of electrical protection for personnel. Additionally, the application of safety standards that focus on safe electrical work practices ensures that personnel working with electrical systems are doing so safely. Safety devices such as circuit breakers, ground fault circuit interrupters (GFCIs), and emergency disconnects must be properly sized, installed, tested, and maintained to ensure personnel safety. GFCIs are required for all electrical services in wet or damp locations. This is particularly critical in pharmaceutical manufacturing operations where process areas are washed with water during routine cleaning or decontamination.

CLEARANCES AND SPACE SEPARATION

All electrical systems generate heat. To prevent premature failure of systems and equipment due to overheating, clear spaces must be maintained around the equipment to permit air circulation. Similarly, adequate clearances must be provided to prevent accidental ignition of ordinary combustible materials. Manufacturers and electrical standards provide specific guidance for these distances. These distances are also necessary to allow safe access for routine and emergency service.

EMERGENCY EQUIPMENT AND RESPONSE

The most important consideration in emergency planning and response equipment selection is the assessment of the risks related to an emergency occurrence. Consideration should be given to the types and quantities of hazardous materials handled and stored, and the equipment used in the facility. Response equipment should then be chosen based on the risk assessment.

EMERGENCY RESPONSE EQUIPMENT

A site must have and maintain an alarm system for personnel. There are different types of alarm systems, based on sound or light. Each area should be evaluated to determine the best alarm for the area and ensure adequate coverage of all areas in the facility. (Alarm systems should comply with the national or local requirements for employee alarm systems.) Areas where hazardous materials

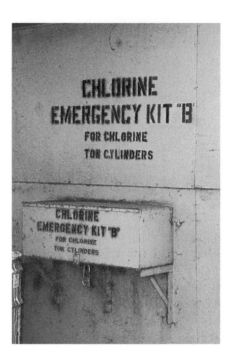

FIGURE 15.7   Emergency spill response kit sign. (From Stonehouse Signs. Available at http://stonehousesigns. com/product/hazardous-chemicals-and-materials-sign-emergency-spill-response-kit)

are used should be equipped with an eyewash and safety shower, spill kits, a first aid kit, a fire alarm, fire extinguishers rated for the hazard, and a fire suppression system. Typically, a high-efficiency particulate air (HEPA) filter vacuum is provided in pharmaceutical facilities where APIs are handled or processed to respond to spills of potent powders (Figure 15.7).

All emergency equipment should be in easily accessible locations that do not block emergency exit routes. In the case of eyewashes and safety showers, quick drenching or flushing of the eyes and body must be provided within the work area at a distance that requires no more than 10 s for personnel to reach. In addition, it must be located on the same level of the hazard, and the path of travel must be free of obstructions that may prevent immediate use of the equipment. Specific details about the placement and design of safety showers and eyewashes are presented in national regulations and consensus standards such as ANSI 358.1.

ERGONOMICS

Ergonomics can be defined in simple terms as fitting the job to the worker. Ergonomics is the study of preventing musculoskeletal disorders (MSDs) in the workplace. This includes the study of human behavior, abilities, and limitations in conjunction with the design of tools, machines, tasks, and the work environment with the goal of a productive, safe, comfortable, and effective interface between the work environment and employee (Figure 15.8).

In the pharmaceutical industry, common ergonomic issues involve strains and sprains from lifting heavy materials, and repetitive motion injuries from improper workstation design or tool design. A focus on ergonomics during the process design and equipment selection can reduce muscle fatigue, increase productivity, and reduce the number and severity of work-related MSDs. MSDs often involve the back, wrist, elbow, and shoulder.

A risk-based approach to prevention of work-related MSDs has been demonstrated to reduce the risk of developing MSDs by evaluating the proposed process and involving employees in review

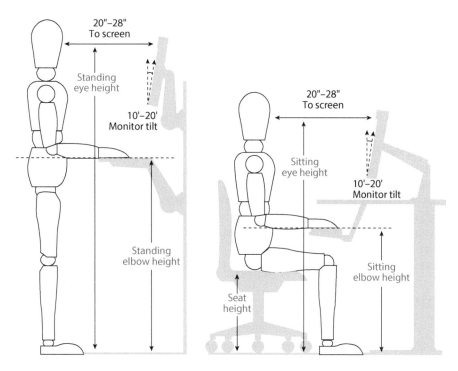

FIGURE 15.8   Ergonomic adjustments. (From JP Office workstations. Available at http://blog.jpofficeworkstations.com.au/2013/03/role-of-ergonomics-preventing-wmsd.html#.VfONGxFVhBc)

of mock workstation design and equipment plans. Reducing exposures involves evaluation of risk factors associated with workstations, tasks, and hand tools.

Risk Factors

Within the pharmaceutical industry, the primary ergonomic risk factors include *awkward posture*, *forceful exertion*, and *repetitive motion*, which affect the back (low back and neck) and upper extremities (arms, hands, wrists, and elbows). The risk factors, if not addressed, may lead to over-exertion and repetitive motion injuries and illnesses.

Awkward postures include reaching overhead or behind the head; twisting at the waist; bending the torso forward, backward, or to the side; squatting; kneeling; and bending the wrist.

Repetitive motion involves repeated motion of the same body part (typically upper extremity and back). The severity of the risks depends on the frequency, speed of the movement, muscle groups involved, and required force.

In evaluation of tasks, equipment, and tools, risk factors such as posture, repetition, and force should be assessed.

Proactive Ergonomics: Principles for Workplace Design

Prevention of work-related MSDs can be accomplished by recognizing, anticipating, and reducing risk factors during the planning stages. Design strategies should include incorporation of principles that reduce risk. These include keeping work close to the body; maintaining arms, shoulders, and wrists in a neutral position (avoid overextension of joints); avoiding bending forward and twisting the trunk and back; avoiding static muscle load (maintaining the same posture for extended periods of time); avoiding tasks above shoulder height (hands and elbows should remain below shoulder level when conducting a task); limiting the weight of a load to be lifted and utilizing mechanical lifting aids; avoiding carrying with one arm; and using transport accessories such as roller convey-ors and mobile platforms.

Hand tool selection and evaluation of handling of small parts and containers should include evaluation of hand grip. A power grip is a grip in which the hand wraps completely around a handle or object and is of lower risk than a pinch grip or pistol grip.

ERGONOMIC PROGRAM ELEMENTS

Prevention includes implementation of an ergonomic process with emphasis on management sup-port, worker involvement, training, risk identification, early reporting of symptoms, solution imple-mentation, and program evaluation.

Tools for evaluation of risk are available through the Federation of European Ergonomics Society (FEES), National Institute of Occupational Safety and Health (NIOSH), Human Factors and Ergonomics Society (HFES), Southeast Asian Network of Ergonomics Societies (SEANES), Union of Latin American Ergonomics Societies (ULAERGO), Center for Registration of European Ergonomists (CREE), and Centers for Disease Control and Prevention (CDC).

FIRE PROTECTION

Within the pharmaceutical industry, compliance with cGMP standards and guidelines supports the overall objectives of a fire protection program. Cleanliness requirements, standardized operat-ing procedures, and access control all contribute to the overall safe operation of a pharmaceutical facility.

The following overview of each of the key elements provides insight into the engineering and management of fire prevention and protection for pharmaceutical manufacturing plants. Engineering criteria are presented in general terms. Detailed design information can only be developed when the specific fire hazards and risks are available. There are many technical resources available to sup-port fire protection engineering efforts. Agencies such as the National Fire Protection Association (NFPA) in the United States, the Health Safety Executive (HSE) in the United Kingdom, and FM Global produce fire protection reference standards and guidelines for use in the pharmaceutical industry. Many engineering firms also employ fire protection engineers who are well versed in the risks and protection needs of the industry.

IDENTIFICATION AND EVALUATION OF FIRE HAZARDS AND RISKS

The overall goal of any fire protection program should be to prevent fires from starting and to minimize the loss impacts of any fire that does occur. Fire prevention requires constant vigilance supported by protective systems, inspections, and fire response plans. The early detection of fire, the safe evacuation of personnel, and prompt actions to control and extinguish the fire are critical to safeguard employees, emergency responders, and the business.

Fire risk assessments must be completed for all sites and operations. The fire hazards must be identified, evaluated, and controlled using a combination of risk elimination, engineering controls, and preventative operating procedures (Figure 15.9).

IDENTIFICATION AND ELIMINATION OF FIRE HAZARDS

Whenever possible, fire hazards should be eliminated. This approach needs to start during the product and process development stage within research and development (R&D). The use of safe and environmentally friendly solvents can play a major role in reducing the combustible loading within a manufacturing plant. Similarly, changing to nonflammable cleaning and decontamination materials eliminates a fire hazard as well.

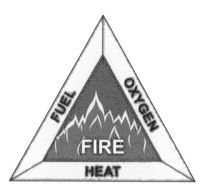

FIGURE 15.9 Oxygen, heat, and fuel. (From Elite Fire. Available at http://www.elitefire.co.uk/news/basics-fire-triangle/)

INSTALLATION AND MAINTENANCE OF PROTECTIVE SYSTEMS

When fire hazards cannot be eliminated, fire-safe construction and protective systems should be provided. Most regulatory building and fire codes require the use of fire-rated construction for occupancy classes, including pharmaceutical manufacturing and storage. The fire ratings for walls, floors, and ceilings and roofs will vary depending on the level of fire hazard (combustible loading), the size of the building or operation, the number of floors in the building, and the fire exposure to other buildings or occupancies. Fire ratings are typically divided into four categories, ranging from 1 to 4 h. Building codes and the insurance and underwriting industry specify fire ratings of various construction assemblies. These ratings can be found in code specifications and consensus standards. When a fire rating is specified, it is critical that all components of the wall or ceiling assembly meet the code requirement. For example, the International Building Code specifies 2-h fire-rated wall construction for laboratories using a moderate volume of flammable liquids. For this occupancy, the wall construction and doors must meet this minimum rating requirement.

Special consideration must be given to the construction of operations that require damage-limiting construction (DLC), such as blast-resistant and pressure-relieving walls and roofs. DLC is typically needed in operations where the potential for an equipment or room explosion hazard exists. Typical examples of these occupancies are pilot plants, chemical processing, flammable liquids and flammable gas processing and storage, combustible powder operations, and larger-scale laboratories. The sizing and design of explosion vents used in combination with pressure-resistant walls and roofs must be based on the explosive characteristics of the materials, quantity of the hazardous material, and hazards of the process.

Process and utility systems should be designed and installed to minimize fire risk. Flammable liquid and gas distribution systems must be installed in accordance with local code and industry best practice. Distribution piping, pump systems, and storage tanks should be provided with remote manual and automatic emergency shutoff devices. The materials of construction should also be closely scrutinized to ensure that the potential for accidental releases is minimized. Gaskets, seals, packing glands, and specialty linings should all be evaluated for their resistance to the materials and atmospheres to which they will be exposed. In some instances, welded or double-wall piping may be necessary to adequately address the risks. Glass piping and process equipment handling flammable liquids and gases should be avoided. Tempered glass and protective wraps can increase the structural integrity of glass systems; however, the potential for a catastrophic spill or release and subsequent fire outweighs the process benefits of glass systems.

All process equipment (including flammable liquid systems, flammable gas systems, process vessels, packaging equipment, ventilation systems, and dryers) should be electrically bonded and grounded (earthed).

FIRE SUPPRESSION SYSTEMS

Automatic sprinkler protection is the most effective and economical method of protecting buildings and processes from fire. It is highly recommended that sprinklers be provided throughout all pharmaceutical manufacturing facilities. Fire loss history within the industry has proven that sprinkler protection is highly reliable and effective at controlling fires in laboratories and warehousing, manufacturing, and support areas. The number of water damage losses from the accidental discharge or leaking of a sprinkler system is very low in the pharmaceutical industry. Alternatively, fire damage in nonsprinklered pharmaceutical occupancies is usually catastrophic.

The authority having jurisdiction (AHJ) (NFPA, local building codes, etc.) and the insurance carrier typically provide sprinkler system design and installation guidelines. Sprinkler designs are determined based on total combustible loading within the protected area. Sprinkler heads can be installed and maintained so that the cGMP requirements are not compromised. For most installations, the use of a standard chrome-plated pendant sprinkler head is the most practical. The ceiling penetrations around the head can be sealed with cGMP-compliant caulking material that provides the required level of cleanness. Pendant heads are easily cleaned using a vacuum, compressed air, or a soft brush and present no greater cleanness risk than most other room components or pieces of production equipment. Recessed or concealed heads can also be used; however, their escutcheon assemblies may hide contaminants and hinder cleaning. Concealed sprinklers should never have their cover plates caulked. This could prevent operation in the event of a fire.

Control valves for sprinkler systems should be readily accessible and well marked. For large buildings, it is advisable to install floor or area isolation valves in addition to system valves. This permits faster system isolation and allows nonaffected areas to remain protected during fire incidents or system renovations.

All sites must have on-site firewater systems consisting of fire hydrants, supply mains, and a dedicated water supply capable of providing water at a flow and pressure adequate for the site's automatic sprinkler and fire hose requirements. This system should be sized based on a credible fire scenario considering the occupancy, construction, and design of the sprinkler systems, as well as the anticipated hose flow required by firefighters. The firewater flow duration must be considered during the design process. The insurance industry and NFPA provide recommended firewater flow duration periods for administration, manufacturing, and storage occupancies. Typically, a flow duration of 90–120 min is used within the pharmaceutical industry.

Where sprinkler protection is not practical due to the incompatibility of water with the occupancy, an alternative automatic fire detection and control system should be provided. Several inert gas chlorinated fluorocarbon (CFC)-free extinguishing systems are now available to the pharmaceutical industry. These systems are typically used within small rooms or equipment where fire suppression is warranted.

MANUAL FIREFIGHTING EQUIPMENT

Portable fire extinguishers should be provided throughout all manufacturing, storage, and support areas. Extinguishers should be selected based on the fire hazards of the protected area. Considerations should also be given to the potential for nonfire damage that can be caused by some types of extinguishing agents. There are several "clean"-agent portable extinguishers currently available that can be used in areas where highly hazardous or flammable materials are not present.

Some fire protection codes require the installation of fire hose connections and hose cabinets for special hazard occupancies (laboratories, warehousing, hazardous materials storage, etc.). When required, it is critical that the equipment selected is compatible with the systems and gear used by the local fire department.

FIRE DETECTION AND ALARMS

Fire detection and alarms are regulatory requirements in most countries. In most jurisdictions, all buildings and process areas must be equipped with an automatic fire detection system that is interfaced with a local audible alarm system. Fire detection can be accomplished using smoke or heat detection or automatic fire suppression (sprinklers, gaseous, etc.). Protection must be installed in all occupied areas, and in concealed spaces where fire hazards exist as a result of either combustible construction or occupancy. For high-value facilities, it is recommended that the automatic fire alarm system be connected to a constantly attended location, such as the site security center or maintenance office, a fire and security monitoring service, or the local fire and police department. For alarm systems that are monitored on-site, a plan must be in place for the immediate notification of the site fire brigade and the local fire department.

Manual fire alarm activation points should be provided throughout all buildings. The location and number of activation points must be determined based on the local code requirements, hazards of the area, congestion, and location of the egress exits. As a minimum, manual activation points should be located at each egress doorway and within 60 m (200 ft) of all points within the protected area.

Each site's emergency alarm system should consist of audible and visual notification devices. Alarms should be audible and visible throughout the protected area. To ensure that audible alarms are heard, they should be at least 15 dBA louder than the ambient noise level. Visual alarms such as strobes should also be provided. All alarm systems should be provided with an uninterruptible power supply (UPS) or backup generator power supply.

CONTROL OF FIREWATER AND HAZARDOUS MATERIAL RUNOFF

Runoff from a fire or hazardous material incident can cause serious property and environmental damage. As a result of several major incidents, many jurisdictions now require emergency containment systems and plans to prevent this type of damage. Firewater runoff must be controlled to prevent environmental impact and the spread of hazardous materials both on-site and into the community. A firewater environmental impact assessment should include a determination of the volume of firewater that would be generated by the most credible fire scenario. Total water flow from automatic sprinkler systems, specialized water spray, and fire hose should be included in the evaluation. A firewater flow duration of 30, 60, 90, or 120 min (based on the severity of the fire hazard) should be used to determine the total fire flow. Large quantities of liquids that may be involved in an incident, such as from a ruptured storage tank or process vessel, should be included in the total aggregate volume when calculating the runoff volume. A determination of the water flow path, accumulation, and final deposition point should be made. The impact should include an assessment of the hazards associated with fire debris and hazardous materials that may be entrapped in the runoff, as well as the potential for exposure to emergency responders. Where the firewater runoff risk presents a serious safety or environmental risk, a specialized drainage and containment system should be provided.

HAZARDOUS MATERIALS

Hazardous materials are defined by their flammability, toxicity, and reactivity characteristics. The handling, use, and storage of hazardous materials in a pharmaceutical manufacturing facility present the potential risk of exposure to personnel, the facility, and the environment. To manage these potential risks, it is critical that facility designers have a thorough understanding of the types of hazardous materials that are planned to be used in the facility, as well as the manner in which they will be handled, used, and stored. Minimum requirements addressing the use and storage of hazardous materials are specified by country-specific regulations and codes. Relevant codes in the United States include

- OSHA regulations contained in 29 CFR 1910, Subpart H
- NFPA
- Building Officials and Code Administrators International (BOCA)

In the United Kingdom, the Health and Safety Executive—Control of Substances Hazardous to Health (COSHH) addresses minimum requirements. In the European Union, Classification, Labelling and Packaging (CLP), and internationally, the United Nations Globally Harmonized System (GHS) of Classification and Labelling of Chemicals specify minimum requirements addressing use and storage of hazardous materials.

It is important that facilities designed to handle hazardous materials meet all of the requirements of the country-specific standards and other best health and safety practices. In addition to meeting these requirements, some jurisdictions may require prior approval before work activities involving hazardous materials are introduced into a new or renovated facility.

HAZARDOUS LOCATIONS

NFPA 70, "National Electrical Code (NEC)," defines hazardous locations as areas "where fire or explosion hazards may exist due to flammable gases or vapors, flammable liquids, combustible dust, or ignitable fibers or flyings." Because electrical equipment can be a source of ignition in a hazardous location, NEC provides detailed recommendations for the construction and installation of electrical equipment and apparatus based on the types of hazards that may be present and the conditions under which those hazards may be present. In the United States, the NEC (NFPA 70) specifies electrical system hazard classifications in Article 500, "Hazardous (Classified) Locations, Classes I, II, III, Divisions 1 and 2."

Class I, Divisions 1 and 2 are those areas where flammable or combustible liquids or gases are used or stored and there is the potential for sufficient vapor to form explosive or ignitable mixtures in air. Division 1 areas contain ignitable concentrations under normal conditions, or are where ignitable concentrations frequently exist due to repair or maintenance operations or where the failure of processing equipment might release concentrations that could be ignited by the simultaneous failure of the electrical equipment. Division 2 areas are those where flammable liquids and gases are used but are normally confined to closed containers and process equipment or where ignitable concentrations are normally prevented by the use of positive mechanical ventilation. Within each of these divisions, there are subgroup classifications for specific materials and hazard characteristics (see NFPA 70, Article 500.6). Within the pharmaceutical industry, examples of Class I areas are solvent storage areas, flammable gas storage, process hood areas where flammable liquids are used, and chemical processing areas.

Class II, Divisions 1 and 2 are areas where combustible dusts are present. Class II, Division 1 areas are those where combustible dust is routinely present under normal conditions in sufficient quantity to form an ignitable mixture in air. This also includes those areas where the failure of equipment or processes could result in the formation of a dust cloud that could be ignited by the simultaneous failure of an electrical apparatus. Dusts that are electrically conductive and are present in hazardous quantities are also included in this classification.

Areas where combustible dust is not normally present in ignitable quantities and where dust accumulations will not interfere with the safe dissipation of heat from electrical equipment are considered Class II, Division 2 locations (see NFPA 70, Article 500.5). Like Class I, Class II also has group-specific classifications for highly volatile materials (see NFPA 70, Article 500.6). Typical pharmaceutical Class II operations are micronizing, powder weigh and dispense, bulk powder handling, blending, and so forth.

Class III locations typically do not occur within the pharmaceutical sector. Class III locations are those that are hazardous due to the presence of easily ignitable fibers, as would typically be seen in the textile and woodworking industries (see NFPA 70, Article 500.5).

In addition to the applicable electric codes, NFPA 5000, "Building Construction and Safety Code"; BOCA National Building Code; and BOCA National Fire Prevention Code establish classifications for building occupancies based on types of hazardous materials that are being handled. These consensus standards provide facility and equipment design criteria for locations in which flammable and combustible liquids are stored, handled, and used.

FLAMMABLE AND COMBUSTIBLE LIQUIDS

Many of the common organic solvents that are used during production, laboratory, and cleaning activities in pharmaceutical manufacturing facilities are considered to be flammable or combustible liquids. The primary hazards associated with flammable and combustible liquids are fire and explosion. Flammable liquids are defined by NFPA as liquids with flash points below 100°F (37.8°C) (Figure 15.10). Flammable liquids, also referred to as Class I liquids, are subdivided into three categories:

1. Class IA liquids have flash points below 73°F (22.8°C) and boiling points below 100°F (37.8°C).
2. Class IB liquids have flash points below 73°F (22.8°C) and boiling points at or above 100°F (37.8°C).
3. Class IC liquids have flash points at or above 73°F (22.8°C) and below 100°F (37.8°C).

Combustible liquids have a flash point at or above 100°F (37.8°C): Class II combustible liquids have flash points at or above 100°F (37.8°C) and below 140°F (60°C), Class IIIA liquids have flash points at or above 140°F (60°C) and below 200°F (93.3°C), and Class IIIB liquids have flash points above 200°F (93.3°C).

When designing flammable and combustible liquid storage areas,

- All inside storage rooms should be designed with a means for containing spills. Options to consider include noncombustible liquid-tight raised sills or ramps that are at least 4 in. in height, designing the floor of the storage area at least 4 in. below the surrounding floor, or installing an open trench in the room that drains to a safe location.
- All door openings should be equipped with self-closing rated fire doors.
- All inside storage rooms should be equipped with appropriate fire protection equipment, such as sprinkler systems or carbon dioxide systems, pursuant to the requirements of the authority having jurisdiction.
- The construction of the walls and wall openings should meet all applicable code requirements for fire resistance. Where necessary, explosion venting should be provided.
- The quantities of flammable and combustible liquids in any given storage room should not exceed those limits established by the appropriate regulatory agency. For example,

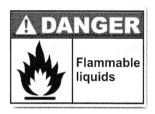

FIGURE 15.10 Danger: Flammable liquids. (From SignsToYou.com. Available at https://signstoyou.com/custom-signs/safety-signs/flammable-explosive/s-1606/)

OSHA and NFPA have established the following requirements for sprinklered inside storage rooms:

- No more than 10 gallons per square foot of floor area with no more than 500 ft^2 of floor area in rooms with walls and wall openings having a fire resistance of at least 2 h
- No more than 5 gallons per square foot of floor area with no more than 150 ft^2 of floor area in rooms with walls and wall openings having a fire resistance of at least 1 h
- There should be no ignition sources present in the inside storage rooms.
- Electrical wiring, equipment, and apparatus installed and used in inside rooms used for the storage of flammable liquids should be approved for Class I, Division 2 locations.
- All inside storage rooms should be equipped with either gravity or mechanical exhaust ventilation to prevent the buildup and accumulation of vapors. OSHA requires that the ventilation provide a minimum of six air changes per hour.
- The layout of inside storage rooms should maintain aisles that are at least 3 ft in width.
- Grounding should be provided for all metal drums, containers, and fixed electrical equipment in storage areas to prevent static electric discharge. NFPA 77, "Recommended Practice on Static Electricity," provides information on measures for reducing hazards due to static electric discharges.
- Class B portable fire extinguishers should be mounted directly outside of each door leading to an inside storage room.
- Reactive materials should not be stored in the same room with flammable and combustible liquids.
- Appropriate eyewash and safety shower equipment should be installed in areas where flammable and combustible liquids are dispensed or in other areas where splashing could occur.
- Climate control should be provided for all storage areas so that flammable and combustible liquids are stored at temperatures below their flash points.

The storage of flammable and combustible liquids should be minimized at the point of use in manufacturing and laboratory areas outside of designated storage rooms. The NFPA limits for quantities of liquids that are located outside of flammable storage cabinets are 600 gallons of Class IA liquids in containers and 800 gallons of Class I, II, or IIIA liquids in containers. OSHA has established the following limits for quantities of liquids that are located outside of an inside storage room or storage cabinet in a building or in any one fire area of a building: 25 gallons of Class IA liquids in containers and 120 gallons of Class IB, IC, II, or III liquids in containers.

Production and laboratory areas in which the incidental use of flammable and combustible liquids is expected to occur should be equipped with an adequate number of suitably sized approved flammable liquid cabinets. Both OSHA and NFPA have established limits of no more than 60 gallons of Class I or Class II liquids and no more than 120 gallons of Class III liquids may be stored in any individual flammable liquid cabinet. Furthermore, NFPA recommends that no more than six flammable liquid cabinets be stored in any single fire area.

TOXICITY

Laboratory and manufacturing operations associated with pharmaceutical manufacturing activities may require the use of chemicals that exhibit both acute and chronic toxicity. Many of these chemicals are standard reagents, including acetone and acetyl nitrile, and may be used in laboratories. In addition, alcohols such as isopropyl alcohol (IPA), ethanol, and methylene chloride may be used in the production process for cleaning or as part of the product blend.

Toxicity indicates that there is statistically significant evidence (based on at least one study conducted according to established scientific principles) that acute or chronic health effects may occur in exposed employees.

Government agencies and professional organizations have established workplace exposure limits for many airborne chemical and physical agents. In addition, many pharmaceutical companies develop exposure limits for their own compounds. The most common type of exposure limit is the 8-h time-weighted average (TWA). Overexposure may occur when 8-h limits or short-term exposure limits are exceeded.

COMPRESSED GASES

Laboratory and manufacturing operations associated with pharmaceutical activities may require the use of compressed gases. The hazards associated with the storage, handling, and use of compressed gases can be serious: some gases may be flammable, reactive, or highly toxic; high concentrations of gases released into a work area can create oxygen-deficient atmospheres; and because the gases are under pressure, there is a potential for explosion or a violent release due to the large amount of potential energy contained in the gas cylinder.

Proper storage is one of the most important design considerations for a facility that will handle compressed gases. Where possible, rooms or areas should be dedicated for compressed gas storage to provide a greater degree of control over potential physical and chemical hazards. All rooms or areas designated for compressed gas storage should be kept free of heat and ignition sources, and the storage of combustible materials should be minimized. All storage areas should also be constructed according to applicable building codes, including NEC electric equipment guidelines for class, division, and group, and equipped with appropriate fire suppression systems.

Because of the extreme physical hazards associated with the potential energy stored in compressed gases, the layout of the facility should take into account the movement of compressed gas cylinders and other hazardous materials throughout the facility in order to minimize travel distances and the movement of cylinders through or adjacent to areas that are not equipped to handle the hazards (e.g., low-hazard areas such as office areas or break rooms). In all cases, cylinders of compressed gases must be securely stored in an upright orientation. Cages or racks are used to store large numbers of cylinders. Straps or bases secured to a wall or other structural member are often used in laboratory areas where single cylinders are used. Cylinder storage should be kept away from high-traffic areas and areas where damage due to contact with moving equipment, such as powered industrial trucks, is minimized. Flammable gases should be segregated from cylinders containing oxygen and reactive gases. A minimum distance of 25 ft should be maintained between flammable gas and oxygen cylinders. As an alternative, a noncombustible barrier of at least 5 ft in height should separate flammable gas and oxygen cylinders. Full cylinders should be stored separately from empty cylinders (Figure 15.11).

Adequate ventilation should be provided in areas in which toxic and flammable gases are being stored and used. It is desirable to maintain cylinders of highly toxic and pyrophoric gases within walk-in fume hoods or other exhausted enclosures. The uncontrolled release of compressed gases can create hazardous atmospheres, including acutely toxic atmospheres, explosive gas– or vapor–air mixtures, or oxygen-deficient (i.e., <19.5% oxygen in air) or oxygen-enriched (i.e., >23.5% oxygen in air) environments. Therefore, it may be necessary to install hardwired toxic gas, flammable gas (i.e., Lower Explosive Limit [LEL]), or oxygen sensors equipped with audible and visual alarms in areas where compressed gases are stored and used. Areas in which the potential for an immediately dangerous to life or health (IDLH) condition could exist due to a release of compressed gases should be equipped with appropriate rescue equipment, including respirators equipped with escape cylinders or self-contained breathing apparatus (SCBA).

All piping systems used for compressed gases should be compatible with the gases that they are designed to hold, and all regulators and outlet connections should be consistent with the guidelines

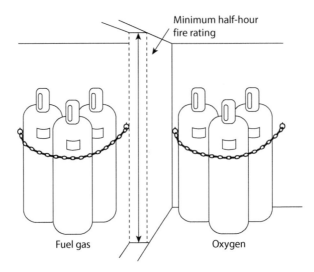

FIGURE 15.11 Gas cylinder storage. (From Canadian Centre for Occupational Health and Safety. Available at http://www.ccohs.ca/oshanswers/safety_haz/welding/storage.html)

established by the Compressed Gas Association (CGA) to help prevent the mixing of gases. Manual shutoff valves with uninterruptible pressure-relief devices should be installed near each point of use of the piping system.

One particular concern among health and safety professionals is the potential for supplied air respirator wearers to connect their breathing air hoses to the outlet connection for another type of gas. Therefore, it is essential that all outlet connections for breathing airlines be designed and installed so that they are unique and wholly incompatible with the outlet connections for all other gas lines. In addition, all lines should be clearly labeled according to the requirements of ANSI A13.1, "Scheme for the Identification of Piping Systems."

CRYOGENIC LIQUIDS

Cryogenic liquids are another class of hazardous materials that require careful consideration during facility planning and design. Some of the hazards associated with cryogenic liquids and gases include severe tissue damage from skin contact with cryogenic liquids and cold equipment surfaces, flammable gas–air or oxygen-deficient atmospheres from the vaporization of cryogenic liquids because relatively small amounts of liquid can create large volumes of gas, the rupture of vessels and piping systems from the rapid expansion of gases, and the embrittlement of the structural materials and condensation of atmospheric oxygen from the extremely cold temperatures.

Many of the safe design considerations for the handling, storage, and use of cryogenic liquid are similar to those for compressed gases: cryogenic liquids should be kept away from heat, ignition sources, and the unnecessary storage of combustible materials; cryogenic liquids should be stored and transported in such a way that equipment will not become damaged; all storage areas should be constructed according to applicable building codes, including NEC electric equipment guidelines for class, division, and group, and equipped with appropriate fire suppression systems; adequate ventilation should be provided in areas where flammable gas–air or oxygen-deficient environments could occur; and hardwired toxic gas, flammable gas (i.e., LEL), or oxygen sensors equipped with audible and visual alarms should be placed in areas where cryogenic liquids are stored and used.

It is critical that all equipment, including tanks, piping systems, and fittings, be specifically designed for use at extreme low temperatures and potentially extreme pressures. All equipment must be equipped with appropriate venting devices and pressure-relief valves. All relief devices should be vented to the outside. To prevent tissue damage due to contact with cold surfaces, all fixed equipment should be thermally insulated. When liquid oxygen or flammable liquids are used, all fixed equipment should be properly grounded and appropriate static dissipative devices should be used with portable equipment and personnel. Because liquid oxygen can cause oxygen to become trapped in porous materials in the event of a spill, only hard-surfaced nonporous materials should be used for room finishing surfaces.

REACTIVE MATERIALS

Reactive materials are those that tend to react spontaneously, react vigorously with air or water, be unstable to shock or heat, generate toxic gases, or explode. There are a variety of different types of reactive materials that can be used in a pharmaceutical manufacturing facility and its associated laboratory spaces, including oxidizers, peroxides and peroxide formers, water-reactive materials, and flammable metals. Although many of the hazards associated with the handling and use of reactive materials can be reduced through prudent work practices by the end users, some important design considerations can be incorporated into the facility design.

In particular, it is critical that reactive materials be stored properly. Both NFPA (including NFPA 430, "Code for the Storage of Liquid and Solid Oxidizers") and BOCA recommend storage and handling guidelines for certain reactive materials and classes of reactive materials. One of the critical issues in storing reactive materials is segregating them from incompatible materials (e.g., oxidizers such as benzoyl peroxide should not be stored with flammable liquids). The storage areas should be constructed according to all applicable building codes, including NEC electric equipment guidelines, and equipped with appropriate fire suppression systems. Because some materials may be water reactive, it may be necessary to design storage areas that are equipped with carbon dioxide or other appropriate fire suppression systems utilizing inert extinguishing agents. In addition, when reactive materials are used, all fixed equipment should be properly grounded and appropriate static dissipative devices should be used with portable equipment and personnel.

Explosive materials should be stored in secured areas that are equipped with appropriate explosion venting devices. Because some reactive materials may be temperature sensitive, refrigerated storage areas may be required. Due to the nature of the materials, the refrigerated areas may need to be equipped with adequate ventilation and hazardous location electrical equipment and apparatus. Other materials that are shock sensitive must be stored in areas where they will not be exposed to damage: they should not be stored above ground level, they should be isolated from vibration-producing equipment, and all rack storage or shelving units should be secured to the foundation and equipped with a means to secure the individual containers to prevent tipping or falling.

The variety of extreme hazards that can exist due to the use of reactive materials punctuates the point that facility designers must have a thorough understanding of the types and nature of the hazardous materials that will be used in the pharmaceutical manufacturing facility and its supporting laboratory and storage facilities to identify the safety principles that need to be incorporated into a facility design to avoid toxic exposures to personnel and potentially catastrophic events in the facility.

MACHINE GUARDING

In any modern pharmaceutical manufacturing facility, there are many examples of production, material handling, utility, and mechanical support equipment that require careful design and installation to ensure safe operation during normal operation, setup, adjustment, and routine service, maintenance, cleaning, and repair. Ensuring personnel safety during these different phases of equipment and machinery operation presents many challenges to the facility design and operations teams.

Many vendors who offer stand-alone equipment have taken the proactive approach of providing machine guarding, safety control systems, and labeling as part of their standard product offerings. These systems are usually well designed, but often they must be evaluated individually in conjunction with the specific use and application of the machinery and equipment.

As with other project elements, careful design and functional specifications are critical to achieve acceptable machine safeguarding arrangements. Development of specific requirements and confirmation of these requirements during equipment and machinery construction and verification are critical. Machine safeguarding should be a standard and documented portion of any equipment or machinery functional specification and a standard part of the functional acceptance test (FAT) conducted at the vendor's facility. Safe equipment and machinery are best achieved while at the vendor's location, rather than after installation in the field.

Employee protection during normal operation of equipment and machinery in the work environment is generally addressed by machine guarding, safety control systems, and labeling of hazardous operations.

Machine hazards are generally categorized into two main groups: power transmission hazards and point-of-operation hazards. Power transmission hazards refer to mechanical components that are designed to transfer mechanical energy or power from one location to another. These types of hazards include rotating or reciprocating machine parts and motions. Point-of-operation hazards refer to the point where machinery is actually performing work on the materials placed within the machine or equipment. This includes cutting, shearing, pinching, and bending actions.

Standard machine guarding configurations include fixed or secure guards over or around hazardous locations that physically prevent personnel access to the hazardous type. Guarding by distance is another concept that allows a machine to perform the required work activity, but is dimensionally configured so that employee body parts are unable to access the hazard point. Perimeter guarding or hostage guarding is a similar concept extensively used on automated equipment. Doors are provided around the perimeter of the equipment or access panel that allow the equipment or machine to operate and hold personnel away from or hostage to the actual machine operation. The perimeter guard doors or barriers may consist of interlocked doors or presence-sensing devices, such as light curtains or pressure-sensitive mats that are designed to keep personnel out of a defined area during machine operation. This type of system is common with a robotic and automated system and can present a challenge when service and maintenance work must be performed while some form of hazardous energy is being released in the equipment or machine. Access to the equipment should be controlled in a manner that allows only one guard door or barrier to be removed at a time and that makes sure the machine comes to an immediate stop upon being opened.

MAINTENANCE AND SUPPORT SERVICES

In the pharmaceutical industry, regular maintenance and support services are essential to keep equipment, machines, and the work environment safe and reliable. Lack of maintenance or inadequate maintenance or servicing can lead to dangerous situations, accidents, and occupational health issues. Maintenance is a high-risk activity with potential for incidents occurring in all areas of a pharmaceutical facility. Therefore, maintenance, support, and service personnel are more likely than other employees to be exposed to various hazards.

Maintenance and support service activities include inspection, testing, measurement, replacement, adjustment, repair, upkeep, fault detection, replacement of parts, servicing, lubrication, and cleaning. Maintenance and servicing is critical to ensure continuous productivity, to produce products of high quality, and to keep the company competitive. Therefore, it is critical that maintenance and service activities required for the start-up and ongoing operation of a pharmaceutical facility, equipment, and utilities be considered in the initial design phase (Figure 15.12).

MAINTENANCE-SPECIFIC HAZARDS AND RISKS

Maintenance operations involve specific risks in addition to the risks associated with any working environment. These include working alongside a running process and in close contact with machinery.

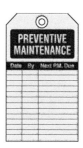

FIGURE 15.12 Preventative maintenance tag. (From Seton. Available at http://www.seton.com/equipment-inspection-tags-preventive-maintenance-50654.html)

During normal operation, automation typically diminishes the likelihood of human error that can lead to accidents. In maintenance activities, contrary to normal operation, direct contact between the worker and machine cannot be reduced substantially—maintenance is an activity where workers need to be in close contact with processes.

Maintenance often involves unusual work and nonroutine tasks, and it is often performed in exceptional conditions, such as working in confined spaces. Maintenance operations typically include both disassembly and reassembly, often involving complicated equipment and machinery. This can be associated with a greater risk of human error, increasing the accident risk.

Maintenance involves changing tasks and working environment. This is especially true in the case of contract workers. Subcontracting is an aggravating factor in terms of safety and health—numerous accidents and incidents relate to subcontracting maintenance. Working under time pressure is also typical for maintenance operations, especially when shutdowns or high-priority repairs are involved.

Because maintenance is carried out in all sectors and areas of the pharmaceutical facility and involves a wide range of tasks, it is associated with potential exposure to various hazards and their associated risks. Basic types of hazards encountered are listed below:

- *Chemical hazards* may include APIs, asbestos, fiberglass, lead paint, vapors, fumes (e.g., asphalt fumes, diesel exhaust, and crystalline silica), dust, and solvents. Typical tasks during which chemical hazards may be encountered include building maintenance, electrical arc welding, carrying out work in confined spaces, and maintenance where hazardous chemicals are present. Potential health outcomes associated with chemical hazards include breathing problems, occupational asthma, allergies, asbestosis, and cancer.
- *Physical hazards* include noise, vibration, excessive heat and cold, radiation (ultraviolet radiation, x-rays, and electromagnetic fields), high physical workloads, and ergonomics-related risks due to poor design of machinery, process, and work environment from the point of view of maintenance, such as difficult-to-reach objects to be maintained, strenuous movements (bending, kneeling, reaching, pushing, and pulling), and working in confined spaces. Typical tasks that may cause exposure to physical hazards include drilling, grinding, filing, sanding, working outdoors, maintenance of the industrial plant (e.g., ovens and furnaces and chilling units), welding, inspection of pipes, and rail maintenance. Potential health outcomes associated with these hazards include hearing problems due to noise, and musculoskeletal disorders.
- *Biological hazards* include bacteria, viruses, mold, and fungi. Typical tasks that may bring personnel in contact with biological hazards include maintenance in waste treatment plants, maintenance where biological agents are handled, such as laboratories, and maintenance in places where bacteria, molds, and fungi are likely to proliferate, such as air conditioning systems. Potential health outcomes from exposure to biological hazards include breathing problems, asthma, allergies, and Legionnaires' disease.

- *Psychological risk factors* include time pressure, shift work (weekend work, night work, on-call work, and irregular working hours), and communication issues arising from working together with staff from contractors. Potential health outcomes are work-related stress, fatigue, and increased accident risk. Many accidents are related to work equipment and machine maintenance, for example, crushing by moving machinery, unexpected start-up, falls from height, accidents involving falling objects, electrocution, electrical shocks, burns, confined spaces, asphyxiation, and explosion or fire.

MEANS OF EGRESS

All facilities must have emergency evacuation paths that lead to safe assembly areas from all buildings and processes. These paths must be properly designed to accommodate the safe and orderly movement of all personnel without impairing emergency responder access to the site or incident area.

Most countries have regulatory codes detailing the design requirements for emergency evacuation routes. However, performance-based designs are becoming much more popular. NFPA 101, "Life Safety Code," is a globally recognized consensus standard that allows for performance-based egress designs (Figure 15.13). At the heart of performance-based designs is a risk assessment.

NFPA 101 provides prescriptive and performance measures that should be incorporated into the design and operation of all new and existing facilities. In general, the evacuation routes must ensure that all personnel, including visitors, are able to reach a safe location, typically known as the assembly area, without incurring any harm from the fire or emergency incident. The following general principles are elements that should be incorporated in prescriptive emergency egress plans or considered in the risk assessment for performance-based designs.

- Has the selection of fire rated or approved materials of construction for structures and internal finishes been included in the design criteria.
- At a minimum, all emergency egress routes should have 1-h fire-resistant construction and automatic sprinkler protection. For high-hazard occupancies, greater fire resistance and DLC may be required.
- Is fire proofing for steel structures included in the design criteria.
- Have the appropriate automatic sprinkler systems, detection systems and alarm notification systems included as part of the design criteria.

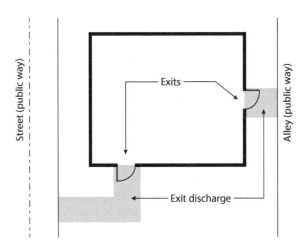

FIGURE 15.13   Egress from multiple exits. (From International Code Council. Available at http://publicecodes. cyberregs.com/icod/ibc/2009f2cc/icod_ibc_2009f2cc_10_sec002.htm)

- The minimum number of exits from any space or room on any floor, story, or mezzanine should be two.
- The number of exits should be increased for higher-occupancy loads and when there are increased life safety hazards, such as hazardous materials processing or storage or congested operations.
- Where multiple exits are required, each exit must be capable of being accessed independently of any other exit. Therefore, an occupant must not be required to travel through one exit to reach a second exit.
- Where more than one exit is required for any room or space, the exits must be remotely located from one another. Egress routes should be direct and as short as practical. The route should always direct personnel through less hazardous areas. For example, it is permissible to have occupants from a laboratory egress through an office area. However, an administrative suite should not egress through a chemical processing area.
- Evacuation routes must be designed to accommodate the safe transport of personnel with physical disabilities (e.g., wheelchair access) and any individuals that may have been injured during an incident. Provisions should be made for transporting physically disabled personnel down stairways in a safe and efficient manner. All stairs should be equipped with nonslip treads and handrails. Elevators are typically not permitted to be used as part of an emergency evacuation plan.
- All emergency evacuation paths must be clearly identified with signs and diagrams indicating the route of travel and the location of the safe assembly area. Doorways along the egress path should be labeled indicating the egress route. Doorways that lead to closed or inaccessible areas should be labeled "No Emergency Exit."
- All emergency evacuation paths must be provided with both primary and emergency lighting of sufficient lumens to allow for the safe movement of personnel. For high-hazard occupancies such as chemical processing, pilot plants, laboratories using flammable materials, warehouses, and hazardous material storage areas, a secondary evacuation route must be provided. The secondary route shall be provided with the same protective features as the primary egress path.
- Exit door width is determined by the number of occupants expected to utilize the doorway during the emergency, but should not be narrower than 32 in. (81 cm).
- All doors located along the evacuation route should open in the direction of travel and should be equipped with panic-type latching hardware. Doors should also operate easily with a minimum force of 133 N (30 lb-ft) required for opening. All doors with automated controls should be designed with the capability to be operated manually in the event of an emergency or power failure.
- All doors required to be fire rated must have an automatic closing device and must not have glass panels of an area greater than 100 in.^{2} (645 cm^2). Fire doors and personnel egress doors should not be blocked open.
- Doors arranged with access control shall be arranged to allow for free egress while maintaining security to prohibit unauthorized entry.
- Stairway width should be determined by the number of occupants expected to utilize it during an emergency. At a minimum, landings must be the same width as the stairway.
- Use of corridors and hallways should be considered to ensure adequate width. The width of any corridor or hallway should be measured by the clear width of the space.

AREAS OF SAFE REFUGE AND ASSEMBLY AREAS

For some occupancies, including high-rise buildings, it may be advisable to direct personnel to a safe area of refuge rather than an outdoor assembly area. An area of refuge is a room or space enclosed with a minimum of 1-h fire-rated construction with self-closing fire doors and automatic sprinkler protection. The area of refuge should be adjacent to a stairway with direct egress outside the building. A means of two-way emergency communication with the emergency response team or fire department must be provided.

EMERGENCY ACCESS

Emergency access to the site, buildings, process areas, and internal spaces should be evaluated during the design, construction, and operation of every pharmaceutical facility. The locations of building equipment, utilities, and access paths should not impede access or egress. Utilities such as gas services, electrical systems, and hazardous material transfer systems should be well marked with emergency shutdown valves and switchgear readily accessible. Emergency system alarm annunciator panels should be located in a main firefighter access or assembly area.

Emergency responder access routes and roads should be provided so that all portions of the facility are within approximately 150 ft of that access road. The access roads should have an unobstructed width of not less than 20 ft and an unobstructed vertical clearance of not less than 13 ft 6 in. The local emergency response agencies should be consulted to ensure that these recommended road clearances are adequate for the emergency response vehicles typically used on-site.

PHYSICAL HAZARDS

HEAT

Heat-generating processes and equipment can cause personnel to experience a variety of heat-related injuries or illnesses that range in severity from discomfort and light-headedness and flushed skin to heat strain and heat stroke. In areas where PPE is required to protect employees from physical or chemical hazards, the potential exposure to heat stress can be exacerbated. Another risk associated with heat is thermal burns from skin contact with hot surfaces. ISO 7243 provides a simple method for assessing and controlling hot environments based on the web bulb globe temperature (WBGT) index. ISO 7933 describes an analytical method of assessment of hot environments based on the human heat balance equation and the calculation of the required sweat rate index (Sreq). A variety of other consensus standards on heat stress include the American Conference of Governmental Industrial Hygienists (ACGIH) threshold limit value (TLV) for heat stress and heat strain, and the NIOSH, "Criteria for a Recommended Standard—Occupational Exposure to Hot Environments."

When designing a facility or process that will utilize equipment that generates heat, it is critical to understand the total heat load that will be introduced into each space. This will help to define the heating and cooling needs for the space in order to maintain occupant comfort during manufacturing operations. All heat-generating equipment should be thermally insulated to reduce the amount of heat that is radiated into the room, to reduce the potential for thermal burns due to skin contact with hot surfaces, and to maximize energy efficiency. Where necessary, local exhaust ventilation (LEV) should be provided for ovens, autoclaves, equipment washers, and other equipment that generate hot exhaust streams. Where radiant heat sources are present, shielding should be used to direct radiant energy away from personnel or critical equipment.

NOISE

Exposure to noise can cause noise-induced hearing loss, as well as interfere with critical audible communications, including face-to-face vocal communications and audible alarms. Noise levels are regulated by both occupational (interior workplace noise) and environmental (noise sources outside of the building, such as exhaust points and generators) agencies. International standards for noise include ISO 13.140, "Noise"; ISO 17.140, "Acoustics and Acoustical Measurements"; and ISO 13.340.20, "Hearing Protection." OSHA has established a permissible exposure limit (PEL) of 90 dBA as an 8-h TWA for noise in 1910.95, "Occupational Noise." Other consensus standards, including ACGIH (*TLVs and BEIs*, TLV for noise, 2014) and NIOSH 98-126 ("Criteria for a Recommended Standard: Occupational Noise Exposure—Revised Criteria"), recommend 85 dBA as a criterion level for noise (Figure 15.14).

Noise is generated from a variety of sources in pharmaceutical manufacturing facilities, including, but not limited to, mechanical noise and impact noise from motors moving equipment, air noise at exhaust points, and noise due to the vibration of equipment and surfaces. In designing a facility and selecting equipment, it is important to understand the types and number of pieces of equipment that will be used in any given area to anticipate the total noise that will be generated in an area and, in turn, to identify appropriate noise controls for that area.

Noise control can be achieved by a variety of different methods, including reducing or eliminating noise at the source, enclosing the noise source, and installing sound absorptive room treatments. The most effective means for reducing noise is to select equipment, such as fans and motors that are quiet by design, based on manufacturer or supplier sound power data. Additional noise control principles to keep in mind include

- Ensure that pumps, motors, and other equipment are properly balanced and mounted to eliminate the sources of vibration and minimize the transfer of vibration to adjacent surfaces and the structure of the building itself.
- Minimize noise from pneumatic systems by operating equipment at the lowest pressures that will enable proper equipment operation and installing regulators on pneumatic systems so that supply air pressures to equipment can be easily controlled by the end user.
- Orient exhaust points and other directional noise sources away from areas in which personnel work.
- Provide silencers for equipment with air intakes and mufflers for exhaust points.
- Minimize noise from piping systems by sizing pipes and selecting valves that are appropriate for the anticipated pressure and flow.
- Design and install ventilation systems with properly sized ducts and select proper hoods, fittings, and other system components that will minimize air turbulence.
- Minimize noise from piping systems and air ducts by installing lagging around the pipes and ducts. If pipe and duct lagging is used in GMP areas, the lagging materials must be nonporous and easily cleanable.

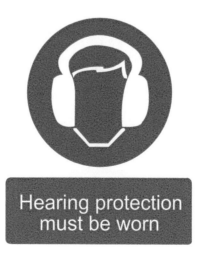

FIGURE 15.14 Noise-level caution sign. (From SafetySupplyWarehouse.com. Available at http://www.safetysupplywarehouse.com/CAUTION_NOISE_LEVEL_GREATER_THAN_85dba_Sign_p/20518.htm)

If excess noise cannot be controlled at the source, enclosures or dedicated rooms should be considered for the noise-producing equipment. For equipment used in manufacturing areas, identify manufacturer or aftermarket acoustical enclosures that can be installed around individual pieces of equipment. In these cases, the materials of construction should be nonporous, easily cleanable, and corrosion resistant. In cases where full enclosures are not feasible, it may be possible to install partial enclosures around equipment or insert partitioning walls between the noise source and the exposed personnel.

VIBRATION

Personnel who interact with vibrating equipment can be exposed to musculoskeletal disorders (MSDs) due to hand–arm vibration (HAV) and whole-body vibration (WBV). A variety of consensus standards, including ISO 2631–1985, "Evaluation of Human Exposure to Whole-Body Vibration"; ANSI S3.18–1979, "Guide for the Evaluation of Human Exposure to Whole Body Vibration"; and the ACGIH TLV for WBV, have been developed to address the potential hazards associated with occupational exposure to WBV.

NONIONIZING RADIATION

Nonionizing radiation is defined as electromagnetic energy with a photon energy of 12.4 eV or less that has insufficient energy to ionize matter such as human tissue. The spectrum of nonionizing electromagnetic energy ranges from optical radiation, which includes ultraviolet (UV), visible, and infrared (IR) radiation with wavelengths of 10 nm to 1 mm, to radiofrequency (RF) and microwave (MW) radiation, with frequencies of about 300 kHz to 300 GHz, to extremely low-frequency (ELF) radiation, with frequencies of 3 kHz or less (Figure 15.15).

In general, optical radiation can cause adverse health effects to the eyes and skin. Lasers may be used in analytical laboratories for particle sizing or in pharmaceutical packaging areas in which bar coding is used. Various consensus organizations, including the American National Standards Institute (ANSI) (ANSI Z136.1, "Safe Use of Lasers," 2000), have established guidelines for the operation of lasers and the design of facilities in which lasers are operated. International laser safety standards include IEC 608 25-1 on the safety of laser products. Lasers are classified according to their output power. In general, lasers used for particle sizing and bar coding are low powered, with output powers of less than 5 mW. The use of these lasers requires standard precautions to be taken

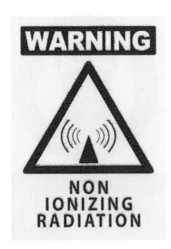

FIGURE 15.15 Warning: Nonionizing radiation. (From Safety online. Available at http://www.safety-online. co.nz/warning-non-ionizing-radiation-sign)

to limit the potential for exposure to laser light. The use of higher-powered lasers with output powers of more than 5 mW requires more rigorous controls. Facility design considerations should be taken into account, including providing nonreflective surface finishing in areas in which lasers will be used to minimize reflection and scattering of laser light, and locating laser equipment so that it is limited to responsible personnel only and potential incidental exposure to bystanders is minimized.

RF and MW radiation-generating equipment in a pharmaceutical manufacturing facility can include equipment that is used for sealing packaging materials and nuclear magnetic resonance (NMR) spectroscopy equipment used in pharmaceutical R&D laboratories. Adverse health effects include heating of the deep tissues, effects on the nervous system, reproductive effects, effects on the eyes, and possible links with cancer. RF and MW equipment is also known to interfere with the function of pacemakers and can cause heating of metal prosthetic devices and other medical implants. Guidelines for exposure to RF and MW radiation have been established by OSHA (29 CFR 1910.97, "Non-Ionizing Radiation") and a variety of consensus organizations, including the International Commission on Non-Ionizing Radiation Protection (ICNIRP), Institute of Electrical and Electronics Engineers (IEEE) (C95.1-1991, "IEEE Standard for Safety Levels with respect to Human Exposure to Radio Frequency Electromagnetic Fields, 3 kHz to 300 GHz"), and ACGIH.

The two most effective methods protecting personnel from exposure to RF and MW radiation are shielding and distancing personnel from RF and MW sources. When selecting and installing RF and MW radiation-generating equipment, it should be equipped with appropriate shielding materials to prevent radiation leakage and penetration. Once installed, the equipment must be electrically grounded. Because the power density of the radiation emitted by an RF or MW source follows an inverse square relationship with distance (i.e., power density decreases by $1/d^2$), distancing personnel from radiation sources can be an effective control strategy. In particular, care should be taken to distance employees from potential exposures by positioning the equipment away from high-foot-traffic areas and providing equipment controls that are remote from the radiation sources.

PROCESS SAFETY MANAGEMENT

Process safety management (PSM) is a risk management tool focused on preventing catastrophic accidents, particularly explosions, fires, and toxic releases, associated with the use of chemicals and other hazardous materials. Although it is primarily applied to chemical API manufacturing, it can also be applied in the design and operation of pharmaceutical finishing facilities. Specific applications can include process unit operations, utility systems (boilers), wastewater systems, tank farms, solvent supply systems, and waste collection systems.

The key provision of PSM is process hazard analysis (PHA), which is a careful review of what could go wrong and what safeguards must be implemented to prevent releases of hazardous materials. PHA evaluations incorporate the concept of risk in determinations of system design criteria. Risk in this setting can be defined as the combination of hazard probability and hazard potential severity, and it is most often expressed in a criticality or risk assessment matrix, as shown in Table 15.1.

PHA methodologies evaluate the risks associated with the operation, design, and potential malfunctions of industrial processes (Figure 15.16). In general, PHAs identify four elements:

1. The source of the hazard
2. The consequence, impact, or effect resulting from the occurrence of the hazard
3. Safeguards, controls, or mitigative features intended to prevent the hazard from occurring or reduce the consequences that result
4. Recommendations if the safeguards or controls are considered inadequate or if none are in place (based on placement of deviation in the criticality matrix)

Many PHA methodologies have been developed. The most popular methodologies are described below.

TABLE 15.1

Risk Assessment Matrix

	Hazard Categories			
	I	II	III	IV
	Catastrophic	Critical	Marginal	Negligible
A. Frequent	1	1	1	3
B. Probable	1	1	2	3
C. Occasional	1	2	2	4
D. Remote	2	2	3	4
E. Improbable	3	3	3	4

Criticality Rating (Risk Classification)	Criticality (Risk Criteria)
1	Unacceptable
2	Undesirable
3	Acceptable with review
4	Acceptable without review

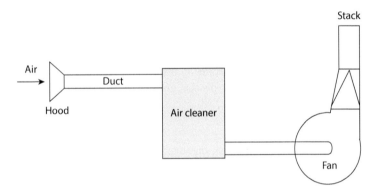

FIGURE 15.16 Example of a process flow diagram. (From Occupational Safety and Health Administration. Available at http://www.intotext.com/OSHA_Safety_Construction/pls/oshaweb/owadispfa8f.html?p_table= STANDARDS&p_id=10648)

The *what-if checklist* is a method of analyzing relatively uncomplicated processes. At each step in the process, "what if" questions are asked and the answers are considered in the evaluation of the effects of the failures of components or errors in the procedures.

A *hazard and operability study* (HAZOP study) systematically identifies every conceivable deviation from the design intent, possible abnormal causes, and adverse hazardous consequences that can occur in a planned or existing process or operation. The HAZOP study focuses on specific portions of the process called nodes. Generally, these nodes are identified from the piping and instrumentation diagram (P&ID) for the process before the study begins. A process parameter is identified, such as *low*, and an intention is created for the node under consideration. Then a series of guidewords are combined with the parameter *flow* to create deviations. For example, the guideword *no* is combined with the parameter *flow* to give the deviation *no flow*. All credible causes of a *no-flow* deviation are then listed, beginning with the cause that can result in the worst possible consequence. Once the causes are recorded, the team lists the consequences, safeguards, and any recommendations deemed appropriate. The process is repeated for the next deviation, and so on, until completion of the node. The process continues with evaluation of the next node.

Failure mode and effects analysis (FMEA) is a method of analyzing a system design or manufacturing process in order to evaluate the potential for failures. It involves identifying all potential failure modes, determining the end effect of each potential failure mode, and determining the criticality of these failure effects. FMEAs are sometimes referred to as FMECAs (failure mode, effects, and criticality analyses). FMEAs are based on standards (both military and commercial) in the reliability engineering industry. These analyses can take many forms, but they are all used to study a particular system and determine how that system can be modified to improve overall reliability and avoid failures. Once this is completed, an FMEA or FMECA can be used to determine the most critical failure modes and then determine how these critical failures can be minimized or eliminated.

Fault tree analysis (FTA) is a method of analyzing system design and performance. It involves specifying a top event to analyze (such as a fire), followed by identifying all of the associated elements in the system that could cause that top event to occur. Fault trees provide a convenient symbolic representation of the combination of events resulting in the occurrence of the top event. Events and gates in FTA are represented by symbols. Fault tree analyses are generally performed graphically using a logical structure of AND and OR gates. Sometimes certain elements, or basic events, may need to occur together in order for that top event to occur. In this case, these events are arranged under an AND gate, meaning that all of the basic events would need to occur to trigger the top event. If basic events alone would trigger the top event, then they are grouped under an OR gate. The entire system, including human interactions, is analyzed when performing an FTA.

Safety integrity level (SIL) determination is the process of determining the amount of risk mitigation required to reduce the risk put forth by a process to a tolerable level. SIL determination is the first step in the development, design, commission, and operation of a safety instrumented system (SIS). SIL determination involves the determination of the SIL for each safety instrumented function (SIF) in an SIS and is dependent on the following factors:

- Corporate standards for the tolerable risk after applying all the layers of protection
- The overall risk from the unprotected hazards that can occur
- The risk reduction provided by all of the non-SIS protection layers

While the HAZOP study identifies and ranks risk hazards, SIL determination focuses on the adequacy of safeguards to mitigate hazards. Furthermore, SIL adds another dimension to safety analysis. Within the framework of a HAZOP, analysts are restricted to the limits of the governing risk matrix (i.e., specific range limits on frequencies of occurrence). In contrast, SIL analysis enables analysts to refine the estimates of frequencies of occurrence to obtain more realistic estimates of risk.

VENTILATION

Industrial ventilation generally involves the use of supply and exhaust ventilation to control emissions, exposures, and chemical hazards in the workplace.

There are five basic types of ventilation systems:

1. Dilution and removal by general exhaust
2. LEV and containment systems
3. Makeup air
4. HVAC (primarily for comfort)
5. Recirculation systems

In a pharmaceutical facility, occupational exposure control is primarily performed utilizing LEV and containment systems. The following is a general overview of the systems available to provide primary containment. Facility design provides a secondary means to contain airborne exposure and surface contamination through a system of personnel and material airlocks, mist showers, and airflows and pressurization.

LOCAL EXHAUST VENTILATION

The principle behind LEV technology is to extract particles before they propagate into a larger volume of air. By reducing the migration of source-generated particulate, the potential for exposure is, in turn, reduced. However, this technology is limited in its ability to control low-exposure levels, and its performance is highly dependent on operator technique. Decay in the device's performance can easily occur if the emission source is slightly outside or moved from the small area designed for capture, operator motions create air turbulence, or the operator obstructs the capture stream. Depending on the specific task being performed, this technology can exhibit control levels in the range of 50 to 100 $\mu g/m^3$. As such, this technology is not recommended for high-containment applications as the primary containment device. The primary use of LEV is for nonpotent and low-potency dust control. However, LEV is sometimes used to supplement other primary high-containment devices. An example of this is the mating of LEV to a split-butterfly valve.

AIRFLOW TECHNOLOGY

Airflow technology (AFT) uses principles similar to those of LEV. However, its effectiveness is dramatically improved. Typical AFT utilizes a directional airstream to sweep source emissions away from the operator's breathing zone. The velocity of the airstream is also designed to minimize particles from settling onto adjacent surfaces. The airstream is cleansed by a filtration system prior to it being recirculated or exhausted. AFT provides a major improvement over LEV, through its ability to control and minimize airborne migration of particles out into the facility. Operator technique still largely affects the performance of this technology. Depending on the specific task being performed, this technology can exhibit control levels in the range of 10 to 100 $\mu g/m^3$. However, one must also realize the issues with decontaminating the equipment following processing.

ISOLATION TECHNOLOGY

The next level of containment is provided through isolation technology. The principle of this technology is to provide a physical barrier between the emission source and the operator and environment. This barrier can be constructed from either soft or rigid materials. Soft-wall isolation technologies range from nonventilated glove bags to ventilated soft-wall isolators, while rigid-wall isolators are generally pressure controlled. Several devices are available to allow items to enter and exit the isolation system, while maintaining isolation integrity. Some examples of these devices include rapid transfer ports (RTPs), split valves, lock chambers, and continuous liner systems. Much like the other two technologies' systems, performance is a function of the specific tasks performed and, in addition, which access devices are installed. The expected range of performance can be anticipated to be between 10 ng/m^3 and 10 $\mu g/m^3$. Industry guidance strongly recommends isolation technology for high-containment applications.

WALKING AND WORKING SURFACES

Walking and working surfaces in a typical pharmaceutical manufacturing facility refer to any interior or exterior surface that is intended for routine or occasional access by personnel. This may include sidewalks, floors, ramps, stairways, elevated platforms and walkways, fixed and portable ladders, and roof-level surfaces. Various building codes and occupational health and safety regulations promulgated throughout the world contain specific specifications for the design and maintenance of walking and working surfaces. These requirements are generally related to the structural design of the surface or the related architectural elements to properly support the required load. This loading must take into consideration personnel, equipment (either permanent or temporary), and materials. Other design requirements include the protection of all open or leading edges where there is a change in elevation, usually greater than 3 ft; the degree of incline or slope for ramps; the elevation transitions between two levels; and the type of floor finishes provided to prevent slippery surfaces. Ice, water, or other liquids, or highly polished or cleanable surfaces can cause slip and fall injuries when surfaces become slippery.

The most opportune time to develop strategies to prevent slip, trip, and fall-related injuries in administrative, production, utility, and maintenance areas is during the design and engineering stages of the project. Key considerations include flooring designs that are sufficient to support the weight of personnel, portable equipment, and materials. Floor loading must take into consideration the weight of both personnel and any other additional loading that process equipment and materials may add. The capacity of elevated platforms or walkways should be clearly posted to prevent potential overloading.

Providing floor surfaces that offer adequate friction or traction is an important consideration in cGMP or clean environments where smooth or highly polished surfaces can often create a hazard or when personnel are required to wear gowning or booties over their shoes. The selection of floor cleaning and gowning garments is an important consideration for clean or aseptic processing areas to prevent serious slip and fall injuries. Special attention should also be given to prevent highly polished surfaces near exterior doors or entranceways. At exterior doors or areas where water moisture or outside debris is routinely present, a well-drained or sloped flooring system with increased traction should be provided to prevent slippery walking surfaces.

Even the slightest changes in elevation are potential points for personnel to misjudge footing and increase their potential for slips and falls. Generally, any surface transition greater than 3/8 in. can result in a potential tripping hazard. A smooth transition with well-identified changes in elevations should be provided. Standard stair designs are often better navigated than sloped or ramped floor surfaces.

Platforms should be provided for any work requiring elevated material handling or equipment operation. Platforms must be designed in accordance with applicable building codes and be of sufficient capacity for the intended loading. Placarding of the platform capacity is often required. Any platform intended for personnel access that is 3 or more feet above surrounding surfaces must be protected with an approved standard barrier or railing on all exposed sides. The standard barrier generally consists of three specific elements: the top rail, midrail, and toe board. The standard railing assembly should be of rigid and durable design capable of withstanding a force of at least 200 lb in any direction. The midrail should be located halfway between the top railing and the toe board. The toe board design is normally a 4 in. high plate that is set off the platform elevation by up to 1/2 in. to allow water to pass beneath. When a vertical ladder is used to access the platform, the point of access to the elevated platform should be protected by a swing gate to prevent personnel from stepping into and falling through the open ladder way.

Industrial stairways should be provided whenever possible for routine access to other elevations and in accordance with applicable building codes. Industrial stairs may be of open or enclosed design. Railings are required and are based on the width of the stairs. Exterior stairs should be designed to be free of ice or snow accumulations in cold climates.

Fixed industrial ladders should only be considered when access to elevations is not required on a continuous basis or by all personnel. Furthermore, industrial ladders are not intended for personnel use if tools and other equipment must be carried or used by personnel while on the ladder. The length and types of vertical ladders fixed to the exterior of buildings or process equipment are governed by various country-specific health and safety standards. Many require the installation of cages or fall-arresting equipment.

Cages are frequently included on exterior ladder ways. They are intended to protect personnel from falling away from the ladder or from contact with objects while climbing. However, personnel can still incur a serious fall while contained within the ladder cage. The length of fixed ladders is restricted to allow personnel to take a break while ascending and to limit the height of the potential fall hazard. Fixed ladder ways restricted to lengths up to 20 ft generally do not require additional fall protection considerations. Fixed ladders of greater length are often equipped with a vertical guide rail system that allows personnel to use fall-arresting equipment. A swing gate that restricts access to the ladder way and only opens outward from the ladder way should protect access to a vertical ladder way.

Any opening in a walking or working surface greater than 6 in. has the increased potential to create a fall hazard and must be barricaded, covered, secured, or otherwise protected. Openings along the edges of platforms should be avoided in the design or must be effectively guarded with a standard railing assembly. Self-closing or double-overhead gates need to be provided where materials are delivered to the edge of an elevated platform or mezzanine also used as a walking or working surface to allow passage of materials without compromising personnel access or safety.

Access to roofs, interstitial spaces, mezzanines, or areas above suspended ceilings in production facilities is often required by maintenance personnel to access mechanical or utility equipment. Frequent access to these levels requires the installation of approved walking and working surfaces, as described above. By design, mechanical equipment should be positioned so that access can be obtained from an approved walking or working surface and never within 6 ft of an unprotected edge. Interstitial spaces present other similar hazards and may require additional features, such as lighting and work platforms with load-bearing surfaces to support the weight of maintenance personnel.

When roofs must be accessed, several potential hazards may exist, including exposure to emissions, non-weight-bearing surfaces, skylights, and unprotected edges. Roofs designed for routine access should be of full weight-bearing capacity and have perimeter protection provided using a standard railing, fall arrest system, or extended exterior parapet wall design. Translucent skylights should also be protected against step-through by physical guarding or the use of a standard perimeter railing.

FURTHER DISCUSSION

1. What are the dangers of working in a confined space, and how can they be mitigated?
2. Why are ergonomics important in the pharmaceutical industry?
3. Describe the safety considerations that limit storage and handling of flammable materials.
4. Why are maintenance personnel more likely to come across hazards than other personnel?

ABOUT THE AUTHOR

George Petroka has more than 30 years of experience in environmental safety and health, industrial hygiene, and process safety working within process industries including Sanofi, Sterling Winthrop, Sunoco, and Pennsylvania Manufacturers Insurance Company (PMA). He has extensive experience in the pharmaceutical industry, having managed environmental health and safety (EHS) for Sanofi and Sterling Winthrop. At IES Engineers (IES), George is a principal responsible for business development and executing and managing EHS Services to the Biopharma Industry. He holds an MS in environmental science and engineering from Drexel University, Philadelphia, and a BS in safety management and a BA in biology from Indiana University of Pennsylvania, Indiana, Pennsylvania. He is both a Certified Industrial Hygienist (CIH) and a Certified Safety Professional (CSP).

16 Sustainability

Asif Syed

CONTENTS

INTRODUCTION

Sustainability, which is important to all sectors of the pharmaceutical industry, is defined as "meeting current needs without compromising the future." In addition to protecting the environment, sustainability offers benefits ranging from operational cost savings to public approval. The cost reduction results from improving efficiency, thereby avoiding the cost of wasteful energy, and the public approval generated by environmental stewardship is a long-term asset. Employee satisfaction is also linked to companies "that do the right thing." Sustainability is simply good business practice that generates innovation beneficial to the company.

Sustainability is applicable to both new development and renovation projects. The facilities and building operations groups are generally responsible for the sustainability goals established and often must demonstrate the sustainable path to top management; thus, facilities and building operations play a major role in the sustainability of the company.

This chapter explains how to structure current sustainable policies in the pharmaceutical industry, that is, how to adopt sustainable practices in product design, design and construction of new facilities, renovation of existing facilities, and ongoing operations. Additionally, key resources for sophisticated sustainable design and operations are identified.

Implementing a sustainable policy, reporting progress, and quantifying achievements are challenging and complex. There are several models used for measuring the sustainability of facilities, such as the rating system of the U.S. Green Building Council's (USGBC) Leadership in Energy and Environmental Design (LEED) and the United Kingdom's Building Research Establishment Environmental Assessment Method (BREEAM). While none of these models are specific to pharmaceutical manufacturing, almost all pharmaceutical companies have at least some commercial office buildings to which the standard model applies. Getting a LEED rating may not necessarily quantify achievements. However, measurable emissions and energy use can be easily quantified by calculating a carbon footprint in tons of carbon dioxide released into the atmosphere and kBTU/year (kW/year), which is a universally accepted measure of energy use by an organization. For existing buildings, after a baseline is established by building performance the first year, subsequent years can demonstrate reduction with energy-efficient measures. For new buildings, the baseline is generally the energy code–mandated energy efficiency measures, and additional sustainable measures can demonstrate a reduction from the baseline.

ISSUES IN SUSTAINABILITY

Generally, sustainable building design aims to reduce the negative impact on the environment and improve the health, comfort, and well-being of the building's occupants. It is achieved by balancing the three P's (i.e., people, planet, and profit). The guiding principles of sustainable buildings are site optimization, reduction of energy consumption, use of environmentally safe materials, reduction of water use, improvement of indoor air quality, and reduction of the ongoing impact to the environment.

AIR QUALITY AND EMISSIONS

The far-reaching benefits of the pharmaceutical industry in enhancing quality of life and preserving life are often overshadowed by environmental issues, such as air pollution. Understanding, documenting, and monitoring the air emissions are generally the first steps toward reducing or managing the emissions. Air emissions include organic and inorganic compounds, which are particulates from manufacturing or formulation. The Clean Air Act classifies the hazardous air pollutants (HAPs). These emissions vary from facility to facility based on the product and process. Air emissions must be identified and contained and require an integrated approach from start to finish. Input from drug designers, manufacturing process engineers, facility design architects and engineers, and local environmental engineers helps to address the issue of HAPs.

ENVIRONMENT

Release of Products

Release of pharmaceutical products into the environment can happen during production, which is under the control of the facilities and operations groups, or postproduction, which is not under the control of the manufacturing facility. Overall, the drug ingredients released postproduction into the environment can be reduced by avoiding overprescribing, patient compliance in drug usage, and proper drug disposal. Postproduction releases are beyond the scope of this book. For designers of pharmaceutical facilities, the most important issue is the release of the drug ingredients or other chemicals into the environment from the facility they design. Though environmental regulations govern specific chemicals, the gold standard of sustainability is not to release any ingredient into the environment, whether or not its effects are known. Processes generate waste and emissions, which depend on the process and materials used.

Water

Pharmaceutical manufacturing facilities often draw attention from the public and environmental groups because pharmaceutical ingredients have contaminated water in local streams, groundwater, or other bodies of water. The greatest concern is the ability of pharmaceutical agents to alter living organisms in these bodies of water. As with air pollution, an integrated approach between all stakeholders, from pharmaceutical developers to facilities designers, such as architects, engineers, and local environmental engineers, is the best for solving the water quality issue. Reduction of water use and water waste greatly contributes to sustainability.

Solid Waste

At pharmaceutical facilities, solid waste is generated from several sources: manufacturing processes, filtration of air and water (i.e., abatement), construction and demolition operations, incineration waste, and excess product. Generally, pharmaceutical solid wastes are generated during formulation, mixing, compounding, and discarding excess. The solid wastes include excess raw materials, spent solvents, reaction residues, air and liquid filter media, and chemical reagents. Most solid wastes are incinerated or disposed off-site.

Compliance with federal, state, and local regulations is required in all solid waste disposal. The regulations are beyond the scope of this chapter. However, solid waste reduction can be integrated into the product design by factoring in the input from the solid waste handling and disposal team. The facility design team must integrate the process of waste reduction and recycling into their overall design.

ENERGY

All pharmaceutical facilities use energy in several different forms, such as electricity for power and light and natural gas to produce heat, steam, and hot water for processing. Liquid fuels, such as diesel, are commonly used as backup fuel sources for generators. While most energy used in the world is directly related to the burning of fossil fuels, there are non–fossil fuel energy sources, such as nuclear, solar, wind, and geothermal. There are several opportunities to reduce energy use in the design, renovation, and operation of pharmaceutical facilities. Reduction of energy leads to lower utility bills for electricity and natural gas, which directly improves the bottom line. The indirect benefit comes from the reduction of the carbon footprint as a result of lower energy use either on-site or at the power plant where the energy is generated.

Generally, pharmaceutical facilities use more energy than other manufacturing practices. The high energy use results from process loads that use steam. While a batch process may operate for a few hours or days of a week, the boiler plant is constantly using energy by staying warm around the clock. In addition, the need for cleanliness, which necessitates a high air-change rate and filtration, is a constant energy drain. The air-change rate, which complies with current Good Manufacturing Practices (cGMPs), varies based on the drug or formulation. The generally accepted industry practices for air-change rates are listed in Table 16.1 [1]. These high air-change rates require fan power to circulate the air, in addition to increasing cooling and heating costs. Careful attention to energy use and costs can lead to reduction in energy preservation of resources, reduction in capital costs, and above all, a reduction in ongoing operational costs, the benefits of which can be reaped year after year.

SUSTAINABLE AND HIGH-PERFORMANCE FACILITIES

High-performance design is generally understood, as defined by the U.S. Energy Independence and Security Act of 2007, as "a building that integrates and optimizes on a life cycle basis, all major high-performance attributes, including energy and water conservation, environment, safety,

TABLE 16.1
Generally Accepted Air-Change Rates for Clean Rooms

FS Clean Room Class	ISO Equivalent Class	Air-Change Rate
1	ISO 3	360–540
10	ISO 4	300–540
100	ISO 5	240–480
1,000	ISO 6	150–240
10,000	ISO 7	60–90
100,000	ISO 8	5–48

Note: FS, Federal Standard; ISO, International Organization for Standardization.

security, durability, accessibility, cost-benefit, productivity, sustainability, functionality, and operational considerations."

The quantitatively measurable aspects of high-performance design are energy and water conservation. The baseline is defined by the governing codes and regulations. The most commonly adopted energy code is ASHRAE 90.1. This standard has a prescriptive methodology of minimum energy efficiency standards, which leads to an annual energy consumption per year in BTU/sf/year (watts/sm/year). Exceeding this value by a percentage, such as 10%, 20%, or 30%, is a good measure of a building's performance in energy efficiency. Similarly, a baseline for water consumption is mandated by the Energy Policy Act of 1992 and 2005.

INTEGRATED PRODUCT DESIGN

Product design plays an important part in sustainability in the pharmaceutical industry. Although the product is paramount, a sustainable design approach and an integrated design process are recommended. An integrated design starts with a design charrette, where everyone involved with the product is invited. The charrette provides an opportunity for all stakeholders to highlight the issues that are important to their role in the life of the product. This process illustrates the different aspects of the product to all parties involved; it eliminates the silos in which groups can sometimes operate. This integrated process improves the production of the product by reducing waste, energy, and especially costs.

SUSTAINABLE ASSESSMENT INITIATIVES FOR BUILDINGS AND PRODUCTS

There are several nonprofit organizations worldwide that promote sustainability in the design, construction, and operation of buildings. These organizations have developed tools that assist designers in tracking and monitoring building sustainability goals that are specific to a building and a site. The USGBC is best known for the development of the LEED rating system. The Green Building Initiative (GBI) is another nonprofit organization that has developed a web-based rating tool called Green Globes. The Energy Star program was developed by the U.S. Environmental Protection Agency (EPA); it rates commercial buildings for energy efficiency and provides a percentile ranking system compared to similar buildings in the United States. The Living Building Challenge offers performance-based standards and a certification program for renovations and new construction.

In addition to these, international organizations include BREEAM in the United Kingdom, European Union, and parts of the Middle East; Building Environmental Assessment Method (BEAM) in Hong Kong; Comprehensive Assessment System for Built Environment Efficiency (CASBEE) in Japan; Green Mark Scheme in Singapore; Green Star in South Africa; and Pearl Rating System in the United Arab Emirates.

SUSTAINABLE BUILDING SYSTEMS

Building systems play a key role in the sustainability of pharmaceutical companies, including manufacturing plants, cGMP facilities, research labs, and administrative office buildings. After a building is built, the systems that keep the building operational are the major users of energy and resources. Well-designed and energy-efficient systems use less energy and generate less waste. Conventional heating, ventilation, and air conditioning (HVAC) systems were designed when the cost of electricity was insignificant compared to the overall cost of doing business. Resources, such as water, were not in short supply. In the last two decades, however, things have changed. The cost of energy has increased dramatically, and developing countries are increasing their demands for limited resources, creating noticeable shortages. Additionally, global warming has been shown to be linked to greenhouse gases.

The HVAC and manufacturing industries have responded to the above changes with new technologies, advanced systems, new design approaches, and operational practices that reduce energy and resource consumption, eliminate waste, and optimize comfort. This change has happened so quickly that many professionals in the industry are just catching up. The old practices and customs are hard to change. The following section introduces several new technologies and advanced systems that are sustainable. This is an introduction to the fundamental concepts that allow designers to identify technologies that are adaptable to pharmaceutical facilities.

RENEWABLE ENERGY PRODUCTION

Solar

Solar energy is the most abundant and clean form of energy available on the planet. Its abundance is such that it could provide 44 quadrillion (4.4×10^{16}) W of power; it would take 44 million large electric power plants, each producing about 1 billion (1×10^9) W of power to equal the energy coming from the sun [2]. The solar energy coming from the sun far exceeds the energy used by humans on the earth. Solar power has zero pollution, no carbon footprint, and no emissions produced by its operation. Solar energy can be captured by thermal or photovoltaic (PV) methods. Thermal energy is captured in the form of heat (hot water) and PV energy in the form of electricity (PV panels). Energy payback estimates for rooftop PV systems are 1–4 years (Figure 16.1); this is the energy that goes into manufacturing PV panels. This should not be confused with the cost payback, which is the cost to install the PV panels at the site, paid back by the reduction in electricity bills. This payback can vary based on the location of the PV installation and the cost of electricity produced from conventional sources, such as coal and natural gas. The cost of electricity varies in different parts of the country. The U.S. Energy Information Administration publishes the electric rates for the different states and regions in the United States, which can vary from 10 to 30 cents per kilowatt-hour (kWh). In addition to this consumption charge, there is also a demand charge, which can vary in different parts of the country. While calculating the cost of electricity, both demand and consumption charges are necessary to compute the total cost.

Approximately 100 W/ft² of useful energy reaches the ground surface of the earth, of which about 15–20 W/ft² can be converted into electricity with PV panels. With solar thermal, about 60–70 W/ft² can be captured in heat. Thus, the efficiency of the thermal system is far higher than that of the PV system. When there is a steady need for hot water in a facility, thermal energy capture is more desirable than PV capture for the same real estate of the roof or ground area.

A PV watts calculator is a web-based tool developed by the National Renewable Energy Laboratory (NREL) and is popular for preliminary studies. It estimates the electricity production potential of a given site. The inputs to the calculator are site location (zip code) and the design of the PV system, such as the PV tilt and direction. The system database includes the cost of grid power for the site location selected. Using these values, a report with estimated monthly and annual electricity production and cost savings is produced. It is recommended that once the decision is made to proceed, a

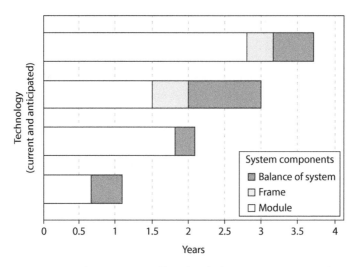

Reaping the environmental benefits of solar energy requires spending
energy to make the PV system. But as this graphic shows, the investment is small.
Assuming 30-year system life, PV systems will provide a net gain of 26–29 years
of pollution-free and greenhouse-gas-free electrical generation.

FIGURE 16.1   Energy payback for rooftop PV panels. (From National Renewable Energy Laboratory, PV FAQs, DOE/GO-102004-1847, U.S. Department of Energy, Office of Energy Efficiency and Renewable Energy, Washington, DC, January 2004. http://www.nrel.gov/docs/fy04osti/35489.pdf)

TABLE 16.2
Sample Output for a Site in New Jersey with a 100 kW System

Month	Solar Radiation (kWh/m²/day)	Alternating Current (AC) Energy (kWh)	Energy Value ($)
January	2.78	7,529	556
February	3.52	8,519	629
March	4.34	11,327	836
April	4.95	12,065	890
May	5.69	13,924	1,028
June	5.86	13,524	998
July	5.73	13,500	996
August	5.47	12,776	943
September	4.91	11,413	842
October	3.99	9,913	732
November	2.68	6,735	497
December	2.35	6,263	462
Annual	4.36	127,488	9,409

professional who is familiar with the system needs to be retained for design and financial analysis, including capital costs, running costs and savings, utility rebates, and grid connections.

The sample output for a site in central New Jersey with a 100 kW system is shown in Table 16.2. The area of roof or ground required for this system can vary based on the type of PV panel chosen. The PV panels can vary from 11 to 16 kW/sf (118 to 172 kW/sm). A 100 kW system will require 9090 to 6250 sf (844 to 580 sm).

Rebates are available from state, federal, and utility suppliers. The Database for State Incentives for Renewables and Efficiency (DSIRE), at http://www.dsireusa.org, is a single source for all available incentives in the United States. The DSIRE is operated by the North Carolina Solar Center at North Carolina State University with support from the Interstate Renewable Energy Council.

Wind Energy

Wind resources vary from state to state based on wind patterns and topography. Approximately 4% of the total power in the United States comes from wind energy [4]. Wind energy resources are available from the NREL. Wind power is available in both utility (large) scale and building (small) scale. Small-scale wind turbines are generally adapted for distributed generation. Distributed renewable energy systems, such as small wind turbines, are combined to work in synchronization with utility power. When there is no demand in the building for the power generated from wind, it is fed into the utility grid for wider distribution.

A wind energy resource assessment particular to the site is the first step toward determining the feasibility of wind power. Wind mapping can be done with maps developed by the National Wind Technology Center (NWTC). Maps are available for all states in the United States and at selected international locations (Figure 16.2).

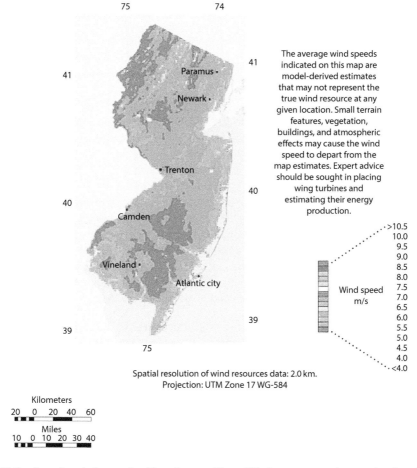

FIGURE 16.2 Sample wind map for New Jersey. (From Wind resource estimates developed by AWS Truepower, LLC. http://www.awstruepower.com. Map developed by NREL.)

To understand the economics of a small wind electric system and decide whether wind energy will work for a particular site, estimates of the following are required:

- Capital cost of turbines, which includes the design cost and installation cost of the turbine and the utility electrical connections.
- Electrical power generated, which is measured in kilowatt-hours (kWh) of power and is offset by costs from the utility company.
- The power (kWh) generated during a building's low-demand times, such as nights and weekends.
- Buyback paid by the utility companies for excess power generated during nights and weekends.
- Building power load profile, which is a reasonably accurate load profile of the building's electrical demand and consumption on an hourly basis for 365 days of the year.
- Wind at the site, which can be measured by software tools that can estimate the annual power generated.
- Cash-flow analysis, which is based on interest on capital, financing, and taxes. A yearly cash-flow profile for the life of the turbines has to be calculated.

Geothermal Heat Pumps

Just a few feet below the ground surface, the temperature of the earth is almost a constant 55°F (12.8°C). In winter, when the outside temperatures are below freezing, there is heat just a few feet below the ground. In summer, when the temperatures are at 90°F (32.2°C), there are cool surfaces just a few feet below the ground. Geothermal energy systems use this resource. Geothermal energy is generally categorized as high, medium, and low, based on the temperature. The constant 55°F (12.8°C) is the lowest form of energy and is abundantly available over almost the entire ground surface of the earth. The higher forms of energy are available at the tectonic plate's active region. A geothermal map of the United States is shown in Figure 16.3.

Geothermal energy is available in high grade (i.e., temperatures higher than 212°F [100°C]), medium grade (i.e., temperatures less than 212°F [100°C]), and low grade (i.e., temperatures of about 55°F [12.8°C]). While the most common form of geothermal energy available is low grade, there are areas where medium and high grades are available. If high-grade heat is available, it can be used to generate electricity; space heating can be accomplished with medium-grade heat. A preliminary investigation of available geothermal energy should be done for the site to determine its feasibility.

A geothermal heat pump is the most common application for areas with low-grade heat. Geothermal heat pumps are basic air conditioners with a reversing valve that makes them heaters in winter. Heat pumps are more efficient than regular air conditioners: (1) The energy required for air conditioning is reduced when the temperature it has to discharge is lower, for example, the 55°F (12.8°C) earth temperature rather than the 95°F (35°C) temperature of summer air. (2) In winter, the warmth of the earth at 55°F (12.8°C) is used to heat the outdoor air from its original temperature, which could be 10°F (−12.2°C). Low-grade heat can be extracted by coupling with the earth in different ways:

1. *Vertical ground loop system.* Wells 100–400 ft deep are drilled in the ground with pipes connected at the bottom with a U-bend to form a loop. The bore is filled with a grout to provide good thermal conductivity between the earth and the pipe. As water flows through the pipes, it gains or loses heat in either the air conditioning or heating process. As a rule of thumb, vertical wells are located 15 ft (4.6 m) on center, or about every 225 ft² (21 m²). Generally, each 200 ft (61 m) of depth produces 1 ton, so a 400 ft (122 m) deep well produces 2 tons. This is a closed-loop piping system, and there is no ground contamination. Parking lots and green lawns are good vertical ground loop locations. The life expectancy of a ground well is generally about 40–50 years.
2. *Horizontal ground loop system.* This system has polyethylene pipes buried in shallow trenches 6 ft (1.8 m) deep. This is most suitable and cost-effective for small projects

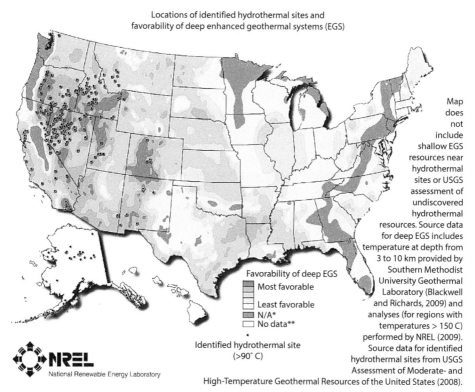

Locations of identified hydrothermal sites and
favorability of deep enhanced geothermal systems (EGS)

Map does not include shallow EGS resources near hydrothermal sites or USGS assessment of undiscovered hydrothermal resources. Source data for deep EGS includes temperature at depth from 3 to 10 km provided by Southern Methodist University Geothermal Laboratory (Blackwell and Richards, 2009) and analyses (for regions with temperatures > 150 C) performed by NREL (2009). Source data for identified hydrothermal sites from USGS Assessment of Moderate- and High-Temperature Geothermal Resources of the United States (2008).

Favorability of deep EGS
Most favorable
Least favorable
N/A*
No data**

Identified hydrothermal site
(>90° C)

NREL
National Renewable Energy Laboratory

*"N/A" regions have temperatures less than 150°C at 10 km depth and were not assessed for deep EGS potential.
**Temperature at depth data for deep EGS in Alaska and Hawaii not available.

FIGURE 16.3 Geothermal map of the United States. (From NREL. Available at http://www.nrel.gov/gis/images/geothermal_resource2009-final.jpg)

with low capacities. Generally, a 400–600 ft (122–182 m) tube loop is required for each ton of air conditioning. The capacity can vary based on the soil conductivity. This is a closed-loop piping system, and there is no ground contamination.

3. *Pond or lake loop system.* This system extracts heat from water in ponds and lakes near the site. The water temperature at the bottom of the pond or lake is cooler than the ambient air in summer and warmer than the ambient air in winter. Coils of polyethylene piping are laid at the bottom of the pond or lake. The system is closed, so there is no cross-contamination of water from the pipes to the water in the pond or lake.

4. *Well water system.* Where a large quantity of water is available in a well, river, lake, aquifer, or sea, a well water system may be used. EPA, state, and federal regulations have to be followed. This is an open-loop system, unlike the three systems described above. Generally, a heat exchanger is added to prevent the water from the well from mixing with the water from the heat pumps. The heat exchanger has multiple benefits: well water is discharged back just as it was taken in, without any additives, which also increases the longevity of the heat pumps and the associated piping and pumping system. The only effect on the well water is that it is discharged at a higher temperature than when it was taken in.

EFFICIENT HVAC SYSTEMS

The HVAC systems are one of the most energy-consuming systems in a building. Only process loads and manufacturing assembly power consumption exceed HVAC energy use. There are several new advanced technologies that are energy efficient, reduce operating costs, and improve indoor air quality and comfort. These technologies should be introduced when the engineering design team is selected, making sure that the engineers have the requisite knowledge and experience. Some of the technologies worth considering are cogeneration, thermal storage, chilled beams, and radiant cooling. These systems are briefly introduced in the sections below. None of these systems have universal adaptability, but each adapts well to certain applications. The design team must look into the benefits of each of these unique systems to see if they apply to their building.

While the above-mentioned systems offer overall system efficiency, the efficiencies of selected equipment should not be overlooked. Equipment efficiencies are mandated by the energy codes; however, the energy codes generally lag behind the latest developments in equipment. Additionally, the project locale (state or country) may not have adopted the latest energy codes. The design team's responsibility is to comply with the codes, and therefore they must research the equipment efficiency of various manufacturers.

COGENERATION

Cogeneration is a process in which fossil fuel–based electrical power is generated, and waste heat is recovered for beneficial purposes. Most fossil fuel–based electrical generators are only 40% efficient. Approximately 60% of the fossil fuel energy is wasted in the form of heat vented through the stack. Cogeneration recovers this heat and uses it for space heating, process heat, and air conditioning, using absorption chillers (Figures 16.4 and 16.5).

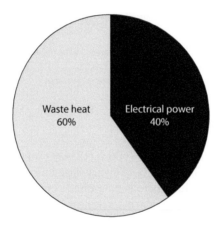

FIGURE 16.4   Conventional power generation.

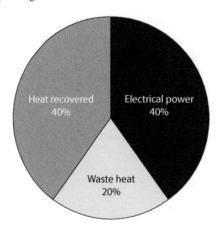

FIGURE 16.5   Cogeneration.

The benefits of cogeneration are high fuel efficiency, low emissions, distributed generation, low distribution losses, low distribution infrastructure and investment, fuel cost savings, high reliability, and resilience.

A reciprocating engine or gas turbine is the most common type of cogeneration used in buildings (Figure 16.6). Electricity is generated by burning a fossil fuel, such as natural gas or diesel. A heat recovery unit is used to generate hot water or steam. In reciprocating engines, both hot water from the engine jacket and steam from the exhaust stack are generated. In gas turbines, the waste gases are hot enough to generate steam.

Cogeneration equipment can vary based on the size of the system and site-specific needs. Cogeneration equipment is available in a variety of sizes. The most common cogeneration systems used in commercial buildings are up to 50 kW fuel cells, 50–250 kW microturbines, 250–4,000 kW reciprocating engines, and 2,000 kW and larger gas and steam turbines. The installed cost of cogeneration is shown in Table 16.3.

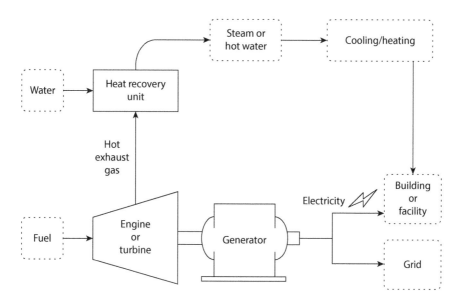

FIGURE 16.6 Engine or gas turbine cogeneration. (From EPA. Available at http://www.epa.gov/chp/basic/index.html)

TABLE 16.3
Installed Cost of Cogeneration

Technology	Installed Cost, $/kW
Reciprocating engine	1,500–2,900
Gas turbine	1,200–3,300
Microturbine	2,500–4,300
Fuel cell	5,000–6,500

Source: U.S. Environmental Protection Agency, Comparison of Combined Heat and Power (CHP) Technology Sizing, Cost, and Performance Parameters, Catalog of CHP Technologies, U.S. Environmental Protection Agency, Washington, DC.

A cogeneration feasibility study is recommended to evaluate the potential for application. It is important to establish and identify the following parameters to get good results:

- Electrical power, space heat, process heat, and air conditioning demand on an hour-by-hour basis for 365 days
- Availability of a reliable source of fuel, such as natural gas
- Cost of fuel and projected cost increases
- Cost of electricity and projected growth
- Incentives and rebates available from state, federal, and utility companies
- First cost of the plant from a contractor familiar with the technology
- Operations and maintenance costs
- Yearly cash flow
- Payback and life cycle costs (LCC)
- Environmental benefits and carbon footprint reduction
- Permit requirements from the state Department of Environmental Protection (DEP)

THERMAL STORAGE

Thermal energy storage is one of the earliest ways to achieve thermal comfort. Early civilizations adopted thermal energy storage from the diurnal (daily) change in temperature at a given location. Temperature variation is one of the most prominent thermal parameters. Diurnal patterns are absorbed in almost all locations, but the most prominent ones are in desert climates, where the nights are cold and days are warm. In building design and engineering systems, there are two types of thermal energy storage systems: building designs that use diurnal patterns and building engineering systems that use the lower cost of electricity at night to produce refrigeration to be used during the day.

The former is truly a renewable or fossil fuel–free energy, while the latter uses fossil fuel. The latter in some applications may use more energy; however, there are some economic benefits and, in some cases, environmental benefits of thermal energy storage. The benefits of chilled water storage (or ice storage) are the primary focus of this discussion. Figure 16.7 shows the times when chilled water (or ice) is produced and the times when the chilled water (or ice) is used.

The most common thermal energy storage in buildings is chilled water (or ice) storage (Figure 16.8). Ice storage plants require less storage volume, but the chillers have to produce ice, which requires more refrigeration or more energy in kilowatts per ton. This system also requires use of glycol in the pipes to avoid freezing. The chilled water storage tanks are generally large, but they

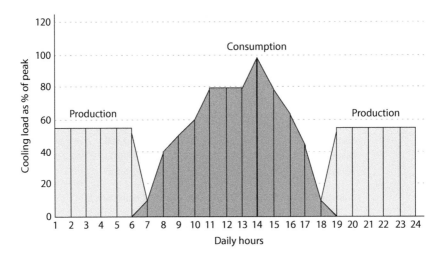

FIGURE 16.7   Chilled water production and consumption over 24 h.

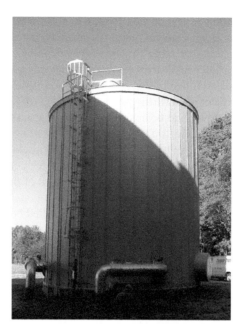

FIGURE 16.8 Chilled water storage tanks at Princeton University, Princeton, New Jersey.

can use regular standard chillers, and water can be used in pipes without the use of glycol. The standard water chillers use less energy (kW/ton) than the ice-making chillers. The economics depends on the differential costs of electricity during day and night. These rates can vary from location to location and among utility companies. A good analysis includes the prediction of energy use and consumption, utility cost structure, available rebates, sound engineering analysis, and simulation of a system close to actual operation.

There are several important benefits of chilled water (or ice) storage systems:

- The cost of electricity is lower at night, so there is cost savings in using energy at night. Electricity produced during peak demand hours is generally the most expensive power.
- The total capacity of the equipment installed can be less than the peak demand (varies by case).
- Using electricity at night reduces the demand for large infrastructure necessary for electric power plants and distributions.
- The nighttime electricity power generation is generally from baseload plants, such as hydro and nuclear, which have lower carbon emissions.
- Nighttime ambient temperatures are lower (due to diurnal effects), which helps chillers operate more efficiently, lowering energy consumption (kW/ton).

CHILLED BEAMS

Chilled beams are becoming popular in the United States with applications in commercial buildings, schools, and science and laboratory buildings. Pharmaceutical manufacturing and buildings that comply with cGMPs in the ancillary spaces can contribute to overall energy reduction and thermal comfort improvement of the facility. Chilled beams were first introduced in Europe. The technology is now produced in the United States, and many contractors have become adept at installation. Chilled beams work on the same principle as induction units, which were popular in the United States in the 1960s and 1970s. Induction units were installed along the perimeter of buildings. Chilled beams are installed in the ceiling. There are two types of chilled beams: active and passive. Active chilled beams are similar to induction units; they work using primary air to induce airflow through a cooling or heating coil. In most applications, except at perimeter locations, a cooling coil is more common. As a rule of thumb, the primary air is one-third and the secondary air is two-thirds of the total; thus, the same amount of water can be chilled with one-third the size of the central system. All chilled beams are water cooling devices and require chilled or hot water connections to the coils. Passive chilled beams do not have induced airflow around the coil. Natural convection over the coil produces airflow (Figure 16.9).

In pharmaceutical buildings, chilled beams can be used in spaces where there is high internal heat gain due to equipment and where 100% outside air is not required. With chilled beams, there is lower energy consumption, and a reduction in fan energy to circulate large quantities of air from central fan systems (large central fans are generally only about 65% efficient), and they can be used in high-ceiling spaces with little ductwork (only about one-third of the ductwork required for conventional variable-air-volume [VAV] systems).

A separate chilled water distribution loop is required for chilled beams, which use chilled water at a higher temperature than conventional 45°F (7.2°C). Chilled water at 55°F–60°F (12.8°C–15.6°C) is used for chilled beams. In some applications, water leaving the air handling unit (AHU) cooling coils can be used.

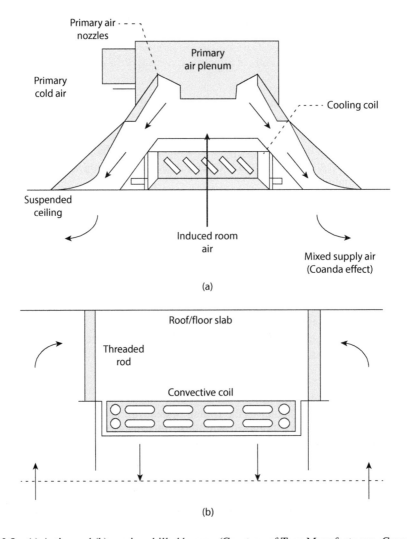

FIGURE 16.9 (a) Active and (b) passive chilled beams. (Courtesy of Taco Manufacturers, Cranston, RI.)

RADIANT COOLING

While radiant heating floors have been used for many years, HVAC radiant cooling floors have been only recently introduced. While radiant cooling panels have been used in hospitals, laboratories, and commercial offices, radiant floors have performed well in some high-profile projects. Radiant cooling has to be carefully analyzed for the right application in pharmaceutical buildings. In spaces where there is a high equipment load and solar load, and the need for a high air-change rate is not required, radiant cooling is a suitable option. The benefits of radiant cooling are (1) energy efficiency, (2) high thermal comfort, (3) small duct systems, (4) high ceiling heights, and (5) small central fan systems.

In a radiant cooling system, chilled water is supplied to the radiant cooling device surface. With radiant cooling systems, large central AHUs can be reduced in size, limited to ventilation rates or minimum air-change rates and latent (removal of moisture from space) cooling. Radiant cooling works on the fundamental physics principle of blackbody radiation, where heat transfer occurs without a medium from a higher-temperature surface to a lower-temperature surface. It is ideal for rooms with equipment and processes that have high-temperature surfaces. In these applications, radiant cooling alone may not be sufficient, but a combination of radiant cooling and a conventional system will be cost-effective and energy efficient. In spaces where there is high solar radiation on the floor due to large skylights, radiant floors are ideal. In a radiant cooling system, heat is transferred directly from the source to the chilled water without the intermediate medium of air, which requires fans for circulation. Fans at best are 65% efficient, and a reduction in their size helps reduce energy and increase efficiency.

There are three different types of radiant cooling technologies:

Radiant panels. These panels are generally ceiling mounted and are typically 2 × 2 ft (600 × 600 mm). The panel construction is generally aluminum, with copper tubes embedded on the back surface of the panel.

Radiant wall and ceiling systems. In radiant wall and ceiling systems, capillary tubes that carry water are embedded in plaster walls and ceilings.

Radiant floors. These floors are the second most common form of radiant cooling after radiant panels. In radiant floors, PEX tubing is used for the underfloor finish in a layer of concrete fill. This adds about 1.5 in. (38 mm) to the floor height. The most common application for radiant floors is in large public spaces (i.e., cafeterias or atriums).

The chilled water in a radiant cooling system has to be above the dew point and is generally in the 60°F–65°F (15.5°C–18.3°C) range. Most chilled water applications use lower temperature chilled water. In almost all radiant cooling systems, a separate loop of higher-temperature chilled water is required. A plate and frame heat exchanger with temperature control valves and circulating pumps are required to form a loop. The space dew point temperature sensor controls the heat exchanger to maintain loop water temperature above the dew point to avoid condensation on the radiant surfaces, which is highly undesirable. Most radiant cooling systems are dual systems with cooling in summer and heating in winter (Figure 16.10).

ENERGY MODELING AND LCC AND ASSESSMENT

ENERGY MODELING

Energy modeling is a computer-based tool used to simulate the building operations of all energy-consuming equipment, such as chillers, boilers, pumps, fans, lighting, plug power, process power, and manufacturing or air handling equipment on an hour-by-hour, day-by-day, week-by-week, and month-by-month basis for 365 days and 8,760 h of the year. The results equal the annual energy

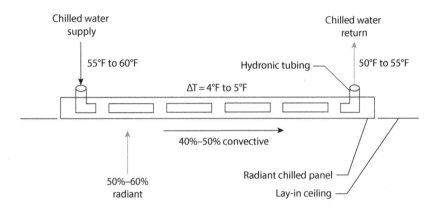

FIGURE 16.10 Radiant cooling panels. (Courtesy of Taco Manufacturers, Cranston, RI.)

use, which is reported in kBTU/sf/year (kW/sm/year) and can be converted to calculate costs. This energy modeling tool allows architects and engineers to assess their designs before they are built. Simple building elements, such as skylights in a space, can be modeled for reduction in lighting energy. Complex building systems, such as radiant cooling, thermal storage, or cogeneration, can also be accurately modeled. This is a very powerful tool to evaluate buildings. The LEED rating system of the USGBC uses energy modeling to measure the energy use of the building and compare it to the baseline (the code minimum). Though counterintuitive, most engineers and architects do not include energy modeling as part of their basic services. It is essential for the facilities team to make sure that energy modeling is included in the fee and this tool is used to evaluate the building designs.

Life Cycle Cost

LCC is an important tool in establishing the suitability and providing a cash-flow model to determine the cost-effectiveness of sustainable technologies and energy conservation measures. The LCC model is used where the annual costs of energy and operations are easily measurable and quantifiable at the building site. Examples of these are electricity, natural gas, and diesel. The LCC accounts for the present cost, recurring costs, life of the products, replacement costs, economic factors, cost of capital, and interest rates. Analysis of LCC is generally used for comparing multiple alternate systems; it provides a present value of all the costs for the life of the system. The life of the system has to be carefully chosen, as it can vary for other systems being evaluated as alternates. Similarly, replacement costs have to be carefully evaluated, estimated, and input into the system.

The LCC analysis is performed in very early phases of the design, generally in the preschematics phase of the project. This presents some unique challenges, as a highly skilled and experienced design team, facilities operations team, and preconstruction team are required. The design team has to conceptualize the design elements accurately so that the preconstruction team can estimate accurate construction costs. The facilities operations team and design team have to estimate the recurring costs, replacement costs, and life of the system accurately. Accurately predicting the cost of utilities in the future for the life of the system is important; therefore, an expert in this field may have to be consulted. The life of the system is generally evaluated for 20–35 years. It is important to note that the life of different systems varies, and accurate replacement costs have to be estimated. Accurate financial information is also required, such as interest rates, cost of capital, and rate of return on capital. It is highly recommended to get the financial team, including the chief financial officer, involved in the LCC analysis.

LIFE CYCLE ASSESSMENT

For products whose annual costs and energy consumption are not easily measurable and quantifiable at the site, the life cycle assessment (LCA) tool is used. Examples of these products are building materials, such as concrete, steel, aluminum, and sheetrock. The LCA is defined [4] as a technique to assess the environmental aspects and potential impacts associated with a product, process, or service by compiling an inventory of relevant energy and material inputs and environmental releases, evaluating their potential environmental impact, and interpreting the results to help make an informed decision [5].

The cradle-to-grave approach is used in LCA for assessing all systems and materials. It starts with raw materials and ends with the final disposal of the material or the finished product, including side streams of raw material waste or diversion. Every step in the life of the product is evaluated. The International Organization for Standardization (ISO) standard for LCA is ISO 14040. The LCA can assist in the material and product selection process by evaluating the impact on the environment of each material. Two competing products or materials can be differentiated after performing an LCA.

ABOUT THE AUTHOR

Asif Syed's 30 years of engineering practice includes large, high-profile projects in the United States, Asia, Europe, Middle East, and South America. His experience includes new and advanced technologies for the LEED gold-rated Hearst Building. Syed has extensive laboratory and pharmaceutical project experience; his major projects include Procter & Gamble, Jansen Pharmaceutical, Stony Brook Graduate Chemistry Building, and Saudi Arabian Food and Drug Authority Buildings. In the renovation of the Biltmore Theater, Syed introduced underfloor air distribution and also designed the mechanical, electrical, and plumbing systems for Zankel Hall at Carnegie Hall and the Newseum in Washington, DC. Syed's current projects include a carbon footprint reduction at St. John's University, a high-performance data center for Princeton University, a LEED mixed-use complex in India, net-zero buildings for the New York School Authority and Stony Brook environmental center, and the LEED gold building for Hilton Realty. He has collaborated with many major architectural firms in the United States. Syed did research at the Building Engineering and Architectural Research Center. He authored a book entitled *Advanced Building Technologies for Sustainability* (John Wiley, New York). Syed is responsible for the design and analysis of mechanical systems, including advanced building technologies, net-zero buildings, energy analysis, life cycle costs, cost-effective energy-saving strategies, and sustainable designs. Syed's high-profile experience on large-scale projects contributes high-value-added expertise from programming to occupancy. Syed is currently at STE Engineers, where he is the founding partner; his previous positions include senior vice president at Flack + Kurtz Consulting Engineers (until 2003) and partner at AKF Engineers (until 2012).

REFERENCES

1. Jaisinghani R, Energy-Efficient, Low-Operating Cost, Cleanroom Airflow Design, presented at the 2003 Conference of the Institute of Environmental Sciences and Technology.
2. National Aeronautics and Space Administration, The Balance of Power in the Earth-Sun System, National Aeronautics and Space Administration, Washington, DC, 2005, https://www.nasa.gov/pdf/135642main_balance_trifold21.pdf.
3. National Renewable Energy Laboratory, PV FAQs, DOE/GO-102004-1847, U.S. Department of Energy, Office of Energy Efficiency and Renewable Energy, Washington, DC, January 2004, http://www.nrel.gov/docs/fy04osti/35489.pdf.
4. American Wind Association, Get the Facts, American Wind Association, Washington, DC, http://www.awea.org/Resources/Content.aspx?ItemNumber=900&navItemNumber=587.
5. Environmental Protection Agency, Life Cycle Assessment (LCA), Risk Management Sustainable Technology, Environmental Protection Agency, Washington, DC, http://www.epa.gov/nrmrl/std/lca/lca.html#define.

17 QA/QC Laboratories and Related Support Spaces

Cassidy Hobbs, AIA

CONTENTS

INTRODUCTION

In pharmaceutical manufacturing facilities, support laboratories play the crucial role of testing the product to verify its quality, safety, and stability at each stage of the manufacturing process, packaging, and product release. These labs are referred to as quality assurance (QA) and quality control (QC) laboratories and exist to support the manufacturing operations of the facility. The design of QA/QC laboratories requires an understanding of the facility; the processes and equipment used in the lab; the hazardous materials present; the heating, ventilation, and air conditioning (HVAC) systems used; and other requirements. Consideration must be given to the safety and protection of lab personnel and the product. Despite their small size relative to the facility at large, QA/QC laboratories are necessary to the operation of the facility, and a thorough understanding of good design practices is necessary to guarantee the efficiency and viability of the facility.

This chapter breaks down the process of programming and designing pharmaceutical support labs and related spaces, such as glass washrooms, sample storage, and stability storage, from initial information gathering through completion of the facility. It explores the key issues in this process for both new facilities and renovations of existing facilities and gives an overview of the components of a lab and the role of QA/QC labs in pharmaceutical manufacturing facilities.

EXECUTIVE SUMMARY

According to the Good Practice Guide *Quality Laboratory Facilities*, from the International Society of Pharmaceutical Engineering (ISPE), "the purpose of the quality laboratory is to support the execution of testing that assures the manufactured products meet the identity, strength, purity, efficacy, and safety as specified in the approved regulatory file" [1]. Testing verifies that no contamination or other problem has occurred in the manufacturing process.

The functions of QA/QC laboratories vary; they are general testing laboratories, sterility testing (microbiology) laboratories, biocontainment laboratories, potent compound laboratories, or other specialty laboratories, such as cold laboratories or laboratories that deal with radioactive substances. General testing laboratories are the most common type of QA/QC laboratory. Microbiology labs test for the presence of microorganisms in sterile products and may also test air and water quality for the facility, so maintaining a sterile, cleanable environment is particularly important. Biocontainment laboratories test biohazardous materials and are rated by the biohazard safety levels of the biological materials they contain, as defined by the National Institutes of Health (NIH) and the Centers for Disease Control and Prevention (CDC). Most QA/QC laboratories can be categorized as either general testing labs or microbiology labs, which may have biocontainment requirements.

The considerations necessary for the design of support labs vary slightly based on the laboratory type, but the key concepts and principles remain the same. In each lab, it is important to understand the necessary equipment and preparation space to help determine the required linear feet of bench space that is needed. Establishing a laboratory module can help to organize the plan. Lab flexibility, the location of offices or write-up space, compliance, and HVAC issues also influence the design of the lab. Recently, the concepts of lean labs, lab culture, and sustainability have grown in popularity, and the owners' attitude toward these will impact the design process.

QA/QC LABS

LABORATORY PLANNING PROCESS

The process of laboratory design follows the path diagrammed in Figure 17.1, from programming through construction and then commissioning. This section will focus on the programming and schematic design phases, as that is when the major decisions relating to lab planning are made.

Laboratory planning can be organized into three stages: problem seeking, analysis, and problem solving (Figure 17.2). In the broadest sense, problem seeking is the task of gathering and organizing

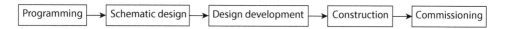

FIGURE 17.1 Design and construction process.

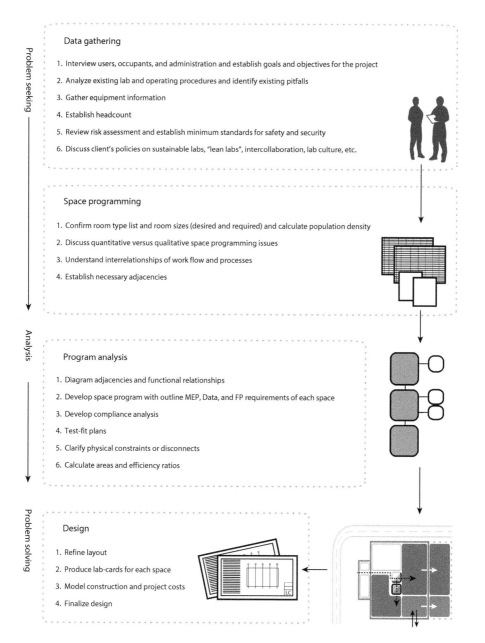

FIGURE 17.2 Problem seeking, analysis, and problem solving.

information, analysis is processing that information, and problem solving is the application of the analysis to get a result. When completed, this is compiled in the basis of design (BOD), a report completed at the end of the schematic design phase that includes all of the information collected, a program of the rooms required, diagrammatic plans laying out the spaces and their relationships, and a lab card for each space. This process applies to all labs, not just QA/QC labs, but in support labs, an understanding of the overall facility is especially important. The QA/QC laboratories may be separate from the main manufacturing areas or may be located near the stage of manufacturing where the tests take place. A single facility may have multiple QA/QC laboratories, depending on the tests that are required.

Problem Seeking

The problem-seeking phase has two parts: data gathering and space programming. Data gathering begins with interviews of lab personnel and the administration to develop goals and objectives for the project and gather information. This process often includes a preinterview survey for the users and a tour of existing facilities if the client has them. It is necessary for the designer to help the users complete the survey, as they may not know their exact needs. The designer may also have to act as referee between conflicting desires of the lab personnel (scientists and technicians) and the facility management or owners. It is also necessary to coordinate with the site's security staff, information technology (IT), and other facility personnel so that facility-wide systems can be integrated.

Data Gathering

The following topics should be covered during the data gathering phase.

Existing Operating Procedures and Facilities

In renovation projects or projects for clients with other facilities, an analysis of the existing facility can provide a wealth of information on the client's needs and existing operating procedures. The analysis can help determine the required amounts of storage and bench space and can help the designer replicate what works well and avoid recreating any existing issues. It is especially important in renovation projects, as there are often missed opportunities of which the client is unaware. Space and resources are often underutilized (e.g., bench space used to store obsolete equipment), and identifying these inefficiencies will allow them to be corrected in a renovation. It is very important for the designer to note how existing hoods are used, and whether storage space is utilized.

The goals of the QA/QC lab can be accomplished through a combination of standard operating procedures (SOPs) and physical design. The methods used by lab personnel when performing tests are defined by SOPs, which can be used to prevent opportunities for contamination of samples; however, it is preferable to prevent problems through the physical design of the lab, rather than SOPs, whenever possible. For example, while waste could be moved through another part of the lab during off-hours in sealed containers, a better solution would be to provide an alternate route directly out of the lab. Various options must be explored, and the SOPs and lab design must work hand in hand. SOPs are laid out in an operations manual for each laboratory, and it is important that laboratory personnel are familiar with the hazards they may encounter in the lab and the SOPs that are in place to protect them and the samples.

Equipment

During the data gathering phase, the design team will begin to identify the types of equipment to be used and the general equipment requirements for space, power, and services. Ultimately, an equipment list will be developed that lists all equipment, along with sizes, services required, electrical requirements, backup power requirements, and in the case of renovations, existing locations and site identification numbers if available. In a renovation, the equipment may be existing or new and may have limits on its relocation. For example, relocating an autoclave or glass washer might necessitate relocating drains in the existing slab, which would unnecessarily add cost to the project. For a new facility, the equipment list is developed by the users and may be modified as the design progresses. Some clients will be able to provide this list, while others will need time and assistance with its development. In a renovation project, this stage may include a survey of the existing equipment. It is important to create the equipment list early in the project, as it will have a large impact on the overall design and schedule. Many pieces of equipment have plumbing or exhaust requirements that must be coordinated with the plumbing engineers (e.g., water sources or drains) and HVAC designers (e.g., exhaust systems). Additionally, many pieces have long lead times, and it is important to make sure they are ordered early enough to arrive in time for installation.

Although they vary by product, general testing laboratories typically contain high-performance liquid chromatography (HPLC) equipment, preparation space (in a fume hood) for mobile phase mixtures for the HPLCs, gas chromatography (GC) equipment, hoods for handling solvents and reagents, and incubators, freezers, and refrigerators for storage. A typical microbiology laboratory might consist of a media prep space with refrigerators, hoods for sampling, and incubators. Table 17.1 shows an example preliminary equipment list. As the project progresses, additional information, such as power requirements and services, is added, and equipment selections are finalized.

1. *Hoods:* There are many types of hoods used in QA/QC laboratories, and often, it is up to the designer to work with laboratory personnel to determine the appropriate type. Often, biosafety cabinets (BSCs), fume hoods, and laminar flow hoods are all referred to as hoods by laboratory personnel, but their uses are very different. It is important to determine hood requirements early in the design process so they are included in the HVAC design.
   - Fume hoods: Fume hoods are used for containment of chemical or biological hazards through negative airflow, which may be exhausted to the outside, connected to the HVAC system, or filtered and returned to the lab.
   - Laminar flow hoods: Laminar flow hoods are used to prevent contamination of samples. High-efficiency particulate air (HEPA) filters remove particulates from the air that is blown over a surface and out into the lab to keep the surface in the hood sterile. Laminar flow hoods come in both vertical and horizontal varieties.
   - Biosafety cabinets: Biosafety cabinets are used to both contain and protect biological materials. They are rated by classification, as shown in Table 17.2.
2. *Incubators:* Incubators are used to store materials at a constant temperature. They are often required to be on emergency power, along with the lab's refrigerators and freezers.

TABLE 17.1
Example Equipment List

		Equipment Schedule		
Keynote	Equipment ID	Manufacturer	Dimensions	Comments
1	3887	Labconco	4 ft 6 in. wide × 36 in. deep	4 ft fume hood
2	3986	TBD	TBD	Incubator
3	3124	Existing	3 ft wide × 3 ft deep × 32 in. high	Incubator—existing
4	3657	VWR	3 ft wide × 3 ft deep × 32 in. high	Incubator
5	3888	TBD	3 ft wide × 3 ft deep × 6 ft high	Refrigerator
6	3754	TBD	3 ft wide × 3 ft deep ×	Refrigerator

Note: TBD, to be determined.

TABLE 17.2
Classification of Biosafety Cabinets

Classification	Biosafety Level	Application
Class I	1, 2, 3	Low to moderate risk
Class II	1, 2, 3	Low to moderate risk
Class III	4	High-risk biological agent

Note: Biosafety levels are discussed later in the chapter.

3. *Gas chromatography units:* GC units are used for separating components of a mixture that can be vaporized. They are deployed on benches and often require a point exhaust at each unit. Exhaust requirements should be determined early in the design process so they can be included in the HVAC design.

4. *High-performance liquid chromatography:* HPLC is a common component of general testing laboratories and is used to separate and identify components in a mixture by pumping the mixture through a column of absorbent material (Figure 17.3). HPLC units are often deployed on benchtops or on rack systems in groups of two to four HPLCs, which are, in turn, associated with a computer workstation where results are received. Ideally, benches or racks for HPLC are lower than the standard 36 in. bench height to allow easy access to the top of the HPLC. Software systems such as Empower allow the workstations to be placed outside of the lab, so that lab personnel can work in greater comfort and safety. This has a cost-saving benefit, since lab space can be reduced and replaced by office space, which is less costly.

5. *Waste:* There are several waste lines attached to each HPLC unit that drain by gravity to a carboy that is often placed in a kneehole or in casework below the bench. This creates a chance for the lines to be knocked out of the carboys, which can lead to spills and can be corrected with a central waste collection system. Ideally, the waste runs to a line in a chase in the center of the bench to a larger carboy in a cabinet at the end, which must be equipped with spill containment and an alarm to prevent overflow if it is not emptied on time. The waste is fed by gravity through small tubing from each section of each HPLC unit to a larger tube, which runs to a drum at the end of each bench. This system prevents lab personnel from knocking the tubing out of the carboys as they walk by. It also facilitates easy waste disposal.

6. *Validation:* Major equipment used in QA/QC laboratories, along with support equipment such as glass washers, autoclaves, and stability chambers, must be validated before use to ensure that they perform accurately. The validation process takes time after installation and must be factored into the schedule. If a piece of equipment does not pass, additional time may need to be spent diagnosing the problem, and in the worst case, new equipment or parts may need to be ordered. See Chapter 7 for further discussion.

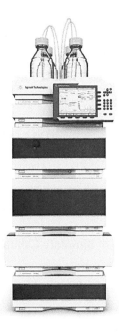

FIGURE 17.3   High-performance liquid chromatography unit. (Photo courtesy of Agilent Technologies, Inc., Santa Clara, CA.)

Risk Assessment

The risk assessment is developed during the problem-seeking phase. Risk assessments are described in more detail in Chapter 7.

Personnel

A headcount of laboratory personnel is needed, along with requirements for write-up space either inside or outside the lab. Locating desks outside the lab is preferable for both safety and convenience; it allows lab personnel to eat at their desks and to work without wearing their lab coats or other protective gear, which results in a more comfortable work environment.

Lab Culture

The interview is also a time to discuss the client's policies on sustainable labs, lean labs, and lab culture. The information gleaned from the interview has an impact on the approach to the lab layout, support spaces, materials, and equipment chosen. Sustainability and lean labs will be discussed later in this chapter.

Space Programming

After the completion of the data gathering phase, space programming can begin.

Confirm Room-Type List and Room Sizes

At this stage, a list of the required rooms and their approximate sizes is compiled, so that the requirements of each space can be explored. The total personnel per net square foot (NSF), which can then be used to generate an estimate for the gross square footage (GSF) of the lab, can be calculated; this can then be used to create an initial cost estimate based on cost per square foot. The size of the lab per person can also be calculated based on the equivalent linear feet (ELF) of bench space required for each person.

Adjacencies and Interrelationships of Workflow and Processes

Before development of a plan can begin, it is necessary to develop the necessary adjacencies between rooms, which are determined by the flow of people and materials, gowning requirements, and shared service spaces. These relationships can be documented with bubble diagrams (Figure 17.4). Components of the laboratory should be laid out when possible to allow for a unidirectional flow of materials. Understanding the flow of materials, personnel, equipment, and waste and the relationships between them is necessary to minimize opportunities for contamination.

Analysis

Diagram Adjacencies and Functional Relationships

During the analysis phase, the adjacencies and flows are diagrammed in a schematic plan (Figure 17.5). In this plan diagram, the program from Figure 17.4 is inserted behind an existing glass wash suite. Note that the autoclave waste must be removed through the glass wash suite, which will necessitate SOPs requiring the waste be moved at night and in sealed containers. SOPs are discussed later in this chapter.

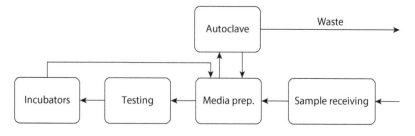

FIGURE 17.4 Bubble diagram showing relationships between spaces.

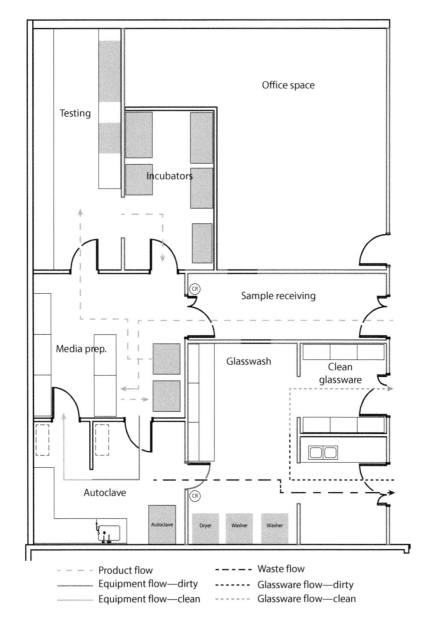

FIGURE 17.5 Schematic plan.

Space Program

The room-type list developed during data gathering is expanded to include finishes, mechanical, electrical, plumbing (MEP) data, fire protection requirements, ceiling heights, services, and other information that relates to each room.

Compliance Analysis

The compliance analysis is developed based on the local and national codes applicable to the facility location and must track types and quantities of potent compounds and solvents or other hazardous materials used in the lab. Code information is discussed in Chapter 13.

Test-Fit Plans

Once equipment and bench space requirements are understood, the designer can lay out a schematic plan of each room to confirm that the allotted square footage is appropriate for the function of the space. The rooms and sizes are then compared to the overall plan to make sure that the program works within the scope of the project.

Problem Solving

It is important that the problem-seeking and analysis phases are complete before problem solving begins, so that all of the criteria are known going into the problem-solving phase. In the problem-solving phase, design of the laboratory begins; the layout is refined and lab cards are produced for each space. At the end of the programming process, the lab cards and the equipment list are compiled together with all of the other information in a final programming report, to be reviewed by the client and then used in the development of construction documents.

Lab Cards

In this phase, a lab card is produced for each space within the lab. The lab card is a plan drawing that includes a layout of the room with all of the necessary equipment, finishes, and electrical and data requirements. It also lists HVAC requirements and services, along with any other room-specific information. Services include compressed air; vacuum; deionized water; hot or cold water; gases, such as nitrogen or helium; steam; and others. The lab cards are reviewed by the users and then used as the basis for the later phases of the design. A sample lab card is included in Chapter 4.

Model Construction and Project Costs

Based on the data gathered, a cost estimate is developed on a cost per square foot basis and included in the programming report.

LABORATORY COMPONENTS

Sample Log-In

When samples are initially brought to the QA/QC lab, they are immediately logged in and stored until they are to be tested. The area dedicated to sample receiving is ideally located close to the entrance of the lab and may include a label printer and write-up space. In-process records may also be stored in this area in secure files for easy reference.

Sample Preparation

An area with open benchtop space is required for the preparation of samples. Often this area is centralized and contains storage shelves, glassware, sonicators, shakers, and centrifuges. If the sample prep is done within the main lab, any sonicators should be located in a separate room, if possible, since they are very loud when in operation.

Weighing

Many labs contain a separate weigh room, which allows for greater control of the temperature and humidity during weighing. A typical weigh room contains several weigh stations with appropriate ventilation and containment for the materials being weighed.

Laboratory Module

Typically, casework is laid out on a 10 or 11 ft module that allows for two 30 in. deep benches with a 5 or 6 ft aisle between. The aisle must allow lab personnel to work back-to-back while still having space for maneuvering carts around the lab. Since typical fume hoods are 3 ft deep, an 11 ft module should be used if they are to be placed facing each other.

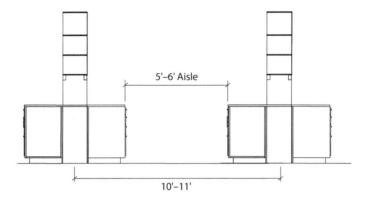

FIGURE 17.6 Casework module.

Figure 17.6 shows the lab module in section. Labs can be open, with shared areas and multiple functions, or small, separated rooms, which are often required for more hazardous operations or for labs with specific needs, such as for light-sensitive materials.

Laboratory casework can be movable or fixed, and a lab can contain any combination of the two, or a combined system of fixed bench with movable cabinets below. Services can be supplied through fixed casework or through the ceiling, so it is important to coordinate the casework type with the strategy for supplying services. Some of the casework may have reagent shelving above, while some may need to stay clear for larger equipment.

Fixed casework has several advantages, including cost, stability, the large amount of storage it provides, and the ability to accommodate sinks and utilities. However, fixed casework is difficult to modify and is not ideal for labs that will need to be reconfigured regularly. Mobile casework has a high up-front cost, but provides greater flexibility. According to research conducted by Jamie Doran for her presentation, "Defining the New Lab of the Future," about 20% of lab users surveyed worked in labs with mobile casework. Several users use the mobility to adjust for multi-project work. Other users expressed concerns about cleanability under the mobile casework [2]. Depending on the lab requirements, either all fixed casework or a mix of fixed and mobile is likely ideal.

Other space planning considerations include the following: (1) Flat island benches should be provided for large equipment. (2) Four-foot doors are necessary for relocating equipment (a fume hood will not fit through 3 ft door). (3) Regulations require appropriate size and space to facilitate cleaning and orderly placement of equipment. (4) Hoods should be located away from entrances or high-traffic areas to minimize disturbance to airflow.

SUPPORT SPACES

Outside of the QA/QC laboratory are additional spaces that exist to support the laboratory's functions, through cleaning of glassware, controlled storage, or facilitation of gowning requirements. In addition to the spaces listed below, gas cylinder storage, locker rooms, stockrooms, office space, and waste handling spaces may be located outside the lab.

GLASS WASH ROOMS

The glass washroom is where glassware for the laboratory is cleaned. Separate glassware washers and dryers may be used and are often seen in older facilities, but combined washer and dryers are much more efficient. Instead of a technician being required to take the glassware from the washer and load it into the dryer, the combined unit will go directly from the wash cycle to the dry cycle. This reduces labor requirements and shortens the cycle time so that more glassware can be cleaned during each shift. Detergent may be stored in small containers and added to the washer by a technician or stored in drums attached to a pump in the machine itself. In addition to the glass washers and dryers, the glass wash room should have space for staging both clean and dirty glassware and a deep sink for washing large glassware items by hand. The room should be large enough to allow carts to move easily and be placed conveniently for loading and unloading. The finishes in the glass wash room should be selected to handle the moisture present, and drainage and ventilation are required.

AUTOCLAVES

Autoclave rooms have the same needs for ventilation, drainage, and finishes as glass wash rooms, with the additional requirement of a steam supply to the autoclave. Autoclaves sterilize equipment, glassware, and media used in biocontainment laboratories. Like glass wash rooms, autoclave rooms require separated spaces for clean and dirty staging and maneuvering room for carts. It is important to size the autoclave with excess capacity, as it is difficult to replace or add to later.

SAMPLE STORAGE

QA/QC laboratories are typically required to retain samples for 1 year after the expiration date or 3 years for over-the-counter (OTC) products with no expiration date. The storage areas should be sized based on the number of samples expected and should be secured and environmentally controlled.

STABILITY CHAMBERS

Stability chambers are rooms designed to maintain a constant temperature and humidity for the storage of samples and materials. A lab may have several stability chambers at different temperatures, depending on the specific needs of the facility. Stability chambers are often prefabricated units made with modular insulated panels with a raised insulated floor and a built-in mechanical system.

SOLVENT STORAGE

Within the lab, solvent quantities are limited by code and often stored in flammable storage cabinets near each fume hood for easy access. Large quantities of solvents must be stored in a fire-rated room, often with a fire suppression system and containment to deal with any spills that may occur.

DRUG ENFORCEMENT ADMINISTRATION STORAGE

If controlled substances are used in a lab, a storage area that complies with the Drug Enforcement Administration requirements must be provided. For schedule I and II drugs, a safe or vault must be provided, depending on the quantities of drugs stored. For schedule III, IV, and V substances, a locked area with controlled access and alarms is adequate. The DEA requirements for controlled substance storage can be found at http://www.deadiversion.usdoj.gov/21cfr/cfr/index.html [3].

LOCKER ROOMS AND GOWNING

Gowning requirements vary by the type of laboratory and materials used; these can be as simple as a lab coat and safety glasses put on at the laboratory entrance, or they may be much more involved, requiring airlocks to enter and exit. A space should be provided for lab coat storage and changing; this area may be incorporated into an airlock if necessary. A detailed description of gowning requirements is outside the scope of this chapter.

COMPLIANCE

During the development of the BOD, the designer reviews the local and national codes and regulations that apply in the jurisdiction where the lab is to be located. A typical code review lists the site address, jurisdiction, applicable codes, use (most laboratories are designated B—business), and specific code requirements that are relevant to the project, along with a plan drawing indicating egress requirements and fire-rated walls and floors. Laboratories should have two exits whenever possible, with doors swinging out in the direction of egress. Requirements for rated walls vary by jurisdiction. See Chapter 13 for further discussion.

The designer must pay special attention to solvents and other hazardous materials that are to be used and stored in the laboratory. The quantity of hazardous materials is governed by control areas, which limit the allowable quantities within different areas of the building. There are limits to the amounts stored overall, and harsher limits to the amounts stored on higher floors, so it is important to understand the implications early in the design.

BIOSAFETY LEVELS

Laboratories designed for biological hazardous materials are rated with biosafety levels defined by the NIH and the CDC, depending on the materials they house. The biosafety level determines the HVAC requirements, security requirements, and type of biosafety cabinets that must be used. Because of the many impacts on the design of the spaces, it is important to know the required biosafety level at the start of the design process.

Biosafety level 1 (BSL-1) is the lowest hazard level. Work at BSL-1 can be performed on benchtops or in chemical fume hoods. These spaces require a minimum of three to four air changes an hour with negative pressure to adjacent spaces.

Biosafety level 2 (BSL-2) represents a moderate hazard level. The BSL-2 labs are required to be locked, with access limited to necessary personnel. Class I and II BSCs are used. The BSL-2 spaces require a minimum of 6–15 air changes an hour with negative pressure to adjacent spaces.

Biosafety level 3 (BSL-3) represents a high-hazard level and is required when dealing with hazards that are potentially lethal by exposure or inhalation. Class I, II, and III BSCs are used. The BSL-3 spaces require a separate HVAC system from the rest of the facility with negative pressure to adjacent spaces that is monitored.

Biosafety level 4 (BSL-4) is the highest level of hazard. All work in BSL-4 spaces is conducted in Class III BSCs. All vent lines are HEPA-filtered, along with the supply and exhaust air from the space. The BSL-4 spaces require a separate HVAC system with monitoring and control of pressurization and with supply fans interlocked to the exhaust system so that the pressurization will not fail in the event of exhaust failure.

POTENT COMPOUNDS

The active pharmaceutical ingredients (APIs) that are used for drugs that treat cancer (i.e., cytotoxic compounds) and myriad other chronic diseases can be incredibly potent, making containment especially important. A risk assessment informs any decisions made about handling the compounds and their containment as the product is handled.

HVAC SYSTEM

The design of the HVAC system for the QA/QC laboratory is largely determined by the level of hazard of the lab. The two main functions are to maintain a comfortable work environment and maintain a safe work environment.

The room temperatures are usually set at 68°F–70°F (20°C–21.1°C). Cooler temperatures may be desired for comfort if lab personnel are in protective clothing. Humidity is usually in the range of 30%–60%. Stronger humidity controls may be required for weigh rooms than for the rest of the lab. Extremely low or high humidity can lead to a number of problems. Low humidity can lead to static discharges and dust. High humidity can lead to moisture problems, condensation, and microbial growth. Humidity that is either too high or too low can lead to equipment malfunctions and can increase the occupants' susceptibility to infection.

The classification level of the lab determines if 100% outside air is required or if some recirculated air may be used, with or without HEPA filtration, and the required air changes per hour. The lab is typically negative to corridors, so that contaminants and fumes are contained within the lab. Redundancy may be desirable so that the system remains functional in the event of failure. In addition to the overall requirements, point exhausts are required at certain equipment that need ventilation or produce heat. This information should be included on the equipment list and lab cards. Fume hoods typically have face velocities of 60–100 cubic feet per minute (CFM) with a hood opening of 18 in. and an exhaust duct velocity of 1,000–3,500 CFM. Chapter 5 contains additional information on HVAC designs.

PROJECT MANAGEMENT ISSUES

Cost

QA/QC laboratories are one of the most expensive parts of a facility to build (per square foot) and operate, as they are high energy users. Renovations within an existing building can be complicated by limited acceptable downtimes and limited accessibility, and costs rise when work must be completed in phases and on nights and weekends to keep facilities operational.

Schedule

Like all parts of the facility with large equipment, long lead times must be factored into the schedule for glassware washers, autoclaves, and other large pieces of equipment. In renovation projects, the schedule is affected by the amount of downtime that is possible without interrupting operations.

QA/QC Lab of the Future

According to "Defining the New Lab of the Future," natural light was rated as a very high priority by lab users, as were views to the outside [2]. Energy efficiency was the third highest priority. Figure 17.7 shows the percentages of users who rated each of 10 criteria as very important, somewhat important, or not important.

Sustainability

Sustainability is not a new trend, but is important to consider in the design of laboratories, especially because of their high energy use. Using hoods efficiently, and providing only the number of hoods needed for operation, can make a difference in terms of both sustainability and operating cost. See Chapter 16 for a discussion of sustainable design in pharmaceutical facilities.

Lean Labs

The concept of a lean lab was developed in Japan and centers around the idea of eliminating waste in both processes and materials through better management of workloads and resources. An activity location analysis tracks the movements of lab personnel throughout a workday to establish the most

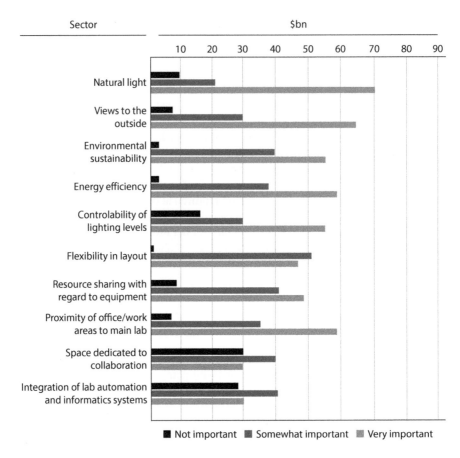

FIGURE 17.7 The ideal lab. (From Doran J, *Defining The NEW Lab of the Future*. Research facilities, May 7–8, 2015, St. Petersburg, FL.)

beneficial adjacencies. An equipment utilization study looks at the use of a piece of equipment by each department and develops a rating of its importance, which is used to determine which pieces can be shared and which must be dedicated to a department. Communication and employee training also play a large role in lean labs, so the location and visibility of visual management boards and other collaborative spaces are important. The main concepts of lean labs as they apply to QC/QA laboratories are as follows: (1) Cellular laboratory workspaces for individual teams or tests minimize travel with easily visible visual management boards to track performance. (2) The integration of write-up, review, and approval areas is in a separate area within the lab. (3) Transportation and motion are minimized by locating the labs close to manufacturing and centrally locating shared services and storage. (4) Equipment requirements are minimized by leveling out the load on the lab to avoid peaks. (5) Resources are shared, rather than owned by any one analyst or team. (6) Flexible bench configurations are used so that efficient adjacencies can be maintained when demands change. Open labs with mobile casework provide the most flexibility. (7) Storage is limited and defined at the point of use, and central lab storage is provided to track use and minimize waste. (8) Communication is enhanced through the use of glazing between offices and labs. (9) Organization is encouraged through the use of open or glass-front cabinets without drawers [4].

WORKSPACE

There has been a movement toward having workspaces for laboratory personnel located outside the lab, because with newer technologies, more of the work can be completed outside the lab. This has allowed for a more comfortable work environment with greater opportunities for natural light and more comfortable finishes, where employees can work without lab coats or other protective equipment and consume food and drink.

FURTHER DISCUSSION

1. What is the role of QA/QC laboratories in pharmaceutical manufacturing facilities?
2. What is the function of a lab card, and what information is included on one?
3. What are the benefits of locating write-up space outside of the lab?
4. What factors must the HVAC designer take into account when designing for a QA/QC lab? How are these different for new buildings versus renovation projects?
5. What steps can the designer take to allow a lab to be more easily adaptable to future changes in users' needs?

ABOUT THE AUTHOR

Cassidy Hobbs joined JacobsWyper Architects in 2012 and has worked on a number of projects, with a focus on lab design. These include several renovation projects for Patheon Pharmaceuticals and the University of Pennsylvania, as well as larger new building projects for McNeil Consumer Products, Regeneron Pharmaceuticals, Ferring Pharmaceuticals, Ashland, Becton Dickinson, and others. Prior to joining JacobsWyper, Hobbs's experience in architecture firms and in the Engineering/Facilities Department at Amtrak provided her with a range of experience, including commercial, residential, historic preservation, facilities, and transportation-related projects. Hobbs is a registered architect and leads the Philadelphia AIA associate committee's monthly study sessions for the architectural exams.

REFERENCES

1. International Society for Pharmaceutical Engineering, *Quality Laboratory Facilities*, Good Practice Guide, International Society for Pharmaceutical Engineering, Tampa, FL, 2012.
2. Doran J, *Defining The NEW Lab of the Future*. Research facilities, May 7–8, 2015, St. Petersburg, FL.
3. Code of Federal Regulations, Title 21, Part 1300, Office of Diversion Control, http://www.deadiversion.usdoj.gov/21cfr/cfr/index.html.
4. Dockery M, Gabardi F, Garay J, Gazvoda J, Kimmel L, Orombelli P, Peytremann C, Reynolds T, Sharton-Kersten T, Shoel G, Sirovatka J, Incorporating Lean Principles into Pharmaceutical QC Laboratory Design, *Pharmaceutical Engineering*, September/October 2014.

18 Packaging and Warehousing

John S. Holton

CONTENTS

INTRODUCTION

This chapter covers good design practices for packaging and warehousing facilities. It discusses the principles that are applied to packaging and warehousing facilities and addresses the critical function of a packaging facility to prevent product mix-ups and cross-contamination. It covers the steps needed to construct a new facility or renovate an existing one, and it describes the function and purpose of packaging and warehousing pharmaceutical product, the multiple levels of packaging areas, critical parameters, and utility system criteria. Chapter 11 specifically addresses sterile packaging, which will not be discussed here. The same hygienic zoning principles (i.e., white, gray, black, transition, and proper gowning techniques) that apply to pharmaceutical processing also apply to pharmaceutical packaging (see Chapter 15 for a description of hygienic zoning principles).

To assist the design engineer and associated team members for a given project, this chapter reviews the initial stages of a project through to the commissioning and qualification and turnover stage. It discusses the items that should be reviewed and documented before initiating a project. The application of risk management is presented to determine the critical components of the project to ensure product and personnel safety and project cost control. The fundamental design principles, the packaging process, and associated space interactions are provided. Facility layout and construction materials are discussed. Design considerations for utility systems (e.g., heating, ventilation, and air conditioning [HVAC] and electrical) are identified, as well as support systems (e.g., compressed air and vacuum). Typical design criteria are described, as well as the mechanism by which to document attainment of certain parameters, such as temperature control.

PACKAGING DEFINED

In its simplest terms, packaging is preparing goods for transport, distribution, storage, retail, and use. Packaging has evolved from simple clay pots and woven bags into the multi-billion-dollar industry that it is today. Primitive packaging was not concerned with the containment, protection, transport, and information or sales functions of modern packaging. Today, demographic studies provide firms with data that help them make smart decisions about packaging design, graphics, and marketing. While navigating regulatory and environmental hurdles, firms are now concerned with the four R's:

- *Reduce:* The amount of packaging material in any given application is minimized without jeopardizing the integrity of the goods within.
- *Reuse:* Whenever possible, packaging systems that can be used over and over again are created.
- *Recycle:* Used packaging materials are collected to be reprocessed into new material.
- *Recover:* Rather than send packaging material to a landfill, it is collected and reused.

IMPORTANCE OF PACKAGING

In the course of packaging operations, preserving the integrity of the drug product and the safety of the patient is of utmost importance. The Food and Drug Administration (FDA) ensures that drug products are suitable for their intended use by making certain that companies that manufacture drug products follow very specific guidelines during the manufacturing process. The same federal regulations that govern the manufacture of drugs apply to the packaging of these products for distribution and sale. From the time the drug product is approved for packaging and distribution until it is prescribed, purchased, and used by the consumer, it is the packaging systems that provide the means to ensure that the safety, efficacy, strength, and purity of the drug product are not compromised. For the purposes of this chapter, only packaging for finished pharmaceutical products, medical devices, and other industry-specific applications (e.g., current Good Manufacturing Practices [cGMPs]) is discussed. The term *drug product* is used to collectively describe the applications in this chapter.

PACKAGING FUNCTIONS

There are four rudimentary packaging functions that must be evaluated during the packaging design process. They are discussed below.

Contain Function

This function is concerned with providing a receptacle to keep some quantity of product together in a single mass. When programming for the contain function, the package designer must consider the physical attributes of the product (e.g., solid, liquid, granular, paste, or discrete item), the product's nature (e.g., corrosive, volatile, flammable, toxic, or pressurized), and the quantity of material to be packaged.

Protect and Preserve Function

All package contents must be protected from cross-contamination and physical damage, such as vibration, abrasion, extreme temperatures, and humidity. Child-resistant, package-opening features are required by law on some drug products. Tamper-proof features have been prevalent since the first Tylenol tampering incident in 1982, and antitheft and anticounterfeit measures may be used as well. The preserve function pertains to stopping or inhibiting chemical degradation of the package contents; for example, oxygen, water vapor, and light are potentially damaging to certain drug compounds, and barriers to these elements are critical to preserving the integrity of the drug product.

Transport Function

The transport function is applicable to unit loads (skid quantities) of goods; however, proper package design for transportation starts at the primary packaging stage. Transportation is always seen as hazardous in some way to the product being moved, so this is an important design feature.

Inform and Sell Function

In clean industry applications, the inform function gives the consumer specific information about the contents of the package. There are regulatory requirements that dictate what information appears on the primary package. Some of this information is preprinted (e.g., drug name, strength, quantity of doses, and drug manufacturer), and some is printed in real time on the packaging line (e.g., lot or batch number and product expiration date). There is printed information at all levels of packaging, even on the drug product itself in the case of tablets and capsules. The drug name, the strength of the dose, the total quantity of doses, and the name and address of the drug manufacturer are absolute minimum requirements for preprinted information. Most printed information appears on the unit of sale, usually the secondary paperboard carton. In the case of prescription medications, there is also preprinted information for the physician or patient in the form of a folded package insert that is placed in the carton with the bottle, pouch, or blister.

Typically, prescription medications have minimalistic packaging because physicians prescribe these medications, so the consumer does not have an opportunity to compare one product to a competitive product. The over-the-counter (OTC) packages, however, compete directly with other medications on the store shelf, and drug manufacturers go to great lengths to differentiate their products from those of their competitors.

LEVELS OF PACKAGING

Primary Packaging

The primary package, the first level of containment, is in direct contact with the finished drug product as a blister card or pouch for tablets or capsules; a glass or plastic bottle for tablets, capsules, powders, or liquids; a glass or plastic syringe, ampule, or vial for injectable drug products; or an aluminum or laminate tube for creams and ointments. This first level is critical to maintain the safety, efficacy, potency, and purity of the drug product. Primary packaging is the level most important to the shelf life of a drug. Some drugs are susceptible to water vapor or carbon dioxide and others to oxygen or light. Certain packaging materials resist these threats, although there is no universal barrier. Some packaging materials use a laminate structure, combining the benefits of two or more materials in a single, multilayer barrier.

The dosage form is directly exposed to the packaging room environment after it is removed from its bulk container and before its introduction to the primary package. This necessitates the use of strict engineering and environmental controls during the primary packaging process to ensure that the drug product is not compromised.

Secondary Packaging

Secondary packaging consists of one or more primary package units contained within a secondary container, usually a paperboard carton or tray. Any supplementary components, such as patient and physician instructions or sales and marketing materials, are added at this level. This level of packaging is the unit of use for prescription products, and for OTC products, it is the package first seen by the consumer on the store shelf; therefore, it is graphics intensive.

Tertiary Packaging

Tertiary packaging is most commonly employed with OTC formulations, usually reserved for bundling together multiple units of use into units of sale at the wholesale level. Examples are stretch banding, shrink bundling, and overwrapping. Tertiary packaging makes it easier to configure distribution loads for shipment and break down distribution loads at the point of sale.

Distributive Packaging

Drug product packaged for sale is usually placed in corrugated shipping containers for distribution. These containers have a prevalent shipping label to comply with regulatory requirements associated with lot number and expiration dating. Corrugated shippers can be palletized into a unit load, or they can be distributed in quantities as small as a single case.

Unit Load

Entire lots of packaged drug product bound for warehouses or distribution centers are usually unitized in pallet quantities. Corrugated cases are stacked, interlocked, and stored in warehouses to await shipment to the consumer.

WAREHOUSING

Warehousing operations should provide appropriate control to prevent contamination or mix-up of materials, containers, closures, packaging, and labels. Storage of finished product or intermediate or raw product materials may need special environmental conditions. Drug products should be stored under appropriate conditions of temperature, humidity, and light so that the safety, identity, strength, quality, and purity of the drug products are not affected.

Specialized, independent storage and handling areas may be needed based on the material considerations identified in the risk analysis, due to environmental health or safety hazards or regulated status as a controlled substance. Controlled access should be employed, as necessary, in the facility.

GENERAL PACKAGING PLANT DESIGN

A pharmaceutical packaging plant can be a stand-alone, dedicated facility or part of a larger manufacturing and warehousing operation. A pharmaceutical company often builds a packaging plant and a warehouse, with future plans to allow packaging to expand into the warehouse area and build additional warehouse space as necessary. Careful consideration must be given to this approach, so that maximum use of vertical warehouse space can be realized when it is converted to packaging space. Adding mezzanine areas for office space and mechanical equipment, such as HVAC systems, is a way to maximize the old warehouse space overhead. Additional general considerations include:

- Areas containing products with potentially hazardous properties that might be released during warehousing (i.e., during sampling, weighing, or dispensing) or primary packaging operations need special consideration. Finishes and environmental conditions for these areas should be equivalent to those used for open processing of exposed products.
- The design should provide adequate lot and material segregation to prevent contamination or mix-ups. Segregation can be implemented by spatial (physical), temporal (time), electronic, or procedural means. The evaluation of segregation requirements is modified based on a review of the risk assessment factors.
- The design should comply with applicable fire and safety codes, accessibility guidelines, and environmental regulations.

Material staging should address the environmental state for the product and raw materials; for example, a product might need staging at 36°F–46°F (2°C–8°C), while labeling materials associated with packaging may need humidity or light controls. Access control and security monitoring of areas may be required.

PRODUCT EXPOSURE

Product exposure is generally classified as nonexposed or exposed.

Nonexposed Products

When product or material is not exposed to the environment, the risk of contamination is minimal (e.g., transfer of finished product by pneumatic transfer, vacuum transfer, or bin transport). Facility requirements, such as architectural, HVAC, and environmental controls, may be reduced.

Exposed Products

When product or material is exposed to the environment, there is potential for contamination of or from the environment. This often requires airlocks and directional airflow, increased ventilation and filtering of air, or heavy reliance on standard operating procedures (SOPs) to reduce potential cross-contamination, such as an operator tracking product or material from one area to another. Increased potency or toxicity of product or material often requires increased levels of protection for the packaging process, primarily to protect personnel and the environment.

USER REQUIREMENTS

Decisions and commitments made in the early phase of project planning are often too costly to change as the project advances to final design and then to execution. Therefore, developing user requirements for the facility before initiating the design process is critical in setting the schedule for the overall delivery for the facility.

To be effective, user requirements should be concise and germane. While it is possible to produce one document that covers the entire scope of a facility, a hierarchy of documents is more effective. User requirements should be well understood and properly applied. Data relevant to developing user requirements should be gathered on the following:

- *Process.* Critical environmental parameters that should be achieved, maintained, and monitored
- *Quality.* Regulatory guidance and quality principles to guide decision making on facility parameters that can affect product quality and patient safety
- *Operations.* Appropriate environment for the working conditions that affect facility design
- *Maintenance.* Critical aspects of the facility design that ensure a low total cost of ownership (TCO) of the specified life of the facility

Within the user requirements, quality requirements should be separated from business or other requirements. The number and titles of these documents will depend on the project size and scope. Documents listing user requirements may include the following:

- *Project charter.* A high-level description of the requirements, including descriptions of the facility capability, the potential for expansion, and corporate architectural requirements.
- *Facility user requirements specifications (URSs).* A concise document that provides the design brief from the organization to the designer, listing any company standards or specifications to be used.

- *System URSs.* A concise document that provides the design brief from an organization to the designer, listing any organization standards or specifications to be used; typically, these are provided for quality-critical systems. The scope of work usually needs designers to develop the design specifications for supporting systems.

User requirements can be stated as performance-based information that describes an operation and sets expectations where critical process parameters (CPPs) are well defined (e.g., temperature or relative humidity) as acceptance criteria (required results) or as expected results where some variation may be acceptable. For performance-based information, the facility designer should gather relevant information and propose expectations that would meet user requirements. Where the rationale for criteria at one facility is well understood, those criteria may be reproduced at a similar facility. Variables involved should be understood, and the facility designer should carefully consider each of these variables when proposing criteria. A formal URS document should provide a vehicle for exchanging information between business units and the design team. The URS should help to:

- Ensure team consensus on project scope, facility use, and functional requirements
- Achieve business objectives for which design options can be assessed and determined
- Generate an understanding of product and process specifications
- Focus design review and design verification and subsequent commissioning efforts

The URSs are a starting point of a process to facilitate compliance with cGMPs and other regulations. Primary regulatory requirements include that "any building or buildings used in the manufacture, processing, packaging, or holding of a drug product shall be of suitable size, construction, and location to facilitate cleaning maintenance and proper operations" (21 CFR 211.42[a]) [1].

Parameter-focused designs decrease the risk of cross-contamination and product and label mix-ups. This chapter defines key parameters to identify and analyze risks to patients, product, and employees, as well as to promote compliance with applicable regulatory requirements. "The design of any such building shall have adequate space for orderly placement of equipment and materials to prevent mix-ups between different components, drug product containers, closures, labeling, in-process materials, or drug products, and to prevent contamination" (21 CFR 211.42[b]) [1].

The facility user requirements can be outlined and incorporated into the design.

Knowing and having a scientific foundation on which products and processes are developed is considered critical to defining the quality aspects and controls needed to design, build, and maintain a compliant packaging and warehousing facility. Once complete, the requirements and product quality aspects that have been identified per product or system should be implemented at each facility producing or processing the same products.

RISK MANAGEMENT

Controlling material mix-ups, contamination, and material storage conditions is a major consideration in designing packaging and warehousing facilities.

Risk management is a systematic application of management policies, procedures, and practices to the task of identifying, assessing, controlling, and monitoring risks. It is typically an iterative process. It should be based on robust science and product and process understanding (i.e., an understanding of critical quality attributes, which are based on and traceable back to the relevant regulatory submission). Qualitative or quantitative techniques may be used. The focus should be on the risk posed to patient safety and product quality. Risk management should reduce risks to an acceptable level. Complete elimination of risk is neither practical nor necessary.

A framework for making risk management decisions should be defined to ensure consistency of application across functions and departments. Such a framework can be effectively implemented when it is incorporated into a comprehensive quality risk management system.

No one tool or set of tools is applicable to every situation in which a quality risk management process is described. International Conference on Harmonisation (ICH) Q9 provides a general overview of and references for some of the primary tools used in quality risk management by industry and regulators and should be referenced in the application of the facility risk assessment [2]. The International Society of Pharmaceutical Engineering (ISPE) Good Practice Guide *Applied Risk Management for Commissioning and Qualification* provides more information on the use of risk assessment for commissioning and verification [3].

A full risk assessment should evaluate all of the systems and their interrelationships, including the facility, utilities, equipment, cleaning, storage, materials, procedures, controls, qualification, validation, maintenance, and records. When starting the risk assessment process, it is critical to define the system boundaries. Once defined, the scope of the project can be defined. The team size should be maintained at about six to eight people and should comprise subject matter experts from manufacturing, operations, engineering, processing, maintenance, quality, customers, and suppliers. In keeping with the focus of patient safety, product quality, and data integrity, the following list includes some of the common hazards for a packaging and warehousing operation: (1) distribution of adulterated product; (2) product mix-ups; (3) label and labeling mix-ups; (4) contamination; (5) misbranded product; (6) legibility and content of the label (e.g., lot number, expiration date, and all bar codes); (7) records integrity; (8) label reconciliation; (9) yield reconciliation; (10) package integrity (package performance); (11) product protection from exposure to detrimental temperature, humidity, or light; and (12) quality system oversight.

Packaging Floor Layout

The packaging plant is laid out with packaging rooms in a grid pattern; the integrated design should satisfy the project specifications and address risk assessment factors, while providing good levels of access for operability, maintenance, cleaning, personnel, product, component raw material, waste, and trash movements. The intent should be to keep all packaging areas as centralized and equidistant from support areas as possible. The material staging specification must address the line clearance philosophy. This staging does not need to be in a separate room, but in a separate area (spatial segregation), which may facilitate production and reduce risks in multiproduct facilities or facilities with high throughput. If there are adjacent packaging lines, there should be adequate control to ensure prevention of mixing up materials, leaflets, or labels. Typically, this control is a barrier that extends to the floor; for example, if a leaflet is dropped, there is no risk of it being transferred to an adjacent packaging line.

Building columns are designed into walls so that the packaging rooms are free and clear for maximum flexibility with respect to equipment layout. Glass can be used to give the plant an open feeling and allow supervisors and inspectors to view the work in process; however, the cost and safety implications must be factored into the final design. Hallways should be large enough to permit the flow of materials and personnel and also to facilitate the movement of packaging equipment. The lengths and widths of the largest machinery used must be determined, and the means by which to move this equipment from the receiving dock to any packaging room and back out to the maintenance and storage areas must be designed into the packaging plant layout.

Raw Material and Finished Goods Warehousing

Maximum throughput is realized when there are dedicated warehouses for raw material and finished goods, and the flow of material is linear. It may appear that these warehouses function in a similar fashion, but they actually operate quite differently. A raw material warehouse is typically high bay, with large volumes of palletized packaging components stored in racks until requested by the packaging floor. Material pulled from the warehouse can be sent to a variety of packaging rooms. There is a great diversity of materials stored in the warehouse—everything from heavy, dense rolls of blister films that can weigh more than 1,000 lb per pallet to very light pallets of flattened, folded, corrugated, shipping cases. Components, such as bottles and caps, take up a lot of warehouse space, and most firms use a just-in-time ordering philosophy with their suppliers to minimize the quantities of these materials that must be stored on-site.

A finished goods warehouse consists of pallet loads of finished product in shipping cases that are ready for distribution. These loads are typically uniform and are floor stacked as many as four pallets high. Trucks are loaded with pallets two units high, so it is efficient to store finished goods two to four units high to minimize fork truck motions. Finished goods usually remain in the warehouse only as long as it takes for the quality assurance department to review the packaging batch record and approve the batch for shipment.

Warehousing operations must provide appropriate control to prevent contamination or a mix-up of materials, containers, closures, packaging, and labels. Storage of finished product or raw product materials may need special environmental conditions and temperature mapping to ensure that conditions in the warehouse meet requirements. Significant changes in humidity may affect the physical properties of cartons, causing variation in line performance (see the "Package Design Principles" section for information relative to temperature mapping requirements). Materials should be stored in a manner that allows for cleaning and inspection.

PACKAGING DESIGN PRINCIPLES

Packaging facilities should be designed to allow product, packaging components, work in process, finished goods, and waste to move through the plant in sequential order. Material flows are designed to prevent cross-contamination. Packaging areas must allow adequate space for materials, equipment, and personnel. In addition, space must be provided for operation, maintenance, and cleaning of packaging equipment. Separate areas are designated for packaging operations, equipment cleaning, storage of clean equipment and tooling, and storage of dirty equipment and tooling. Exposed product processing that requires a controlled environment may need personnel gowning, airlocks, high-quality room finishes, and a cleaning regimen to protect the product. Restrooms and other personnel convenience areas should not open directly into primary or secondary packaging areas. Exposed wood pallets and other wood products should not be used in primary packaging areas where direct product exposure is possible. All HVAC systems should be designed to prevent cross-contamination and infiltration of extraneous matter. Proper filtration must be provided in areas where contamination is a possibility. Architecturally, horizontal surfaces should be avoided (e.g., use sloped sills) to minimize the collection of particulate matter.

Packaging Process Assessment

Before undertaking a detailed facility design, a thorough study is necessary of the current and potential future packaging process parameters. The results of this assessment should be contained within the facility and system user requirements. The following outline can be used in this assessment:

- *Product.* Toxicity, sensitivity, drug classification, number of stock keeping units (SKUs), stability requirements, dosage form, package format, packaging materials, and labeling
- *Production.* Campaign, changeovers, product mix, scale, clinical versus commercial, batch size, number of lots, throughput speeds, and number of lines
- *Quality assurance.* SOPs, validation, reject rates, quality inspections, exception handling, pest control, and cleaning procedures
- *Equipment.* Dedicated and multiuse, primary, secondary, tertiary, fixed and portable, changeovers, automation, accumulation, backup, redundancy, tooling, and spare parts
- *Personnel.* Accessibility, flow, training, biometrics or passwords, gowning, and workstations
- *Logistics.* Fork trucks, battery charging, storage racks, cold storage, quarantine, hazardous materials, and controlled substances

- *Environment and safety.* Occupational Safety and Health Administration (OSHA); Environmental Protection Agency (EPA); personal protective equipment; SOPs; confined space; environmental monitoring; lighting levels; sound levels; and fire safety, including possible containment of water used to extinguish a fire
- *Support facilities.* Restrooms, locker rooms, break rooms, cafeteria, nurses' station, label storage, and retained sample storage
- *Utilities.* Compressed air, electricity, vacuum, and specialty gases

PACKAGING SPACE LAYOUT

In designing packaging space for pharmaceutical and medical device applications, care must be taken to protect the integrity of the product. The cGMP regulations state that operations should be performed within specifically designed areas of adequate size (21 CFR 211.42[c]) and that procedures should be in place for prevention of mix-ups and cross-contamination by physical or spatial separation from operations on other drug products (21 CFR 211.130[a]). Care must be taken in providing facility design to mitigate or completely eliminate these risks.

Packaging areas are typically located adjacent to manufacturing areas, the raw material warehouse, and the finished goods warehouse. Ideally, drug product and packaging components flow into one end and finished goods out of the other end of the process. The waste streams created by the packaging process must also be considered. Before a detailed design is created, a flow diagram of the packaging process is constructed to show all process inputs and outputs and all points of operator intervention. During the design stage, the design and engineering firm must have access to accurate electronic drawings of the packaging processes, including plan views, equipment elevations, and utility connection points. Packaging suites are relatively clean areas with high levels of activity, noise, and movement. This is the opposite of processing areas where most of the work takes place out of sight from operating personnel in closed systems. Thus, most firms want packaging areas to include large viewing windows where packaging processes can be viewed from an area where gowning is not required.

Spatial Requirements

Packaging areas require adequate floor space for equipment, personnel, and materials. Entrances to packaging areas must be properly sized so that the largest piece of equipment needed for a given process can be moved into and out of the space without building modifications or service interruptions. A minimum of 5 ft should be provided between equipment and packaging area partitions to provide access to power panels, allow for the movement of equipment and materials, and provide safe egress for personnel in the event of an emergency. In a well-designed packaging process, all operator interventions should take place from one side of the line. This includes regular adjustments; charging the line with raw materials, such as bottles, caps, labels, foil and film, folding cartons, and package inserts; and removing finished goods from the line. Dimensionally, packaging spaces should be designed to maximize equipment use while minimizing space.

Safe Egress

Because of the linear nature of automated packaging processes, the complete line layout, including skids of packaging components, must be factored into safety plans. Some automated lines can be as long as 150 ft or more, and equipment could possibly compromise paths to emergency exits. Additional exits may be needed, or line crossovers can be used as necessary.

Ceiling Height

In most applications, in both primary and secondary packaging suites, ceiling height should not be less than 10 ft. In instances where drug product is fed from above, a ceiling height of 14 or even 16 ft may be applicable. In every case, the equipment manufacturer or packaging line integrator must be consulted to determine the maximum height needed for the equipment.

Lighting

Lighting fixtures should be accessible to allow proper maintenance, such as changing bulbs and repair or replacement of the ballast. Lighting fixtures used in exposed protection areas should allow for cleaning and be able to withstand the pressure and temperature of any water streams used for washdown. Lighting levels between 60 and 75 foot-candles are generally sufficient for most packaging operations. Some areas may need higher foot-candles if there is an online inspection task, for example, to be performed, or perhaps lower foot-candles if there is a backlit automatic machine-based inspection. Most of the automated inspection areas tend to be shrouded, and adjustment of local lighting levels is not required.

Packaging Space, Equipment and Process Relationships

Primary packaging operations are followed in-line by any number of secondary and tertiary processes (i.e., it is a linear process). Individual machines are linked to each other by a series of conveyors, and logical process controls and buffer zones provide an integrated packaging operation. Some processes are highly automated, with minimal operator intervention, while others are entirely manual, with operators performing all machine functions. The factors that dictate the degree of automation include equipment costs, operating costs, labor rates, desired throughput, and the duration of the packaging campaign.

Packaging lines are usually arranged either in a U-shape, with the beginning of the line and the end of the line located in the same general vicinity, or straight through, with the beginning and end of the packaging process located at opposite ends of the packaging area. The design method is impacted by the general plant layout, but there are distinct advantages and disadvantages to each method. In a U-shaped design, the packaging area tends to be operator-centric, with the man–machine interface located on the inside of the U. The operation can be centrally supervised, and one operator can manage multiple machine stations. All staged packaging components, such as foil, cartons, and package inserts, are also located on the inside of the U. Supervisors have a central vantage point to manage the entire operation. In a straight-through configuration, operations are process-centric, with multiple operators located at different machine stations along the length of the line. Operators and packaging components are staged on one side of the line. Regardless of the line layout, material and personnel flows must be properly designed to avoid mix-ups.

HVAC

The packaging and warehouse facility designer must be familiar with industrial HVAC, as defined in various documents by the American Society of Heating, Refrigerating, and Air-Conditioning Engineers (ASHRAE) and the American Conference of Governmental Industrial Hygienists (ACGIH). Knowledge of local construction codes, National Fire Protection Association (NFPA) standards, environmental regulations, and OSHA regulations is also assumed. The HVAC system must comply with these and all applicable building, safety, hygiene, and environmental regulations. The design of the HVAC system should consider critical parameters, product exposure, and processes.

Critical parameters for the room environment, which are those that could potentially present a high risk to product quality and patient safety, may include temperature, humidity, and viable and nonviable airborne contaminants, depending on the application. Contamination from viable particles may be a particular risk if an exposed product has microbial limits. Space lighting levels may be a critical parameter, depending on product sensitivity. Room volume air changes and room pressure may be critical parameters when handling exposed products or materials with defined exposure limits. The relative direction of airflow between spaces may be a critical parameter if airborne particles or vapors could have a detrimental effect on product or material in an adjacent space [4].

The classification of product exposure is an important consideration in the design and specification of the HVAC system. The level of protection required must consider if the air is being supplied for exposed or nonexposed product. Operating ranges should be considered in establishing design criteria. The concepts of alert and action points also apply to HVAC monitoring systems. To satisfy cGMP regulations, critical parameters should be monitored, alarmed, and recorded [4].

Room Temperature

Room temperature may be a critical parameter for both open and closed operations. Most products, materials, and processes can handle a wide range in temperatures. However, the width of this range decreases as the exposure time increases. Product stability and personnel comfort must be considered in establishing room temperature requirements. Product requirements are often defined by controlled room temperature, as defined by the United States Pharmacopoeia (USP) General Notices and Requirements [5]: "a temperature maintained thermostatically that encompasses the usual and customary working environment of 68°F to 77°F (20°C to 25°C), that results in a mean kinetic temperature calculated to be not more than 77°F (25°C), and that allows for excursions between 59°F and 86°F (15°C and 30°C) [found] in pharmacies, hospitals, and warehouses." Provided the mean kinetic temperature remains in the allowed range, transient spikes up to 104°F (40°C) are permitted provided they do not exceed 24 h. Articles may be labeled for storage at controlled room temperature or up to 77°F (25°C), or other wording based on the same mean kinetic temperature. The mean kinetic temperature is a calculated value that may be used as an isothermic storage temperature that simulates the nonisothermal effects of storage temperature variations. Specifying tighter requirements than those actually required will result in a system that is more expensive to purchase and maintain.

Relative Humidity

Room relative humidity may affect exposed product or materials that are sensitive to water vapor. Relative humidity levels generally have negligible effects on sealed containers or aqueous product; however, liquid product can lose moisture to a low-humidity room over an extended period of time. Relative humidity levels can also affect equipment and product storage. Typically, if there are no specific product requirements, humidity is controlled between 30% and 55% relative humidity. This range is selected based on increased problems with static electricity at levels lower than 25% and the increased potential for mold growth at levels greater than 60%. Wide variations in relative humidity in packaging facilities can affect equipment operations and throughput due to changes in material characteristics. It should be noted that specifying tighter requirements than those actually required will not necessarily result in a better-designed HVAC system, but will generally result in a system that is more expensive to purchase and maintain.

Care should be taken with equipment selection, whether for humidification or dehumidification purposes, to ensure that it does not promote microbiological contamination or provide a potential breeding ground for microbiological contamination. If humidification is needed, boiler water additives should not make breathing air unsafe, in conformance with ASHRAE 62 indoor air quality (IAQ) guidelines and any locally applicable codes. Site steam may be used for humidification; clean steam or pure steam is not necessarily required. Boiler water additives (e.g., chelating agents) should not be used, as they can make occupant breathing air unsafe. Products may be sensitive to boiler additives (see the "Site Steam and Condensate" section below).

If dehumidification is provided, the system selected should not have the potential to contaminate the product adversely. Cooling coil-type systems generate large amounts of condensate that must be drained properly and cleaned periodically to avoid microbial contamination. Liquid and dry desiccant systems should be evaluated for potential carryover of desiccant into the supply air system and its effect on the exposed product.

If relative humidity control is required, the boundary of the space to be controlled should be analyzed for potential moisture ingress, through air movement or moisture migration. Vapor barriers or construction materials having low-moisture permeability should be considered.

Airborne Contaminants

The requirements for filtration of air supply depend on the level of protection, but as a minimum should meet ASHRAE 62.2 for IAQ [6]. In nonexposed product areas, no air filtration is required. Air filtration is recommended to protect coils in air handling units (AHUs), both for occupants and to facilitate housekeeping. A minimum of MERV 8 (30% ASHRAE dust-spot efficiency/EN 779 G4) filtration is suggested; however, some sites may need higher filter efficiency and dust-holding capacity as a result of natural local airborne materials, such as pollen, coal, quarry dust, and a combustion exhaust particulates, or to meet ASHRAE 62.2.

In exposed product areas, a minimum of MERV 12 (85% ASHRAE dust-spot efficiency/EN 779 F8) filters is recommended. If air is returned to the HVAC system, a minimum of an H13 (per EN 1822) high-efficiency particulate air (HEPA)–grade filter in the supply or return duct system normally provides adequate protection against cross-contamination between exposed products and materials. If the HEPA filter is critical to deterring cross-contamination, it should be regularly leak tested (see ISO 14644-3), monitored, repaired, or replaced, as required [7]. The area is typically monitored periodically to confirm satisfactory performance. If a failure of the primary HEPA filter would jeopardize product integrity or potent compounds are present, a secondary in-line HEPA filter should be considered; however, HEPA filtration is not adequate for airstreams carrying hazardous or detrimental vapors. It should be noted that an H13-grade filter will not necessarily be suitable for a full-face leak test (ISO 14644-3 B6.2.5), unless it is specified as requiring one [7]. An H14-grade filter is normally suitable for a full-face leak test (ISO 14644-3 B6.2.5), but will typically have a slightly higher pressure drop [7]. Where a HEPA filter is used to control contamination, filter changing during routine or unexpected maintenance should be considered for contamination control. Where potent compounds are present, a safe change or "bag in–bag out" system may be required.

Although there are no airborne particulate classification requirements for packaging and warehouse facilities, such as those that exist for aseptic processing, the design of primary packaging areas should be treated similarly to the last stage of manufacturing. There is no requirement to validate these spaces to this level of cleanliness. Sampling and weighing facilities within a packaging facility require qualification to a standard matching the related manufacturing area. If it requires grade 8 (ISO 8, 0.5 µm particle size) at rest, cleanliness levels have been successfully achieved with 95% dispersed oil particulate (DOP) (MERV 16/EN 1822 H11) filter banks installed in the AHU. The use of terminal HEPA filters is not normally a regulatory requirement, but they may be used where there is exposed product.

If HEPA filters are used on the supply air system, periodic testing is recommended to confirm installation integrity. This testing, generally, can be the total penetration method (i.e., scan testing of the entire filter face would not normally be required). An alternative approach would be routine monitoring of the supply air particle count. Provision of permanent test connections in the air handling equipment or ductwork may be considered. Typically, the testing may be on an annual basis supported by a visual inspection of the filter for damage every 6 months.

In a facility where multiple products are exposed concurrently, dedicated air handlers and ductwork may be more practical and cost-effective than filtration of return air or the use of once-through air. Capital costs will be higher, but filter maintenance and ongoing testing costs should be lower. The efficiency of the chosen air filtration should reflect the potential for cross-contamination as determined by a formal assessment of the risk to product quality and patient safety.

Contamination can originate from both the internal and external environment. In all air handling systems, the filtration should be evaluated for adequate arrest of external particulates.

In recirculation systems, the filtration should be specified based on the risk of cross-contamination of product and level of control of both recirculated and incoming particulates. For exposed product areas, if the facility is multiproduct and some of the products have no cross-contamination tolerance with other products, air should not be returned (even if HEPA filtered). A once-through system may be required. Although microbiological control is not normally a consideration, if air intakes are downwind from a high-density source of organisms (e.g., waste treatment facilities), microbial control filtration (e.g., HEPA) may be appropriate.

Relative Pressure

Room relative pressure may be a critical parameter if product is exposed and if it is in a multiproduct building, where some or all products are in dry form, exposed to room air without barriers or capture, or can become airborne and migrate to other product areas. The same applies for products in vapor form where vapor migration could have a detrimental effect on other products or materials.

If airborne concentrations of product, materials, or contaminants are high enough to pose an exposure threat to operating personnel, then air relative pressure may be an issue. When this occurs, both personnel and products exposed in the facility could be at risk. Adjacent spaces are uncontrolled, so that airborne migration of particles in either direction is possible, presenting the risk of cross-contamination. It is also a common practice to maintain a building at slightly positive pressure to minimize the potential for ingress of external particulates, by keeping the supply air volume slightly greater than the extract volume.

While there are no quantified requirements for relative pressurization, in a packaging and warehousing facility, typical design and operational pressure differentials of about 0.02 or 0.03 in. water gauge (wg) are specified. The velocity and direction of airflow between spaces should be adequate to prevent counterflow of airborne particulates or vapor contaminants for spaces where airborne cross-contamination is a concern. Relative pressure gradients should be designed to prevent airborne particulates from passing from a given primary packaging space to an adjacent primary packaging space or from passing from any other adjacent space into primary packaging spaces.

Airlocks or buffer zones are often used to separate production areas from adjacent common corridor and staging areas, noncontrolled areas, and potent drug manufacturing areas. To provide protection, when the doors are closed, positive or negative pressure differentials should be monitored. Time-delay interlocks or alarms that operate if both doors are open simultaneously may be used for added control. Consideration should be given to an emergency override capability when such interlocks are employed. Pressured airlocks may have either positive or negative relative pressure, depending on the situation.

Airflow variations from dust collecting, vacuum, or process systems and their effect on pressurization must be considered in the design and operation of the HVAC system. Before air balancing, rooms should be inspected for obvious leakage paths and architectural integrity, which may have a significant effect on the room air-balance requirements (and associated operating costs), the maintenance of differential pressure, or the ability of particulates to enter or leave the space. Routine monitoring, maintenance, and calibration or air pressure differential devices should be established.

Systems Design Criteria

Table 18.1 provides typical systems design criteria for an HVAC system in a packaging and warehouse facility. Specific product requirements may alter these criteria. In general, the temperature and humidity criteria are provided to satisfy personnel comfort.

Air-Change Rates

Air-change rates are defined as the number of theoretical times the air in a room changes based on the supply air volume and the room volume (less any significant fixed equipment). The exhaust air volume also may be used for this calculation if the room is kept at negative pressure. There is no regulatory requirement for the rate of air changes per hour (ACH).

TABLE 18.1
Typical System Design Criteria

	Packaging, Dispensing, and Sampling	Labeling, cGMP Warehouse
Product protection	Exposed	Not exposed
Temperature (personnel comfort)	68°F–77°F (20°C–25°C)	68°F–77°F (20°C–25°C)
Temperature (product)	59°F–86°F (15°C–30°C)	59°F–86°F (USP 15°C–30°C ≤ 25°C MKT)
Humidity (% RH)	30–55	30–55
(These figures are typical; product or stored material stability data will be an overriding factor in the definition of these criteria.)		
Filtration	MERV 12 (85% ASHRAE dust-spot efficiency/EN 779 F8)	MERV 8 (30% ASHRAE dust-spot efficiency/EN 779 G4)
Room pressure (in wg range)	0.02 (5 Pa) to 0.05[1] (12.5 Pa)	Positive[2]

Source: International Society for Pharmaceutical Engineering, *Packaging, Labeling, and Warehousing*, ISPE Good Practice Guide, International Society for Pharmaceutical Engineering, Tampa, FL, 2012.

Note: (1) Airflow is provided to control potential risk of contamination or cross-contamination.

(2) Space is slightly positive relative to less critical areas and to the outside, typically verified by air balance. Differential pressure-monitoring gauges are not normally considered necessary for these areas, where product is not exposed. MKT, mean kinetic temperature; RH, relative humidity; MERV, minimum efficiency reporting value.

Airflow into and out of a space should be based on providing the required cooling, heating, relative humidity, pressurization, particulate control, dilution ventilation, and recovery time from a spill or dust emission. These factors generally result in 4–20 ACH. The application of 15 ACH or greater, in conjunction with the use of filtration equal to or greater than 95% DOP may assist in meeting grade 8 (ISO 8) criteria.

Monitoring

Regular monitoring of critical parameters should indicate to the user when requirements exceed preset operational limits. Assistance in determining the location of the critical points being monitored should come from the temperature mapping process. An alert will indicate when a monitored parameter is beginning to drift out of control. The values of critical parameters include the following:

- *Design condition.* The specified range or accuracy of a controlled variable used by the designer to determine the performance requirements for an engineered system.
- *Normal operating range.* A range that may be selected as the desired acceptable value for a parameter during normal operations. This range should be within the normal operating range, which defines the alert limits, beyond which investigation is indicated.
- *Operating range.* The range of validated critical parameters (acceptance criteria) within which acceptable product can be manufactured. The operating range defines the limits at which action must be taken.

The relationships among the design condition, normal operating range, and the operating range, including the alert and action limits, are shown in Figure 18.1.

Worker Comfort

Maximum and minimum room temperatures and humidity should be within OSHA or local health guidelines (see ASHRAE 55 and ISO 7730 for requirements and guidelines). Conditions may need to be adjusted for workers in protective clothing. A range of 30%–60% relative humidity is

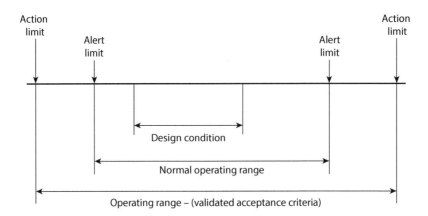

FIGURE 18.1 Values of critical parameters for a system.

recommended for worker comfort where occupancy is continuous. However, since some facilities have 100% outdoor air systems, the need and cost of comfort dehumidification and humidification where humidity will not affect the product should be assessed. Low humidity can lead to an increase in (1) the potential for static discharges, (2) dust clinging to surfaces, (3) particulate generation from dry skin, and (4) corrosion and microbial growth in spaces and building materials [4].

Workplace noise levels should be addressed, especially where local or portable dust collection systems are used. Applicable OSHA and local regulations should be followed [4].

Ventilation for Hazardous Environments

Recirculation of flammable vapors is not recommended unless the recirculation system includes appropriate means to detect and remove those vapors. Areas where flammable materials are stored or exposed will usually be served by once-through air systems. Local spot exhaust is recommended at points of flammable and toxic material exposure.

Building electrical hazard classification and static grounding should be applied to HVAC components and instrumentation, in accordance with national and local codes.

When dilution ventilation is used to control flammable vapors, the threshold limit value for the material drives the dilution air volume, not the lower explosive limit. Airborne flammables can lead to very large air handling volumes, increased operating costs, and health problems in workers.

Permissible product and constituent airborne concentrations depend on material toxicity, as determined by the facility user. The handling of potent or toxic materials should rely first on product containment, then capture (as in a hood or isolator), and finally dilution. A process that is contained (e.g., a glove box) requires less HVAC energy, creates less risk to workers, and poses less cross-contamination potential than traditional open processes. The designer and user should agree on the level of protection required for the process, as well as the protection for personnel provided by the process equipment.

Electrical

Most major pieces of packaging equipment have a central control panel with a single-power connection point. Large machines are usually three-phase loads. In most cases, on primary packaging machines, heat sealers, and shrink tunnels, there is a substantial resistive load associated with heaters and sealing bars. Any subsystems with different voltage requirements are usually fed from step-down transformers within the primary integral panel. There are exceptions to this with add-on auxiliary systems, such as vacuums, printers, and other single-phase loads. Care must be taken to quantify the existing packaging equipment load and estimate all potential future equipment loads that could be added at a later date due to the inherent flexibility of secondary packaging operations. Primary electrical distribution and low-voltage wiring for machine controls from machine to machine are usually run in raceways underneath the framework of the equipment. This can be in a conduit or, in the case of integrated bottle packaging lines, custom wire raceways designed and provided by the equipment manufacturer. It is customary to provide convenience outlets as required around the perimeter of packaging spaces. A data port should be located near the supervisor's area if required.

The design of the facility should also consider the pressurization of rooms with respect to adjacent space and the related impact on the potential for contamination. Pressurization requirements for contamination control may conflict with requirements for hazardous area electrical classification of adjacent rooms. These conflicts should be resolved in combination with the HVAC and architectural design. To address such conflicts, techniques to minimize air leakage, such as sealed conduits and openings or sealed lighting fixtures, ideally with maintenance access from the service area, are used. While the power system is not critical, reliability could be important to business operations. The effects of loss of power or poor power quality on a critical piece of equipment or instrument should be considered and the resulting failure conditions examined [4].

Compressed Air

Some packaging equipment consumes large amounts of compressed air. Air quality should be pharmaceutical grade whenever compressed air directly contacts the drug product or the drug product contacts surfaces of packaging materials and equipment. Component-orientating equipment, such as vibratory bowls and bottle unscramblers, use small microjets to orient parts or propel parts around rails during the packaging process. Venturi systems use compressed air to generate a vacuum for suction cups that are used to pull cartons and inserts from magazines. Bottle cleaners use blasts of compressed air to blow dust and other particles from bottles before filling. Collectively, these loads can be substantial.

Total compressed air volume, pressure, and peak loads must be understood before properly sized compressed air supply systems can be designed. It may be necessary to provide more than one supply point for a given packaging line and install surge tanks as necessary, depending on peak load requirements. Compressed air quality for machine operation should meet or exceed the packing equipment manufacturer's requirements. Compressed air that comes in direct contact with drug product or primary packaging material product contact surfaces should be clean, dry, pharmaceutical-grade air. The nature of the fluid being conveyed should be considered when selecting materials for storage and distribution systems.

Chilled Water

Many packaging operations use arrays of electric cartridge-style heaters and sealing tooling to create certain package features. Sealing stations on many machines use chilled water to control sealing temperatures precisely; some machines are compact by design to ensure that the heat from the sealing bars does not migrate into other machine stations. In most cases, this chilled water is provided by a local stand-alone chiller located within the packaging area.

Site Steam and Condensate

Where site steam is used for humidification of process areas with exposed product, there may be special requirements (e.g., permissible boiler additives should be food grade; see 21 CFR 173.310 [8] or the ISPE Good Practice Guide on HVAC [9]). Other options to consider for humidification include local electric boilers; atomizing nozzle systems, using compressed air; and ultrasonic nozzles. If close control is required, then a close control–type unit with dual chambers should be specified. The potential for microbial growth when the system is not in use should be considered.

Other Utility Requirements

Dust collection is usually required for powder fill and uncoated tablet-filling applications. Depending on the level of control required, dust control can be an integral part of a balanced HVAC system or a localized stand-alone feature at the point of use.

Nitrogen and other specialty gases are used in several different ways in packaging processes, most notably to displace oxygen in primary packaging for oxygen-sensitive products. Depending on the quantity required, the gas can be provided in cylinders or piped into the packaging area from a remote source.

A vacuum can be provided in three ways: (1) induced by compressed air and Venturi, (2) supplied by a vacuum pump that is integral to the packaging system (preferred), or (3) provided by a remote vacuum-generating system. System design considerations should address the potential for cross-contamination if the blower fails, the potential effect on the HVAC balancing, and the cleaning and disposal of system equipment [4].

For fire protection, the sprinkler system is usually selected to be recessed with flush mounting caps for ease of ceiling cleaning. In areas where toxic products may be handled or exposed, a system to retain the sprinkler discharge, such as a water tank or door sills, may be required for environmental reasons [4].

PRIMARY PACKAGING AREAS

Primary packaging rooms should have the same critical design criteria as pharmaceutical manufacturing suites. Primary packaging areas are usually designated as white zones, accessed through a transition zone designed to facilitate proper gowning procedures. When handling nontoxic products, room pressure gradients typically cascade away from the primary room, through the airlock or transition zone, and into secondary packaging and other support areas to ensure that contaminants are not transferred. When toxic products are handled, the preferred practice is to have the airlocks (for both gowning and de-gowning) under a slightly positive pressure to the primary packaging area. The use of automated misting showers in the first step of the de-gowning area should also be strongly considered. The misting shower room should be under slight negative pressure to act as a sink to both the primary packaging area and the second stage of the de-gowning space.

Typical primary packaging processes consist of horizontal blister machines, bottle-filling equipment, vertical and horizontal pouch-filling equipment, and other processes where the drug product or medical device is exposed to the general room environment for some period of time. The drug product can be a tablet, capsule, liquid, cream, powder, or other dosage form. Drug product is exposed when bulk drug containers are opened, when the bulk drug product is transferred to the product hoppers or tanks on the filling equipment, and when the drug product has been transferred to the primary package, but before the package is completely sealed. This is the case with blister packaging before top web seal, horizontal pouch applications before final top seal, and bottling operations before capping.

Finishes

Finishes in primary packaging areas should be as smooth, durable, and monolithic as possible to provide maximum cleanability and prevent areas where dirt could accumulate. Penetrations of the primary packaging boundary should be sealed, with silicon sealant or similar material, to maintain the pressure and containment integrity. Ceilings should be seamless with a smooth finish and coated with epoxy paint. Lay-in ceiling tiles are acceptable in some instances, provided they are washable, nonshedding, and use clips and gaskets to hold them in place. Walls should be monolithic, with coves at the sills and base to facilitate proper cleaning. Wall finishes should take into account the potential degrading effect room sanitizers may have. Some means of impact resistance should be provided to prevent damage from pallets and material handling equipment in areas susceptible to such damage. Stainless steel panels and corner guards are preferred. Floors should be monolithic systems, such as epoxy terrazzo, troweled epoxy, or seamless welded vinyl.

Equipment

Primary equipment tends to be fixed, in that once the packaging process is defined, there will be no major changes to the primary equipment. There will be tooling changes from lot to lot and put-up to put-up, but the machine footprint, staging requirements for raw materials, and utility requirements, in most instances, will not change. Auxiliary systems, such as chillers, printers, and vacuums, should be scrutinized for clean operation.

Utilities

Utility service for packaging equipment in primary areas should stub up through the floor to maintain clean, uncluttered walls and prevent conduit or pipe drops from the ceiling. Where primary packaging equipment transitions to the secondary process through a dividing wall, it is acceptable to bring utility services to the machine at the point where the primary discharge conveyor passes through the wall.

Materials Staging

Only material quantities for the current lot should be staged in primary packaging areas. This includes drug product and packaging components. Total material staging requirements are usually not more than two pallets for each component due to the storage density of the drug product and the rolls of foil in blister-forming operations. Bottling operations are a special case. Bottle staging and bottle unscrambling should take place in a secondary area because of the space taken up by unit loads of bottles and caps.

SECONDARY AND TERTIARY PACKAGING AREAS

Secondary packaging areas are usually designated as gray zones. The drug product or medical device is contained within the primary package, and the risk of exposure to product or operator is minimal. The space must be configured to support flexible operations. It is not necessary to totally enclose secondary and tertiary areas. Segregation between packaging lines must be maintained, preferably by solid partitions at least 4 ft high. It is acceptable practice to provide air conditioning for an entire secondary packaging gallery by the same air handling system.

Finishes

Finishes in secondary packaging areas should be durable and cleanable. Ceilings at a minimum should be lay-in ceiling tiles that are washable and nonshedding. Walls should have coves at the sills and base to facilitate proper cleaning. An epoxy-coated concrete masonry unit is acceptable. Some means of impact resistance should be provided to prevent damage from pallets and material handling equipment in areas susceptible to damage. Stainless steel panels and corner guards are preferred. Floors can be troweled epoxy, vinyl tile, or epoxy paint. The level of fork truck traffic is a primary determinant for which floor system to use.

Equipment

Where primary equipment tends to be fixed, secondary and tertiary equipment tend to be more flexible. Typical secondary and tertiary operations consist of check weighing, cartoning, labeling, hand packing, bundling, banding, overwrapping, case packing, and palletizing. There are numerous auxiliary operations that typically take place in secondary areas, such as printing, coding, and package inspection. Maintenance and calibration procedures, associated storage, and areas with a specified function for parts storage, including cleaning and changeovers, should be considered.

Utilities

Because of the flexible nature of most secondary and tertiary packaging operations, stubbing up through the floor is not practical. Packaging equipment should be fed from strategically located stainless steel or extruded aluminum power poles that extend up into the suspended ceiling and can be relocated as necessary as packaging process layouts change. Attempts must be made to minimize individual ceiling drops, and cords and conduits must be kept off of the floor.

Materials Staging

Lot quantities of secondary packaging components can take up considerable floor space, depending on package complexity and lot size. Typically, when a packaging process is programmed, space for a single pallet of each packaging component is allotted on the packaging floor. As material is expended, more material is signed into the area. Each process must be assessed on a line-by-line basis, however, because high throughput may require more than one pallet of certain components on hand.

SUPPORT AREAS AND ADJACENCIES

Overflow Materials Staging

For high-volume or large-lot-sized packaging operations, it is customary to provide a staging area adjacent to the packaging area for packaging components. In most instances, rack storage is not necessary. Packaging materials are staged in pallet quantities on the floor, usually single stacked so that the material can be easily moved with a pallet jack when it is needed. It is necessary to provide segregated staging for each individual packaging line to prevent mix-ups. These areas should be treated as secondary packaging areas from a facility design standpoint.

Wash Areas

Packaging equipment must be cleaned between lots and especially between products. Most packaging equipment is not designated as clean-in-place; therefore, it is practical to clean equipment and tooling in a centrally located area. In most instances, it is only necessary to clean product contact surfaces, such as product hoppers and filler parts in the central wash area. Parts and tooling can be cleaned manually in specially designed wash basins or automatically in commercial part washers. It is necessary to understand exactly what is to be cleaned so that the appropriate wash basins or automated equipment is selected. Depending on the cleaning method chosen, proper hot and cold water service, drainage, and electrical service must be provided. Some cleaning procedures require elevated water temperatures or a purified water rinse, and this must be considered during the design phase of the project. A properly designed wash area will have separate, defined staging areas for "dirty" equipment to be cleaned and for equipment that has been designated as clean and ready for use.

Equipment Storage

It is necessary to provide space for excess equipment in any packaging facility plan. Although it makes good business sense to keep as much equipment as possible fully used, there still needs to be equipment storage space available. Storage areas should be located near the maintenance shop. Although most machine maintenance is done in place on the packaging floor, there are instances where major modifications or complete rebuilds are undertaken, and this work typically takes place in the shop. Machines may be staged for a period of time on the way to be serviced and possibly back out to the packaging floor. Equipment storage areas should be large enough to handle this modification and rebuild volume, spare machinery, and other equipment as necessary. Due to the weight and size of packaging machinery, floor storage is most appropriate. Some rack storage is appropriate for small auxiliary equipment, such as printers, scanners, and other devices. Spare parts, subassemblies, and smaller equipment can be stored in shelving units.

Tooling Storage

Tooling presents some special storage requirements over and above typical equipment storage parameters. Tooling describes the product-specific parts required to change a packaging machine to run different products or formats. Tooling can be product contact parts on a primary packaging machine, such as slats and funnels on a tablet-filling machine or timing screws on a bottle-filling machine. There is also tooling in secondary applications, such as the tuckers, plows, and folding rails on a cartoning machine or sealing tooling on a pouch machine. Regardless of the application, the following special conditions apply to tooling storage: (1) controlled temperature and humidity to minimize corrosion on untreated surfaces; (2) condensed storage, as some tooling sets can be quite small; (3) segregated storage, so parts for a given format can be stored together and not get mixed up with other sets; and (4) special protection for sensitive machined tools, such as seal tooling, forming dies, and punches, to prevent nicks and other marks.

When planning a tooling storage area, it is important to understand the types of packaging equipment that will be used and the total sets of tooling for each packaging machine. It is not unusual for a single blister-forming machine to have 10 or more individual sets of tooling. As most tooling is quite expensive, it usually goes into storage when a given product run is completed.

Maintenance Shop

Adequate space should be provided for a maintenance and engineering area to support packaging operations. There are various levels of machine maintenance, from minimal daily maintenance checks to manufacturing machine tooling in-house. Firms make business decisions about how much maintenance to perform using in-house personnel and how much to perform using contracted or original equipment manufacturer resources. These decisions have a direct bearing on the size of the maintenance area that needs to be designed. Packaging equipment maintenance can function as a stand-alone support unit, or it can be merged with a manufacturing machinery maintenance unit if these functions are required in a multifunctional plant. Both are cGMP functions, but the major difference is that most manufacturing maintenance occurs in the manufacturing plant, while packaging equipment maintenance occurs in the maintenance area. Care should be taken, however, to keep facilities maintenance and equipment maintenance areas separate to comply with cGMP regulations.

Label Room

Labeling is perhaps the most intensive cGMP parameter associated with packaging. Printed materials are always present in packaging areas, and the FDA insists that the creation, storage, and use of printed materials be managed in a controlled fashion. There are preprinted materials, such as cartons, blister foils, pouch films, physician and patient inserts, and other high-volume (skid quantity) materials that must be managed under cGMP guidelines, but these items are typically stored in a warehouse and retrieved as needed. The label components that require an extra level of security are batch- or lot-specific labels with lot number and expiry information and small unit-of-use labels that contain detailed product information. Typically, unprinted stock is stored in the warehouse, and lot quantities are brought into the label room for printing. Labels are usually quite dense from a storage perspective, so lot quantities may be a case or two or may be as much as an entire skid, but rarely more. Labels are printed as needed and placed in a locked, rolling cart after inspection and approval.

Printed labels are transferred to the packaging floor for use on the secure carts. The size of the label room is completely dependent on the size and complexity of the packaging operation. The end user must be consulted about the details of the packaging process to ensure that a properly sized labeling area is designed. As a minimum, finishes, space conditioning requirements, and light levels should be the same as for secondary packaging. Space must be provided for raw label storage, finished label storage, cart storage, label printers, inspection machines, records, and printing inks. Depending on the chemical composition of the inks, special storage cabinets and ventilation may be required. Labeling materials may be sensitive to temperature or humidity and need appropriate storage conditions. Additionally, security measures, such as card access and security cameras, are usually required.

Testing Labs and Other Quality Control Areas

Depending on the type of packaging process, some in-process testing of packages is required. Most tests are concerned with the integrity of the seals on the primary package. Leak testing equipment and pull-strength testers are the principal pieces of equipment used for in-process testing. Most test equipment is benchtop, with a few exceptions. Casework with adequate linear benchtop space is required with cabinetry for storage of test materials. A means to temporarily stage packages to be tested is also required.

Office Space

Typically, office space is provided for packaging supervisors and managers in the gray or black areas. Space must be provided for operations personnel, such as first-line supervisors, area managers, and administrative support. Some firms also want the planners, buyers, and other analysts close to the packaging operations, and if this is the case, space must be provided for them. There are other support functions, such as engineering and document control, that must be assessed and provided for as necessary. It is also important to understand the proposed hours of operation, as a multiple-shift operation requires additional office space or a shared office plan.

SPECIAL DESIGN CONSIDERATIONS

TEMPERATURE MAPPING

Temperature mapping should be performed in areas where product will be stored in a significant quantity, within a space, such as a warehouse or environmental chambers, to identify the locations that are representative of the environmental extremes within the space and determine where the permanent area monitoring sensors should be placed. The duration of any mapping should, at a minimum, cover a representative period at the extremes of the external environmental conditions (e.g., coldest winter and hottest summer days). Some mapping should also be done with different amounts of material stored in the area.

The temperature mapping sensor locations may become permanent or be used to map the facility and provide supporting data to identify the sites for fewer permanent sensors, which give readings representative of the worst-case conditions, typically for high and low temperatures. Usually, fewer humidity sensors are required than temperature sensors, as the absolute moisture content is normally consistent within a facility. Typically, there will not be systems generating significant amounts of moisture within a warehouse or chamber. As the relative humidity varies with temperature, a minimum relative humidity is monitored where the temperature is likely to be the lowest.

FLAMMABLE MATERIALS STORAGE

Some printing inks and other substances used in the packaging process are flammable and require special storage. The design firm needs to understand the nature of the flammable materials, as well as the total maximum quantity of materials required to be stored at the facility. If the packaging area is a part of a larger multiuse facility with other flammable material storage requirements, it may be appropriate to use a small storage cabinet for lot-sized quantities of flammable materials in the packaging area and store the larger quantities of flammable materials in a centralized storage area.

CONTROLLED SUBSTANCES

There are very specific storage requirements for controlled substances, as defined by the U.S. Drug Enforcement Administration (DEA). Section 1301.72 of the Code of Federal Regulations permits small quantities to be stored in a safe or steel cabinet and large quantities to be stored in a specially constructed vault with controlled access and alarm capability [10]. The noted section provides all of the required construction details for compliance.

REFRIGERATED OR FROZEN STORAGE

Some biologics and other drug formulations need to be stored in a refrigerated or frozen state. Drug products may need to be protected as raw materials, finished goods, or both. The maximum quantities of drug product that are required to be stored as a raw material and as finished goods must be known for proper sizing of the environmentally controlled area. Typically, the required storage area for finished goods is many times that of the raw material of the same drug product because of the different densities of drug product per pallet. There may also be multiple products that need to be stored. Cold storage areas should be properly designed to provide uniform temperature distribution across all levels. There will be major differences in system and supporting facility design to consider, depending on whether the requirement is for refrigerated storage (typically 2°C–8°C) or frozen storage (typically –25°C or more). Most applications can use prefabricated systems, consisting of gasketed sheet metal–encased foam panels and doors. A safety allowance of 25% (at least) should be factored into the square footage calculations for growth. Some other typical requirements for cold storage areas include (1) a temperature monitoring system, (2) alarms for overtemperature or undertemperature, (3) redundant mechanical systems for backup in the event of mechanical failure and for defrost cycle allowance, (4) emergency generator backup, (5) temperature mapping and validation, (6) a secondary source of cooling water (if the refrigeration system condensers are water cooled), and (7) a preaction fire suppression system.

PROJECT MANAGEMENT ISSUES

COSTS

Generally speaking, packaging facilities are typically built to the same standards and finishes as nonsterile manufacturing facilities. Facility construction costs per square foot of packaging space tend to be somewhat lower than costs for manufacturing space, because there are fewer unusual design features. Costs range from $125 to $250 per square foot (or more), depending on geographical region and level of finish selected. Special environmental conditioning for sensitive products or special construction for hazardous products can greatly increase costs. Specialized HVAC equipment to maintain tight temperature, humidity, and room pressure tolerances adds to the total cost. The cost of ongoing operations can be substantial as well. Packaging equipment notoriously consumes compressed air, and the usage needs to be understood to determine the total cost of operating the packaging plant accurately.

Packaging equipment can be very expensive, especially for custom-built, one-of-a-kind machines. High machine output also translates directly to high machine cost. Prices run from less than $10,000 for a very rudimentary carton erector to as much as $5 million for a top-of-the-line, highly automated, fully integrated, ultra-high-speed bottle line. It is important to note that there is no standard budgetary rule of thumb to try to compute the cost of packaging equipment. It is incredibly variable, depending on the package format, desired throughput, level of automation, machine flexibility, and other factors. In clean industries, certainly all primary packaging equipment and most secondary packaging equipment purchased are qualified and validated. There is a cost associated with the formal documentation required to specify, purchase, install, qualify, and validate packaging equipment. In this case, there is a general rule of thumb that can be used for planning purposes. Building systems' commissioning and qualification costs are, on average, 3%–5% of building construction costs. Packaging equipment qualification and validation costs are, on average, 8%–15% of total costs.

SCHEDULES

There is a natural progression to finish packaging areas after manufacturing areas and before warehousing. Construction crews use the roughed-in packaging areas for staging for the finished work in

TABLE 18.2
Typical Timeline for a Custom Packaging Line

Project Task	Duration (Months)	Cumulative (Months)
Develop user requirements specification	1	1
Develop functional and design specifications	1	2
Prototyping and proof of concept	2	4
Approval to proceed	Milestone	
Detailed design	4	8
Drawing release	Milestone	
Parts and subsystems procurement	4	12
Assembly	3	15
Testing and debugging	1	16
Factory acceptance testing and shipping	1	17
Commissioning and qualification	1.5	18.5
Validation	1.0	19.5
Approved for use	Milestone	

the manufacturing areas and then move staging into the roughed-in warehouse to finish the packaging area. Equipment installation and commissioning and validation activities follow the same natural set of sequences. Packaging equipment lead time needs to be factored into the master project timeline. Lead time varies with the cost and complexity of the equipment, and complex, high-speed equipment can take as long as 18 months to deliver. Table 18.2 shows what a typical timeline for a custom packaging line might be.

FUTURE DEVELOPMENTS: PACKAGING TRENDS

Although solid dosage forms are still the obvious volume leader, advances in biotechnology are making parenterals (i.e., vials, syringes, and cartridges) more and more common. These products are typically very expensive, and they usually require special temperature considerations. Most have a 2°C–8°C storage requirement and can be out of refrigeration for a very limited time during labeling, packaging, and shipping operations. Others are actually frozen products at –25°C and below; freeze safe containers are becoming a very big business. Properly designed refrigeration in proximity to the packaging lines is critical. The need to ensure sterility throughout the packaging and labeling operation is also extremely important (e.g., container or closure integrity for vials, syringes, and cartridges). As advances in biotechnology lead to increased numbers of products gaining FDA approval, these issues will become more and more crucial.

Most new prescription drug products are higher in cost than they were 10 or even 5 years ago. This has led to a changing philosophy by major pharmaceutical firms that now spend more on packaging to protect the product, as well as make the packaging more convenient for the physician, pharmacist, nurse, and patient. This is evident with unit-dose packaging (e.g., blisters for oral solid dosage forms and syringes or cartridges for parenterals). This trend also addresses the increasing attention to medication errors, most of which can be traced to the repackaging or reconstitution of products. Since many of the biotech products are intended for self-medication by patients, the only way to ensure compliance with dosing regimens is to have a unit-dose package that is ready to use. The downside of this for manufacturers and packagers is the tremendous increase in total packaged volume that results from unit packages (e.g., 1 vial vs. 10 syringes). Also, most biotechnology companies with home-use kits on the market are including alcohol swabs, needles, and reconstitution aids in the package to make administration simpler and more convenient. All of this increased complexity in packaging is putting renewed emphasis on the proper design of packaging facilities and critical support equipment. This is also creating some divergence of packaging operations toward generics (cheaper and faster) versus newly approved products (expensive and more complex).

SPECIAL DISCUSSION: RADIOFREQUENCY IDENTIFICATION

Radiofrequency identification (RFID) is a technology that has been around since the 1940s. It uses radio waves to read information from and write information to special chips or tags that can be embedded in standard label stock or directly applied as self-adhesive devices. Regular users of toll roads, for example, often have an E-ZPass transponder in their car, which is very close to the RFID technology. In the last decade, it has made inroads into the packaging industry. Wal-Mart, for example, informed all of its top suppliers that they must begin using RFID technology at the pallet level by 2005. Other concerns, such as the Department of Defense, Tesco (a British retailer), CVS, and the Red Cross, are working on pilot RFID applications. The intent is to move the use of this technology even further down the supply chain, all the way to the unit of use. One of the principal benefits of this technology is that no direct line-of-sight scanning is required, as with bar code systems, so entire skid loads can be scanned without unloading the pallet. The RFID technology is also capable of reading and writing anywhere in the supply chain, so information can be upgraded in the field if necessary. The most promising application in packaging is the incorporation of the RFID tag into a label. Many cut label suppliers are looking into ways to incorporate the "smart tag" into their label-making processes. There are also several label printer and applicator machine manufacturers that will be offering a unit capable of printing readable labels and writing data to embedded chips, using RFID technology. At first glance, RFID seems like a "cannot miss" proposition. In the laboratory, the technology performs flawlessly, reading and writing information at incredible speeds in a controlled environment.

Developmental shortcomings aside, RFID is a very promising technology. It will permit scan-free (compared to current bar coding technology) data acquisition on a grand scale, with expectations approaching 1,000 tags/s. It will play a major role in manufacturing and packaging logistics, point-of-sale transactions, and inventory control. Full-scale implementation of RFID technology for packaging is not a question of if, but when.

Costs

In the field, the performance is hampered by cost. There is a cost associated with the tags themselves, and a one-time cost associated with the hardware and software. Sophisticated tags can cost up to $1.00 each, although for most applications, the cost is around $0.30 apiece. It is anticipated that as demand increases, the cost will drop further to less than $0.10 each. Readers can cost from $500 to $10,000; magnified over a multiunit operation, these costs could be prohibitive. These costs will be spread out between the manufacturers and converters, which will ensure the tag is present and properly encoded, and the distribution centers, wholesalers, and retailers, which will interpret information from the tags.

Speed and Operational Effectiveness

The best case is an entire pallet load of individually tagged units that could be read at once. There are many factors that prohibit this from happening, such as the degree of RFID penetration to the center of the pallet, the orientation of the tag to the reader, and the packaging materials used. Metals and foils reflect RFID waves, and liquids tend to absorb them.

Tag Durability

The tag manufacturing process needs to be properly monitored to ensure that the tags are robust before application. In the course of secondary processing and application, the tags need to be handled properly to ensure that they are not damaged. Many secondary operations include embedding the RFID tag into label stock, which is sent to the user in roll form. The tag must endure the stresses associated with the radius imparted on the label as it is wound onto the roll. Estimates of the number of tags that do not work right out of the box run as high as 10%.

INDUSTRY STANDARDS

The technology at its current stage of development is reminiscent of bar coding technology 25 years ago. There really are no industry standards that dictate how the units should be built or how information is written or read. Different retailers have different requirements, and different suppliers have different capabilities, but just as industry demand led to accelerated development of standards for bar coding, the same forces will have very similar effects on RFID standards development. There is a not-for-profit organization called EPCglobal that is spearheading the standards effort. It is a joint venture between the European group EAN International and the Uniform Code Council. Its goal is to develop and commercialize the Electronic Product Code Network, which it hopes will become the global standard for RFID.

ABOUT THE AUTHOR

John S. Holton, pharmaceutical engineer, has more than 40 years of experience in the HVAC industry. In the first 20 years of his career, he was involved in the design of HVAC systems for nuclear power plants and industrial facilities. The last 21 years have been focused on pharmaceutical and biotechnology facilities. He was the director of engineering for Worldwide Facilities and Operations for Cephalon, Inc., an international biopharmaceutical company with corporate headquarters located in Frazer, Pennsylvania. He is affiliated with the North American ISPE, Delaware Valley Chapter, and is a past president and past member of the membership and program committees. He also was chairman of the North American–South American Affiliate Council of ISPE. His involvement also includes active participation, on the national level, as a cowriter of the released *Packaging, Labeling, and Warehousing* Good Practice Guide. He was responsible for the preparation of the chapter on HVAC and provided significant input to the electrical and instrumentation and controls section of the guide. Holton received a BS degree in mechanical engineering from the New York Institute of Technology, Old Westbury campus.

REFERENCES

1. Code of Federal Regulations, cGMP in Manufacturing, Processing, Packing, or Holding of Drugs and Finished Pharmaceuticals, 21 CFR 210 and 211.
2. International Conference on Harmonisation, ICH Q9: Quality Risk Management, Technical Requirements for Registration of Pharmaceuticals for Human Use, International Conference on Harmonisation, Geneva.
3. International Society for Pharmaceutical Engineering, *Applied Risk Management for Commissioning and Qualification*, ISPE Good Practice Guide, International Society for Pharmaceutical Engineering, Tampa, FL, 2011.
4. International Society for Pharmaceutical Engineering, *Packaging, Labeling, and Warehousing*, ISPE Good Practice Guide, International Society for Pharmaceutical Engineering, Tampa, FL, 2012.
5. U.S. Pharmacopeial Convention, USP General Notices and Requirements: Preservation, Packaging, Storage and Labeling, United States Pharmacopeial Convention, Rockville, MD, www.usp.org/uspnf
6. American Society of Heating, Refrigerating, and Air-Conditioning Engineers, ASHRAE 62.2: Ventilation and Acceptable Indoor Air Quality in Low-Rise Residential Buildings, American Society of Heating, Refrigerating, and Air-Conditioning Engineers, Atlanta, GA, 2013.
7. International Organization for Standardization, ISO 14644-3: Cleanrooms and Associated Controlled Environments, Part 3: Test Methods, International Organization for Standardization, Geneva.

8. Code of Federal Regulations, Secondary Direct Food Additives Permitted in Food for Human Consumption, 21 CFR 173.

9. International Society for Pharmaceutical Engineering, *Heating, Ventilation and Air Conditioning (HVAC)*, ISPE Good Practice Guide, International Society for Pharmaceutical Engineering, Tampa, FL, 2009.

10. Code of Federal Regulations, Physical Security Controls for Non-Practitioners; Narcotic Treatment Programs and Compounders for Narcotic Treatment Programs; Storage Areas, 21 CFR 1301.72.

Appendix I: Novel Drug Delivery

Edward J. Tannebaum, AIA

INTRODUCTION

Novel drug delivery is an extremely important aspect of the development of a drug product. New methods of drug delivery have been developed to both improve the drug's entry into the body and extend the life of the drug's financial viability through extending its patent. This article describes unique developments in forms of drug delivery, and provides an overview of drug delivery resources.

A drug delivery method has multiple goals: to simplify the actual delivery by improving the ease of use, to minimize the side effects of introduction into the body, to direct the introduction of the product to its specific location of need, and to manage the dosage delivery from immediate to sustained or extended release accurately. Many drugs require unique processing to develop means of achieving the most direct method of applying the active chemical compound to its intended delivery point. At the same time, due to patent expirations, new methods of physical delivery may provide an extension of the drug's life span as a proprietary product within a drug manufacturer's portfolio. The combination of improving delivery options and the financial implications of improved uniqueness has dramatic effects on both the product's position in the marketplace and its long-term benefit to the patient.

The design of facilities with compliant construction and meeting regulatory requirements poses a variety of challenges. The design of facilities for these novel drug delivery products ranges from utilizing existing processes to the invention and utilization of newer processes that may have been used formerly for other industries and must be modified to work within a Good Manufacturing Practice (GMP) environment. Starting with the early stages of development, the project progresses from a careful analysis of the risk-based approach to scale-up and commercialization, meeting the intent of regulatory agency submissions and their clinical trial stages.

EXECUTIVE SUMMARY

MANUFACTURING PROCESSES

The development of unique molecules that are competitive to produce and approvable by the worldwide regulatory agencies is a primary objective when developing novel drug delivery methods.

As worldwide drug manufacturing has become more subject to counterfeiting, along with the abuse of drug forms, it has become necessary to reformulate existing drugs in unique ways to make the drugs more difficult to counterfeit or to reformulate finished forms into illegal forms of concentration, especially with controlled substances. New methods to produce molecules that are not reproducible have become a valuable addition to drug development. Inherent molecule processes that destroy an active chemical when the particle's composition is altered dramatically reduce the possibilities for counterfeiting and limit the use of active ingredients for illicit purposes.

New, convenient methods of drug delivery that improve the security of accurate dosing, extended-release capabilities, and dermatological to transmucosal delivery are among the many delivery systems being added to product formulations. High-impact tablet formulations that resist tampering will extend the life of existing controlled substance products due to their ability to limit adulteration; these will become more prominent in the coming years. Electronic, PC-based system implants are among the newer forms of delivery that will ensure accurate, timely dispensing of drugs, for both inpatient and outpatient use.

The following forms of delivery for drug products are an example of these unique developments:

- Advanced controlled-release technologies
- Bioavailability enhancement
- Insoluble actives
- Unstable actives
- Potent and toxic actives
- Small-molecule delivery
- Taste masking (for liquid and solid presentations)

Contract development and manufacturing organizations (CDMOs) are in the forefront of the creation and development of these unique delivery platforms. Development firms concentrate their efforts on a narrow band of patentable delivery platforms focused on differing delivery needs.

Some of the primary delivery platforms are categorized below:

- Patient-friendly delivery systems (e.g., transdermal patches, transmucosal sprays, dissolvable films, and mini-tablets)
- Needle-free delivery systems (e.g., coated tablets with tiny needles that are exposed in the gastrointestinal tract, microfluidic atomization, refillable sprayers, microneedle technology, and jet injectors)
- Release delivery systems (e.g., immediate release [IR], controlled release [CR]—pediatric and adult, and osmotic delivery)
- Focused site delivery systems (e.g., focused ultrasound delivery, implantable pumps, and MRI-directed microbubbles)

DRUG DELIVERY RESOURCES

The following list of development organizations provides a sampling of the unique novel drug delivery companies that are currently striving to bring new solutions to the market, for either curing varied disease types or bringing improved efficacy to existing drug products. The major contributors to these novel drug delivery organizations are small, science-based companies, created and sustained by investors or major pharma funding to advance their research and clinical applications of their respective products. The scientific expertise of these companies grows as offshoots of major pharma organizations, where these novel approaches cannot be financially justified within the research and development programs focused on major drug programs for higher-volume drugs.

Company	Location	Business Type
Oncolytics Biotech	Calgary, Alberta	Human reovirus delivery
Meros Polymers	Edmonton, Alberta	Polymer-assisted drug delivery
Soluble Therapeutics	Birmingham, Alabama	Protein formulation technology
QRxPharma	North Sydney, New South Wales, Australia	Abuse prevention drug technology
Innate Immunotherapeutics	Sydney, Australia	Delivery system for immune triggers
Vaxxas Nanopatch	Sydney, Australia	Vaccine patch delivery system
Austrianova Biotechnology	Maria Enzersdorf, Austria	Bioinert polymer encapsulation
PolyPid	Santa Clara, California	Polymer lipid encapsulation matrix, ophthalmic therapies

Continued

Company	Location	Business Type
Icon Bioscience	Sunnyvale, California	
Medallion Therapeutics	Valencia, California	Targeted delivery solutions for pharmaceuticals and biologic therapies
MannKind	Danbury, Connecticut	Inhalable biologics, gene therapy
Egalet	Vaerlose, Denmark	Extended release
Prometheon Pharma	Alachua, Florida	Needle-free method for passive delivery of large-molecule drugs
GeNO	Cocoa, Florida	Nitric oxide generation and delivery
Clearside Biomedical	Alpharetta, Georgia	Ocular drug delivery technology, lipid nanoparticle (LNP)
Arcturus Therapeutics	San Diego, California	siRNA drug delivery systems
ViaCyte Aviva Biosciences	Athens, Georgia San Diego, California	Stem cell therapies, drug screening technology
Osmotica Pharmaceutical	Marietta, Georgia	Drug delivery, antibody conjugates
Concortis Biosystems	San Diego, California	
MedGenesis Therapeutix	Mannheim, Germany	Neurologic treatment—convection-enhanced delivery, drug
CRISI Medical Systems	San Diego, California	delivery technology
Leukocare Biotechnology	Martinsried, Germany	Biologic formulation, extracellular matrix
Halozyme Therapeutics	San Diego, California	
Toxikon	Sankt Ingbert, Germany	Medical devices, drug delivery touchscreen insulin pump
Tandem Diabetes	San Diego, California	
Prometheon Pharma	Alachua, Florida	Needle-free method for passive delivery of large-molecule drugs
GeNO	Cocoa, Florida	Nitric oxide generation and delivery
Accu-Break Pharmaceuticals	Plantation, Florida	Breakable tablets
Clearside Biomedical	Alpharetta, Georgia	Ocular drug delivery technology
ViaCyte	Athens, Georgia	Stem cell therapies
Osmotica Pharmaceutical	Marietta, Georgia	Drug delivery
MedGenesis Therapeutix	Mannheim, Germany	Neurologic treatment—convection-enhanced delivery
Leukocare Biotechnology	Martinsried, Germany	Biologic formulation
Toxikon	Sankt Ingbert, Germany	Medical devices, drug delivery
NeuroDerm	Ness Ziona, Israel	Reformulations of established drugs

ABOUT THE AUTHOR

Edward J. Tannebaum has more than 45 years of experience as an architect, construction manager, and corporate facilities lead, primarily focused on the pharmaceutical industry. A graduate of the College of Architecture, Planning and Design at Kansas State University, Manhattan, Ed has been a lead figure in the design and construction of solid dosage facilities throughout the world. As the head of facility design and construction for Johnson & Johnson, McNeil Consumer Healthcare Division, he was responsible for the planning and execution of facilities, both domestically and abroad. His comprehension of the OSD business from the owner's, designer's, and constructor's perspectives has provided him with a unique perspective into operational issues that are critical to address in these projects. His knowledge of domestic and international statutes and trends has become a larger and larger focus in recent years of consulting. As a senior principal of Integrated Project Services (IPS) for many years, he led design and build efforts and many conceptual design activities related to OSD and novel drug delivery facilities. For many years, he was a frequent speaker at International Society for Pharmaceutical Engineering educational programs related to design and project facilitation. His role as a principal of Strategic Planning Initiatives, LLC, provides him with a platform of expertise to continue assisting pharmaceutical management with strategic master planning to coincide with their business needs. Tannebaum was the author of the OSD chapter for the first edition of *Good Design Practices* and has provided input to bring the publication to its current level of information, authoring Chapter 9 of this edition.

Appendix II: Biopharmaceutical Factories of the Future

Mark A. Butler

INTRODUCTION

You do not have to look far to see the advancements in technology that impact the way we work and live. Advancements in automation, digital technologies, communication, data management, three-dimensional printing, the creative commons, and the Internet of Things (IoT) are just a few examples that are reshaping the way we work and the way work gets done in manufacturing plants. These advancements, along with others, are pushing manufacturing into a new age of productivity and efficiency. Some refer to this as the fourth industrial revolution, or industry 4.0.

Industry 4.0 is a collective term for technologies and concepts that see manufacturing as an interconnected system or value chain. This revolution in manufacturing is largely based on technology and connected systems enabled by the IoT. The result of this convergence brings us smarter manufacturing plants. This revolution is not the result of one individual trend, but rather the result of a broad range of interconnected elements operating together as a system. For example, on the factory floor, embedded sensors and real-time dynamic data collection can span the entire supply chain of a product or process and provide new levels of visibility, flexibility, and autonomy in production lines. Advanced analytics and data management are also creating new opportunities for competitive advantage and manufacturing optimization. Analysis of selected data enables companies to have insight into production and real-time information that allows greater visibility into the supply chain and manufacturing life cycle. In addition, embedded sensors can provide real-time monitoring of machinery, indicating when equipment may be at risk of failure and when maintenance or preventative maintenance is required. This intelligence can be used to eliminate potential outages before they happen and increase equipment reliability and efficiency. When embedded sensors are combined with modular construction, modular equipment skids, and process systems, the connected equipment and processes create smart, mobile unit operations or mini-factories that can be transported anywhere in the world to provide decentralized manufacturing. The combined impact of these technologies is transforming manufacturing to more agile, efficient, fast, flexible, and responsive manufacturing networks.

In the biopharmaceutical manufacturing arena, other technological advancements are evolving, such as three-dimensional printing, process intensification, higher yields, single-use technologies, and continuous processing, that are changing the way biopharmaceutical products are manufactured. The area of diagnostics and treatment is being powered by the convergence of connectivity and analytics. New tools, tests, and apps are being developed that bring diagnostic information right to a patient's bedside and, in some cases, provide real-time information about the patient.

INTERNET OF THINGS

At the center of this convergence is the IoT. The McKinsey Global Institute recently issued a report predicting that the IoT will offer nearly $11 trillion in annual economic impact by 2025 [1].

In McKinsey's list of nine areas where economic value could accrue, the largest potential area for growth is manufacturing and factories. The report indicates that, as a direct result of the IoT, operations and equipment optimization in manufacturing have the most potential to improve performance. Technology suppliers are ramping up their IoT business plans and creating strategies for the design, implementation, and operation of complex systems to collect data from the physical world and deploy capabilities to control, capture, and analyze data in real time.

To illustrate how connected we have become, we just have to look at the number of objects that are connected. Between 2007 and 2008, the number of objects or things connected to the Internet exceeded the number of people on our planet. Cisco predicts that by the year 2020, the number of connected things on the Internet will top 50 billion connected objects [2]. This equates to approximately nine connected objects per person living on the planet. The more connected objects we deploy, the more innovations that will be developed to process and handle the data coming from all the connected objects in the physical world. Connected processes, products, and machines will enable optimization of production and will require the integration of building systems and equipment. Sensor-driven production lines and product components will enable factories to react in real time to changes in the market and supply chain. Data collection and analytics will allow more rapid and responsive manufacturing where products and production processes can adapt to changes in demands. This exponential explosion of connectivity and its projection into the future will continue to result in people being connected to objects in ways we have yet to imagine and more automation in manufacturing that will improve quality, reduce cost, and increase efficiency.

IMPACT ON FACILITIES

In parallel to this technological explosion, the biopharmaceutical industry has had to deal with pressures from many different sources, including drug shortages, product recalls, patent expirations, and generic and biosimilar drugs. These pressures, and others, are impacting the industry at an ever-increasing pace and forcing new creative innovations to deliver lower-cost, high-quality products. In addition, there has been a significant shift in product portfolios for many biopharmaceutical companies to include personalized medicine in their product mix. Personalized medicine may be thought of as a tailored treatment specifically for the individual characteristics and needs of a patient, and it sometimes uses the patient's own cells. The number of personalized products in cell therapy, plus targeted high-potency products and complex biologics such as antibody drug conjugates (ADCs), has risen in the last few years and is forecasted to increase in the years to come. To meet the requirements of these new products, processes need to be developed and deployed that are aligned with the manufacturing profile that includes smaller batch sizes, limited production runs, and high levels of containment.

This portfolio shift is driving process architects and design professionals to think about new ways to design and build manufacturing facilities to accommodate these changes, and to design facilities that are more flexible and agile. In the past, it was common for a launch facility to be designed to support a single product, so future modifications were not very easy to achieve. Large, fixed, stainless steel vessels; process equipment; and high-purity piping systems with clean-in-place (CIP) and sterilize-in-place (SIP) systems have given way to smaller-scale, single-use systems and "plug-and-play" equipment with disposable bags and tubing. Designing and building these smaller, modular, and flexible facilities is a radical shift from the way facilities were designed and built in the past. These new facilities offer smaller footprints, require less energy and water, are more sustainable, and have a lower cost, and therefore a lower financial barrier to entry for start-up companies.

Enabling technologies will continue to lead the way for manufacturers to advance biomanufacturing into the future. New innovative technologies are improving economics, flexibility, and quality to benefit both the manufacturers and patients alike. Some of these new enabling technological advancements are

1. *Modularization.* Modularization provides transportable facilities and process skids to improve speed to market, flexibility, and quality.
2. *Continuous manufacturing with process analytical technology (PAT).* Continuous manufacturing with PAT requires a smaller footprint than batch processing and fewer setup and cleaning cycles, and allows for quicker scale-up from clinical phase, speed to market, reduced offline quality control and analysis, less maintenance, lower energy use, and less product loss.
3. *Single-use systems (SUSs).* SUSs are available throughout nearly every step of the production process, have lower capital costs than built-in-place stainless steel systems, facilitate quicker changeovers for multiproduct facilities, provide increased flexibility, and reduce water and energy use.

These examples show that the fourth industrial revolution is well underway, enabling manufacturing to improve efficiency and reduce costs.

CLOUD-BASED COLLABORATION

Another technological advancement is cloud-based collaboration. The ability to access data and control operations remotely on mobile devices utilizing cloud computing and connectivity provides us the ability to be connected to processes and equipment anywhere in the world. Through cloud computing, we have the ability to access and analyze large volumes of data to make quicker, more informed decisions. This enabling technology will help to transform biopharmaceutical manufacturing into a flexible and more agile manufacturing unit.

As we look into the future and see more connected objects and new technologies, it is clear that biopharmaceutical companies will need to train and hire specialized workers who possess experience and skills in programming and information technology (IT) to manage huge amounts of data from all the connected objects on the plant floor. In addition to the impact on the biopharmaceutical companies, architectural and engineering design firms will need to hire and train specialized personnel so they are well versed in the technological advancements and can design adaptive, connected, compliant, and flexible facilities. Finally, builders and contractors will also need to hire and train personnel that understand the technologies so they can construct and commission these complex and highly automated and connected facilities. The convergence of connected objects and biopharmaceutical manufacturing will continue to evolve, bringing us smarter factories and opportunities to rethink the way we design and conduct current operations.

ABOUT THE AUTHOR

Mark A. Butler is a senior vice president and principal for Integrated Project Services (IPS) located in Blue Bell, Pennsylvania. IPS is a global design, construction, commissioning, and qualification company serving the life sciences industry. Mark Butler has more than 30 years of experience in the design, construction, and operations of biopharmaceutical manufacturing facilities. In addition to his design experience, Mark managed capital projects for Pfizer and was a program manager for a $350 million research and development program. His experience includes program management, strategic planning, consulting, and project management for both new and renovation projects. Mark is a graduate of both Pennsylvania State University, University Park, and Ferris State University, Big Rapids, Michigan, holding degrees in heating, ventilation, and air conditioning, and solar thermal technology. He was awarded the Penn State "Outstanding Alumni Award" in 1996 and holds a patent pending for ultraviolet sterilization in cold-mist humidifiers. He is a frequent speaker, author, and member of the International Society for Pharmaceutical Engineering (ISPE); American Society of Heating, Refrigerating, and Air-Conditioning Engineers (ASHRAE); and American Society of Mechanical Engineers (ASME).

FURTHER READING

EvaluatePharma, Orphan Drug Report 2014, EvaluatePharma, October 2014.
Hessman T, The Dawn of the Smart Factory, *Industry Week*, February 14, 2013.

REFERENCES

1. McKinsey Global Institute, The Internet of Things: Mapping the Value Beyond the Hype, McKinsey Global Institute, June 2015.
2. Evans D, The Internet of Things, How the Next Evolution of the Internet Is Changing Everything, Cisco Internet Business Solutions Group, San Jose, CA, April 2011.

Index